Neurobiology of Panic Disorder

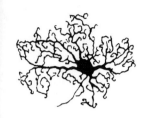

Frontiers of Clinical Neuroscience

Series Editors

Ivan Bodis-Wollner, M.D.
Mt. Sinai School of Medicine
New York

Earl A. Zimmerman, M.D.
Oregon Health Sciences University
Portland

Frontiers of Clinical Neuroscience
VOLUME 8

NEUROBIOLOGY OF PANIC DISORDER

Edited by
JAMES C. BALLENGER, M.D.
Department of Psychiatry and Behavioral Sciences
Medical University of South Carolina
Charleston, South Carolina

Wiley-Liss
New York

Address all Inquiries to the Publisher
Alan R. Liss, Inc., 41 East 11th Street, New York, NY 10003

While the authors, editors, and publisher believe that drug selection and dosage and the specifications and usage of equipment and devices, as set forth in this book, are in accord with current recommendations and practice at the time of publication, they accept no legal responsibility for any errors or omissions, and make no warranty, express or implied, with respect to material contained herein. In view of ongoing research, equipment modifications, changes in governmental regulations and the constant flow of information relating to drug therapy, drug reactions and the use of equipment and devices, the reader is urged to review and evaluate the information provided in the package insert or instructions for each drug, piece of equipment or device for, among other things, any changes in the instructions or indications of dosage or usage and for added warnings and precautions.

Library of Congress Cataloging–in–Publication Data

Neurobiology of panic disorder / edited by James C. Ballenger.
    p. cm. — (Frontiers of clinical neuroscience ; v. 8)
    Companion v. to: Clinical aspects of panic disorder.
    Includes bibliographies and index.
    ISBN 0–471–56210–6
    1. Panic disorders. 2. Biological psychiatry. I. Ballenger,
James C. II. Clinical aspects of panic disorder. III. Series.
    [DNLM: 1. Biological Psychiatry. 2. Fear—physiology. W1
FR946DM v. 8 / WM 178 N494]
RC535.N483 1989
616.85'22—dc20
DNLM/DLC
for Library of Congress   89–12404
                                       CIP

Contents

ANIMAL MODELS

PRECLINICAL STUDIES

GENETICS

POSTULATED BRAIN MECHANISMS
FOR PANIC ANXIETY

CHALLENGE STRATEGIES

BRAIN IMAGING STUDIES

ANXIETY AND DEPRESSION

IMMUNOLOGY AND SLEEP ABNORMALITIES

Contributors

Asaf Aleem, Department of Psychiatry, Wayne State University, Detroit, MI 48207; and Veterans Administration Hospital, Allen Park, MI 48101; present address: Department of Psychiatry, Emory University, Wesley Woods Geriatric Hospital, Atlanta, GA 30029-5102 [107]

Raymond F. Anton, Department of Psychiatry and Behavioral Science, Medical University of South Carolina, Charleston, SC 29425 [349]

James C. Ballenger, Department of Psychiatry and Behavioral Sciences, Medical University of South Carolina, Charleston, SC 29425 [xiii]

Richard Balon, Department of Psychiatry, Wayne State University, Lafayette Clinic, Detroit, MI 48207 [107]

Joseph Biederman, Department of Psychopharmacology, Massachusetts General Hospital, Harvard University School of Medicine, Boston, MA 02114 [71]

Harry A. Brandt, Unit on Eating Disorders, Section on Biomedical Psychiatry, Laboratory of Clinical Sciences, National Institute of Mental Health, Bethesda, MD 20892 [313]

Dennis S. Charney, Clinical Neuroscience Research Unit, Connecticut Mental Health Center, and Department of Psychiatry, Yale University School of Medicine, New Haven, CT 06508 [91,205]

Raymond R. Crowe, Department of Psychiatry, University of Iowa College of Medicine, Iowa City, IA 52242 [59]

Mark A. Demitrack, Section on Clinical Neuroendocrinology, Biological Psychiatry Branch, Laboratory of Clinical Sciences, National Institute of Mental Health, Bethesda, MD 20892 [313]

Sandra E. File, Psychopharmacology Research Unit, UMDS, University of London, and Division of Pharmacology, Guy's Hospital, London SE1 9RT, England [31]

Thomas D. Geracioti, Section on Clinical Neuroendocrinology, Biological Psychiatry Branch, Laboratory of Clinical Sciences, National Institute of Mental Health, Bethesda, MD 20892 [313]

Michelle Gersten, Child Study Center, Yale University School of Medicine, New Haven, CT 06510; present address: Department of Psychiatry, Mount Sinai Medical Center, Box 1228, New York, NY 10029 [71]

Jane Gibbons, Department of Psychology, Harvard University, Cambridge, MA 02138; present address: Nine Sterling Road, Waltham, MA 02154 [71]

William M. Glazer, Clinical Neuroscience Research Unit, Connecticut Mental Health Center, and Department of Psychiatry, Yale University School of Medicine, New Haven, CT 06508 [91]

Vivette Glover, Department of Chemical Pathology, Bernhard Baron Research Laboratory, Queen Charlotte's and Chelsea Hospital, London W6 OXG, England [143]

Philip W. Gold, Clinical Neuroendocrinology Branch, Laboratory of Clinical Sciences, National Institute of Mental Health, Bethesda, MD 20892 [313]

Wayne K. Goodman, Clinical Neuroscience Research Unit, Connecticut Mental Health Center, and Department of Psychiatry, Yale University School of Medicine, New Haven, CT 06508 [91]

Jack M. Gorman, Department of Psychiatry, Columbia University College of Physicians and Surgeons, New York NY 10032 [187]

George R. Heninger, Clinical Neuroscience Research Unit, Connecticut Mental Health Center, and Department of Psychiatry, Yale University School of Medicine, New Haven, CT 06508 [91]

Maureen O. Johnson, Department of Psychology, Harvard University, Cambridge, MA 02138 [71]

Jerome Kagan, Department of Psychology, Harvard University, Cambridge, MA 02138 [71]

Konstantine Kalogeras, Section on Clinical Neuroendocrinology, Biological Psychiatry Branch, Laboratory of Clinical Sciences, National Institute of Mental Health, Bethesda, MD 20892 [313]

Charles Kellner, Department of Psychiatry and Behavioral Sciences, Medical University of South Carolina, Charleston, SC 29425 [271]

Mitchel A. Kling, Section on Clinical Neuroendocrinology, Biological Psychiatry Branch, Laboratory of Clinical Sciences, National Institute of Mental Health, Bethesda, MD 20892 [313]

Michael R. Liebowitz, New York State Psychiatric Institute and Department of Psychiatry, College of Physicians and Surgeons, Columbia University, New York, NY 10032 [155]

Jan Lerbinger, McLean Hospital, Belmont, MA 02178 [321]

Roy T. Mathew, Department of Psychiatry, Duke University Medical Center, Durham, NC 27710 [281]

Thomas A. Mellman, Section on Anxiety and Affective Disorders, Biological Psychiatry Branch, National Institute of Mental Health, Bethesda, MD 20892 [365]

Aurelio Ortiz, Department of Psychiatry, Wayne State University, Lafayette Clinic, Detroit, MI 48207 [107]

Laszlo A. Papp, Department of Psychiatry, Columbia University College of Physicians and Surgeons, New York, NY 10032 [187]

J.C. Pecknold, Department of Psychiatry, Douglas Hospital, Research Center, Verdun, Quebec H4H 1R3, Canada [121]

Teresa A. Pigott, Section on Clinical Neuropharmacology, Laboratory of Clinical Sciences, National Institute of Mental Health, Bethesda, MD 20892 [313]

Robert Pohl, Department of Psychiatry, Wayne State University, Lafayette Clinic, Detroit, MI 48207 [107]

Lawrence H. Price, Clinical Neuroscience Research Unit, Connecticut Mental Health Center, and Department of Psychiatry, Yale University School of Medicine, New Haven, CT 06508 [91]

Eric M. Reiman, Department of Psychiatry, Washington University School of Medicine, St. Louis, Missouri 63110; present address: Department of Psychiatry, University of Arizona School of Medicine and Center for Brain and Behavioral Studies, Samaritan Health Services, Phoenix, AZ 85006 [245]

J. Steven Reznick, Department of Psychology, Yale University, New Haven, CT 06510 [71]

Jerrold F. Rosenbaum, Department of Psychopharmacology, Massachusetts General Hospital, Harvard University School of Medicine, Boston, MA 02114 [71]

Peter P. Roy-Byrne, Department of Psychiatry and Behavioral Sciences, University of Washington School of Medicine, Seattle, WA 98195 [271]

Diana P. Sandberg, New York State Psychiatric Institute and Department of Psychiatry, College of Physicians and Surgeons, Columbia University, New York, NY 10032 [155]

Merton Sandler, Department of Chemical Pathology, Bernhard Baron Research Laboratory, Queen Charlotte's and Chelsea Hospital, London W6 OXG, England [143]

Alan F. Schatzberg, McLean Hospital, Harvard University School of Medicine, Belmont, MA 02178 [321]

M. Katherine Shear, Department of Clinical Psychiatry, The New York Hospital-Cornell Medical Center, New York, NY 10021 [173]

David V. Sheehan, Department of Psychiatry, University of South Florida School of Medicine, Tampa, FL 33612 [321]

Nancy Snidman, Department of Psychology, Harvard University, Cambridge, MA 02138 [71]

Marvin Stein, Department of Psychiatry, Mount Sinai School of Medicine, City University of New York, New York, NY 10029-6574 **[333]**

Svenn Torgersen, Center for Research in Clinical and Applied Psychology, Department of Psychology, University of Oslo, 0315 Oslo 3, Norway **[51]**

Robert L. Trestman, Department of Psychiatry, Mount Sinai School of Medicine, City University of New York, New York, NY 10029-6574 **[333]**

Thomas W. Uhde, Section on Anxiety and Affective Disorders and 3-West Clinical Research Unit, Biological Psychiatry Branch, National Institute of Mental Health, Bethesda, MD 20892 **[3,219,365]**

Susan R.B. Weiss, Section on Psychobiology, Biological Psychiatry Branch, National Institute of Mental Health, Bethesda, MD 20892 **[3]**

William H. Wilson, Department of Psychiatry, Duke University Medical Center, Durham, NC 27710 **[281]**

Scott W. Woods, Clinical Neuroscience Research Unit, Connecticut Mental Health Center, and Department of Psychiatry, Yale University School of Medicine, New Haven, CT 06508 **[91,205]**

Vikram Yeragani, Department of Psychiatry, Wayne State University, Lafayette Clinic, Detroit, MI 48207 **[107]**

Preface

Although twenty-five years ago the anxiety and phobic disorders occupied a relatively minor place in psychiatry, they currently represent a major focus of research and clinical interest in the field. This shift in importance can probably be attributed first to the increased understanding of the differential diagnosis of the anxiety disorders, which culminated in the almost revolutionary changes in The American Psychiatric Association Diagnostic and Statistical Manual III (DSM-III). In DSM-III, the recognition of the central aspect of panic attacks in the diagnosis of panic disorder became widely accepted, particularly in the United States. However, the centrality of panic attacks in clarifying the differential diagnosis of all the anxiety disorders had its greatest impact in DSM-III-R in which anxiety disorders were divided into those with and without panic attacks.

Certainly the increased clarity of both the diagnosis and clinical picture of the panic disorders could not have resulted in the widespread interest in this area were it not for the epidemiologic evidence that the syndrome is not rare but actually quite common. Panic disorder and panic disorder complicated by phobic avoidance have a six-month prevalence rate of three to seven percent of the population in the United States (Myers et al., 1984). With apparently similar prevalence rates around the world, the anxiety disorders are now recognized as probably the most common psychiatric disorders (Epidemiologic Catchment Area Survey) and the psychiatric disorders which most frequently lead to medical attention.

Interest in panic disorder was also stimulated by the remarkable advances in effective treatments over this same period. Evidence that panic disorder is responsive to pharmacologic treatments began evolving in the early 1960s and has accelerated rapidly since that time. Similarly, behavior therapy and, more recently, cognitive therapy have also been shown to be effective in this syndrome, and there is lively interchange between multiple therapeutic viewpoints and modes of approach.

Until it was demonstrated in the early 1960s that the symptoms of panic disorder were responsive to antidepressants, the anxiety disorders, including panic disorder, were thought to be psychological syndromes. However, the symptom picture of panic attacks seemed to many observers to have a ''biological'' character, and thought turned to whether there might be biological factors involved. Panic attacks begin explosively and involve marked tachycardia, palpitations, shortness of breath, chest pain, headache, trembling, GI symptoms, and other autonomic nervous system symptoms. The view that panic attacks and panic disorder might substantially involve neurobiological substrates, etiologies, and pathophysiologies seemed revolutionary to some. In many respects the anxiety disorders have been previously considered to be the psychiatric problems least likely to be biological in nature. Since anxiety is universal and so many of the anxiety symptoms that we experience are clearly related to our cognitions and experiences, anxiety symptoms were thought by most to be ''purely psychological.'' Certainly most of the treatments had been psychological and involved psychotherapy, psychoanalysis, or behavior therapy.

Over the last decade, the pace of research into biological aspects of panic disorder has increased rapidly, and biological research is now active in many psychiatric research centers around the world. Whereas research in this area in the 1960s and early 1970s was restricted to a few sites, most major psychiatric research centers are now involved in the study of panic disorder in some capacity, and are quite frequently engaged in biological studies of panic disorder. In recognition of the growing importance of biological research in panic disorder, the *American Journal of Psychiatry* in 1986 devoted a special section to the biological aspects of panic disorder. I had the pleasure of being invited to write the editorial introducing these seven excellent papers. In that editorial (Ballenger JC: Biological aspects of panic disorder) I proposed that there was growing and converging evidence to suggest a potentially understandable "biology of anxiety." Although the studies were, and in many ways still are, preliminary and nondefinitive, they provided considerable promise that we will gain important new understandings of the biological aspects of these disorders in the relatively near future.

This volume and its companion to follow (*Clinical Aspects of Panic Disorder*) were designed to capture the excitement of this rapidly evolving field. Interest in this field and the researchers involved have become international in scope. These volumes attempt to be inclusive, covering as much of the field as possible. To my knowledge, this is the first comprehensive book devoted to the broad neurobiological aspects of panic disorder. Because most of the work in this area has been performed during the last five years, much of it remains unpublished. We have assembled in this volume some of that unpublished data, in order to highlight in one place much of the work in this field, and to stimulate interest, research, and interchange about the issues raised.

This book begins with an extensive and well organized chapter by Weiss and Uhde, who review what we know of the animal models of anxiety. The second chapter, by File, is a comprehensive review of preclinical studies of brain systems thought to be involved in anxiety. Many readers may be surprised at the extent of evidence that there is an "anxiety system" in the central nervous system, and this area is excellently reviewed in these two chapters.

Torgersen and Crowe review the familial and genetic marker studies suggesting genetic inheritance of panic disorder in humans. Although there is no definitive evidence of genetic inheritance for any single anxiety disorder at this point, these chapters present the evidence from familial, twin, and genetic marker studies that suggest that we are near such a demonstration.

Chapter 5 explores what might be inherited in people who go on to develop panic disorder. Kagan's demonstration of an apparent inborn propensity to anxiety, particularly on separation from mother or in response to novel or strange situations, is a dramatic and important finding. The report of his research with Rosenbaum on the children of adult panic disorder patients demonstrates early but fascinating evidence that this childhood behavioral pattern may be related to the development of panic disorder in adults. These early studies of potential childhood antecedents of panic disorder are quite important, since this group of children has the highest likelihood of subsequently developing panic disorder as adults.

The book then shifts to presentation of the specific brain neurotransmitter substrates that have been implicated in the etiology or pathophysiology of anxiety and panic disorder. Following the elegant work of Redmond and his colleagues at Yale, the noradrenergic system, primarily located in the central bilateral midbrain nucleus, the locus ceruleus (LC), appears to be involved in the central anxiety system and perhaps provides an excellent model for panic anxiety. The chapter by Charney and colleagues is a direct attempt to explore the validity of this model in panic disorder patients as is the chapter by Pohl and colleagues, although from a different perspective. The contribution by Pecknold reviews the evidence that the serotonin system may be involved in either the pathogenesis, pathophysiology, or treatment of panic disorder. Glover and Sandler then review evidence of a molecule called tribulin that appears to be present in increased amounts in anxious humans, and they review its potential role in human anxiety disorders.

The next section reviews various challenge strategies that have been employed in attempts to understand the pathophysiology of panic disorder. The strategy of utilizing challenges that stress various biological systems has become increasingly popular in psychiatry. Often a biological system will appear normal at rest, but under challenge will demonstrate significant abnormalities. For instance, the demonstration that the IV infusion of sodium lactate induced panic attacks in patients with panic disorder but not in normals has stimulated a great deal of theoretical speculation and research into the potential mechanisms of lactate's induction of panic. This field has become well-developed over the last decade and is reviewed by Sandberg and Liebowitz. Dr. Shear's chapter reviewing nonpharmacologic aspects of the lactate infusion is an excellent review of the impact of nonbiological measures such as cognition on biological phenomena. The chapter by Gorman and colleagues explores the observation that panic can also be induced by carbon dioxide challenge. This work has also been provocative and helpful in exploring potential biological mechanisms of panic. This work also serves as the background for the potential evolution of clinically useful diagnostic tests with CO_2. Potentially, a CO_2 challenge could be simply administered in a practitioner's office, and if it could assist in the differential diagnosis of anxiety disorders, the CO_2 provocation test could become the first clinically useful challenge test in this area. The chapter by Woods and colleagues outlines the first studies of biological responses that occur in panic disorder patients when they are exposed to natural phobic stimuli. Although this strategy is crucial in our attempts to understand the neurobiology of panic disorder, the difficulties involved have limited investigations in this area and make the work of this group particularly important. Uhde then presents the research demonstrating that caffeine can also stimulate panic attacks in panic disorder patients and reviews studies of the biological systems involved, including the adenosine system.

The book then explores the three most commonly used brain-imaging techniques in this area and reviews what anatomic evidence of a neurobiology of panic disorder exists. Although positron emission tomography (PET) work in panic disorder patients is mostly limited to the work of Reiman and colleagues, PET has already provided exciting insights into the potential anatomic circuitry involved in the expression of, if not initiation of, panic anxiety, and he reviews this area in his chapter. The chapters by Kellner and Mathew review the CT/MRI and cerebral blood flow studies in panic patients.

Panic disorder and depression appear to share multiple overlapping features. Certainly depression is a common occurrence in panic disorder patients, with probably two-thirds of this population experiencing depression sometime during their lifetimes. There also appear to be overlapping genetic influences for the two syndromes. The chapters by Gold and colleagues and Shatzberg explore the relationships of the two syndromes by looking at biological measures and techniques which have been useful in understanding the biology of depressive illness. These include various neuroendocrine measures and the study of the hypothalamic-pituitary-adrenal axis. Stein's chapter explores the recent research concerning the relationship of the immunologic system to anxiety and, potentially, panic disorder. Similarly, the chapter by Anton explores the provocative early suggestion of abnormalities in the prostaglandin system. The chapter by Mellman and Uhde on sleep disorders in panic explores the important biological parameter of sleep for clues to the pathophysiology of panic disorder and its relationship to depressive illness.

The companion volume to follow in this series (*Clinical Aspects of Panic Disorder*) takes the next step in this area of clinical research. In that volume, we start from the biological models, techniques, and issues summarized herein and explore them as they relate to the clinical aspects of panic disorder. We hope the reader finds both volumes useful and enjoyable.

James C. Ballenger

American Psychiatric Association (1980): "Diagnostic and Statistical Manual of Mental Disorders." (Third Edition). Washington D.C.

Ballenger JC (1986): Biological aspects of panic disorder (editorial). *Amer J Psychiatry* 143(4):516–518.

Ballenger JC (1990) (ed):"Clinical Aspects of Panic Disorder." New York, Wiley-Liss.

Myers JK, Weissman MM, Tischler GL, Holzer GE III, Leaf PJ, Orvaschel H, Anthony JC, Boyd JH, Burke JD, Kramer M, Stoltzman R (1984): Six-month prevalence of psychiatric disorders in three communities: 1980–82. *Arch Gen Psychiatry*, 41:959–970.

Animal Models

Animal Models of Anxiety

SUSAN R.B. WEISS, PhD, AND THOMAS W. UHDE, MD

Section on Psychobiology (S.R.B.W.) and Section on Anxiety and Affective Disorders and 3-West Clinical Research Unit (T.W.U.), Biological Psychiatry Branch, National Institute of Mental Health, Bethesda, Maryland 20892

INTRODUCTION

Anxiety is a state in humans that is subjectively experienced as unpleasant or threatening and that is often accompanied by physiological changes (e.g., increases in sympathetic tone; increased plasma catecholamines, cortisol, and growth hormone) as well as a set of behavioral responses generally aimed at avoiding or escaping the situation associated with the anxiety. An analogous state can be produced in other species, in which similar physiological responses can be measured and in which behaviors characterized as "fight or flight" are evoked. The survival value of an escape or avoidance response to a dangerous situation is obvious. However, the importance of the subjective feelings of anxiety in the production of this response is less obvious. This distinction cannot, however, be readily addressed through animal studies, so the focus of animal research has been on behavioral and physiological measures that resemble those observed in human anxiety or on behavioral procedures that permit the identification of pharmacological agents that specifically reduce or eliminate pathological anxiety. The former allow the determination of causal events and concomitant biochemical and physiological alterations associated with anxiety; the latter allow the elucidation of pharmacologic and environmental manipulations that can modify anxiety.

Anxiety-related disorders in humans can be usefully conceptualized as an overgeneralized or exaggerated anxiety response to stimuli that are not actually threatening. In addition, some forms of pathological anxiety (e.g., spontaneous panic attacks) are often observed in the absence of any apparent environmental influences. Three forms of anxiety-related pathologies defined by the DSM III include phobias, generalized or chronic anxiety, and panic disorder. Phobias are defined as persistent and recognizably irrational fears of a particular object or a situation. A phobic response includes significant distress and a compelling desire to avoid that object or situation. Chronic anxiety/generalized anxiety disorder is defined as a more or less continuous state of anxiety lasting for at least 1 month. The symptoms of generalized anxiety include motor tension, autonomic hyperactivity, apprehensive expectations, and vigilance and scanning. Panic disorder is characterized by the occurrence of sudden, intense, spontaneous episodes of terror without a clearly identifiable environmental precipitant. The attacks are characterized by a sense of impending doom or a fear of "going crazy," accompanied by tachycardia, chest discomfort, hyperventilation, diaphoresis, and other signs of physiological arousal. Context-predisposed panic attacks also may emerge over the course of the illness in situations when escape might be impaired. These differ from specific phobias in which the panicky feelings inevitably occur when the patient is exposed to the feared objects (spiders, cats) or situations (riding an elevator). Frequently, panic disorder is also associated with agoraphobia, a fear of any place or situation in which help or support would not be readily available upon sudden incapacitation. Many investigators (Freud, 1895; Klein, 1964; Uhde et al., 1985a) believe that the onset of agoraphobia is preceded by the experience of unexpected panic attacks. As a result

Neurobiology of Panic Disorder, Pages 3–27
Published 1990 by Alan R. Liss, Inc.

of these panic attacks, patients subsequently attempt to avoid any place or situation in which panic attacks might occur. Frequently, these are previously neutral places where spontaneous panic attacks have been inconsistently experienced. A pattern of multiple phobias emerges, which may even result in the patient's self-imposed confinement to his/her home. The fears typically associated with agoraphobia (e.g., crowded stores, public places, bridges, tunnels) may themselves trigger context-predisposed panic attacks. Thus, agoraphobia may be the learned consequence of panic attacks, since the unpredictability and spontaneity of the panic attacks might reduce the likelihood that the environmental provocation would be confined to any one particular situation. This, combined with the intensity of the experience, might cause an overgeneralization of anxiety to a wide range of situations.

It should not be surprising that animal models of anxiety disorders are not complete veridical matches to human anxiety, since the pathogenesis of and linkage among the human disorders remain unclear. Moreover, the specific biological concomitants of human anxiety vary among individuals or over time, and some of the more reliable and marked symptoms are relatively nonspecific. A variety of animal models, therefore, must be used in examining the many different features of both normal and pathological anxiety. For example, taste aversions (Garcia and Koelling, 1966; Seligman, 1970, 1972) and snake fear in monkeys (Hebb, 1946; Murray and King 1973; Yerkes and Yerkes, 1936) may model some simple or specific phobias, and behavioral sensitization paradigms, which examine the effects of repeated exposure to stimuli, may mimic certain aspects of chronic anxiety (Kandel, 1983). Animal models of spontaneous or unpredictable panic attacks are not currently available, although the intense protest response of primates, observed immediately following separation from a parent or peer, offers many behavioral parallels to panic attacks (Suomi et al., 1981). Additionally, investigators can chemically induce an apparent state of intense fear in animals by means of chemical agents such as beta-carbolines or yohimbine (Crawley et al., 1984a; File et al., 1982; Ninan et al., 1982; Skolnick et al., 1984). These drugs, as well as caffeine and lac-

tate, have also been used to study anxiety and panic disorder in humans (Boulenger et al., 1984a,b, 1986; Charney and Heninger, 1985-a,b; Charney et al., 1983, 1985; Holmberg and Gershon, 1961; Liebowitz et al., 1984, 1985; Rainey et al., 1984; Uhde et al., 1984a, 1985b, 1989).

Animal models of human disorders have been used for many years to help identify etiological factors, concomitant biochemical and behavioral abnormalities of the disease state, and effective treatment strategies. This chapter discusses some of the current animal models of anxiety, with particular attention to the applicability and/or limitations of these models for our understanding of anxiety in humans.

PHARMACOLOGICAL PROBES

The recent observation that certain pharmacological agents can produce behavioral and physiological changes that resemble those seen in severe human anxiety, as in, e.g., panic attacks, has opened a whole new area of investigation. This research is focused on the relationship between the effects of these drugs on the nervous system and the underlying biochemical and physiological basis of anxiety in humans. Needless to say, exogenous administration of a drug to produce a set of behavioral and physiological responses that resemble those seen in human anxiety is not proof that the system upon which the drug acts is normally involved in anxiety. However, the similarity of the drug response to the behavioral syndromes of panic and anxiety in man makes these drug challenges intriguing. In particular, beta-carbolines, yohimbine, and caffeine may provide a wealth of data and are currently being studied in humans and other species.

Benzodiazepine–Gamma-Aminobutyric Acid (GABA) Systems

Since the benzodiazepines are the most commonly used agents in the treatment of generalized or anticipatory anxiety in humans, it seemed reasonable to suppose that understanding their mechanisms of action and observing their effects might provide clues to the more general nature of anxiety. The development of three classes of compounds that interact with benzodiazepine binding sites in the brain (Mohler and O'Kada, 1977) in specific and opposing fashions has further enhanced the usefulness of these drugs. Benzodiazepine agonists, inverse agonists, and antagonists that can be differentiated on a number of biochemical, behavioral, and physiological measures have been synthesized. In general, agonists, of which diazepam is the prototype, are anxiolytics, anticonvulsants, sedatives, and muscle relaxants. Inverse agonists, such as the beta-carboline derivatives, appear to produce behavioral effects opposite to those of the agonists; i.e., they are anxiogenic (Dorow et al., 1983; Peterson et al., 1983) and proconvulsant (Braestrup et al., 1982; Corda et al., 1983; Cowen et al., 1981; Petersen, 1983; Peterson et al., 1983). Antagonists, such as Ro 15-1788 (Hunkeler et al., 1981; Mohler and Richards, 1981), are relatively free of behavioral and physiological effects when administered alone (Bonetti et al., 1982) but will reverse the effects of either agonist or inverse-agonist drugs (Nutt et al., 1982; Polc et al., 1982; Schweri et al., 1982). The benzodiazepine binding site has been postulated to be part of a supramolecular complex that includes a GABA receptor and a chloride ionophore (Olsen, 1981; Tallman et al., 1980). Agonist effects are generally associated with enhanced GABA-ergic transmission (Costa, 1982), whereas inverse agonists are associated with decreased GABA function (Braestrup et al., 1983). The role of GABA in the anxiolytic effects of benzodiazepines, however, has recently been questioned (Sanger, 1984; Sepinwall and Cook, 1978). GABA agonists, e.g., show variable effects in animal models of anxiety and in human trials (Sanger, 1985), and GABA antagonists unreliably reverse benzodiazepine effects in animal models, often only at convulsant doses (Sepinwall and Cook, 1978). The possibility is thus suggested that a non-GABA-coupled benzodiazepine receptor site is involved in the mediation of the anxiolytic effects of the benzodiazepines. The anxiolytic potency of benzodiazepine compounds, both in humans and as predicted from animal models, is significantly correlated with the binding potency of these compounds at the benzodiazepine receptor site (Cook, 1982; Cook and Davidson, 1973; Cook and Sepinwall, 1975a), suggesting a pharmacological role, at least of this receptor, in anxiety modulation.

Based on these considerations, Ninan and associates (1982) investigated the effects of an intravenously administered benzodiazepine inverse agonist, ethyl-B-carboline-3-carboxylate (B-CCE), in chair-adapted rhesus monkeys. The monkeys showed profound signs of fear, such as struggling in the chair, head and body turning, vocalization, immobilization, defecation and urination, and decreased food and water intake. These monkeys also demonstrated increased sympathetic and hypothalamic-pituitary-adrenal axis activity as evidenced by increased adrenocorticotrophic hormone (ACTH), cortisol, and beta-endorphin levels in plasma. All these effects were prevented by pretreatment with the benzodiazepine antagonist Ro 15-1788, suggesting a specific benzodiazepine receptor-mediated process. These investigators (Crawley et al., 1984a; Skolnick et al., 1984) then examined the effects of coadministration of B-CCE and one of the following commonly used or experimental anxiolytic medications: clonidine, an alpha-2-adrenergic agonist (which, at low doses, acts presynaptically on the autoreceptors of locus ceruleus neurons to decrease their firing); propranolol, a beta-adrenergic receptor antagonist; cyproheptadine, a serotonin antagonist; diazepam, a benzodiazepine agonist; and 4,5,6,7-tetrahydroisoxazolo-[5,4-C]pyridine-3-ol (THIP), a GABA agonist. The behavioral effects of B-CCE in the monkeys were blocked by clonidine, diazepam, cyproheptadine, and THIP, and the heart rate and blood pressure changes were blocked by clonidine, diazepam, and propanolol. The increased levels of ACTH and beta-endorphin were blocked completely by diazepam and to a more limited extent by clonidine and propranolol. The different spectrum of effects of the various antianxiety drugs on the behavioral vs. autonomic concomitants of B-CCE administration may reflect the differential effectiveness of these agents in the treatment of specific symptoms of anxiety or in different types of anxiety disorders. Curiously, the autonomic effects of the drugs and their role in the reduction of anxiety are of some theoretical import; James (1884, 1890) and Lange (1885) speculated long ago on the importance of interoceptive cues produced by the autonomic nervous system in the attribution of emotional value to a given situation. In particular, they suggested that we feel anxious because of physical sensations, e.g., our heart is beating rapidly, and not vice versa. The implication, then, is that, if the autonomic cues of the rapid heartbeat could be reversed, then the anxiety would also be relieved.

The beta-carboline-induced state is a particularly compelling model of anxiety (including perhaps panic attacks) for both its behavioral and physiological concomitants as well as its pharmacologic responsivity. Indeed, corroboration is obtained from consideration of a small sample of humans (N = 5), two of whom experienced profound and intense anxiety similar to panic attacks following the administration of a beta-carboline derivative (FG 7142) (Dorow et al., 1983).

Noradrenergic System

The relationship between stress, anxiety, and catecholamine release and turnover has been the focus of research since the early part of this century. The basic hypothesis has been that pathological anxiety is related to episodes of increased catecholaminergic activity. The importance of the noradrenergic system in particular has been suggested by work arising from the chemical induction of anxiety in humans (Charney and Heninger, 1985a,b; Liebowitz et al., 1985; Rainey et al., 1984; Uhde et al., 1984b, 1985b) and manipulation of the locus ceruleus in other species (Redmond, 1981; Redmond and Huang, 1979). The locus ceruleus provides noradrenergic input to the limbic cortex, amygdala, and hippocampus, all of which have been linked to fear and anxiety in animal models and human pathology.

Electrical stimulation of the locus ceruleus in monkeys is associated with intensity-related struggling movements, vigilance/scanning, lip-smacking, teeth-grinding, chair-grasping, hair-pulling, yawning, and hand-wringing (Redmond, 1981; Redmond and Huang, 1979). Many of these behaviors are normally expressed responses to threatening stimuli in the environment. A similar behavioral profile can be produced through pharmacological manipulations that increase locus ceruleus firing and noradrenergic output (Redmond, 1981; Redmond and Huang, 1979). Moreover, bilateral lesions of the locus ceruleus decrease the responsiveness of monkeys to threatening conditions (e.g., human confrontation) (Redmond, 1981; Redmond and Huang, 1979), a finding that may also be relevant to human pathologies in which a lack of appropriate anxiety is a prominent feature (e.g., hypomania and antisocial personality disorder).

Human studies of the pharmacology of the noradrenergic system have shown that some drugs that increase locus ceruleus firing (e.g., yohimbine and caffeine) may have anxiogenic effects in man (Boulenger et al., 1984a,b, 1986; Elam et al., 1981; Gorman et al., 1964; Uhde and Boulenger, 1986), whereas others (e.g., buspirone and carbamazepine) do not (Olpe and Jones, 1983; Uhde et al., 1984c). Drugs that decrease locus ceruleus firing (e.g., benzodiazepines, ethanol, morphine, and clonidine) generally have anxiolytic and/or sedative effects (Aghajanian, 1977; Bird and Kuhar, 1977; Korf et al., 1974; Pohorecky and Brick, 1977; Strahlendorf and Strahlendorf, 1981). Overall, studies of locus ceruleus function suggest that the noradrenergic system might play a role in a spectrum of arousal states ranging from disinterest in normal fear-producing stimuli, through increased arousal and alertness, to hypervigilance and panic ("fight and flight" behaviors). Further studies will be required to elucidate the role of this neurotransmitter system and others in the etiology and neurobiology of anxiety.

BEHAVIORAL SUPPRESSION PROCEDURES

Punishment Procedures

Of the several procedures commonly used to screen for new anxiolytic agents, the most widely used is what has been referred to as the conflict procedure (Geller and Seifter, 1960). This model has been shown to be highly selective to antianxiety agents and has been tested in a great variety of species [e.g., goldfish (Geller et al., 1974), pigeons (McMillan, 1973; Morse, 1964), rats (Cook and Davidson, 1973; Geller, 1962), cats (Jacobsen, 1957; Yen et al., 1970), pigs (Dantzer, 1975; Dantzer and Roca, 1974), and monkeys (Beer and Migler, 1975; Cook and Catania, 1964; Holtzman and Villarreal, 1973)]. In general, the paradigm involves repeated, alternating exposure to two different experimental contingenices. In the presence of one stimulus, the subject's responses occasionally produce reinforcement, e.g., food or milk. In the presence of a second stimulus, responses in addition produce a noxious stimulus, such as electric shock. Consequently, the rate of response differs in the two situations, higher rates being generated when only reinforcement is present and lower rates occurring when both punishment and reinforcement are present. The behavioral suppression or decreased response rate that occurs when the shock is presented simultaneously with the positive reinforcement, i.e., in the "conflict" component of the schedule, has been demonstrated to be reversed by drugs with clinical anxiolytic effectiveness (Cook and Davidson, 1973; Cook and Sepinwall, 1975a,b). These include benzodiazepines, barbiturates, meprobamate, ethanol, and buspirone (see Sepinwall and Cook 1978 for review). In contrast, amphetamine and several other drugs without anxiolytic effects are generally ineffective in increasing the rate of occurrence of punished behavior (Sepinwall and Cook, 1978). In addition, a good correlation has been demonstrated in this paradigm between clinical efficacy and response-increasing potency of many anxiolytic drugs (Cook and Davidson, 1973). The reliability of the behavioral baselines, once established, makes this a useful procedure for the repeated testing of the same or different drugs. However, not all drugs with at least some antianxiety properties, e.g., morphine or clonidine (Hoehn-Saric et al., 1981), reliably reverse the behavioral suppression (Sepinwall and Cook, 1978). This procedure also carries the drawback that considerable time is necessary to train the animals and to determine appropriate levels of shock for each animal. In addition, rates of responding in the punished components are commonly quite low, making detection of propunishment (and therefore possibly anxiogenic) effects of drugs difficult to document (but see Glowa et al., 1986, for an exception).

Recently, the usefulness of the conflict paradigm has been extended to include the elucidation of neuroanatomical and neurochemical substrates of the anxiolytic effects of benzodiazepines on punished behavior. Intra-amygdaloid injections of midazolam (a benzodiazepine agonist) or muscimol (a GABA agonist) have been shown to increase punished responding, and this effect was blocked by the coadministration of a GABA antagonist (Petersen and Scheel-Kruger, 1982). In contrast, injections of GABA into the dorsal raphe nuclei did not increase punished behavior, although intra-raphe chlordiazepoxide did (Thiebot et al., 1984). Taken together, these data further emphasize the controversy over the role of GABA in the benzodiazepine antianxiety effects but also suggest that the conflict may be resolved by studying benzodiazepine effects on different brain structures.

A similar but more convenient procedure has been developed by Vogel and associates (1971), in which water-deprived animals are given access to a water bottle from which both water and shock are simultaneously delivered to the animal when it attempts to drink. A principal advantage of this procedure is that the behavior to be punished is already well established in the subjects. Again, benzodiazepines and other anxiolytic drugs increase responding when shock is present but not when shock is absent (Lippa et al., 1979; Vogel and Principi, 1971). Furthermore, this procedure can be used to screen for propunishment or anxiogenic compounds: By manipulating the shock level appropriately, intensities can be found that do not suppress drinking under control conditions but that do following the administration of anxiogenic compounds (e.g., beta-carbolines) (Corda et al., 1983).

The beta-carboline-induced suppression of water intake can be reversed by benzodiazepine antagonists or diazepam, again suggesting mediation by the benzodiazepine receptor (Corda et al., 1983). This procedure has also been used to characterize behaviorally the recently isolated endogenous peptide diazepambinding inhibitor (DBI), which acts at the benzodiazepine receptor site (Gupta and Holland, 1969). DBI appears to be anxiogenic in this conflict procedure, which is consistent with its other biochemical and physiological properties (Costa, 1982).

The pharmacological specificity of this paradigm has not yet been investigated adequately with regard to anxiogenic compounds, and the additive nature of the low-intensity shock and anxiogenic compounds might also be worthy of study. It could be useful to understand how two very different stimuli are translated by the animal into a summed overt behavioral suppression.

Conditioned Suppression

Another procedure based on the suppression of behavior by noxious stimulation is the conditioned suppression procedure. Also known as the conditioned emotional response (CER) or Estes-Skinner procedure, it was suggested at its introduction as an experimental model of anxiety (Estes and Skinner, 1941) and was one of the earliest behavioral baselines for the assessment of drug effects (Brady, 1956). Most frequently, this procedure superimposes upon an ongoing appetitive baseline brief presentations of a previously neutral stimulus ending in unavoidable shock. Despite continued availability of positive reinforcement, behavior nevertheless becomes suppressed during the preshock stimulus, only to resume promptly after the delivery of the unavoidable shock. The clearly counterproductive loss of reinforcers in the face of an inevitable event offered strong appeal as a model of anxiety. However, this paradigm has not proved as reliable a screen for drugs as the punishment procedure (Capell et al., 1972; Ray, 1964; Sepinwall and Cook, 1978; but see Lavener, 1963; Metlot and Deutsch, 1984; and Miczek, 1973; for examples of successful antisuppressant effects of anxiolytics in the CER paradigm).

One potentially important difference between the conflict and CER paradigms is the contingent vs. noncontingent nature of the noxious stimuli. This issue has been addressed by studies using yoked pairs of animals trained to respond for food. One of the pair received response-contingent shock and the other received noncontingent shock on the same schedule as its partner. Benzodiazepines selectively increased punished responding in the animals receiving contingent shock and not in those receiving noncontingent shock (Huppert and Iversen, 1975; McMillan and Leander, 1975).

Several general criticisms have been made concerning the conflict and CER models of behavioral suppression. First, benzodiazepines have been shown to increase consummatory responses (Cooper and Estall, 1985; Randall et al., 1960) and thus may increase responding because of an enhancement of the reinforcement value of the food or water rather than because of a specific effect on suppressed behavior per se. If so, then there is little utility in a punishment or CER procedure, since consummatory responses can be more easily measured, and the animal could be spared the aversive experience. This criticism is seriously weakened by the work of Margules and Stein (1968) and Cook and Davidson (1973), who tried to mimic the effects of anxiolytics on punished responding by increased food deprivation. No increases in punished responding resulted. A second criticism concerns the use of noxious stimuli in these procedures, which may confound antianxiety properties of drugs with their analgesic effects. However, morphine's inconsistent effects in the conflict procedure (Sepinwall and Cook, 1978) suggest that analgesia is not sufficient to reverse reliably the behavioral suppression (and, in addition, corresponds to the opiate's inconsistent anxiety-reducing effects in humans). A third and more telling criticism is that the specificity of the conflict procedure may be limited to certain classes of anxiolytic agents and thus may produce false negatives in drug screening procedures. This, of course, is of potential clinical import in any drug screening procedure.

Even with these criticisms in mind, the usefulness of the punishment, or conflict, paradigm cannot be overestimated from the standpoint of anxiolytic drug screening. However, the value of these paradigms for our understanding of human anxiety is less apparent. The idea of conflict created by simultaneous presentation of reinforcing and punishing stimuli has a certain face validity, but that may be where its utility ends. For example, the benzodiazepine-produced increases in punished responding and not in unpunished responding may be explained, at least in part, on the basis of rate dependency (see Sanger and Blackman, 1976; Robbins, 1981; Spealman, 1978). That is, in many experimental situations, the behavioral effects of drugs have been shown to be dependent on the ongoing rate of the behavior in the absence of drug administration (Dews, 1958; Kelleher and Morse, 1968; Robbins, 1981; Schiller, 1952). In particular, many drugs have been shown to increase low rates of responding while not affecting or decreasing higher rates of responding. These effects have been demonstrated in single experimental sessions in the same animals, ruling out any possibility of individual differences accounting for the differential drug effects. Similarly, in the conflict procedure, benzodiazepines increase low rates of responding (in the punished component) while not affecting higher rates of responding (in the nonpunished component). Thus the differential effects on punished behavior may be, in part or in toto, attributable to differential effects on baselines of differing response rates, regardless of whether punishment is employed. Caution, then, is required in interpreting the drug effects on punished behavior as representing pharmacologic manipulation of fear or anxiety.

Species-Relevant Paradigms

Other models of behavioral suppression or inhibition attempt to make use of species-relevant "anxiety-producing" situations. The simplest of these is the *open-field paradigm*, in which rodents are exposed to a large, open arena, usually well illuminated, in which fecal boli, locomotor activity, and appetitive responses are measured (Broadhurst, 1957; Hall, 1934). In general, high rates of defecation and an inhibition of exploratory activity and consummatory responses are observed. However, following habituation to the environment or the administration of anxiolytic drugs, these behaviors may be modified.

Crawley and associates (Blumstein and Crawley, 1983; Crawley, 1981; Crawley and Goodwin, 1980) used a modification of the open-field paradigm that takes into account rodents' avoidance of brightly lit areas to evaluate behavioral suppression and drug effects. Their apparatus contained a dark and a bright side, and the relevant measure was the number of crossings each subject made to each side. In addition, overall locomotor activity was measured separately to rule out any nonspecific sedating properties of drugs. Crawley et al. (1984b) employed this model to evaluate the effects of both anxiolytic and anxiogenic substances and found it simple to use and fairly specific for anxiolytic substances (which increase the number of crossings). It appears, however, to be less sensitive to anxiogenic compounds, a limitation it shares with most other procedures.

Disruption of social interaction has also been used to model anxiety, the assumption being that, in rodents at least, social behavior decreases in aversive situations. File (1980) and Geller (1962) exposed pairs of same-sexed rats to environments that contained greater or lesser degrees of "fear-provoking" stimulation and then measured the rats' social contact (e.g., licking and grooming). The variables of which these behaviors were a function were familiarity with the test environment and ambient lighting, with the most behaviorally suppressing situation being one with low familiarity and bright illumination. Under these conditions, social behavior was suppressed, and the effects of anxiolytics could be measured (File and Hyde, 1978). Under conditions of high familiarity and dim lighting, extensive social interaction occurred, and the effects of anxiogenic compounds became manifest (File et al., 1982; File and Lister, 1983). Again, this model offers a fairly simple and quick way to assess drug effects. However, it has the disadvantage of being sensitive to nonspecific sedating or activating properties of drugs, the extent of which requires separate evaluation.

The *acoustic startle reflex* is a reliably elicited and quantifiable behavior. Furthermore, the response can be augmented by pairing the eliciting stimulus with a conditioned stimulus that had previously been presented with foot shock. This is known as the potentiated startle response paradigm, which has been shown to be highly sensitive to the effects of anxiolytic agents (Davis, 1980). Similarly, *defensive burying* is a behavior observed in rodents in response to conditioning with an aversive stimulus (Treit et al., 1981). Rats that received shock through a metal prod will subsequently bury the prod when given access to it in their home cages. Tests with other stimuli showed a high degree of stimulus control by the conditioned stimulus. Suppression of the defensive burying behavior has also been found following the administration of anxiolytic but not other drugs (Treit, 1985). Finally, *isolation-induced behavioral alterations*, especially aggression, can be observed in rodents (usually mice) and can be modified by anxiolytic drugs (Garattini and Valzelli, 1981).

Although these procedures are of interest in relation to their ability to differentiate different classes of drugs, their relation to anxiety is not completely clear. The effects of illumination on the behavior of rodents is of some interest in view of reports of sensitivity to light in some panic disorder patients (Hobbs et al., 1984). Analogies between social interaction and social withdrawal or social phobias in man can also be drawn. However, anxious patients in general do not show increased startle responses or overt aggression, although treatment with benzodiazepines has been associated with an increase in hostile verbal content and "disinhibited" behaviors in several patient populations. Defensive burying behavior could also be viewed as somewhat analagous to the avoidance of fearful objects and stimuli in man. Many assumptions must be made in the interpretation of the animal's behavior and its precipitants to consider these as models of human anxiety. Nevertheless, they may prove to be simple and useful tools for drug screening.

Phobias may develop following a single instance or few instances of exposure to the stimulus, or they may be learned by observation of other individuals. Although phobias to a wide variety of stimuli occur, most typically they are associated with certain stimuli and not others (e.g., spiders and snakes vs. kittens and refrigerators). In the *taste aversion procedure*, a novel food or drink (e.g., saccharin-flavored water) is paired with illness as a result of coadministration of an unconditioned toxic stimulus (e.g., lithium chloride or ionizing radiation). On subsequent presentations of the previously novel flavor, little or no consumption occurs (Garcia and Koelling, 1966). It is important to note that the avoidance response can occur after a single exposure to the stimulus and despite an interval of several hours between exposure to the novel flavor and the effect of the unconditioned stimulus. The behavior can also be highly resistant to extinction (i.e., repeated exposure to the novel stimulus without the consequent illness-producing effect weakens the avoidance only slowly). In addition, there appears to be a species-typical preparedness for the kinds of stimuli to which an animal will develop an aversion. Rats, e.g., will avoid a substance by its taste (Garcia and Koelling, 1966), whereas pigeons will make use of its visual properties (Glowa and Barrett,

1983). These various qualities of taste aversion in animals, and its uniqueness among animal learning paradigms, make it an intriguing phenomenon, especially with respect to its relevance to human phobic responses (Seligman, 1971; Seligman and Hager, 1972).

Intense fear and avoidance of snakes have been demonstrated in monkeys reared in the wild (Hebb, 1946; Yerkes and Yerkes, 1936) and can be acquired by laboratory-reared monkeys through observation of their conspecifics' response (Mineka et al., 1984). Additionally, these responses are difficult to diminish by extinction (Mineka and Keir, 1983; Mineka et al., 1980) even with the presentation of reinforcement in the presence of the "phobic" stimulus. This model in primates holds great promise for examining the development and plasticity of phobic responses in humans.

DRUG DISCRIMINATION

Another behavioral analogue of anxiety attempts to use the interoceptive cues produced by "anxiogenic" substances in drug discrimination trials (Lal and Emmett-Oglesby, 1983). In these paradigms, a subject may be exposed to a two-choice situation in which pressing one lever will produce food and pressing the other lever will not. The lever associated with reinforcement in a particular session is determined by the drug treatment of the subject prior to the session. For example, pentylenetetrazol (PTZ) administration may be associated with correct right-lever responses, whereas saline pretreatment is associated with reinforced left-lever responses. No other cues are available to the subject other than the presession administration. Following training with a particular drug and dose, testing can be conducted to evaluate generalization to other doses of the same drug or to related drugs. Drugs that antagonize the effects of the training drug can also be assessed. In essence, the animal is revealing something about its subjective drug experience and the relation of one drug to another. PTZ has been used as a model anxiogenic drug in drug discrimination studies for several reasons (Lal and Emmett-Oglesby, 1983). First, it has been shown to produce anxiety in humans. Second, it can be given repeatedly at low doses with no evidence of development of sensitization or tolerance to its discriminative stimulus properties. Third, it has few peripheral side effects (unlike yohimbine, for example), increasing the likelihood that the central action of the drug forms the basis of the discrimination.

Animals trained to discriminate PTZ from saline show marked generalization to anxiogenic drugs such as the beta-carbolines, yohimbine, and high but not low doses of cocaine (Lal and Emmett-Oglesby, 1983; Shearman and Lal, 1981). This latter finding is of some interest in that cocaine shares its chemical properties with two classes of drugs: stimulants, which may be associated with cocaine's euphoriant properties, and local anesthetics, which may be linked to its proconvulsant and anxiogenic effects. In similar drug discrimination studies, the effects at high doses of cocaine were shown to be blocked by diazepam but not haloperidol, whereas the effects of low doses of cocaine were blocked by haloperidol but not diazepam (Shearman and Lal, 1981). Generalization to PTZ is also produced by precipitated and nonprecipitated withdrawal from diazepam (Lal and Emmett-Oglesby, 1983). Anxiolytic compounds block the PTZ-based discriminations in a dose-related manner, and drugs that are most effective clinically are also the most effective in blocking the PTZ discriminative cues. A high correlation exists between a drug's minimal effective dose generated in the conflict procedure and the drug's ED50 dose in PTZ discrimination (R = 0.96, P < 0.01) (Lal and Shearman, 1981). The advantages of this paradigm over the conflict procedure include a sensitivity to anxiogenic drug or environmental conditions and a lack of dependence on rate of responding and hence a wider range of dose-response relationships that can be examined (Lal and Emmett-Oglesby, 1983).

GENETIC MODELS

Recent evidence indicates that panic attacks and agoraphobia show a fair degree of heritability, similar to that reported for other psychiatric disorders (Crowe et al., 1983). The degree of genetic relatedness of phobic or generalized anxiety disorders is less clear, and it may be that the syndromes are genetically tied to less specific factors, e.g., physiological responsiveness or unusual susceptibility to certain types of conditioning. (These less specific factors, of course, may operate in panic disorder as well.) Nevertheless, the development of animal models of anxiety or emotionality have been attempted on the basis of selective breeding experiments.

Maudsley Rats

Maudsley high-reactive rats have been bred since 1954 on the basis of their high rates of defecation in an open-field situation (Broadhurst 1957, 1960, 1962, 1975). After 15 or more generations, groups of rats have been identified that respond with greater degrees of emotionality or behavioral impairment on tests as diverse as avoidance conditioning (Broadhurst, 1966; Joffe, 1964), maze learning (Weldon, 1967), and stress-induced polydipsia (Imada, 1972). The utility of such models is in characterizing the differential responsiveness of these animals to drugs with specific actions in the brain and in searching for specific related anatomical or biochemical alterations or adaptations. Differences have been described in the reactive strain in thyroid and adrenal gland function (Broadhurst and Eysenck, 1965; Feuer, 1969), in their responsiveness to psychomotor stimulants (Gupta and Holland, 1969; Satinder, 1971), and in their preference for alcohol (Brewster, 1969). In addition, reactive rats have been shown to have lower levels of norepinephrine in many of their peripheral tissues (e.g., adrenal glands, spleen, and heart) (Liang and Blizard, 1978). Finally, decreased numbers of benzodiazepine receptors in the reactive rats have been reported (Robertson et al., 1978), although this finding has not been replicated in a more recent study (Tamborska et al., 1986).

Nervous Dogs

A "nervous" line of pointer dogs has also been bred since the early 1970s on the basis of behavioral abnormalities initially observed in a single pointer female (Murphree, 1973; Murphree et al., 1977). This particular animal had been used for many years as a hunting dog until on one particular occasion she experienced a "nervous breakdown," from which she never completely recovered. She was bred, and her offspring were studied along with the offspring of another, more stable dog of the same line. All the nervous mother's pups showed the nervous syndrome that she exhibited. Behaviorally, the nervous line of pointers demonstrate their abnormalities most predominantly in the presence of humans. The nervous dogs can be interactive and playful with other dogs, and they breed and care for their young normally. However, when exposed to humans, the dogs show such signs of fear as freezing, trembling, urination, defecation, and catatonic immobility. Normal responses to threat, such as aggression, vocalization, or escape, are noticeably absent in these animals except when they are placed in unfamiliar environments or, in some cases, after diazepam administration (Uhde and Weiss, unpubished observations). The development of these abnormal behaviors reliably follows a time course beginning when the dogs are 3 months of age and continuing to the full-blown state by 1 year of age (Murphree et al., 1974a,b). Attempted environmental interventions at any point in the development of these dogs have not modified their ultimate behaviors, although in some cases temporary ·shifts towards friendliness were seen (Murphree et al., 1974; Reese, 1978). Biochemical studies of the cerebrospinal fluid (CSF) and plasma have shown few dissimilarities between the nervous and normal strains (DeLuca et al., 1974). There are higher levels of cholinesterase in the spinal fluid of nervous dogs compared to the normals, and there appears to be a hyporesponsiveness to external stressors such as food deprivation, exercise, epinephrine injection, and foot shock, as measured by levels of creatine phosphokinase (CPK) in the plasma. Measures of noradrenergic and serotonergic metabolites in the CSF and of plasma lactate levels, lymphocytes, monocytes, hematocrit, and hemoglobin were not different for the two strains (DeLuca et al., 1974). No differences in brain ^{3}H-yohimbine binding were observed between the nervous and normal lines of pointer dogs (Klein et al., 1988). The nervous dogs do show an increased susceptibility to atrioventricular block and, in certain environments, to mange. The nervous pointers can be trained to bar press for food while under the influence of benzodiazepines (Murphree et al., 1969), but their behaviors to date have been relatively resistant to single-dose diazepam treatment and unresponsive to administration of the benzodiazepine antagonist Ro 15-1788 (Uhde, 1986). This latter finding argues against the hypothesis of an innate benzodiazepine inverse agonist as the principal pathogenesis of nervous behaviors in this genetic model. It remains to be determined whether chronic treatment might be more helpful. Interestingly, "spontaneous" (i.e., not based on selective breeding) abnormal behaviors in purebred beagles, including patterns similar to those found in the nervous pointer dogs, are significantly reduced with chronic imipramine treatment. Moreover, the time course of this response parallels that seen with imipramine treatment of panic disorder.

One general caution for experiments designed to breed animals for a particular trait concerns the difficulty in knowing exactly what trait is being selected. For example, we have recently determined that, in a small sample of the pointer dogs (25 nervous and 15 normals), 72% of the nervous dogs and none of the normals were deaf according to an auditory evoked response assessment. Further investigation of these animals revealed that the behavioral abnormalities of the nervous dogs were present in both the normally hearing and the deaf animals (Klein et al., 1988). However, the lesson for experimenters carrying out breeding experiments remains, namely, that the interpretation of the etiology and extent of behavioral abnormalities in animals must be made very cautiously.

Apart from this obvious example of the difficulties that can be encountered in breeding experiments is another, more subtle, yet theoretically important problem, that of analagous vs. homologous behaviors. The ability to develop an avoidance response to stimuli that are potentially dangerous would be of obvious importance for survival and thus may be very primitive in phylogentic origin. As such, there may be common biological underpinnings to these behaviors in a variety of species. Alternatively, however, the importance of these responses in a great range of environments may mean that, despite common pressures for these behaviors to develop, their ultimate emergence could have followed different evolutionary paths in their respective biological substrates.

An example is the nonhomologous development of digits on the anterior appendages of man and raccoons. Despite great superficial similarities, these developments do not share a common evolutionary ancestry. That is to say, they are structurally analogous but not homologous. This difficulty cannot be directly addressed by breeding experiments but should be kept in mind with regard to extrapolations from the data.

MOLECULAR BASIS OF ANXIETY

In an elegant set of experiments, Kandel and associates (Kandel, 1983, 1985; Walters et al., 1979, 1981) have begun to explore the molecular basis of anxiety using sensitization and classical conditioning of the gill withdrawal reflex in aplysia. Aplysia are sea mollusks that, despite the simplicity of their nervous system, have been shown to exhibit behaviors similar to those described in man as learning, memory, and anxiety. Furthermore, the simplicity of the aplysia's nervous system has provided an opportunity to work out the details of the neural circuitry of several of the behavioral responses (Kandel, 1983; Kandel and Schwartz, 1982). Chronic anxiety was modeled using a sensitization paradigm, in which increased behavioral responsivity follows repeated exposure to an unconditioned aversive stimulus in the absense of an explicit conditioned stimulus. Anticipatory anxiety was modeled with a classical aversive conditioning procedure, in which a conditioned stimulus immediately preceded an unconditioned aversive stimulus (Kandel, 1983; Walters et al., 1979, 1981). The behavioral responses produced by these procedures include increased defensive reactions (head and siphon withdrawal, escape locomotion, and inking) and decreased appetitive responses. This method of study has been very fruitful. Kandel and associates (1983) demonstrated that sensitization occurs through changes in the sensory neurons and facilitatory interneurons activated by the aversive stimulus. These interneurons synapse on the presynaptic terminals of the sensory neurons and release a serotonin-like neurotransmitter that activates cyclic adenosine monophosphate (cAMP) and enhances the transmission of the sensory neuron. This enhancement occurs by a series of steps that produce an increased-dura-tion action potential and cause the release of more neurotransmitter by the sensitized neuron. With sufficient repetitions of this event, the serotonin-activated cAMP migrates to the nucleus of the cell and can alter transcription of m-RNA to make this process a more permanent one within the cell. Classical conditioning, at least in the short term, seems to occur through cellular mechanisms similar to those of sensitization, but with a much greater response enhancement in the sensory neuron following fewer training trials (Kandel, 1985). This increased response appears to be a function of the activation of the sensory neurons associated with the conditioned stimulus just prior to the activation of those neurons associated with the unconditioned stimulus (see Kandel, 1983, 1985, for a detailed description of the molecular events underlying these processes).

Kandel speculates that similar learning mechanisms may be involved in the development of anxiety and that these would then be reversible by counterconditioning or psychotherapy, which could reverse the changes in mRNA transcription that occurred with conditioning. It remains to be established whether parallel processes operate in the development of sensitization or classical conditioning in aplysia and anxiety in humans. It seems likely, however, that the fundamental principles of learning may be consistent across species (see Razran 1971).

INTEGRATIVE MODELS

In the discussion that follows, attention is given to several behavioral models of anxiety in which an integration of genetics and environmental precipitants is considered. The complexity of this interaction in the development of behavioral pathology will become readily apparent and will be a major focus of the conclusion.

Learned Helplessness

Learned helplessness is a model that has been more traditionally associated with depression than with anxiety. However, the overlap and coincidence of these symptoms in human pathology are significant and may be associated with common etiological factors and biological underpinnings. In fact, the most effective treatments for panic disorder at present are tricyclic antidepressants, monoamine oxidase inhibitors, and alprazolam, which is a triazolobenzodiazepine with reported antidepressant effects (Ballenger et al., 1988; Klein, 1964; Sheehan et al., 1980, 1984). The learned helplessness model is one in which animals are exposed to uncontrollable aversive events (usually electric shock) and are then tested for their ability to acquire new behavior in either positive or negative reinforcement procedures (Overmier and Seligman, 1967; Seligman and Maier, 1967). Often, the comparison is made between subjects with control over the termination of a noxious event and those with no control but equivalent exposure to the noxious stimuli (a yoked-control procedure). Hence, subsequent behavioral or biochemical alterations can be analyzed with respect to control over the environment and not just to exposure to aversive events. Impaired acquisition of appetitive and escape tasks (Brown and Jacobs, 1949; Dinsmoor, 1958; Dinsmoor and Campbell, 1956; Maier and Seligman, 1976; Morse, 1964; Seligman, 1975; Seligman and Hager, 1972), decreased aggression (Coromi and Thurmond, 1977; Maier et al., 1972), hypercortisolemia (Swenson and Vogel, 1983), alterations in noradrenergic and serotenergic function (Weiss et al., 1975; Petty and Sherman, 1982), increased ulceration (Weiss, 1970, 1971), and analgesia (Grav et al., 1981; Jackson et al., 1979; Maier et al., 1982) are among the effects reported in animals subjected to uncontrollable but not controllable stress. These effects can be reversed by the administration of antidepressants chronically, but not acutely, following exposure to uncontrollable stress (Anisman et al., 1980; Leshner et al., 1979; Petty and Sherman, 1980; Sherman et al., 1982). Prophylaxis with chronic antidepressant or acute anxiolytic administration has also been reported (Sherman et al., 1979).

Recently, a behavioral impairment similar to that seen following exposure to uncontrollable shock was reported in animals treated 24 hr earlier with a benzodiazepine inverse agonist (Drugen et al., 1985). These data were interpreted as suggesting that similar interoceptive cues may be produced by exposure to uncontrollable shock or administration of an anxiogenic drug and that the drug effects were trans-

lated into a behavioral deficit similar to that produced by electric shock. (Note the similarity here to the additivity of propunishment drugs with electric shock in the conflict procedure; see above.) Although these data are provocative, the fact that no other drugs have been examined in this procedure leaves unanswered questions concerning the pharmacological specificity of the effect. Additional study of these findings would certainly be worthwhile.

For some time, investigators studying the learned helplessness phenomenon, especially in rats, have been aware of the difficulties related to the reliable induction of a behavioral impairment in certain strains of rats (Petty, 1985), in different rats from the same litter (Doty et al., unpublished observations), and even at particular times of the year (Henn, 1985). These individual differences have become a source of interest; they may be reflective of different predispositions of animals toward certain behavioral pathologies. As a consequence, various experimenters have been breeding rats according to their performance in the learned helplessness paradigm (Henn, 1985). It remains to be seen how well these differential performances can be produced through breeding experiments, especially in such already inbred strains.

Individual differences between rats of the same litter may also be observable in more natural settings, in which the rats are allowed to develop normal social interactions and hierarchies. Perhaps those rats that are more dominant are also more resistant to the effects of exposure to uncontrollable stress. This may be the result of differential biochemical or endocrine factors and may also involve some degree of learning. For example, dominant rats could develop a greater sense of control over their environment, since their behavior is more effective than that of less dominant rats in either obtaining reinforcers (e.g., access to food) or avoiding aversive consequences (e.g., offensive attacks). In a fascinating set of experiments, Mineka et al. (1985) demonstrated that monkeys given control over the delivery of food, water, and treats in their environment were much less fearful and more exploratory in stressful situations than those without such control. This suggests that control per se and not just control over aversive events can exert profound effects on subsequent behavior. Mineka and Kihlstrom (1978) also suggest that loss of control, especially in an environment in which previous control was established, may be detrimental to subsequent behavior, although Weiss and Glazer (1975) have shown that experience with control over shock will protect rats from the effects of subsequent helplessness training. Which of these findings is the more general is subject to verification and may depend on the amount of protection and/or the degree of loss of control.

An additional advantage of the breeding studies for the learned helplessness paradigm is that control over or manipulation of the early environment can also be accomplished. Perhaps the strain and litter differences seen by investigators in this field can be accounted for by differences in numbers of animals cohoused, temperature variations in the colony, or changes in diet or personnel. Most of these possibilities are difficult to address because rats usually are purchased from breeding colonies, and this information is not readily available. "Helplessness" (i.e., a deficit in the acquisition of new behavior) has been demonstrated in adult rats that received exposure to uncontrollable aversive events as weanlings (Brookshire et al., 1961; Levine et al., 1956), strengthening this argument even more. Furthermore, these differences in individuals or in litters may become more profound or more obvious when the animals are exposed to aversive events or other kinds of challenge situations (see below).

Primate Separation and Intrusion Studies

Over the years, beginning with the work of Harry Harlow (Seay et al., 1962), various monkey separation studies have been conducted. These have included isolation from mothers, surrogate mothers, peers, and all conspecifics. The resultant behavioral and physiological aberrations bear a marked resemblance to those seen in human reactive depression. Although the separation model has typically been used to study depression, it may serve equally well as a model of anxiety and has recently been considered in this capacity (Suomi et al., 1981). An initial protest response occurs immediately following separation, perhaps similar to what occurs in man during a panic attack or exposure to a phobic stimulus. This response is characterized by extreme agitation, increased vocalization (which has not been demonstrated in adult humans), and sympathetic crisis (increased heart rate, blood pressure, temperature, and cortisol and catecholamine levels). Note, however, that, in contrast to panic attacks in man, the protest behaviors in a monkey are likely to be highly adaptive in a nonexperimental environment, resulting in the primate's reunion with its lost family member or peer (Bowlby, 1969, 1973; Engel, 1962). In addition, panic attacks early in the course of panic disorder usually occur without a direct environmental precipitant, although many patients recalling their first panic attack note that it occurred at a time when they were experiencing a major life stress (Faravelli, 1985; Roy-Byrne et al., 1986a,b; Uhde et al., 1985a). In primates, a depressive response follows the separation by several days and is characterized by decreased activity, abnormal sleep patterns, increased self-mouthing and self-mutilation, decreased cortisol suppression following exogenously administered dexamethasone, and decreased noradrenergic and serotonergic turnover (Suomi et al., 1981). Both the initial "anxiety" response and the later "depressive" response have been shown to be alleviated by the administration of chronic antidepressants (Suomi et al., 1981). Interestingly, research in panic disorder patients suggests that major separations (e.g., death of a loved one) increase the risk for a subsequent major depression without increasing the frequency of panic attacks or the severity of phobic avoidance (Roy-Byrne et al., 1986a).

Monkeys that have experienced some form of separation also show abnormal behavior patterns when introduced to their normal environment. They are inclined toward enhanced contact following reunion (well above preseparation levels), greater responsivity to fear-eliciting stimuli (e.g., novel environments), and spontaneous or unprecipitated signs of "anxiety" (e.g., self-directed behaviors). This latter anxiety response can also become conditioned to a stimulus that had been paired with the initiation of a separation (Baysinger and Suomi, 1978). The admixture of "depression" and "anxiety" behaviors in the separation paradigms of monkeys is reminiscent of the influence and possible genetic linkage (Leckman et al., 1983) of depression and anxiety seen in panic disorder (Breier et al., 1984; Uhde et al., 1985a). The primate separation model, therefore, may provide a useful tool for identifying those biological substrates common to major depressive illness and panic disorder.

Another means of inducing "anxiety" in rhesus monkeys is exposing them to a group of unfamiliar monkeys who are in turn all familiar with each other. Studies of this sort enclose the initiate in a wire mesh cage to protect it from harm. Nevertheless, the monkeys show signs of great distress, including agitation, vocalization, and increased sympathetic activity. Again, a long-lasting sensitivity to other anxiety-producing stimuli is seen in these animals, along with decreased exploratory activity (Suomi, 1986).

In the course of these studies, a great deal of individual variability in monkeys was seen in response to the experimental manipulations, especially in the longer-latency behavioral consequences. This has been seen for both the anxiety-like reactions and the depressive response, which in some animals is completely absent. Recently, breeding experiments have been undertaken to examine the genetic relatedness of these behaviors as well as their susceptibility to modification by early environmental factors (e.g., nurturant vs. rejecting mothers) (Suomi, 1986).

Two strains of animals have been bred, which can be described as high- and low-reactive, based on their responses in various situations (Suomi, 1986). High-reactive monkeys show an increased responsiveness to separation, marked by expression of the depressive syndrome. High-reactive monkeys are much less investigative of novel stimuli in their environment, and the females tend to be more rejecting mothers. The low-reactive animals are less disrupted by environmental stressors and usually do not show a depressive response following separation. The reactiveness of individual monkeys can be detected at a very early age through the use of a variety of classical neurological tests (at 1 week of age) (Schneider, 1984), cortisol responses to mild stressors (at 1 month of age) (Suomi, 1986), and a measure of autonomic responsiveness (change in heart rate response following conditioning) (at 2 months of age) (Suomi et al., 1981). These measures have been shown to correlate significantly with anxiety- or depression-related behaviors (mainly self-directed behaviors, e.g., self-mouthing) observed later in life following exposure to an environmental stressor (Suomi, 1983, 1984; Suomi et al., 1981).

This model may provide a wealth of information but is still in its early stages. One of the main advantages of the study of monkeys is the ability of experimenters to identify anxiety-like behaviors on occasions other than when a specific noxious stimulus is present. The initial effects of separation are interesting and profound, but of greater import may be the longer-latency responses, such as self-mutilation, self-mouthing, or increased contact with the mother or peers upon reunion. The observation of these behaviors in lieu of a predisposing past history and without a specific environmental precipitant is much more similar to what is observed in human anxiety, especially pathologically. However, for this model to be of use, a thorough knowledge of the normal behavioral repertoire of the monkeys is necessary (Harlow and Harlow, 1969, 1971; Suomi et al., 1981). In addition, these experiments demonstrate the necessity of using challenge situations to bring out pathological states that may be reflective of underlying genetic propensities and environmental conditioning: In familiar, nonthreatening situations, the high- and low-reactive monkeys appear similar; it is only following a separation or intrusion experience that the individual differences in responsiveness become manifest (Suomi, 1984). This may be similar to anxiety-disordered patients who can function quite normally under many circumstances but show a decreased level of tolerance to certain internal or external stressors.

The data from the primate studies raise several important issues concerning the development of pathological anxiety. The influence of genetic factors seems to be important, in that different baseline sensitivities to fear-producing stimuli are observed. Second, the effect of early experience may be important, especially with regard to maternal care. The differences between rejecting and nurturant mothers may be important in determining whether early stresses produce sensitization to or protection from the effects of later stresses. Other factors as well may contribute to overall effects of stress, including predictability, controllability, and intensity of the stressor. Lack of predictability of either aversive events or safety might result in sensitization to the effects of external stressors, whereas the predictability and controllability of such events could result in tolerance. These primate separation and intrusion models of anxiety, apart from providing us with useful drug and/or biochemical assays, may also give us clues to the development and nature of anxiety.

In this respect, sensitization and tolerance may be useful ideas to consider regarding the development of anxiety. A study that illustrates this point rather dramatically involved a repeated 4 day separation of peer-reared monkeys following 3 days of reunion (Mineka et al., 1980). Initially, the animals displayed the normal protest reaction to the separation, followed by a depressive response in some animals. With repeated cycles, the monkeys began to display increasingly protest-related behaviors during progressively earlier periods of their reunion, even while their response during the actual separation was becoming less dramatic. This development of "anticipatory anxiety" is similar to sensitization in that the behaviors are occurring with earlier onset. At the same time, tolerance may be developing in the anxious or depressive response seen during separation, illustrating the importance of both of these phenomena and their interaction in behavioral pathology.

One further example of the importance of sensitization in the development of panic disorder is that of a human patient who gradually developed panic attacks following repeated self-administration of cocaine (Post et al., 1987). The anxiogenic effects of the drug increased, and eventually full-blown panic attacks occurred. Later, spontaneous panic attacks developed even though the patient had ceased cocaine use for many months. Thus, once established, episodes of panic continued to occur without contact with the provoking stimulus.

NEUROANATOMICAL SUBSTRATES OF ANXIETY

The following discussion centers on one particular theory of anxiety, which focuses on some of the neuroanatomical and neurochemical substrates of anxiety. This is not meant to be an exhaustive review; several brain areas that probably play an important role in the neurobiology of anxiety are not discussed (e.g., the amygdala and the forebrain dopamine systems). However, the usefulness of this theory is apparent in that it provides a conceptual framework from which to begin examining the biological substrates of anxiety-related behaviors.

Gray and colleagues (Gray, 1983, 1985; Gray et al., 1981) have attempted to incorporate the data gathered from animal models of anxiety and studies of mechanisms of antianxiety drug action into a coherent theory of anxiety in which certain brain areas and several neurotransmitters are specifically implicated. The model Gray proposes depends on several ideas. He defines anxiety-producing stimuli as those associated with punishment, nonreward, or novelty. When any of these stimuli impinge on the nervous system, a set of behavioral responses are produced that include behavioral inhibition (of behaviors such as exploration, feeding, and sex), increased arousal (or sympathetic activation), and hypervigilance. This coordinating of input and output is accomplished by the "behavioral inhibition system," upon which antianxiety agents exert their effects. Gray has mapped this system onto several brain structures, including the septal area, the hippocampus, the locus ceruleus, and the raphe nuclei. The septal-hippocampal system functions as a comparator, which determines whether or not incoming stimuli fall into the category of "anxiety-provoking." If so, then the behavioral inhibition system is activated, and normal motor programs are temporarily aborted and the behaviors described above are produced. Whereas the hippocampus and septum function in this comparator role, the locus ceruleus acts to modulate the sensitivity of the system, and the raphe may also act in a modulatory rule. The data upon which this theory rests are discussed below.

Locus Ceruleus

As was mentioned above, Redmond and co-workers (Redmond, 1981; Redmond and Huang, 1979) have shown that electrical and pharmacological activation of the locus ceruleus results in increased fear responses in monkeys, and lesions or pharmacological inhibition of the locus ceruleus are associated with decreased fear behaviors. Although these findings are controversial (Mason and Fibiger 1979), Weiss and associates (1982) have also claimed that increased firing of the locus ceruleus underlies the behavioral impairment observed following exposure to uncontrollable stress, which, they speculate, is most similar to "anxious depression." They speculate that total depletion of norepinephrine in the locus ceruleus is a consequence of massive release occurring during a stressful event. This depletion is by approximately 20%, which may represent the functional pool of norepinephrine (Glowinski 1975). The loss of norepinephrine results in an understimulation of the presynaptic alpha-2-adrenergic autoreceptors and hence a net increase in the activity of the locus ceruleus neurons. Weiss et al. (1982) note that the time course of the behavioral depression follows the time course of the norepinephrine depletion and that the recovery of the performance deficit occurs when synthesis of norepinephrine is increased sufficiently to replenish the loss. The increased norepinephrine synthesis is accomplished by greater tyrosine hydroxylase activity. In addition, repeated exposure to stressors (15 days) increases tyrosine hydroxylase activity and prevents the induction of the behavioral impairment. Pretreatment with a monoamine oxidase inhibitor (MAOI) during exposure to uncontrollable stress prevents the development of the behavioral deficit, presumably by decreasing the breakdown of norepinephrine and preventing the depletion. Local injections of clonidine, an alpha-2-adrenergic agonist that stimulates the autoreceptors of the locus ceruleus neurons, reverse the effects of exposure to uncontrollable shock. Administration of yohimbine, an alpha-2-adrenergic antagonist, produces a behavioral depression similar to that seen following exposure to uncontrollable stress.

Although these data strongly support a role of the locus ceruleus in the behavioral impairment produced by exposure to uncontrollable stress, they do not rule out an equally important role for other brain systems in this behavior as well. The vast interconnections between the locus ceruleus and the limbic system suggest that further investigation is warranted into the role of other brain structures and neurotransmitter and/or neuropeptide systems in behaviors resulting from exposure to inescapable stress.

Raphe Nuclei

The role of the raphe nuclei and serotonin (5-HT), in particular, in anxiety has been most difficult to elucidate. The data are as yet unclear regarding whether increases or decreases in 5-HT function are associated with reductions in anxiety. Some of the possible reasons for these discrepancies are presented below.

Chemical lesions of the raphe nuclei, which result in destruction of 5-HT-ergic neurons (Geller and Blum, 1970; Hartman and Geller, 1971; Stein et al., 1973), and treatment with 5-HT antagonists (Schoenfield, 1976; Sepinwall and Cook, 1978; Stein et al., 1973) produce increases in punished responding. Furthermore, the anxiolytic actions of the benzodiazepines may be related to their effects on 5-HT-ergic neurons (Stein, 1981). Benzodiazepines produce a decrease in the turnover of 5-HT in brain (Jenner et al., 1975; Saner and Pietscher, 1979) as well as an inhibition of firing of 5-HT-containing neurons (Laurent et al., 1983; Pratt et al., 1979; Preussler et al., 1981). The decrease in turnover is also seen for catecholamines (Corrodi et al., 1971; Haefely et al., 1981). However, the decrease in catecholamine turnover is associated with tolerance, whereas the effect on 5-HT is not (Wise et al., 1972). Since the anxiolytic effects of the benzodiazepines do not diminish with repeated administration, this would suggest that benzodiazepine effects on 5-HT neurons are more relevant for their anxioltyic actions. In contrast, tolerance develops to the sedative effects of the benzodiazepines and thus may be more closely tied to their effects on catecholamines (Stein, 1981).

If the anxiolytic effects of the benzodiazepines are mediated, at least in part, by their abilities to decrease 5-HT-ergic function, then increases in 5-HT should produce behavioral effects similar to those observed in fear-provoking situations (Wise et al., 1972). These effects have been more difficult to demonstrate, although a number of factors may account for this. 5-HT administration, peripherally or centrally, produces an indiscriminate behavioral depression (Gerson and Baldessarinni, 1980). This may be a reflection of activation of brainstem and spinal cord pathways that are involved in motor behavior but not in anxiety-related behavior. In addition, there appear to be different 5-HT receptor sites. These have only recently been characterized and are now being studied with more selective ligands. In support of the importance of 5-HT systems in the actions of benzodiazepines, intraventricular 5-HT injections have been shown to reverse the effects of benzodiazepines on punished behavior (Wise et al., 1972). Local injections into the region of the raphe increased punished responding in one study but also decreased the activity of the 5-HT-containing neurons (Thiebot et al., 1984). However, local injections of 5-HT into the amygdala decreased neural firing (Wang and Aghajanian, 1977), an effect also seen with local injections of midazolam and muscimol (which can also produce increases in punished responding) (Petersen and Scheel-Kruger, 1982).

In an interesting series of studies, Ellison (1977) reported that 5-HT-depleted rats placed in a novel environment exhibited behaviors characteristic of increased fear (e.g., decreased exploration, agitation, freezing, and hypervigilance). However, if the 5-HT-depleted rats previously had been group-housed in an environment rich with rat playthings, then they were less fearful and more dominant than controls or norepinephrine-depleted rats. These results emphasize strongly the importance of the testing situation for determining drug effects.

These results are reminiscent of the effects described for arousal on human cognitive function: Very low or very high levels are associated with submaximal performance, whereas moderate levels are linked to better performance. If decreased 5-HT levels cause an increase in arousal, then the combination with a highly stressful or novel situation could result in behavioral dysfunction, e.g., freezing or agitation. In a less stressful environment, however, the increased arousal might be associated with more effective behaviors.

Septum-Hippocampus

Evidence for a role of the septum and hippocampus in Gray's theory of anxiety comes from two sources. One is the observation of a high density of benzodiazepine receptors in these brain regions (although benzodiazepine receptors are widely distributed in brain); the second concerns the effects of lesions of the septum and hippocampus on several behavioral measures that Gray and others suggest are a reflection of anxiety-related processes (Gray et al., 1981). These behavioral paradigms assess resistance to the effects of extinction and punishment. Both these procedures produce decreases in the rate of occurrence of some ongoing behavior. Extinction does this by omitting the consequences of previously effective responses; punishment operates by providing an additional consequence, such as electric shock. An animal's precise response to these contingencies depends, in part, on its experimental history. For instance, an animal that has been exposed to intermittent reinforcement (in which, say, only every tenth response produces food) will initially be more resistant to the effects of extinction than will an animal whose every response was reinforced. Similarly, if the reinforced behavior of an animal is also occasionally punished during training, there will be less suppression when the animal later is tested with punishment for every response than if punishment had never been administered.

Gray and colleagues (1981) have reported that anxiolytic treatment during training on either procedure will eliminate the differential effects seen during subsequent testing. That is, in the extinction procedure, animals trained on intermittent reinforcement but also receiving anxiolytic drugs show no greater resistance to subsequent (drug-free) extinction tests than animals whose every response was reinforced. Likewise, in the punishment procedure, training under anxiolytics eliminates the differences between intermittent punishment and no punishment when the animals are subsequently tested (again, drug-free) by punishing every response. Note that differential effects of experimental history were eliminated only when a drug was given during the training phase of the two procedures. If anxiolytics were given only during the subsequent testing phase of either procedure, then, despite response rate increases, the effects of the differential training nevertheless emerged. If anxiolytics were given during training and testing, then both effects resulted: Response rate increases in testing were found and the effects of differential training were eliminated.

Lesions of the septum and hippocampus have been observed to produce behavioral effects in these paradigms that are similar to those produced by benzodiazepines (Gray et al., 1981). Medial and lateral septal lesions can be differentiated in the same way as benzodiazepines given during training vs. testing. That is, lateral septal lesions abolish the differential responsiveness to extinction or punishment afforded by prior exposure to intermittent reinforcement or punishment, whereas medial septal lesions increase responding during extinction or punishment while leaving the effects of prior training undisturbed. Hippocampal lesions produce the combined behavioral effects of benzodiazepines given during training or during testing. Gray explains these results on the basis of the known anatomical connections of these structures. The medial septal nuclei project to the hippocampus. The major subcortical outflow of the hippocampus is to the lateral septal nuclei. According to Gray, incoming signals of nonreinforcement or punishment reach the medial septal nuclei and are conveyed to the hippocampus, which activates the "behavioral inhibition system." Lesions of the medial septal nuclei would thus prevent behavioral inhibition and increase responding during extinction or punishment irrespective of previous training while not interfering with the effects of such training. Gray further postulates that the hippocampus acts as a comparator to determine the "meaning" of the signals of nonreinforcment or punishment. In the situation in which an animal has been given intermittent reinforcement or punishment, the best behavioral strategy for the animal is to continue responding to obtain the intermittently presented reinforcers. Thus the hippocampus, upon making this determination, must alter its subsequent output and does so by signalling the lateral septal nuclei, which then alters the input of the medial septal nuclei to the hippocampus. Thus, lesions of the lateral septal nuclei produce a failure of the system to use the information obtained by the prior training experiences. The behavioral results obtained following such a lesion would be comparable to giving benzodiazepines during training. Lesions of the hippocampus, according to this model, should produce effects similar to the combined lesions, and the behavioral data obtained by Gray support this conclusion.

One implication of Gray's results that warrants further discussion concerns the effect of benzodiazepines given during training. The effects of the training are diminished under these circumstances. Gray considers the effect of the training in untreated animals to be like a "toughening-up" process, which decreases the susceptibility of these animals to the disruptive effects of anxiety-producing stimuli (Gray, 1985). Similarly, Weiss et al. (1982) demonstrated a prophylactic effect of repeated exposures to stress on the behavioral impairment produced by a single exposure to uncontrollable stress (and suggest the importance of noradrenergic mechanisms in the process). If these findings are relevant to human anxiety, then the use of benzodiazepines clinically might warrant further deliberation. If anxiolytics interfere with the development of appropriate coping skills for subsequent life stressors, then perhaps they ought to be prescribed only with great hesitancy. If, on the other hand, a sensitization process underlies the development of pathological anxiety, then the use of benzodiazepines at an early point in the development of the syndrome might actually be prophylactic. These issues need to be kept in mind clinically and point up the importance of developing good animal models for the etiology of anxiety, not just for the ability to screen antianxiety agents.

Although Gray's theory affords a certain degree of internal consistency and does account for his and others' data, it should still be considered rather cautiously. For one thing, Gray's theory is heavily dependent on his interpretation of the tasks he uses as productive of a state of anxiety. In addition, some of the drug or lesion effects may have alternative explanations, unrelated to anxiolysis. For example, the effect of benzodiazepines given during training is to abolish the effects of the training. These results may be related to the well established memory-impairing properties of benzodiazepines rather than to their anxiolytic effects. A similar argument can be made for the effects of hippocampal lesions. Overall, this theory offers an interesting conceptualization of the neuroanatomical substates of anxiety, but further study will be necessary to demonstrate the relevance of the behavioral paradigms to human anxiety and to incorporate other brain structures of known relevance to anxiety into the model.

CONCLUSIONS

Animal models of anxiety have been useful in conceptualizing the possible biological substrates and neurotransmitter systems underlying both normal and pathological human anxiety. Current animal models offer multiple approaches, each with distinct advantages for clarifying one or another aspect of anxiety. Most abundant are models for the identification and characterization of pharmacological agents with anxiolytic or anxiogenic potencies. The recent discovery of agents with relatively selective biochemical effects (e.g., the beta-carbolines) that can produce, in nonhuman species, behavioral and physiological responses analagous to those seen in human anxiety offers new opportunities for the study of the specific neurochemical and neuroanatomical underpinnings of anxiety. In addition, the work of Kandel and associates on the molecular basis of neuronal plasticity, particularly in what may be considered behaviors analogous to those observed in anxiety-provoking situations, holds great promise for our understanding of the molecular mechanisms involved in the development and maintenance of anxiety-related patterns of responding. Gray has provided a start, but further work is necessary to integrate the data from a multiplicity of experimental approaches into a cogent theory of the neuroanatomical, neurochemical, and neurophysiological substrates of anxiety. What are needed most, however, are models in which the overlap of genetics and environment can be studied and in which a wide range of behaviors are available for modification. In such a setting, factors such as controllability, predictability, and early experiential effects could be evaluated for their role as determinants of subsequent behavior. Furthermore, the characterization of the importance of repeated exposures to stressful life events in the development of behavioral pathology or coping strategies could be studied. Currently, the primate separation and intrusion studies offer the best opportunity to consider these various factors. Furthermore, recent work with cross fostering of newborn primates should be of particular relevance to the importance of early maternal care. Although only a few laboratories have the facilities to conduct these studies, their importance for our understanding of human anxiety cannot be overemphasized and we eagerly await their results.

REFERENCES

Aghajanian G (1977): Tolerance of locus coeruleus neurons to morphine and suppression withdrawal response by clonidine. Nature 276:186–187.

Anisman H, Suissa A, Sklar LS (1980): Escape deficits induced by uncontrollable stress: antagonism by dopamine and norepinephrine agonists. Behav Neural Biol 28:34–51.

Ballenger JC, Burrows GD, DuPont RL Jr, Lesser IM, Noyes R Jr, Pecknold JC, Rifkin A, Swinson RP (1988): Alprazolam in panic disorder and agoraphobia: Results from a multicenter trial. Arch Gen Psychiatry 45:413–422.

Baysinger CM, Suomi SJ (1978): Abstr Am Soc Primatol 1:2–3.

Beer B, Migler B (1975): Arch Int Pharmacodyn Ther 212:221–292.

Bird S, Kuhar M (1977): Iontophoretic applications of opiates to the locus coeruleus. Brain Res 122:523–533.

Blumstein LK, Crawley JN (1983): Further characterization of a simple, automated exploratory model for the anxiolytic effects of benzodiazepines. Pharmacol Biochem Behav 8:37–40.

Bonetti EP, Pieri R, Cumin R, Schaffner R, Pieri M, Gamzu ER, Muller RKM, Haefely W (1982): Benzodiazepine antagonist RO 15-1788: Neurological and behavioral effects. Psychopharmacology 78:8–18.

Boulenger J-P, Bierer L, Uhde TW (1986): Anxiogenic effects of caffeine in normal controls and patients with panic disorder. In Shagass C (ed): "Biological Psychiatry, 1985" New York: Elsevier, pp 454–456.

Boulenger J-P, Uhde TW, Marangos PJ, Salem N Jr, Post RM (1984a): Psychopathological effects of caffeine: Possible involvement of the adenosine system in anxiety disorders. Clin Neuropharmacol 7:426–427.

Boulenger J-P, Uhde TW, Wolff EA, Post RM (1984b): Increased sensitivity to caffeine in patients with panic disorders: Preliminary evidence. Arch Gen Psychiatry 41:1067–1071.

Bowlby J (1969): "Separation and Loss: Vol. 1, Attachment." New York: Basic Books.

Bowlby J (1973): "Separation and Loss: Vol. 2, Loss." New York: Basic Books.

Brady JV (1956): Behavioral stress and physiological change comparative approach to experimental analysis of psychosomatic problems. Science 123:1033–1034.

Braestrup G, Honore C, Nielsen M, Petersen EN, Jensen LH (1983): Benzodiazepine receptor ligands with negative efficacy: Chloride channel coupling. Adv Biochem Psychopharmacol 38:29–36.

Braestrup G, Schmiechen R, Neef G, Nielsen M, Petersen EN (1982): Interaction of convulsive ligands with benzodiazepine receptors. Science 216:1241–1243.

Breier A, Charney DS, Heninger GR (1984): Major depression in patients with agoraphobia and panic disorder. Arch Gen Psychiatry 41:1129–1135.

Brewster DJ (1969): Ethanol preference in strain of rats selectively bred for behavioral characteristics. J Genet Psychol 115:217–227.

Broadhurst PL (1957): Determinants of emotionality in the rat. I. Situational factors. Br J Psychol 48:1–12.

Broadhurst PL (1960): Experiments in psychogenetics. In Eysenck HJ (ed): "Experiments in Personality, Psychogenetics and Psychopharmacology, Vol. 1." London: Routledge and Kegan Paul, pp 1–120.

Broadhurst PL (1962): A note on further progress in psychogenetic selection experiment. Psychol Rep 10:65–66.

Broadhurst PL (1966): Behavioral inheritance, past and present. Cond Reflex 1:3–15.

Broadhurst PL (1975): The Maudsley reactive and nonreactive strains of rats. A survey. Behav Genet 5:299–319.

Broadhurst PL, Eysenck HJ (1965): Emotionality in the rat: A problem of response specificity. In Banks C, Broadhurst PL (eds): "Stephanos: Studies in Psychology, Presented to Cyril Burt." London: University of London Press, pp 205–221.

Brookshire KH, Littmann RA, Stewart CN (1961): Residual of shock-trauma in the white rat: A three factor theory. Psychol Monogr 75(10):1–32.

Brown J, Jacobs A (1949): The role of fear in motivation and acquisition of responses. J Exp Psychol 39:747–759.

Capell H, Ginsberg R, Webster CD (1972): Amphetamine and conditioned 'anxiety.' Br J Pharmacol 45:525–531.

Charney DS, Heninger GR (1985a): Noradrenergic function and the mechanism of action of antianxiety treatment. I. The effect of long-term alprazolam treatment. Arch Gen Psychiatry 42:458–467.

Charney DS, Heninger GR (1985b): Noradrenergic function and the mechanism of action of antianxiety treatment II. The effect of long-term imipramine treatment. Arch Gen Psychiatry 42:473–481.

Charney DS, Heninger GR, Jatlow PI (1985): Increased anxiogenic effects of caffeine in panic disorders. Arch Gen Psychiatry 42:233–243.

Charney D, Heninger GR, Redmond DE Jr (1983): Yohimbine induced anxiety and increased noradrenergic function in humans: Effects of diazepam and clonidine. Life Sci 33:19–29.

Cook L (1982): Animal psychopharmacological models: Use in conflict behavior in predicting clinical effects of anxiolytics and their mechanisms of action. Prog Neuropsychopharmacol Biol Psychiatry 6:579–583.

Cook L, Catania AC (1964): Effects of drugs on avoidance and escape behavior. Fed Proc Fed Am Soc Exp Biol 23:818–835.

Cook L, Davidson AB (1973): Effects of behaviorally active drugs in a conflict-punishment procedure in rats. In Garattini E, Mussini E, Randall LO (eds): "The Benzodiazepines." New York: Raven Press, pp 327–345.

Cook L, Sepinwall J (1975a): Behavioral analysis of the effects and mechanisms of action of benzodiazepines. In Costa E, Greengard P (eds): "Mechanism of Action of Benzodiazepines." New York: Raven Press, p 1028.

Cook L, Sepinwall J (1975b): Psychopharmacological parameters and methods. In Levi L (ed): "Emotions—Their Parameters and Measurement." New York: Raven Press, pp 379–404.

Cooper SJ, Estall LB (1985): Behavioral pharmacology of food, water and salt intake in relation to drug action at benzodiazepine receptors. Neurosci Behav Rev 9:5–19.

Corda MG, Blaker WD, Mendelson WB, Guidotti A, Costa E (1983): B-carbolines enhance the shock-induced suppression of drinking in the rat. Proc Natl Acad Sci USA 80:2072–2076.

Coromi CR, Thurmond JB (1977): Effects of acute exposure to stress on subsequent aggression and locomotion performance. Psychosom Med 39:436–443.

Corrodi H, Fuxe K, Lindbrink P, Olson L (1971): Minor tranquilizers, stress and central catecholamine neurons. Brain Res 29:1–6.

Costa E (1982): Coexistence of putative neuromodulators in the same axon: Pharmacological consequences at receptors. In "Co-Transmission." London: Macmillan Press, Ltd.

Cowen PJ, Green AR, Nutt DJ, Martin IL (1981): Ethyl B-carboline carboxylate lowers seizure threshold and antagonizes flurazepam-induced sedation in rats. Nature 290:54–55.

Crawley JN (1981): Neuropharmacologic specificity of a simple animal model for the behavioral action of benzodiazepine. Pharmacol Biochem Behav 15:695–699.

Crawley JN, Goodwin FK (1980): Preliminary report of a simple animal behavior model for the anxiolytic effect of benzodiazepines. Pharmacol Biochem Behav 13:167–170.

Crawley JN, Ninan PT, Pickar D, Chrousos GP, Skolnick P, Paul SM (1984a): Non-human primate models of anxiety, behavioral and pharmacological correlates with human anxiety. Psychopharmacol Bull 20:403–407.

Crawley JN, Skolnick P, Paul SM (1984b): Absence of intrinsic antagonist action of benzodiazepine antagonists on an exploratory model of anxiety in the mouse. Neuropharmacology 23:531–537.

Crowe RR, Noyes R, Paul DL, Slymen D (1983): A family study of panic disorder. Arch Gen Psychiatry 40:1065–1069.

Dantzer R (1975): Activity of psychotropic drugs on punished behavior in pigs. J Pharmacol (Paris) 6:323–340.

Dantzer R, Roca M (1974): Tranquilizing effects of diazepam in pigs subjected to a punishment procedure. Psychopharmacologia 40:235–240.

Davis M (1980): Neurochemical modulation of sensory-motor reactivity: Acoustic and tactile startle reflexes. Neurosci Biobehav Rev 4:241–263.

DeLuca DC, Murphree OD, Angel C (1974): Biochemistry of nervous dogs. Pavlov J Biol Sci 9:136–148.

Dews PB (1958): Studies in behavior. IV: Stimulant actions of metamphetamine. J Pharmacol Exp Ther 122:137–147.

Dinsmoor J (1958): Pulse duration and food deprivation in escape from shock training. Psychol Rep 4:531–534.

Dinsmoor J, Campbell SL (1956): Escape-from-shock training following exposure to inescapable shock. Psychol Rev 2:43–49.

Dorow R, Horowski R, Paschelke G, Amin M, Braestrup D (1983): Severe anxiety induced by FG-7142, a B-carboline ligand for benzodiazepine receptors. Lancet 2:98–99.

Drugen RC, Maier SF, Skolnick P, Paul SM, Crawley JN (1985): An anxiogenic benzodiazepines receptor ligand induces learned helplessness. Eur J Pharmacology 113:453–457.

Elam M, Yoa J, Thoren P, Svensson TH (1981): Hypercapnia and hypoxia: chemoreceptor-mediated control of locus coeruleus neurons and splanchnic sympathetic nerves. Brain Res 222:373–381.

Ellison GD (1977): Animal models of psychopathology: The low norepinephrine and low serotonin rat. Am Psychol 32:1036–1045.

Engel GL (1962): Anxiety and depression-withdrawal: The primary effects of unpleasure. Int J Psychoanal 43:89–136.

Estes WK, Skinner BF (1941): Some quantitative properties of anxiety. J Exp Psychol 29:390–400.

Faravelli C (1985): Life events preceding the onset of panic disorder. J Affect Disord 9:103–105.

Feuer G (1969): Difference in emotional behavior and in function of the endocrine system in genetically different strains in albino rats. In Bajusz E (ed): "Physiology and Pathology of Adaptation Mechanisms." Oxford: Pergamon, pp 214–233.

File SE (1980): The use of social interaction as a method for detecting anxiolytic activity of chlordiazepoxide-like drugs. J Neurosci Methods 2:219–238.

File SE, Hyde JR (1978): Can social interaction be used to measure anxiety? Br J Pharmacol 62:19–24.

File SE, Lister RG (1983): Interactions of ethyl-B-carboline-3-carboxylate and RO 15-1788 with CGS 8216 in an animal model of anxiety. Neurosci Lett 39:91–94.

File SE, Lister RG, Nutt DJ (1982): The anxiogenic action of benzodiazepine antagonists. Neuropharmacology 21:1033–1037.

Freud S (1895): In Strachey JA (ed): "The Complete Works of Sigmund Freud, Vol. III, Standard Edition." London. Hogarth Press and Institute of Psycho-Analysis.

Garattini S, Valzelli L (1981): Is the isolated animal possible model for phobia and anxiety? Prog Neuropsychopharmacol Biol Psychiatry 5:159–165.

Garcia J, Koelling R (1966): Relations of cue to consequence in avoidance learning. Psychon Sci 4:123–124.

Geller I (1962): "Use of Approach-Avoidance Behavior (Conflict) for Evaluating Depressant Drugs." Philadelphia: Lea & Febiger.

Geller I, Blum K (1970): The effects of 5-HTP on parachlorophenylalanine (P-CPA) attenuation of "conflict" behavior. Eur J Pharmacol 9:319–324.

Geller I, Croy DJ, Ryback RS (1974): Effects of ethanol and sodium phenobarbital on conflict behavior of goldfish (Carassius auratus). Pharmacol Biochem Behav 2:545–548.

Geller I, Seifter J (1960): The effect of meprobamate, barbiturates, d-amphetamine, and promazine on experimentally induced conflict in rats. Psychopharmacologia 1:482–494.

Gerson SC, Baldessarinni RJ (1980): Motor effects of serotonin in the central nervous system. Life Sci 27:1435–1451.

Glowa JR, Barrett JE (1983): Response suppression by visual stimuli paired with post session d-amphetamine injections in the pigeon. J Exp Anal Behav 39:165–173.

Glowa JR, Skolnick P, Paul SM (1986): Effects of the ethyl ester of B-carbolne-3-carboxylic acid and diazepam on non-suppressed and suppressed responding in the rhesus monkey. Eur J Pharmacol 129:39–47.

Glowinski J (1975): Properties and functions of intraneuronal monoamine compartments in central aminergic neurons. In Snyder SH, Iverson SD (eds): "Handbook of Psychopharmacology, Vol. 3." New York: Raven Press, pp 139–167.

Grant S, Huang Y, Redmond D Jr (1980): Benzodiazepines attenuate single unit activity in the locus coeruleus. Life Sci 27:2231–2236.

Grav JW, Hyson RL, Maier SF, Madden IV J, Barchas JD (1981): Long-term stress-induced analgesia and activation of the opiate system. Science 213:1409–1411.

Gray JA (1983): A theory of anxiety: The role of lymbic system. Encephale IX:161B–166B.

Gray JA (1985): Issues in the neuropsychology of anxiety. In Tuma AH, Maser JD (eds): "Anxiety and the Anxiety Disorders." Hillside, NJ: Lawrence Erlbaum, pp 5–26.

Gray JA, Davis N, Feldon J, Nicholas J, Rawlins P, Owen SR (1981): Animal models of anxiety. Prog Neuropsychopharmacol Biol Psychiatry 5:143–157.

Gupta BD, Holland HC (1969): An examination of the effects of stimulant and depressed drugs on escape/avoidance conditioning in strains of rats selectively bred for emotionality/nonemotionality. Psychopharmacologia 14:95–105.

Haefely, W Pieri L, Polc P, Schaffner R (1981): General pharmacology and neuropharmacology of benzodiazepine derivatives. In Hoffmeister F, Stille G (eds): "Handbook of Experimental Pharmacology, Vol. 55, Part II." Berlin: Springer-Verlag, pp 13–262.

Hall CS (1934): Emotional behavior in the Rat I. Defecation and urination as measures of individual differences in emotionality. J Comp Psychol 18:385–403.

Harlow HF, Harlow MK (1969): Effects of various mother-infant relationships on rhesus monkey behaviors. In Foss BM (ed): "Determinants of Infant Behavior, Vol. 14." London: Methuen, pp 15–36.

Harlow HF, Harlow MK (1971): Psychopathology in monkeys. In Kimmel H (ed). Experimental Psychopathology in Monkeys." New York. Academic Press, pp 203–229.

Hartman RJ, Geller I (1971): P-Chlorophenylananine effects on a conditioned emotional response in rats. Life Sci 10:927–933.

Hebb DO (1946): On the nature of fear. Psychol Rev 53: 259–276.

Henn F (1985): Address given at the National Institute of Mental Health, Bethesda, Maryland.

Hobbs WR, Wilkinson EC, Peterson GA, Laraia M, Cox D, Ballenger J (1984): The Psychophysiology of agoraphobia. In Ballenger J (ed): "Biology of Agoraphobia." Washington, DC: American Psychiatric Press, Inc., pp 66–80.

Hoehn-Saric R, Merchant A, Keyser M, Smith V (1981): Effects of clonidine on anxiety disorder. Arch Gen Psychiatry 28:1278–1282.

Holmberg G, Gershon S (1961): Autonomic and psychic effects of yohimbine hydrochloride. Psychopharmacologia 2:93–106.

Holtzman SG, Villarreal JE (1973): Operant behavior in the morphine-dependent rhesus monkey. J Pharmacol Exp Ther 184:528–541.

Hunkeler W, Schaffner R, Haefely W (1981): Selective antagonists of benzodiazepines. Nature 290:514–516.

Huppert FA, Iversen SD (1975): Response suppression in rats—Comparison response contingent and noncontingent punishment of effect of minor tranquilizer chloradiazepoxide. Psychopharmacology 44:67–75.

Imada H (1972): Emotional reactivity and conditionability in four strains of rats. J Comp Physiol Psychatr 79:474–480.

Iorio LC, Eisenstein N, Brody PE, Barnett A (1983): Long-term analgesic effect of inescapable shock and learned helplessness. Pharmacol Biochem Behav 18: 379–382.

Jackson RL, Maier SF, Coon DJ (1979): Long-term analgesic effect of inescapable shock and learned helplessness. Science 206:91–93.

Jacobsen E (1957): The effects of psychotropic drugs under psychic stress. In Garattini S, Ghetti V (eds): "Psychotropic Drugs." Amsterdam: Elsevier, pp 119–124

James W (1884): What is emotion? Mind 19:188–205.

James W (1890): "The Principles of Psychiatry," New York: Holt, Rinehart, & Winston (reprinted, New York: Dover Press, 1950).

Jenner P, Chadwick D, Reynolds EH, Marsden DC (1975): Metabolism with chlorazepam, diazepam and diphenylthydantoin. J Pharm Pharmacol 27:707–710.

Joffe JM (1964): Avoidance learning and failure to learn in two strains of rats selectively bred for emotionality. Psychon Sci 1:185–186.

Kandel ER (1983): From metapsychology to molecular biology: Explorations into the nature of anxiety. Am J Psychiatry 140:1277–1293.

Kandel ER (1985): Cellular mechanisms of learning and biological basis of individuality. In Kandel ER, Schwartz JH (eds): "Principles of Neural Science." Amsterdam: Elsevier Science Publishing Co.

Kandel ER, Schwartz JH (1982): Molecular-biology of learning modulation of transmitter release. Science 218:397–408.

Kelleher RT, Morse WH (1968): Determinants of the specificity of behavioral effects of drugs. Ergebnisse Der Physiologie 60:1–56.

Klein DF (1964): Delineation of two drugs-responsive anxiety syndromes. Psychopharmacologia 5:397–408.

Klein E, Lennox RH, Uhde TW (1988): Alpha-2 adrenergic receptor binding in platelets and brains of nervous and normal pointer dogs. Psychiatr Res 22:241–247.

Klein E, Steinberg S, Matthews D, Weiss SRB, Uhde TW (1988): The relationship between genetic deafness and fear-related behaviors in nervous pointer dogs. Physiol Behav 43:307–312.

Korf J, Bunney A, Aghajanian G (1974): Noradrenergic neurons—Morphine inhibition of spontaneous activity. Eur J Pharmacol 25:165–169.

Lal H, Emmett-Oglesby MW (1983): Behavioral analogues of anxiety. Neuropharmacol 22:1423–1441.

Lal H, Shearman G (1981): Discriminative stimulus properties of cocaine related to an anxiogenic action. Prog Neuropsychopharmacol Biol Psychiatry 5: 57–63.

Lange K (1885): Translated by Haupt IA (1922) for K Dunlap (ed): "The Emotions." Baltimore: Williams & Wilkins.

Laurent J-P, Margold M, Hembel H, Haefely W (1983): Reduction by 2 benzodiazepines and pentobarbital at the multiunit activity in substantia nigra, hippocampus, nucleus, locus coeruleus and nucleus raphe dorsalis of encephale-isole rats. Neuropharmacology 22: 510–512.

Lavener H (1963): Condition suppression in rats and the effect of pharmacological agent thereon. Psychopharmacologia 4:311–316.

Leckman JF, Weissman MM, Merikangas KR, Paul DL, Prusolff BA (1983): Panic disorder and major depression—Increased risk of depression, alcoholism, panic and phobic disorders in families of depressed probands with panic disorder. Arch Gen Psychiatry 40: 1055–1060.

Leshner AI, Remler H, Biegnon A, Samuel D (1979): Desmethylimipramine (DMI) counteracts learned helplessness in rats. Psychopharmacology 66:207–208.

Levine S, Chevalier J, Korchin S (1956): The effects of early shock and handling on later avoidance learning. J Personality 24:475–493.

Liang B, Blizard DA (1978): Central and peripheral norepinephrine concentrations in rat strains selectively bred for differences in response to stress—Confirmation and extension. Pharmacol Biochem Behav 8:75–80.

Liebowitz MR, Fyer AJ, Gorman JM, Dillon D, Appleby IL, Levy G, Anderson S, Levitt M, Palij M, Davies SO: Lactate provocation of panic attacks. I. Clinical and behavioral findings. Arch Gen Psychiatry 41:764–770.

Liebowitz MR, Gorman JM, Fyer AJ, Levitt M, Dillon D,

Levy G, Appleby IL, Anderson S, Palij M, Davies SO, Klein DF (1985): Lactate provocation of panic attacks. II. Biochemical and physiological findings. Arch Gen Psychiatry 42:709–719.

Lippa AS, Wash R, Greenblatt E (1979): Preclinical neuro-psychopharmacological testing procedures for anxiolytic drugs. In Fielding S, Lal H (eds) In: Anxiolytics: New York: Pergamon Press, pp 41–73.

Maier SF, Anderson C, Lieberman SA (1972): Influence of control of shock on subsequent shock-elicited aggression. J Comp physiol Psychol 81:94–100.

Maier SF, Drugan RC, Grau JW (1982): Controllability, coping behavior, and stress induced analgesia in the rat. Pain 12:47–56.

Maier SF, Seligman MEP (1976): Learned helplessness: Theory and evidence. J Exp Psychol Gen 105:3–46.

Margules DL, Stein L (1968): Increase of "anti-anxiety" activity and tolerance of behavioral suppression during chronic administration of oxazepam. Psychopharmacology 13:74–80.

Mason S, Fibiger H (1979): Current concepts. I. Anxiety: the locus coeruleus disconnection. Life Sci 25:2141–2147.

McMillan DE (1973): Drugs and punished responding. I: Rate-dependent effects under multiple schedules. J Exp Anal Behav 19:133–145.

McMillan DE, Leander JD (1975): Drugs and punished responding. V: Effects of drugs on responding suppressed by response dependent and response independent electric shock. Arch Int Pharmacodyn Ther 213:22–27.

Metlot C, Deutsch R (1984): The effect of diazepam on a conditioned emotional response in the rat. Pharmacol Biochem Behav 20:459–499.

Miczek KA (1973): Effect of scopalamine amphetamine and benzodiazepines or conditioned suppression. Pharmacol Biochem Behav 1:401–411.

Mineka S, Davidson M, Cook M, Keir R (1984): Observational conditioning of snake fear in rhesus monkeys. J Abnorm Psychol 93:355–372.

Mineka S, Gunnar M, Champoux M (1985) Cited in Tuma AH, Maser JD (eds): Anxiety and the Anxiety Disorders, New Jersey: Lawrence Erlbaum Assoc, pp 212–242.

Mineka S, Keir R (1983): The effect of flooding on reducing snake fear in rhesus monkey: Six month follow-up and further flooding. Behav Res Ther 21:517–535.

Mineka S, Keir R, Price V (1980): Fear of snakes in wild-reared and laboratory-reared rhesus monkeys (Macaca mulatta). Anim Learn Behav 8:653–663.

Mineka S, Kihlstrom JF (1978): Unpredictable and uncontrollable events: A new perspective on experimental neurosis. J Abnorm Psychiatry 87:256–271.

Mineka S, Suomi SJ, DeLizio RD (1980): Multiple separations in adolescent monkey: an opponent-process interpretation. J Exp Psychol 110:56–85.

Mohler H, Okada T (1977): Benzodiazepine receptor: Demonstration in the central nervous system. Science 198:849–851.

Mohler H, Richards JG (1981): Agonist and antagonist benzodiazepine receptor interaction in vitro. Nature 294:763–765.

Morse WH (1964): Effect of amobarbital and chlorpromazine on punished behavior in the pigeon. Psychopharmacolgia 6:286–294.

Murphree OD (1973): Inheritance of human aversion and inactivity in two strains of the pointer dog. Biol Psychiatry 7:23–29.

Murphree OD, Angel C, DeLuca DC, Newton JEO (1977): Longitudinal studies of genetically nervous dogs. Biol Psychiatry 12:573–576.

Murphree OD, Angel C, DeLuca DC, Newton JEO, Farris DVM Jr (1974a): Nervous dogs: a partial model for psychiatric research. Lab Anim. 3:16–19.

Murphree OD, DeLuca DC, Angel C (1974b): Psychopharmacologic facilitation of operant conditioning of genetically nervous pointer dogs. Pavlov J of Biol Sci 9:17–24.

Murphree OD, Peters JE, Dykman RA (1969): Behavioral comparisons of nervous, stable, and crossbred pointers at age 2, 3, 6, 9, and 12 months. Cond Reflex 4: 20–23.

Murray S, King J (1973): Snake avoidance in feral and laboratory reared squirrel monkeys. Behavior 47:281–289.

Ninan PT, Insel TM, Cohen RM, Cook JM, Skolnick, Paul SM (1982): Benzodiazepine receptor-mediated experimental anxiety in primates. Science 218:1332–1334.

Nutt DJ, Cowen PJ, Little HJ (1982): Unusual interactions of benzodiazepine receptor antagonists. Nature 295: 436–438.

Olpe H, Jones R (1983): The action of anti-convulsant drugs on the firing of locus coeruleus neurons, selective activating effects of carbamazepine. Eur J Pharmacol 91:107–110.

Olpe H, Jones R, Steinmann M (1983): The locus coeruleus: Action of psychoactive drugs. Experientia 39: 242–249.

Olsen RW (1981): GABA benzodiazepine-barbiturate receptors interactions. J Neurochem 37:1–13.

Overmier JB, Seligman MEP (1967): Effects of inescapable shock upon subsequent escape and avoidance learning. J Comp Physiol Psychol 63:23–33.

Petersen EN (1983): A potent convulsive benzodiazepine receptor ligand. Eur J Pharmacol 94:117–124.

Petersen EN, Jensen LH, Honore T, Braestrup C (1983): Costa E, Biggio G (eds): Differential pharmacological effects of benzodiazepine receptor inverse agonists. In: "Advances in Biomedical Psychopharmacology" vol. 38. New York: Raven Press, p 57–64.

Petersen EN, Scheel-Kruger J (1982): The GABAergic anticonflict effect of intra-amygdalaloid benzodiazepines. Demonstration by a new water-lick paradigm. In Spiegelstein MI, Levy A: "Behavioural Models and the Analysis of Drug Action. (Proc. of the 27th OHOLO Conf)." Amsterdam: Elsevier, pp 467–473.

Petty F (1985): IV World Congress of Biological Psychiatry, Abstract 225.6.

Petty F, Sherman A (1980): Reversal of learned helplessness by imipramine. Psychopharmacology 3:371–373.

Petty F, Sherman A (1982): A neurochemical differentiation between exposure to stress and the development of learned helplessness. Drug Dev Res 2:43–45.

Pohorecky L, Brick J (1977): Activity of neurons in the

locus coeruleus of the rat: Inhibition of ethanol. Brain Res 131:174–179.

Polc P, Bonetti EP, Schaffner R, Haefely W (1982): A three-state model of benzodiazepine receptors explaining the interactions between benzodiazepine antagonist RO 15-1788, benzodiazepine tranquilizers, B-carbolines and phenobarbitone. Arch Pharmacol 321: 260–264.

Post RM, Weiss SRB, Pert A, Uhde TW (1987): Chronic cocaine administration: Sensitization and kindling effects. In Fisher S, Raskin A, Uhlenhuth EH (eds): "Cocaine: Clinical and Biobehavioral Aspects." London/New York: Oxford University Press, pp 109–173.

Pratt J, Jenner P, Reynolds EH, Marsden CD (1979): Clonazepam induces decreased serotonergic activity in the mouse brain. Neuropharmacology 18:791–799.

Pruessler DW, Howell GA, Frederickson CJ, Trulson ME (1981): Raphe unit activity in freely moving cats: Effects of benzodiazepines. Soc Neurosci Abstr 7:923.

Rainey JM, Pohl RB, Williams, M, Knitter E, Freedman RR, Ettedgui E. (1984): Lactate and Isoproterenol anxiety states. Psychopathology 17[Suppl]:74–82.

Randall LO, Schallek W, Heise GA, Keith EF, Bagdon R (1960): The psychosedative properties of methaminodiazepoxide. J Pharmacol Exp Ther 129:163–171.

Ray OS (1964): The effects of tranquilizers on positively and negatively motivated behavior in rats. Psychopharmacologia 4:311–316.

Razran G (1971): "Mind in Evolution." Boston; Houghton Mifflin.

Redmond DE Jr (1981): Clonidine and the primate locus coeruleus: evidence suggesting anxiolytic and antiwithdrawal effects. In Lal H, Fielding S (eds): "Psychopharmacology of Clonidine." New York: Alan R. Liss, Inc., pp 147–163.

Redmond DE Jr, Huang YH (1979): New evidence for a locus coeruleus-norepinephrine connection with anxiety. Life Sci 25:2149–2162.

Reese A (1978): Familial vulnerability for experimental neurosis. Pavlov J Biol Sci 13:169–173.

Robbins TW (1981): Behavioral determinants of drug action role-dependency revisited. In Cooper SJ (ed): "Theory in Psychopharmacology, Vol. 2." New York: Academic Press, pp 2–63.

Robertson HA, Martin IL, Candy JM (1978): Differences in benzodiazepine receptor-binding in Maudsley reactive and Maudsley non-reactive rats. Eur J Pharmacol 50:455–457.

Roy-Byrne PP, Geraci M, Uhde TW (1986a): Life events and the course of illness in patients with panic disorder. Am J Psychiatry 134:1033–1035.

Roy-Byrne PP, Geraci M, Uhde TW (1986b): Life events and the onset of panic disorder. In Shagass C, Josiassen RC, Bridger WH, Weiss KJ, Stoff D, Simpson GM (eds): Biological Psychiatry 1985." New York, Elsevier Publishing Co., 457–459.

Saner A, Pietscher A (1979): Effect of diazepam on cerebral 5-hydroxytryptamine synthesis. Eur J Pharmacol 55:315–318.

Sanger DJ (1985): GABA and the behavioral effects of anxiolytic drugs. Life Physiol Psychol 76:359–364.

Sanger DJ and Blackman VE (1976): Rate-dependent ef-

fects of drugs: A review of the literature. Pharmacol Biochem Behav 4:76–83.

Satinder KP (1971): Genotype dependent effects of d-amphetamine sulphate and caffeine on escape avoidance behavior in rats. J Comp Physiol Psychol 76:359–364.

Schiller PH (1952): Innate constituents of complex responses in primates. Psychol Rev 59:177–191.

Schneider ML (1984): Neonatal Assessment in Rhesus Monkeys. MS thesis, University of Wisconsin at Madison. Cited in Gittleman R (ed): "Anxiety Disorders of Childhood." New York: Guilford Press.

Schoenfield RI (1976): Sergic Acid Deithylamide-and mesacaline-induced attenuation of the effect of punishment in the rat. Science 192:801–803.

Schweri, M, Cain M, Cook J, Paul S, Skolnick P (1982): Blockade of 3 carbomethoxy-B-carboline induced seizures by diazepam and the benzodiazepine receptor antagonists RO-15-1788 and CGS 8216. Pharmacol Biochem Behav 17:457–460.

Seay B, Hansen EW, Harlow H (1962): Mother-infant separation in monkeys. J Child Psychol Psychiatry 3: 123–132.

Seligman MEP (1970): On the generality of the laws of learning. Psychol Rev 77:408–418.

Seligman MEP (1971): Phobias and preparedness. Behav Ther 2:307–320.

Seligman MEP (1972): Seligman MEP and Hager J (eds): "Biological Boundaries of Learning." New York: Appleton-Century-Crofts.

Seligman MEP (1975): "Helplessness: On Depression, Development and Death." San Francisco, Freeman.

Seligman MEP, Maier SF (1967): Failure to escape traumatic shock. J Exp Psychol 74:1–9.

Sepinwall J, Cook L (1978): TITLE In Iverson LL (ed): "Handbook of Psychopharmacol, 13." New York: Plenum Press, pp 345–393.

Shearman GT, Lal H (1981): Discriminative stimulus properties of cocaine related to an anxiogenic action. Prog Neuropsychopharmacol Biol Psychiatry 5:57–63.

Sheehan DV, Ballenger J, Jacobson G (1980): Treatment of endogenous anxiety with phobic, hysterical and hypochondriacal symptoms. Arch Gen Psychiatry 37: 51–59.

Sheehan DV, Coleman JH, Greenblatt DJ, Jones KJ, Levin P, Orsulak PJ, Peterson M, Schildkraut JJ, Uzogora E, Watkins D (1984): Some biochemical correlates of panic attacks with agoraphobia and their response to a new treatment. J Clin Psychopharmacol 4:66–75.

Sherman AD, Allers GL, Petty F, Henn FA (1979a): A neuropharmacologically relevant animal model of depression. Neuropharmacology 18:891–893.

Sherman AD, Allers GL, Petty F, Henn FA (1979b): Specificity of the learned helplessness model of depression. Pharmacol Biochem Behav 16:449–454.

Skolnick P, Ninan P, Insel T, Crawley J, Paul S (1984): A novel chemically induced animal model of human anxiety. Psychopathology 17[Suppl 1]:25–36.

Spealman RD (1978): Comparisons of drug effects on responding punished by pressurized air or electric shock delivery in squirrel monkeys. Pentobarbitol, chlordiazepoxide, d-amphetamine and cocaine. J Pharmacol Exp Ther 209:309–315.

Stein L (1981): Behavioral pharmacology of benzodiazepines. In Klein DF, Rabkin J (eds): "Anxiety: New Research and Changing Concepts." New York: Raven Press.

Stein L, Wise CD, Berger BD (1973): Antianxiety action of benzodiazepines: Decrease in activity of serotonin neurons in the punishment system. In Garatini S, Muscini E, Randall LO (eds): "Benzodiazepines." New York: Raven Press, 299–326.

Strahlendorf J, Strahlendorf H (1981): Soc Neurosci Abstr 7:312.

Suomi SJ (1983): Social development in rhesus monkeys: Consideration of individual differences. In Oliverio A, Zappella M (eds): "The Behavior of Human Infants." New York: Plenum Press.

Suomi SJ (1984): The development of affect in rhesus monkeys. In Fox N, Davidson R (eds): "The Psychobiology of Affective Development." Hillsdale, NJ: Lawrance Erlbaum, pp 19–159.

Suomi SJ (1986): Anxiety-like disorders in young nonhuman primates. In Gittleman R (ed): "Anxiety Disorders of Childhood." New York: The Guilford Press.

Suomi SJ, Kraemer GW, Baysinger CM, Delizio RD (1981): Inherited and experimental factors associated with individual differences in anxious behavior displayed by rhesus monkeys. In Klein DF, Rabkin J (eds): "Anxiety: New Research and Changing Concepts." New York: Raven Press, pp 179–200.

Swerson RM, Vogel WH (1983): Plasma catecholamine and corticosterone as well as brain catecholamine change during coping in rats exposed to stressful foot shock. Pharmacol Biochem Behav 18:689–693.

Tallman JF, Paul SM, Skolnick P, Gallager DW (1980): The age of anxiety-pharmacology of the benzodiazepines. Science 107:274–281.

Tamborska E, Insel T, Marangos PJ (1986): Peripheral and central type benzodiazepine receptors in Maudsley rats. Eur J Pharmacol 126:281–289.

Thiebot, MH, Hamon M, Soubrie P (1984): Serotonergic neurones and anxiety related behavior in rats. In Trimble MR, Zorifan E (eds): "Psychopharmacology of the Limbic System." New York: Wiley, pp 164–173.

Treit D (1985): Animal models for the study of anti-anxiety agents: A review. Neurosci Biobehav Rev 9: 203–222.

Treit D, Pinel JPJ, Fibiger HC (1981): A new paradigm for the study of anxiolytic agents. Pharmacol Biochem Behav 15:619–626.

Uhde TW: Animal models of anxiety. Paper presented at the 25th Annual Meeting of the American College of Neuropsychopharmacology, Dec. 10, 1986, Washington, DC.

Uhde TW, Boulenger J-P (1989): Caffeine model of panic. In Lerer B, Gershon S (Eds); "New Directions in Affective Disorders." New York: Springer-Verlag.

Uhde TW, Boulenger J-P, Jimerson DC, Post RM (1984a): Caffeine: Relationship to human anxiety, plasma MHPG and cortisol. Psychopharmacol Bull 20:426–430.

Uhde TW, Boulenger J-P, Post RM, Siever LJ, Vittone BJ, Jimerson DC, Roy-Byrne PP (1984b): Fear and anxiety relationship to noradrenergic function. Psychopathology 17(3):8–23.

Uhde TW, Boulenger J-P, Roy-Byrne PP, Geraci MF, Vittone BJ, and Post RM (1985a): Longitudinal course of panic disorder: Clinical and biological considerations. Prog Neuropsychopharmacol Biol Psychiatry 9: 39–51.

Uhde TW, Post RM, Ballenger JC, Boulenger J-P (1984c): Carbamazepine in the treatment of neuropsychiatric disorders. In Emrich HM, Okuma T, Miller A (eds): "Anticonvulsants in Affective Disorders." Amsterdam: Excerpta Medica, International Congress Series 626.

Uhde TW, Roy-Byrne PP, Vittone BJ, Boulenger J-P, Post RM (1985b): Phenomenology and neurobiology of panic disorder. In Tuma AH, Maser JD (eds): "Anxiety and the Panic Disorders." Hillsdale, NJ Lawrence Erlbaum, pp 557–576.

Vogel JR, Beer D, Clody DE (1971): A simple and reliable conflict procedure for testing anti-anxiety agents. Psychopharmacologia 21:1–7.

Vogel JR, Principi K (1971): Effect of chlordiazepoxide on depressed performance after reward production. Psychopharmacologia 21:8–12.

Walters ET, Carew TJ, Kandel ER (1979): Classical conditioning in aplysia. Proc Natl Acad Sci USA 76: 6675–6679.

Walters ET, Carew TJ, Kandel ER (1981): Associate learning in aplysia-evidence for conditioned fear in an invertebrate. Science 211:504–506.

Wang RY, Aghajanian GK (1977): Inhibition of neurons in the amygdala by dorsal raphe stimulation: Mediation through a direct serotonergic pathway. Brain Res 120:85–102.

Weiss JM (1970): Somatic effects of predictable and unpredictable shock. Psychosom Med 32:397–409.

Weiss JM (1971): Effects of coping behavior in different warning signal conditions on stress pathway in rats. J Comp Physiol Psychiatr 77:1–13.

Weiss JM, Bailey WH, Goodman PA, Hoffman LJ, Ambrose MJ, Salman S, Charry JM (1982): A model of neurochemical study of depression. In Spiegelstein MY, Levy A (eds): "Behavioral Models and the Analysis of Drug Action" Amsterdam: Elsevier Scientific Publishing Co, pp 195–223.

Weiss JM, Glazer HI (1975): Effects of acute exposure to stressors on subsequent avoidance-escape behavior. Psychosom Med 37:499–521.

Weiss JM, Glazer HI, Pohorecky LA, Brick LA, Miller NE (1975): Effects of chronic exposure to stressors on avoidance-escape behavior and on brain norepinephrine. Psychosom Med 37:522–534.

Weldon E (1967): An analogue of extraversion as a determinant of individual differences in behavior in the rat. Br J Psychol 58:253–259.

Wise CD, Berger BD, Stein L (1972): Benzodiazepines: Anxiety-reducing activity by reduction of serotonin turnover in the brain. Science 177:180–183.

Yen HCY, Krop S, Mendez HC, Katz MH (1970): Effects of some psychoactive drugs on experimental "neurotic" (conflict induced) behavior in cats. Pharmacology 3:32–40.

Yerkes RM, Yerkes A (1936): Nature and conditions of avoidance (fear responses in chimpanzee). J Comp Psychol 21:53–66.

Preclinical Studies

2

Preclinical Studies of the Mechanisms of Anxiety and Its Treatment

SANDRA E. FILE, PhD, DSC

Psychopharmacology Research Unit, UMDS Division of Pharmacology, University of London, Guy's Hospital, London SE1 9RT, England

INTRODUCTION

The preclinical studies described in this chapter have focused on three main areas of inquiry. The first concerns the neurochemical pathways modulating anxiety, including the role of the gamma-aminobutyric acid (GABA)-benzodiazepine receptor complex as well as aminergic and peptidergic pathways. A secondary consideration is whether animal tests can detect pro- and anti-panic compounds and whether the neurochemical changes in panic and anxiety can be distinguished. The second main area is the evidence from animal tests of a nonsedative anxiolytic. The third area is still very much under investigation; it concerns the possible mechanism of benzodiazepine dependence and therefore the changes underlying the enhanced anxiety manifested during benzodiazepine withdrawal.

ANIMAL TESTS OF ANXIETY

In all our existing animal tests, the animal's response to the test situation is adaptive. The tests are, therefore, measuring a physiological, rather than a pathological, state. However, as long as the biochemical changes in physiological and pathological anxiety are the same, differing only in intensity and frequency, these tests should have predictive value for the pathological state. The possible links between anxiety and panic are considered in a later section. Animal tests of anxiety can generally be considered in three main classes. In the first, tests are based on conflict or conditioned fear; in the second, anxiety is generated by novel situations; in the third, anxiety is chemically induced.

The two most widely used conflict tests are the Geller-Seifter and the Vogel punished drinking test. In the Geller-Seifter test, the rat receives food reward for pressing a lever but also receives an electric foot shock. This punished schedule alternates with an unpunished schedule during which lever-pressing is still rewarded but no shock is given. In the Vogel test, the rat is thirsty and is able to drink water but also receives an electric shock through the water spout or the bars of the floor. In these tests, it is assumed that it is the anticipation of punishment that causes a reduction in responding and that drugs that reduce anxiety will therefore result in an increased rate of responding. In the Vogel test, as in the Geller-Seifter test, it is also important to include a measure of unpunished responding, so that any nonspecific stimulant or sedative drug effects, or any changes in food or water intake, can be detected. In both these tests, benzodiazepines enhance the rate of responding in the punished periods, without increasing the rate of unpunished responding. Although these tests have face validity, no attempt has been made to validate them other than pharmacologically. A newer test is that of punished locomotion; a mouse receives foot shock whenever it crosses from one metal plate to another. A measure of unpunished crossing can also be obtained. Although less widely investigated, this test has proved sensitive to drug-induced increases and decreases in anxiety.

Neurobiology of Panic Disorder, Pages 31–48
© 1990 Alan R. Liss, Inc.

The social interaction test of anxiety exploits the uncertainty and anxiety generated by placing rats in an unfamiliar or brightly lit environment. The dependent variable is the time pairs of male rats spend in active social interaction (mostly social investigation), and both the familiarity and the light level of the test arena are varied. Undrugged rats show the highest level of social interaction when the test arena is familiar and is lit by low light. Social interaction declines if the arena is unfamiliar to the rats or is lit by bright light; anxiolytic drugs prevent this decline. The overall level of motor activity is also measured so that the specificity of changes in social behavior can be assessed. This is one of the few animal tests of anxiety that has been validated behaviorally and physiologically as well as pharmacologically (see File and Hyde, 1978, 1979; File, 1980, 1985a). To validate the test behaviorally, measures indicative of anxiety and stress such as defecation, self-grooming, and displacement activities were correlated with the reductions in social interaction, and other causes of response change (e.g., exploration of the environment, odor changes) were excluded. To validate the test physiologically, changes in adrenocorticotropic hormone (ACTH), corticosterone, and hypothalamic noradrenaline were measured.

A second test of anxiety that exploits the anxiety generated by a novel situation is the elevated plus-maze. In this test, the anxiety is generated by placing the animals on an elevated open arm; in this case, it is the height, rather than the light level, that is crucial for generating behavioral and physiological changes. The apparatus is in the shape of a plus sign, with two open and two enclosed arms. The rat has free access to all arms, and anxiolytics increase the percentage of time the animals spend on the open arms and the percentage of all entries made into the open arms. This test has also been validated behaviorally and physiologically (Pellow et al., 1985a; Pellow and File, 1986a).

Strictly speaking, the tests that fall into what was called the third group are not tests of anxiety. These tests explore the nature of the state produced by a drug or by electrical stimulation of the brain. In the drug discrimination paradigm, rats are trained to lever press on one le-

ver in the presence of drug treatment and to select a different lever after vehicle injections. If the training drug were to have one specific action only, that of increasing or decreasing anxiety, then this would be a test for selecting similar anxiolytic or anxiogenic compounds. However, it measures the overall stimulus effect of a drug, which is an amalgam of all its neurochemical and behavioral effects. In a second test, a specific place (e.g., a distinctive compartment in a two-compartment chamber) is associated with drug experience, and a different place is associated with vehicle injections. The rat is then allowed to choose between the two places. The assumption is that a choice of the drug-associated place implies that the cues associated with the drug were rewarding; of course, this may not be the same as anxiety reduction, and it is probably a better reflection of the abuse potential of a drug. Finally, it is possible to allow rats to self-stimulate electrically in brain areas that have both rewarding and aversive effects and then to determine the effects of drugs on this self-stimulation. This test is extremely sensitive to the rewarding effects of drugs, but it may also be able to detect changes in anxiety (see Liebman, 1985, for review).

The experiments described in this chapter have used the two tests of anxiety that have been most extensively validated and that do not use deprivation and electric shock, i.e., the social interaction and the elevated plus-maze tests. In general, there has been excellent agreement between all the tests of anxiety in the classification of anxiolytic and anxiogenic compounds. However, recent experiments on pro- and anti-panic compounds indicate that the tests may differ in the type of anxiety that they generate. In particular, the elevated plus-maze, in which the height of the maze is the anxiogenic stimulus, may be more sensitive than the social interaction test to agents that modulate panic.

ROLE OF THE GABA-BENZODIAZEPINE RECEPTOR COMPLEX

Since the discovery of binding sites for the benzodiazepines, our knowledge of the neurochemistry of these sites has developed rapidly. We now know that they occur on a supramolecular complex with GABA receptors and with other binding sites in an area or domain associated with a transmembrane chloride ionophore. The benzodiazepines exert their functional effects by enhancing the action of GABA to open the chloride channel (see Chapter 9, this volume). Other drugs, such as the barbiturates, act at a site on the domain of the chloride ionophore and also exert their functional effect by enhancing the effects of GABA.

Benzodiazepine Site

The benzodiazepines have proved effective in tests of anxiety of all three classes, and, in at least two of them (the Geller-Seifter test and the social interaction test), their effects are more marked after a few days of administration than they are acutely (File and Hyde, 1978; Margules and Stein, 1968; Cook and Sepinwall, 1975), similar to their clinical effects.

The full importance of the benzodiazepine binding site for mediating changes in anxiety emerged with the discovery that a new compound acting at this site, ethyl-β-3-carboxylate (β-CCE), had the behavioral effect of *enhancing* anxiety (File et al., 1982). This effect was first shown in the social interaction test, where an anxiogenic action is revealed in a specific decrease in active social interaction, without a concomitant drop in motor activity. At about the same time as the discovery of these "anxiogenic" ligands for the benzodiazepine binding site, a third class of ligand was discovered. The first example of this was the imidazodiazepine flumazenil (Ro 15-1788) (Hunkeler et al., 1981), which has the ability to antagonize the actions of the benzodiazepines. We showed that this compound, in addition to being able to antagonize the anxiolytic effects of the benzodiazepines, was also able to antagonize the anxiogenic effects of β-CCE (File et al., 1982).

After the initial demonstration of the anxiogenic effect of β-CCE, anxiogenic effects of other beta-carbolines were demonstrated in human volunteers (Dorow et al., 1983), in the social interaction test (File and Pellow, 1984a; File et al., 1984; Hindley et al., 1985), in a modified Geller-Seifter test (Prado de Carvalho et al., 1983), in the Vogel punished drinking test (Corda et al., 1983; Petersen et al., 1982, 1983), in punished locomotion (Stephens and Kehr, 1985), and in the elevated plus-maze (Pellow and File, 1986a). However, not all beta-carbo-

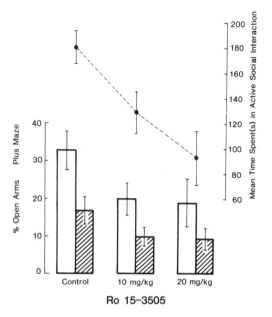

Fig. 2–1. Effects of the partial inverse agonist Ro 15-3505 in two tests of anxiety. Ro 15-3505 significantly (*P* < 0.05) decreased social interaction between pairs of rats tested in a low light, familiar arena (at top) and significantly (*P* < 0.05) decreased the percent entries made on the open arms of the plus-maze (open columns). The decrease in percent time spent on the open arms (hatched columns) was not significant.

lines are anxiogenic, and several with anxiolytic properties have now been synthesized (see File and Baldwin, 1987a, for review). Thus the chemical class of the compound does not predict the direction of its behavioral effect.

Although most of the benzodiazepines are anxiolytic, compounds with a benzodiazepine structure can be anxiogenic, as with the imidazodiazepine Ro 15-3505 in the social interaction test and the elevated plus-maze (see Fig. 2–1). In the social interaction test, the rats were tested in a low-light, familiar arena. Ro 15-3505 produced a significant reduction (*P* < 0.05) in active social interaction and no decrease in motor activity. This is the profile produced by other anxiogenic compounds, but the effects are only mild. This is in accord with the classification of this compound as a partial inverse agonist. In the elevated plus-maze, Ro 15-3505 decreased the percentage of entries made onto the open arms (*P* < 0.05) but did not significantly reduce the percentage of time spent on the open arms. Once again, these results indicate a mild anxiogenic effect.

One beta-carboline, ZK 93426, has properties similar to those of flumazenil in that it can antagonize both the anxiolytic effects of benzodiazepines and the anxiogenic effects of other beta-carbolines (Jensen et al., 1984). Interestingly, like flumazenil, it also has anxiogenic effects in the social interaction test (File et al., 1986a). If these compounds are true antagonists, i.e., compounds that bind to the benzodiazepine site but lack efficacy, then they would not be expected to have any behavioral effects. Any such effects could therefore indicate the presence of an endogenous ligand for the benzodiazepine "receptor," i.e. the behavioral changes result from displacing an endogenous ligand. So far, flumazenil has been shown to have anxiogenic effects in the social interaction test (File et al., 1982; File and Lister, 1983a; File and Pellow, 1984b), in the Vogel punished drinking test (File and Pellow, 1985a), and in tests of food and water consumption in a novel environment (Hoffman and Britton, 1983; File and Pellow, 1985a). ZK 93426 has anxiogenic effects in the social interaction test (File et al., 1986) and in the Vogel punished drinking test (Petersen et al., 1983). However, some of the animal tests of anxiety have failed to detect any action of these antagonists, e.g., the elevated plus-maze (Pellow and File, 1986a) and the punished locomotion test (Stephens and Kehr, 1985). This could reflect simply the relative sensitivity to anxiogenic drug effects of the various tests. Alternatively, it could mean that each test differs in the baseline level or the type of anxiety it produces and therefore in the extent to which one or more endogenous ligand is released. This question has been discussed in greater length elsewhere (File and Pellow, 1986a,b), and in general the behavioral evidence favors the existence of one or more endogenous ligands.

The Chloride Ionophore

Dihydropicrotoxinin was the first ligand discovered to bind to a site associated with the chloride channel. Other ligands have since been developed, and it seems that there may be several binding sites on a domain associated with the chloride channel. Barbiturates and pyrazolopyridines are thought to act at sites on this domain (Olsen, 1982; Goldberg et al., 1983). Barbiturates have anxiolytic effects in all the three classes of animal tests, and the pyrazolopyridine tracazolate has anxiolytic effects in the social interaction test, in the Vogel punished drinking test (File and Pellow, 1985d; Patel and Malick, 1982), and in the elevated plus-maze (Pellow and File, 1986a), although it is inactive in the Geller-Siefter conflict test (Patel and Malick, 1982). Binding sites on the domain of the chloride channel can also support anxiogenic actions of subconvulsant doses of picrotoxin, pentylenetetrazole (File and Lister, 1984), and the convulsant benzodiazepines Ro 5-3663 and Ro 5-4864 (File and Pellow, 1983; File and Lister, 1983b).

Benzodiazepines, as well as antagonizing anxiogenic effects of beta-carbolines (Corda et al., 1983; File and Pellow, 1984a), are also able to antagonize the anxiogenic effects of drugs acting on the domain of the chloride channel. Thus they can antagonize the effects of picrotoxin, pentylenetetrazole, Ro 5-3663, and Ro 5-4864 (File and Lister, 1984; File and Pellow, 1983, 1985b). The behavioral consequences of combining the benzodiazepine antagonist flumazenil and drugs acting on the domain of the chloride channel are different from those seen with the combination of flumazenil and anxiogenic ligands acting at the benzodiazepine site. Flumazenil *enhances* the anxiogenic effects of picrotoxin and pentylenetetrazole (File and Pellow, 1985c).

Benzodiazepine Dependence

Whereas tolerance develops very rapidly to some of the effects of benzodiazepines, e.g., the sedative and anticonvulsant properties, there is considerable controversy over whether tolerance develops to the anxiolytic effects (for review, see File, 1985c). The problem of assessing tolerance to anxiolytic effects in clinical studies is that anxiety is a disorder that shows natural waxing and waning. In animal studies, the anxiolytic effects are still found in all tests after 5 days of treatment, but, with longer treatment, tolerance has been found in the punished crossing test (Stephens and Schneider, 1985), in the Vogel conflict test (Brown et al., 1984), in defensive burying of a shocked probe (Treit, 1985), in eating in a novel environment (Cooper et al., 1981), and in the social interaction and elevated plus-maze tests (Vellucci and File, 1979; File et al., 1987a). In general, it has been found that it takes 2–3 weeks of treatment before tolerance is found to the anxiolytic effects. However, the rate of development of tolerance may also be test-specific. Thus it can be detected in the punished crossing test after only 6 days of treatment (Stephens and Schneider, 1985), whereas in the Geller-Seifter test it was not detected after 22 days (Margules and Stein, 1968).

Lader and File (1987) have recently suggested that chronic treatment with benzodiazepines induces a state of drug dependence. The underlying changes are manifest by tolerance to the behavioral effects of benzodiazepines and by the incidence of withdrawal responses when the drug is discontinued. It is likely that there are several different mechanisms of dependence, since tolerance develops at different rates to different behavioral effects of the benzodiazepines, and, on drug withdrawal, there is a different time course for the appearance of different symptoms. Increased anxiety is one of the cardinal features of benzodiazepine withdrawal in patients (Hollister et al., 1961; Ladewig, 1984). Our interest was therefore to determine whether the development of tolerance of anxiolytic effects was linked to the occurrence of increased anxiety on withdrawal of the drug. A second interest was to determine treatment that would reverse this withdrawal anxiety.

In the social interaction test and in the elevated plus-maze, a test dose of chlordiazepoxide (CDP; 5 mg/kg) still had significantly anxiolytic effects after 5 days of pretreatment with either 5 or 20 mg/kg/day (File et al., 1987a; Baldwin et al., 1987). When rats were tested 24 hr after their last dose of CDP, there was no significant increase in anxiety compared with controls. However, when the rats were tested in the plus-maze or in the social interaction test after 21 days of pretreatment with CDP, there was tolerance to the effects of a probe dose of CDP, and when these rats were tested 24 hr later they showed significant increases in anxiety (File et al., 1987a) (Fig. 2–2). It therefore seemed that, after 3 weeks of benzodiazepine treatment, neurochemical changes had occurred such that CDP was no

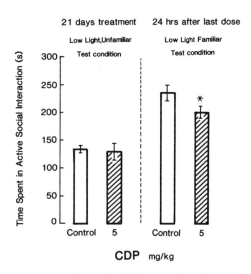

Fig. 2–2. Mean time(s) spent in active social interaction by pairs of rats tested 1) in a low light, unfamiliar arena after 20 days of injections of water (control group) or CDP (5 mg/kg) and 30 min after an injection of water or CDP, respectively, and 2) in a low light, familiar arena 24 hr after their last injection, following 21 days of water or CDP (5 mg/kg).

longer anxiolytic, and, on its removal, an increased anxiety could be detected.

The next experiments investigated possible treatments for this withdrawal anxiety. Rats that were treated for 21 days with CDP (10 mg/kg/day) showed enhanced anxiety when tested in the elevated plus-maze 24–30 hr after the last dose. This effect could be completely reversed by the benzodiazepine antagonist flumazenil (Ro 15-1788 4 mg/kg) (File and Baldwin, 1987b). Flumazenil was without effect in the vehicle-treated control rats and has previously been found to lack effects in the plus-maze at doses up to 20 mg/kg (Pellow et al., 1985a). Although in high doses flumazenil has been reported to have some partial agonist actions (see File and Pellow, 1986a, for review), there have been no reports of anxiolytic activity at doses less than 20 mg/kg, so it is unlikely that a partial agonist action can explain our withdrawal reversal. When the animals in withdrawal were challenged with the inverse agonist FG 7142, rather than an enhancment of the withdrawal, there was partial reversal of the anxiogenic effects. However, the rats in withdrawal when treated with FG 7142 did not differ significantly from either the controls or the withdrawal group.

Do these experiments shed any light on the mechanism of benzodiazepine dependence induced by 3 weeks of treatment? There is no evidence that 3 weeks of treatment with low doses of chlordiazepoxide induces any changes in benzodiazepine binding (see File, 1985c). One possibility is a decrease in the effect of GABA. This could result from a decrease in GABA release, a change in GABA binding, or a decrease in the coupling between the GABA binding site and the chloride ionophore. It is not obvious how a benzodiazepine antagonist would reverse any of these changes. However, a single injection of flumazenil (4 mg/kg), either immediately or 22 hr before electrophysiological recording, was able to reverse the subsensitivity to GABA that resulted from 3–4 weeks of diazepam (5 mg/kg) treatment in the rat (Gallager et al., 1984; Gonsalves and Gallager, 1985). An alternative explanation is that there is an endogenous ligand for the benzodiazepine binding site with anxiolytic properties. Various candidates have been proposed (see Mohler, 1981, for review), and recently an endogenous benzodiazepine has been found in mammalian brain (DeBlas and Sangameswaran, 1987). If such a ligand were present in control animals and if chronic benzodiazepine treatment suppressed the production of this ligand, then the rats in withdrawal would be more anxious than the controls. This would also explain tolerance to the anxiolytic effects of the benzodiazepines since the controls would have ligand plus CDP and the chronically treated group only CDP. Were this the mechanism, one would expect that 1) tolerance would be only partial and 2) the scores of both the control rats and those chronically treated with CDP would be the same after administration of the benzodiazepine antagonist. One might also expect that FG 7142 would potentiate withdrawal. The results from our experiment thus seem to exclude this possibility. A third alternative is that tolerance develops to the anxiolytic effects of CDP because of enhanced production and release of an endogenous anxiogenic ligand. Such a mechanism could well take a considerable length of time and would be consistent with our finding

of no changes after only 5 days of treatment. The rats in withdrawal would then show enhanced anxiety because of the production of this ligand, and the benzodiazepine antagonist would reverse withdrawal anxiety by blocking the action of the ligand. FG 7142 is only a partial inverse agonist, and, if the endogenous ligand was a full inverse agonist, then FG 7142 would act as an antagonist in its presence and partially reverse withdrawal or would have no significant effects. This possibility is consistent with our experimental results. A candidate endogenous anxiogenic ligand has been identified (Costa and Guidotti, 1985), and increased concentrations have been found after chronic diazepam treatment (Guidotti, 1987).

Flumazenil seems to have the ability to reverse benzodiazepine withdrawal responses, whether it is given 8 or 24 hr after the last dose of benzodiazepine (Gonsalves and Gallager, 1985; File and Baldwin, 1987). Furthermore, the intermittent administration of flumazenil during the course of chronic (2 weeks) diazepam treatment prevented the development of tolerance to the sedative effects and reduced the severity of withdrawal responses in primates (Gallager et al., 1986). Baldwin and File (1989) have recently found that a single administration of flumazenil, during the course of chronic CDP treatment, and 6 days before the drugs was withdrawn, was sufficient to prevent the increased anxiety normally seen during withdrawal.

Overall these results suggest a possible clinical treatment for benzodiazepine withdrawal. Although a benzodiazepine would reverse the withdrawal anxiety, it would also serve to maintain the underlying changes of dependence; in contrast, it seems that flumazenil has the ability to restore the GABA-benzodiazepine receptor complex to its drug-naive state. The benzodiazepine antagonist properties of flumazenil are retained at least after 5 days of treatment (File et al., 1986b), and the animal data suggest that intermittent treatment is sufficient. Flumazenil is already in clinical use in emergency treatment of benzodiazepine overdose. However, it is possible that at least some of the responses seen in withdrawal, for example, signs of increased autonomic arousal, reflect changes in nonbenzodiazepine pathways, such as the noradrenergic system. Such

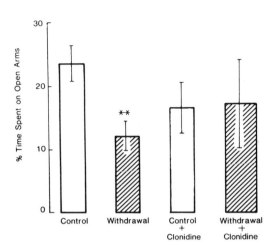

Fig. 2–3. Percent time spent on the open arms of the elevated plus-maze by rats tested 24 hr after their last injection, following 20 days of water (control) or CDP (10 mg/kg); half of each group was tested 30 min after water injection, and half were tested 30 min after clonidine (0.02 mg/kg).
**$P < 0.01$ spontaneous withdrawal group vs. controls.

marked autonomic changes could also indirectly result in increased anxiety. It is therefore possible that drugs acting on nonbenzodiazepine pathways could also reduce benzodiazepine withdrawal responses. Clonidine has been used clinically to treat benzodiazepine withdrawal, and Figure 2–3 shows the effect of clonidine in the plus-maze when it is given to control animals and to those in spontaneous withdrawal, tested 24 hr after their last dose of CDP (previously given 10 mg/kg/day for 20 days). It can be seen in Figure 2–3 that there was a tendency for clonidine to reduce the withdrawal response, but this effect was not significant. A more effective treatment might have been a beta-blocker.

OTHER SITES OF ACTION OF ANXIOGENIC DRUGS

As was reviewed above, drugs acting at two sites on the GABA-benzodiazepine receptor complex can act either to increase or to decrease anxiety, and it is thought that their initial action is to reduce or to enhance, respectively, the action of GABA. The next stage in the sequence, however, is largely unknown. It

remains necessary to identify the pathways influenced by the GABA-ergic neurons. This task has been approached in two ways. Early preclinical studies manipulated candidate pathways by lesions or by drug treatments and sought to determine whether these manipulations produced anxiolytic effects in animal tests (for review, see File, 1984). A more recent approach has been to study the sites of action of anxiogenic drugs that do not act on the GABA-benzodiazepine receptor complex.

Noradrenergic Sites

The main evidence for a noradrenergic site for anxiogenic drugs comes from the effects of yohimbine (see Chapter 6, this volume). This drug causes anxiety in humans (Holmberg and Gershorn, 1961; Charney et al., 1983) and in animal tests (Handley and Mithani, 1984a,b; Pellow et al., 1985a,b). It was not possible to reverse significantly the anxiogenic effect of yohimbine with acute chlordiazepoxide in the social interaction test (Pellow et al., 1985b) or in the elevated plus-maze (see Fig. 2–4). However, chronic treatment with CDP did reverse the effects of yohimbine in the elevated plus-maze test (see Fig. 2–4), as did administration of sodium phenobarbital (Johnston and File, 1989a). These reversals could be purely functional, i.e., strong anxiolytic action counteracting an anxiogenic action, and the results do not provide information on the site of action of yohimbine.

Yohimbine acts at alpha-2-adrenoceptors and at higher doses acts at alpha-1, dopamine, and 5-HT sites as well. The question is whether yohimbine's anxiogenic effects are mediated solely by an action at alpha-2-adrenoceptors. Certainly, yohimbine's effects can be reversed by clonidine (Pellow et al., 1985b), in doses low enough to be acting at alpha-2-adrenoceptors. However, other, specific alpha-2 agonists (BHT 920 and guanfacine) have not significantly reversed yohimbine's effects in the plus-maze (see Table 2–1). The role of alpha-2 receptors is further called into question by our finding that the more specific alpha-2 antagonist idazoxan was not anxiogenic in either the social interaction test or the elevated plus-maze (File, 1987). The situation is further complicated by the finding that the alpha-2 agonist guanfacine significantly

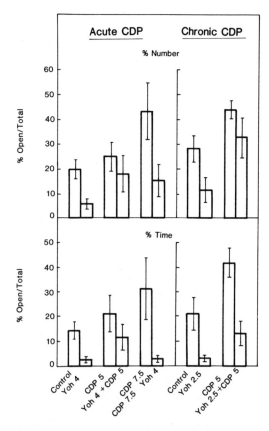

Fig. 2–4. Percent number of entries onto open arms **(top)** and percent time spent on open arms **(bottom)** by rats injected with water (control) or yohimbine (Yoh; 4 mg/kg) or with an acute injection of chlordiazepoxide (CDP; 5 or 7.5 mg/kg) alone or in combination with yohimbine (left). The histograms at right show the effects of 5 days of injections with water (control) or CDP (5 mg/kg/day); half of each group was tested 30 min after an ip injection of water, and the other half were injected with yohimbine (2.5 mg/kg). In all cases, yohimbine significantly reduced the scores compared with controls. The only significant reversal of this effect was after chronic treatment with CDP.

reduces the percentage of time spent on the open arms, indicating an anxiogenic action (Johnston et al., 1988). Thus it is possible that yohimbine's anxiogenic effects arise from its simultaneous actions on several transmitter pathways. Support for this possibility comes from the partial reversal of yohimbines's anxiogenic effects in the elevated plus-maze by the

5-HT$_1$ agonist RU 24969 and the trend to reversal by the 5-HT$_2$ antagonist ritanserin (Pellow et al., 1987) and by apomorphine (Johnston and File, 1989b). It is therefore possible that complete reversal of yohimbine's effects can be achieved only with a drug that also acts on multiple transmitter pathways.

5-HT Sites

A link between 5-HT and the anxiolytic action of benzodiazepines has been suggested for some time (Stein et al., 1975; Cook and Sepinwall, 1975; (see Chapter 8, this volume), stemming from the finding that benzodiazepines reduce 5-HT turnover. It would therefore be expected that drugs that enhanced 5-HT function would be anxiogenic. The effects of compounds that inhibit the reuptake of 5-HT have been investigated, but in general no consistent effects have been found (see File, 1984; Johnston and File, 1986). The possible role of 5-HT in anxiety is discussed below in the section on novel anxiolytics.

A recent approach to studying the neurochemical basis of anxiety has been to administer an anxiogenic drug and to study the correlation between the behavioral changes it induces and the in vivo release of neurotransmitters (File et al., 1987b). Rats with dialysis loops implanted in the dorsal hippocampus were injected with anxiogenic doses of pentylenetetrazole and the dialysate was collected over a period of 30 min. Immediately after this period, each rat was tested in the elevated plus-maze. On the basis of their scores in this test, the rats were divided into an "anxious" group (those that spent 0% of their time on the open arms) and a "nonanxious" group. The anxious group showed significantly less 5-HT and glycine release. Although pentylenetetrazole also reduced the release of noradrenaline, this was not significantly related to the differences in behavior in the elevated plus-maze.

These results suggest that *decreased* 5-HT function in the hippocampus might be related to *increases* in anxiety. This is consistent with the postsynaptic 5-HT agonist effects of buspirone in the hippocampus (Rowan and Anwyl, 1986) and suggests that anxiety-related changes in 5-HT function in the hippocampus might be in the opposite direction from changes in other brain regions, e.g., in the dor-

TABLE 2–1.
Effects of Alpha-2 Agonists, Alone and in Combination with Yohimbine (Yoh), in the Elevated Plus-Maze†

Drug group	Percent time on open arms	Drug group	Percent time on open arms
Controls	33.3 ± 5.1	Controls	17.5 ± 3.1
Yoh 2.5	8.6 ± 2.5	Yoh 2.5	7.8 ± 2.1
Clonidine 0.01	29.4 ± 5.3	BHT 920 0.025	18.0 ± 2.6
Clonidine 0.01 + Yoh 2.5	23.0 ± 5.4*	BHT 0.025 + Yoh 2.5	12.2 ± 6.5
Controls	22.9 ± 4.6	BHT 920 0.1	20.0 ± 1.7
Yoh 2.5	5.2 ± 2.4	BHT 920 0.1 + Yoh 2.5	2.3 ± 1.4
BHT 933 1	15.7 ± 5.3	Guanfacine 0.25	10.5 ± 3.4
BHT 933 1 + Yoh 2.5	4.9 ± 2.4	Guan 0.25 + Yoh 2.5	2.8 ± 1.4
BHT 933 10	21.7 ± 5.4	Guanfacine 1	9.6 ± 1.7
BHT 933 10 + Yoh	1.6 ± 0.8	Guan 1 + Yoh	7.4 ± 3.8

†The scores are the mean ± SEM percent time spent on the open arms, and all doses are in mg/kg.
*$P < 0.05$ significantly different from the group given yohimbine alone. In all cases, the yohimbine group differed significantly from controls

sal raphe. We are currently investigating the effects on in vivo transmitter release in the amygdala following administration of pentyle-netetrazole and in vivo transmitter release in the hippocampus following administration of other anxiogenic compounds. In each case, we will divide the animals on the basis of their behavior in the elevated plus-maze, so that we can determine which changes in neurotransmitter release are related to changes in anxiety.

Peptidergic Modulation

ACTH has long been suggested to have general arousing and fear-inducing properties (de Wied, 1977) (see Chapter 18, this volume), and in the social interaction test it has anxiogenic effects that can be antagonized by chlor-diazepoxide (File and Vellucci, 1978). This behavioral effect is not secondary to the release of corticosterone; the shorter fragment $ACTH_{4-10}$, which has no steroid-releasing action, also has an anxiogenic effect (File, 1979). An anxiogenic action could also be demonstrated with intracerebroventricular (icv) (File and Clarke, 1980) and with intraseptal (Clarke and File, 1983) administration of $ACTH_{4-10}$. With the absence of specific ACTH antagonists, it was not possible to identify further the site of action of these effects.

Recently, icv corticotropin-releasing factor (CRF) has been shown to reduce punished lever pressing in the Geller-Seifter test, although the specificity of this effect is in question, because unpunished lever pressing was also decreased (Thatcher Britton et al., 1983). CRF also reduces eating in a novel environment (Britton, 1984); specifically, reduces social interaction (Dunn and File, 1987) and reduces the percent of time spent on the open arms in the elevated plus-maze (File et al., 1987c) (see Fig. 2–5). These results suggest that this peptide might have an anxiogenic effect (see Chapter 18, this volume). The anxiogenic effects were antagonized by chlordiazepoxide, but this may not indicate a benzodiazepine site of action, since flumazenil (Ro 15-1788, 1 mg/kg) failed to reverse the effects of CRF in the elevated plus-maze (File et al., 1987) or in the social interaction test (see Fig. 2–5).

It is not possible to determine whether these effects are due to an action of CRF itself or are secondary to the release of ACTH. Some support for the former possibility comes from the fact that icv CRF, but not ACTH, increased motor activity of the rats in the social interaction test. It is also possible that other explanations can be found for the effects of CRF in animal tests. For example, it could be that CRF has a

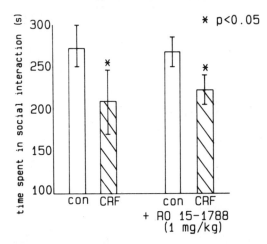

CRF (100ng/rat) and RO 15-1788 in the social interaction test

Fig. 2–5. Time(s) spent in active social interaction by pairs of rats tested in a low light, familiar arena after icv injection of vehicle (CON) or CRF, plus an ip injection of water (left) or flumazenil (Ro 15-1788; right). $*P < 0.05$ vs. control.

direct effect to reduce social investigation. This action would be consistent with the elevation of CRF in socially withdrawn, depressed patients (Nemeroff et al., 1984). So far, there have been no reports of elevated CRF in anxious patients. With the increased use of CRF challenge in psychiatry, it will be interesting to determine whether patients experience increased anxiety following administration of CRF.

NOVEL ANXIOLYTICS

The search for novel anxiolytics continues, not because the benzodiazepines lack anxiolytic efficacy but in the hopes of finding an anxiolytic with fewer additional effects. One of the main problems associated with the use of benzodiazepines for the treatment of daytime anxiety is that they are also sedative. A nonsedative anxiolytic would have considerable clinical advantage. There is also the hope of finding an anxiolytic with less risk of inducing dependence. There have been several candidates for a nonsedative anxiolytic, among both the drugs acting at the GABA-benzodiazepine receptor complex and those with nonbenzodi-

azepine sites of action. New compounds will be reviewed both as regards their efficacy in animal tests of anxiety and with respect to their sedative actions.

Drugs Acting at the GABA-Benzodiazepine Receptor Complex

The first candidate for a nonsedative anxiolytic was CL 218,872, a triazolopyridazine that displaces benzodiazepines from their binding sites, but was selective for a subtype of benzodiazepine receptor, in contrast to classical 1,4-benzodiazepines, which have equal affinity for the two receptor subtypes (Lippa et al., 1979). It was claimed that CL 218,872 was effective in animal tests of anxiety and was without sedative effects. Although the first half of the claim has been supported by other workers in several tests of anxiety (e.g., File, 1982; Oakley et al., 1984; Pellow and File, 1986a), the second part has been consistently refuted. Several workers have shown that the sedative effects of CL 218,872, revealed by reductions in spontaneous motor activity, are just as marked as those of the benzodiazepines (Oakley et al., 1984; File et al., 1985; McElroy et al., 1985). Thus, unfortunately, the possibility of finding a functional role for the two subtypes of central nervous system (CNS) benzodiazepine receptors was not realized, and behaviorally there is nothing to distinguish CL 218,872 from the 1,4-benzodiazepines.

Two other candidates were the phenylquinolines PK 8165 and PK 9084, which displace benzodiazepines from their binding site in vitro (LeFur et al., 1981), although they may not do so in vivo (Keane et al., 1984). They were claimed to have anxiolytic activity because they enhanced punished drinking in the rat and were claimed to lack sedative effects on the basis of failure to potentiate barbiturate sleeping time and because the dose that reduced spontaneous activity in mice was twice the dose of chlordiazepoxide that reduced activity (LeFur et al., 1981). Once more, other workers have failed to replicate these findings. Neither quinoline was really effective in five different animal tests of anxiety (File and Lister, 1983c; Keane et al., 1984; Pellow and File, 1986a), and, although an increase in punished drinking was replicated, there was also an increase in unpunished drinking (Pellow,

1985). Thus the anxiolytic efficacy of these compounds must be seriously questioned, and the claim that these compounds are nonsedative must also be questioned. They potentiate the hypnotic effects of benzodiazepines (Mizoule et al., 1984), reduce spontaneous motor activity in rats (File, 1983; File and Pellow, 1984c), and produce drowsiness and lethargy in volunteer subjects (von Frenckell et al., 1986).

More encouraging results have been found for the pyrazoloquinoline CGS 9896, which acts at the benzodiazepine binding site (Yokoyama et al., 1982). The evidence that CGS 9896 is anxiolytic in conflict tests is not unequivocal, and for some reason it may work only after oral administration (Bennett and Petrack, 1984; File and Pellow, 1986c). The compound has a good anxiolytic profile in the social interaction and elevated plus-maze tests (File and Pellow, 1986c), and it has a benzodiazepine-like effect on electrical self-stimulation of the brain (Bernard et al., 1985). It has been claimed to have little sedative potential, because it has no muscle-relaxant or ataxic effects (Bernard et al., 1985). However, it must be asked whether muscle relaxation and ataxia are relevant to the question of clinical sedation, which is reflected in drowsiness. This latter effect is better measured in animals by the reduction of spontaneous motor activity. CGS 9896 reduces the spontaneous motor activity of mice at doses between 30 and 300 mg/kg (Bernard et al., 1985), and in the rat it reduces motor activity at 10 mg/kg and reduces rears at 3 mg/kg (File and Pellow, 1986c). Some doubt must therefore remain regarding whether this drug is nonsedative. Of course it is possible that factors other than sedation will reduce spontaneous activity, only electroencephalogram (EEG) measures or clinical evidence will finally settle the question.

The pattern of results found with this compound raises the possibility that the relative lack of sedative effect may be accompanied by a less widespread anxiolytic activity. It is possible that the effects of CGS 9896 are due to its being a partial agonist at the benzodiazepine receptors, i.e., to its having a lower maximum effect compared with benzodiazepines. So far, the evidence needed to support this, i.e., a lower receptor occupancy to achieve an anxi-

olytic effect than to achieve sedation, is lacking. However, with the proliferation of novel compounds acting at the benzodiazepine site, it should be possible to determine behaviorally whether at least a clear separation of anxiolytic and sedative doses can be achieved.

A similar pattern of results has been found for the beta-carboline ZK 91296, which has anticonflict activity at doses of 3–30 mg/kg in the Geller-Seifter conflict test (Petersen et al., 1984) and in the punished locomotion test (Stephens and Kehr, 1985) and anxiolytic activity in the social interaction test at 5 mg/kg (Pellow and File, 1986b). It does not reduce spontaneous motor activity at doses lower than 40 mg/kg (Pellow and File, 1986b). However, this clear separation of anxiolytic and sedative doses is again accompanied by a failure to find anxiolytic action at all doses in the social interaction test (e.g., no effect at 15 mg/kg) and by a failure to have a positive effect in the Vogel conflict test or in the elevated plus-maze (Petersen et al., 1984; Pellow and File, 1986b).

Some of the newer putative anxiolytics, rather than acting at the benzodiazepine receptor, and hence displacing benzodiazepine binding, have the effect of enhancing binding. One of these compounds is the pyrazolopyridine tracazolate, which enhances the binding of benzodiazepines through an action at a site associated with the chloride channel (Malick et al., 1984). Tracazolate has somewhat limited effects in animal tests of anxiety. It is ineffective in the Geller-Seifter conflict test but has an anxiolytic action in the Vogel conflict test (Patel and Malick, 1982); at 5 mg/kg, it has an anxiolytic effect in the social interaction test and the elevated plus-maze, but these effects disappear at higher doses (File and Pellow, 1985d; Pellow and File 1986a). It was initially claimed to be nonsedative on the basis of results on barbiturate sleeping time and rotarod performance (a measure of muscle relaxation and ataxia) (Malick et al., 1984); on measures of spontaneous motor activity in rats, it was not sedative below 25 mg/kg (File and Pellow, 1985d). The 3,4-benzodiazepine tofisopam does not displace benzodiazepines from their binding site but enhances their binding (Saano and Urtti, 1982). There have been clinical reports that tofisopam is a nonsedative anxiolytic, and, if this can be confirmed, it will have important implications for animal tests of anxiety. None of the tests has detected an anxiolytic-like effect with tofisopam (for review, see Pellow and File, 1986c).

Drugs Acting at 5-HT Receptors

An alternative strategy in the search for a nonsedative anxiolytic is to find a drug that exerts its anxiolytic action "downstream" from the benzodiazepine receptors. If different neurochemical pathways mediate the sedative effects of benzodiazepines from those mediating their anxiolytic effects, then this approach should be promising.

Because benzodiazepines reduce 5-HT turnover, it might be expected that 5-HT antagonists would also have an anxiolytic profile. However, their effects in animal tests are inconsistent (see Johnston and File, 1986; Pellow et al., 1987, for reviews), and metergoline, a 5-HT antagonist, has even been found to increase anxiety in volunteers (Graeff et al., 1985). It is possible that the lack of clear effects is in part due to the nonspecificity of the available compounds.

With the development of new drugs acting more specifically at 5-HT receptor subtypes, it has been possible to reinvestigate the role of 5-HT in anxiety. Ceulemans et al. (1985) reported that the 5-HT$_2$ antagonist ritanserin reduced anxiety in patients with generalized anxiety disorder. The evidence from animal tests is conflicting with anxiolytic and anxiogenic and no effects reported (Pellow et al., 1987; Johnston and File, 1988a). The results with 8-OHDPAT, a 5-HT$_{1A}$ agonist, and with ipsapirone, which also acts at 5-HT$_{1A}$ receptors (although it is not clear whether as an agonist or antagonist), are also conflicting. There is no strong pattern to the results dependent on the type of animal test that was used, but there is an indication that the plus-maze test is relatively insensitive to the effects of novel 5-HT ligands, whereas some changes in social interaction have been reported (see Johnston and File, 1988a, for a review of these data).

Buspirone is a nonbenzodiazepine that has been found to have anxiolytic action in some patients (Wheatley, 1982), although it did not significantly reduce anxiety in other studies (Olajide and Lader, 1987). A recent study found that buspirone was effective only in female patients and only in patients that were also benzodiazepine-naive (Pecknold et al., 1985; Schweizer et al., 1986); it was also less effective and took longer to work than diazepam. It was originally thought that the effects of buspirone were mediated through actions on dopaminergic pathways (Stanton et al., 1981; Taylor et al., 1982; Wood et al., 1983), but more recently it has been found to bind with 5-HT$_{1A}$ receptors (Peroutka, 1985; Eison et al., 1986). Buspirone has been reported to have few sedative effects clinically (Taylor et al., 1984), so it may prove similar to other new compounds in having both less sedative effect as well as weaker anxiolytic effects than the benzodiazepines. Buspirone has very little effect in animal tests of anxiety, although there is some evidence of an anxiolytic effect at a low dose in the social interaction test (for review, see File, 1985b). One reason why it may have proved difficult to detect the anxiolytic effects of buspirone in animal tests is that it increases ACTH concentrations (Gilbert et al., 1987). Since ACTH has the effect of reducing social interaction, this would counteract any tendency for the anxiolytic action to enhance social interaction. If buspirone proves clinically effective, this will provide a very real challenge to our animal tests.

Recently a 5-HT$_3$ receptor antagonist was reported to have an anxiolytic action in the social interaction test but not in the Vogel conflict test (Jones et al., 1987; Tyers et al., 1987), and 5-HT$_3$ binding sites have been identified in the CNS (Kilpatrick et al., 1987). The elevation of social interaction scores was found in the high light, unfamiliar test condition. We therefore investigated the effects of three 5-HT$_3$ antagonists on the social interaction of pairs of male, hooded Lister rats, tested in a brightly lit, unfamiliar test arena. GR 38032F (0.01–1 mg/kg) was without significant effect; BRL 43694A (1 mg/kg) and ICS 205930 (0.1 mg/kg) significantly increased social interaction, by an amount similar to that seen with chlordiazepoxide (CDP; 7.5 mg/kg) (Johnston and File, 1988b). CDP had an anxiolytic action in the plus-maze, but the 5-HT$_3$ antagonists were without effect (Johnston and File, 1988b). To investigate whether the increased social interaction really reflected an anxiolytic action, we examined the effects of two of the 5-HT$_3$ an-

TABLE 2–2.
Mean (±SEM) Time(s) Spent in Active Social Interaction by Pairs of Rats Tested in a High Light, Unfamiliar Arena (HU); a High Light, Familiar Arena (HF); a Low Light, Unfamiliar Arena (LU), or a Low Light, Familiar (LF) Arena†

	HU	HF	LU	LF
Control	103.0 ± 7.3	193.4 ± 13.6	103.9 ± 7.0	189.8 ± 10.9
CDP 7.5**	140.4 ± 13.8	217.1 ± 18.7	168.4 ± 15.6	201.8 ± 19.2
GR 38032F				
0.1 mg/kg	92.7 ± 4.1	188.3 ± 12.3	86.5 ± 8.7	175.9 ± 15.5
1 mg/kg	81.4 ± 2.8	202.4 ± 6.9	101.0 ± 9.9	165.5 ± 8.6
BRL 43694				
0.1 mg/kg	99.3 ± 8.3	164.9 ± 11.9	100.0 ± 12.6	178.2 ± 15.5
1 mg/kg	104.7 ± 9.1	164.7 ± 10.2	94.5 ± 11.7	174.1 ± 15.5

†The rats were tested 1 hr after oral dosing with water (control), chlordiazepoxide (CDP; 7.5 mg/kg), GR 38032F (0.1 or 1 mg/kg), or BRL 439694 (0.1 or 1 mg/kg).
**$P < 0.01$ vs. controls.

tagonists in all four of the test conditions in the social interaction test. Once again CDP (7.5 mg/kg, orally) significantly increased social interaction ($P < 0.01$), but neither GR 38032F (0.1 and 1 mg/kg) nor BRL 43694A (0.1 and 1 mg/kg) had a significant effect (see Table 2–2). It therefore seems to be premature to conclude on the basis of animal experiments that 5-HT$_3$ antagonists have an anxiolytic action. It does seem that they are able to increase social interaction, but this was not as robust an effect as the elevation produced by CDP, and it was found only at restricted doses with two of the antagonists. Therefore, it is possible that these drugs have some more direct effect on social interaction.

LINK BETWEEN ANXIETY AND PANIC

In 1980, changes were made to the DSM III, and clear distinctions were made between generalized anxiety, agoraphobia, social and simple phobias, and panic disorder. The distinction between generalized anxiety and panic disorder arose primarily from the work of Donald Klein (1981). He distinguished between the two on the basis of symptoms and natural history of the diseases and on the basis of the most effective treatment. He had found that his patients suffering from panic attacks received little benefit from benzodiazepines but that the incidence of attacks was greatly reduced by treatment with antidepressants. However, both the clinical separation of the diseases and their different treatments have since been subject to considerable criticism.

First, the clinical distinctions specified in the DSM III do not seem to be as clear as was proposed by Klein; the problems with overlapping symptoms and history of the conditions has been recently reviewed by Tyrer (1986). There is overlap between agoraphobia and panic, anxiety and panic, depression and panic, and anxiety and depression. It seems that the clinical picture may be returning to a view of a general neurotic disorder in which patients exhibit one or more of the symptoms of anxiety, depression, phobia, or panic in different episodes of their illness (Tyrer, 1986).

Second, the evidence for the most effective drug treatments is also controversial. The initial reports that benzodiazepines were effective only in generalized anxiety and antidepressants were effective only in depression and panic disorder have recently been challenged. There are now studies in which high doses of benzodiazepines *have* been found to be effective in treating panic attacks (Beaudry et al., 1985; Noyes et al., 1984), and recent studies have found that antidepressants were more effective than benzodiazepines in reducing anxiety, phobias, and depression in neurotic patients (Johnstone et al., 1980; Tyrer et al., 1980; Kahn et al., 1986; Lipman et al., 1986). The triazolobenzodiazepine alprazolam is effective in treating panic disorder (see, e.g., Von Voigtlander and Straw, 1985), but this does not really help to elucidate the underlying neurochemical changes. It could be effective either because of its potent action at benzodiazepine receptors or because it possesses additional actions on the noradrenergic system.

If panic is to be regarded as severe anxiety, then the animal tests that have proved sensitive to anxiogenic and anxiolytic agents should also be sensitive to pro- and anti-panic agents. Certainly, the triazolobenzodiazepines are effective in animal tests of anxiety (File and Pellow, 1985e), but this could be because of their benzodiazepine-like effect and not necessarily reflecting an antipanic action. The efficacy of antidepressants in preventing panic attacks has not been questioned, but animal tests of anxiety have not detected anxiolytic activity of antidepressant drugs (Johnston and File, 1987). Clonidine has been used to treat panic attacks but has no anxiolytic action in the social interaction test (Pellow et al., 1985b) or in the plus-maze (Johnston and File, 1988). We have also been unable to detect any effects of panic-inducing agents in the social interaction test (Johnston and File, 1987). However, there is some evidence that the elevated plus-maze can detect effects of the panic-promoting agents yohimbine and isoproteronol (Johnston and File, 1988c). It is thus possible that the nature of the anxiety provoked by elevation is more akin to panic, and the changes induced by unfamiliarity and bright light are more akin to a state of generalized anxiety. However, the general insensitivity of animal tests to antipanic compounds does suggest that mechanisms underlie the actions of these drugs different from those of the benzodiazepines and other anxiolytics acting at the GABA-benzodiazepine receptor complex.

ACKNOWLEDGMENTS

The author is supported by a Wellcome Trust Senior Lectureship.

REFERENCES

Baldwin HA, File SE (1989): Flumazenil prevents the development of chlordiazepoxide withdrawal in the social interaction test of anxiety. Psychopharmacology 97:424–426.

Baldwin HA, File SE, Aranko K (1987): Evidence that the incidence of withdrawal responses to benzodiazepines is linked to the development of tolerance. Soc Neurosci Abstr 13:452.

Beaudry P, Fontaine R, Chouinard G, Annable L (1985): An open clinical trial of clonazepam in the treatment of patients with recurrent panic attacks. Prog Neuropsychopharmacol 9:589–592.

Bennett DA, Petrack B (1984): CGS 9896: a nonbenzodiazepine, nonsedating potential anxiolytic. Drug Dev Res 4:75–82.

Bernard PS, Bennett DA, Pastor G, Yokoyama N, Liebman JM (1985): CGS 9896: Agonist-antagonist benzodiazepine receptor activity revealed by anxiolytic, anticonvulsant and muscle relaxation assessment in rodents. J Pharmacol Exp Ther 235:98–105.

Britton DR (1984): Studies with CRF in an animal model of anxiety. Clin Neuropharmacol 7:S96.

Brown CL, Jones BJ, Oakley NR (1984): Differential rate of tolerance to the sedative, anxiolytic and anticonvulsant effects of benzodiazepines. Abstracts 14th CINP Congress, p 243.

Ceulemans DLS, Hoppenbrouwers MLJA, Gelders SYG, Reyntjens AJM (1985): Serotonin blockade or benzodiazepines? Pharmacopsychiatry 18:303–305.

Charney DS, Heninger GR, Redmond DE (1983): Yohimbine induced anxiety and increased noradrenergic function in humans: Effects of diazepam and clonidine. Life Sci 33:19–29.

Clarke A, File SE (1983): Social and exploratory behaviour in the rat after septal administration of ORG 2766 and ACTH$^{4-10}$. Psychoneuroendocrinology 8:343–350.

Cook L, Sepinwall J (1975): Behavioral analysis of the effects of and mechanisms of action of benzodiazepines. In Costa E, Greengard P (eds): "Mechanism of Action of Benzodiazepines." New York: Raven Press, pp 1–28.

Corda MG, Blaker WD, Mendelson WB, Guidotti A, Costa E (1983): β-Carbolines enhance shock-induced suppression of drinking rats. Proc Natl Acad Sci USA 80:2072–2076.

Costa E, Guidotti A (1985): Endogenous ligands for benzodiazepine recognition sites. Biochem Pharmacol 34:3399–3403.

DeBlas A, Sangameswaran L (1987): Demonstration and purification of an endogenous benzodiazepine from the mammalian brain with a monoclonal antibody to benzodiazepines. Life Sci 39:1927–1936.

De Wied D (1977): Peptides and behavior. Life Sci 20:195–204.

Dorow R, Horowski R, Paschelke G, Amin M, Braestrup C (1983): Severe anxiety induced by FG 7142, a β-carboline ligand for benzodiazepine receptor function. Lancet ii:98–99.

Dunn AJ, File SE (1987): Corticotropin-releasing factor displays an anxiogenic action in the social interaction test. Hormones Behav 21:193–202.

Eison AS, Eison MS, Stanley M, Riblet LA (1986): Serotonergic mechanisms in the behavioral effects of buspirone and gepirone. Pharmacol Biochem Behav 24:701–707.

File SE (1979): Effects of ACTH$^{4-10}$ in the social interaction test of anxiety. Brain Res 171:157–160.

File SE (1980): The use of social interaction as a method for detecting anxiolytic activity of chlordiazepoxide-like drugs. J Neurosci Methods 2:219–238.

File SE (1982): Animal anxiety and the effects of benzo-diazepines. In Usdin E, Skolnick P, Tallman J, Greenblatt D, Paul SM (eds): "Pharmacology of Benzodiazepines." London: MacMillan Press, pp 355–364.

File SE (1983): Sedative effects of PK 9084 & PK 8165, alone and in combination with chlordiazepoxide. Br J Pharmacol 79:219–223.

File SE (1984): Neurochemistry of anxiety. In Burrows GD, Norman T, Davies B (eds): "Drugs in Psychiatry." New York: Elsevier Biomedical Press, Vol 2, pp 13–30.

File SE (1985a): Animal models for predicting clinical efficacy of anxiolytic drugs: social behaviour. Neuropsychobiology 13:55–62.

File SE (1985b): Models of anxiety. Br J Clin Pract 39:15–19.

File SE (1985c): Tolerance to the behavioral actions of benzodiazepines. Neurosci Biobehav Rev 9:113–122.

File SE (1987): The contribution of behavioural studies to the neuropharmacology of anxiety. Neuropharmacology 26:877–886.

File SE, Baldwin HA (1987a): Effects of β-carbolines in animal models of anxiety. Brain Res Bull 19:293–299.

File SE, Baldwin HA (1987b): Flumazenil: A possible treatment for benzodiazepine withdrawal anxiety ? Lancet ii:106–107.

File SE, Baldwin HA, Aranko K (1987a): Anxiogenic effects in benzodiazepine withdrawal are linked to the development of tolerance. Brain Res Bull 19:607–610.

File SE, Baldwin HA, Dunn AJ (1987c): Decreased social interaction induced by ACTH and CRF: Interactions with chlordiazepoxide and flumazenil. Neuroendocrinol Lett 9:160.

File SE, Clarke A (1980): Intraventricular ACTH reduces social interaction in male rats. Pharmacol Biochem Behav 12:711–715.

File SE, Curle PF, Baldwin HA, Neal MJ (1987b): Anxiety in the rat is associated with decreased release of 5-HT and glycine from the hippocampus. Neurosci Lett 83:318–322.

File SE, Dingemanse J, Friedman HL, Greenblatt DJ (1986b): Chronic treatment with Ro 15-1788 distinguishes between its benzodiazepine antagonists, agonists and inverse agonist properties. Psychopharmacology 89:113–117.

File SE, Hyde JRG (1978): Can social interaction be used to measure anxiety? Br J Pharmacol 62:19–24.

File SE, Hyde JRG (1979): A test of anxiety that distinguishes between the actions of benzodiazepines and those of other minor tranquillisers and of stimulants. Pharmacol Biochem Behav 11:65–69.

File SE, Lister RG (1983a): Interactions of β-CCE & Ro 15-1788 with CGS 8216 in an animal model of anxiety. Neurosci Lett 39:91–94.

File SE, Lister RG (1983b): The anxiogenic action of Ro 5-4864 is reversed by phenytoin. Neurosci Lett 35:93–96.

File SE, Lister RG (1983c): Quinolines and anxiety: Anxiogenic effects of CGS 8216 and partial anxiolytic profile of PK 9084. Pharmacol Biochem Behav 18:185–188.

File SE, Lister RG (1984): Do the reductions in social interaction produced by picrotoxin and pentylenetetrazole indicate anxiogenic actions? Neuropharmacology 23:793–796.

File SE, Lister RG, Maninov R, Tucker JC (1984): Intrinsic behavioural actions of propyl β-carboline-3-carboxylate. Neuropharmacology 23:463–466.

File SE, Lister RG, Nutt DG (1982): The anxiogenic action of benzodiazepine antagonists. Neuropharmacology 21:1033–1037.

File SE, Pellow S (1983): The anxiogenic action of a convulsant benzodiazepine: reversal by chlordiazepoxide. Brain Res 278:370–372.

File SE, Pellow S (1984a): The anxiogenic action of FG 7142 in the social interaction test is reversed by chlordiazepoxide and Ro 15-1788 but not by CGS 8216. Arch Int Pharmacodyn Ther 271:198–205.

File SE, Pellow S (1984b): The anxiogenic action of Ro 15-1788 is reversed by chronic, but not by acute, treatment with chlordiazepoxide. Brain Res 310:154–156.

File SE, Pellow S (1984c): Behavioural effects of PK 8165 that are not mediated by benzodiazepine receptors. Neurosci Lett 50:197–201.

File SE, Pellow S (1985a): The benzodiazepine receptor antagonist Ro 15-1788 has an anxiogenic action in four animal tests of anxiety. Br J Pharmacol 84:103P.

File SE, Pellow S (1985b): The anxiogenic action of Ro 5-4864 in the social interaction test: effects of chlordiazepoxide, Ro 15-1788 and CGS 8216. Neuropsychobiology 14:193–197.

File SE, Pellow S (1985c): Does the benzodiazepine antagonist Ro 15-1788 reverse the actions of picrotoxin and pentylenetetrazole on social and exploratory behaviour? Arch Int Pharmacodyn Ther 277:272–279.

File SE, Pellow S (1985d): The anxiolytic, but not the sedative, properties of tracazolate are reversed by the benzodiazepine receptor antagonist Ro 15-1788. Neuropsychobiology 14:193–197.

File SE, Pellow S (1985e): The effects of triazolobenzodiazepines in two animal tests of anxiety and the holeboard. Br J Pharmacol 86:729–736.

File SE, Pellow S (1986a): Intrinsic actions of the benzodiazepine receptor antagonist Ro 5-1788. Psychopharmacology 88:1–11.

File SE, Pellow S (1986b): Do the intrinsic actions of benzodiazepine receptor antagonists imply the existence of an endogenous ligand for benzodiazepine receptors? In Biggio G, Costa E (eds): "Advances in Biochemical Pharmacology: GABAergic Transmission and Anxiety." New York: Raven Press, pp 187–201.

File SE, Pellow S (1986c): Behavioral pharmacology of the pyrazoloquinoline CGS 9896, a novel putative anxiolytic. Drug Dev Res 7:245–253.

File SE, Pellow S, Jensen LH (1986a): Actions of the β-carboline ZK 93426 in an animal test of anxiety and in the holeboard: Interactions with Ro 15-1788. J Neural Transmiss 65:103–114.

File SE, Pellow S, Wilks LJ (1985): The sedative effects of CL 218,872, like those of chlordiazepoxide, are reversed by benzodiazepine antagonists. Psychopharmacology 85:295–300.

File SE, Vellucci SV (1978): Studies on the role of ACTH and of 5-HT in anxiety using an animal model. J Pharm Pharmacol 30:105–110.

Gallager DW, Heninger K, Heninger G (1986): Periodic benzodiazepine antagonist administration prevents benzodiazepine withdrawal symptoms in primates. Eur J Pharmacol 132:311–338.

Gallager DW, Lakoski JM, Gonsalves SF, Rauch SL (1984): Chronic benzodiazepine treatment decreases postsynaptic GABA sensitivity. Nature 308:74–77.

Gilbert F, Dourish CT, Stahl SM (1987): Correlation between increases in food intake and plasma ACTH levels after administration of 5-HT$_{1A}$ agonists in rats. Neuroendocrinol Lett 9:176.

Goldberg ME, Salama AI, Patel JB, Malick JB (1983): Novel non-benzodiazepine anxiolytics. Neuropharmacology 22:1499–1504.

Gonsalves SF, Gallager DW (1987): Time course for development of anticonvulsant tolerance and GABAergic subsensitivity after chronic diazepam. Brain Res 405:94–99.

Graeff FG, Zuardi AW, Giglio JS, Lima Filho EC, Karniol IG (1985): Effects of metergoline on human anxiety. Psychopharmacology 86:334–338.

Guidotti A (1987): An octadecaneuropeptide (ODN) derived from DBI as a putative endogenous ligand of benzodiazepine recognition sites. Abstracts 10th IUPHAR Congress, Sydney, Australia, S113.

Handley SL, Mithani S (1984a): Effects of αadrenoceptor agonists and antagonists in a maze-exploration model of "fear" motivated behaviour. Naunyn-Schmiederbergs Arch Pharmacol 327:1–5.

Handley SL, Mithani S (1984b): Effects on punished responding of drugs acting at αadrenoceptors. Br J Pharmacol 82:341P.

Hindley SW, Hobbs A, Paterson IA, Roberts MHT (1985): Microinjection of methyl-β-carboline-3-carboxylate into nucleus raphe dorsalis reduces social interaction in the rat. Br J Pharmacol 86:753–761.

Hoffman DK, Britton DR (1983): Anxiogenic-like properties of benzodiazepine antagonists. Soc Neurosci Abstr 9:129.

Hollister LE, Motzenbecker FP, Degan RO (1961): Withdrawal reactions from chlordiazepoxide (Librium). Psychopharmacologia 2:63–68.

Holmberg G, Gershon S (1961): Autonomic and psychiatric effects of yohimbine hydrochloride. Psychopharmacologia 2:93–106.

Hunkeler W, Mohler H, Pieri L, Polc P, Bonetti EP, Cumin R, Schaffner R, Haefely W (1981): Selective antagonists of benzodiazepines. Nature 290:514–516.

Jensen LH, Petersen EN, Braestrup C, Honore T, Kehr W, Stephens DN, Schneider H, Seidelman D, Schmiechen R (1984): Evaluation of the β-carboline ZK 93426 as a benzodiazepine receptor antagonist. Psychopharmacology 83:249–256.

Johnston AL, File SE (1986): 5-HT and anxiety: Promises and pitfalls. Pharmacol Biochem Behav 24: 1467–1470.

Johnston AL, File SE (1987): Pro- and anti-panic treatments and measures of anxiety in the rat. Soc Neurosci Abstr 13:452.

Johnston AL, File SE (1988a): Effects of ligands for specific 5-HT receptor sub-types in two animal tests of anxiety. In Lader MH (ed): "Buspirone: A New Introduction to the Treatment of Anxiety." London: RSM Services, pp 31–42.

Johnston AL, File SE (1988b): Effects of 5-HT$_3$ antagonists in two animal tests of anxiety. Neurosci Lett S32: S44.

Johnston AL, File SE (1988c): Can animal tests of anxiety detect panic-promoting agents? Hum Psychopharmacol 3:149–152.

Johnston AL, File SE (1989a): Sodium phenobarbitone reverses the anxiogenic effects of compounds acting at three different sites. Neuropharmacology 28:83–88.

Johnston AL, File SE (1989b): Yohimbine's anxiogenic action: evidence for noradrenergic and dopaminergic sites. Pharmacol Biochem Behav 32:151–156.

Johnston AL, File SE, Koening E, Cooper T (1988) A comparison of the effects of rilmenidine with those of guanfacine and clonidine in the holeboard and elevated plus-maze. Drug.

Johnston AL, Koening-Berard E, Cooper TA, File SE (1988): A comparison of the effects of clonidine, rilmenidine and guanfacine in the holeboard and elevated plus-maze. Drug Dev Res 15:405–414.

Johnstone EC, Cunningham Owens DG, Frith CD, McPherson K, Dowie C, Riley G, Gold A (1980): Neurotic illness and its response to anxiolytic and antidepressant treatment. Psychol Med 10:321–328.

Jones BJ, Oakley NR, Tyers MB (1987): The anxiolytic activity of GR 38032F, a 5-HT$_3$ receptor antagonist, in the rat and cynomolgus monkey. Br J Pharmacol 90: 90P.

Kahn RJ, McNair DM, Lipman RS, Covi L, Rickels K, Downing R, Fisher S, Frankenthaler LM (1986): Imipramine and chlordiazepoxide in depressive and anxiety disorders: 2. Efficacy in anxious outpatients. Arch Gen Psychiatry 43:79–85.

Keane P, Simiand J, Morre M (1984): The quinolines PK 8165 and PK 9084 possess benzodiazepine-like activity in vitro but not in vivo. Neurosci Lett 45:89–93.

Kilpatrick GJ, Jones BJ, Tyers MB (1987): identification and distribution of 5HT$_3$ receptors in rat brain using radioligand binding. Nature 330:746–748.

Klein DF (1981): Anxiety reconceptualized. In Klein DF, Rabkin JG (eds): "Anxiety: New Research and Changing Concepts." New York: Raven Press, pp 235–263.

Lader MH, File SE (1987): The biological basis of benzodiazepine dependence. Psychol Med 17:539–547.

Ladewig D (1984): Dependence liability of the benzodiazepines. Drug Alcohol Depend 13:139–149.

LeFur G, Mizoule J, Burgevin MC, Ferris O, Heaulme M, Gauthier A, Gueremy C, Uzan A (1981): Multiple benzodiazepine receptors: evidence of a dissociation between anticonflict and anticonvulsant properties by PK 8165 and PK 9084 (two quinoline derivatives). Life Sci 28:1439–1448.

Liebman JM (1985): Anxiety, anxiolytics and brain stimulation reinforcement. Neurosci Biobehav Rev 9:75–86.

Lipman RS, Covi L, Rickels K, McNair DM, Downing R, Kahn RJ, Lasseter VK, Faden V (1986): Imipramine and chlordiazepoxide in depressive and anxiety disorders: 1. Efficacy in anxious outpatients. Arch Gen Psychiatry 43:68–77.

Lippa AS, Coupet J, Greenblatt EN, Klepner CA, Beer B (1979): A synthetic non-benzodiazepine ligand for benzodiazepine receptors: A probe for investigating neuronal substrates of anxiety. Pharmacol Biochem Behav 11:99–106.

Malick JB, Patel JB, Salama AI, Meiners BA, Giles RE, Goldberg (1984): Tracazolate: a novel nonsedative anxiolytic. Drug Dev Res 4:61–73.

Margules DL, Stein L (1968): Increase of antianxiety activity and tolerance to behavioural depression during chronic administration of oxazepam. Psychopharmacology 13:74–80.

McElroy JF, Fleming RL, Feldman RS (1985): A comparison between chlordiazepoxide and CL 218,872—a synthetic nonbenzodiazepine ligand for benzodiazepine receptors on spontaneous locomotor activity in rats. Psychopharmacology 85:224–226.

Mizoule J, Rataud J, Uzan A, Mazadier M, Daniel M, Gauthier A, Ollat C, Gueremy C, Renault C, Dubroeucq MC, LeFur G (1984): Pharmacological evidence that PK 8165 behaves as a partial agonist of brain type benzodiazepine receptors. Arch Int Pharmacodyn Ther 271:189–197.

Mohler H (1981): Benzodiazepine receptors: Are there endogenous ligands in the brain? Trends Neurosci 5: 116–118.

Nemeroff CB, Wederlov E, Bissette G, Walleus H, Karlsson I, Eklund K, Kilts CD, Loosen PT, Vale W (1984): Elevated concentrations of CSF corticotropin-releasing factor-like immunoreactivity in depressed patients. Science 226:1342–1344.

Noyes R, Anderson DJ, Clancy J, Crowe RR, Slymen DJ, Ghoneim MM, Hinrichs JV (1984): Diazepam and propranolol in panic disorder and agoraphobia. Arch Gen Psychiatry 41:287–292.

Oakley NR, Jones BJ, Straughan DW (1984): The benzodiazepine receptor ligand CL 218,872 has both anxiolytic and sedative properties in rodents. Neuropharmacology 23:797–802.

Olajide D, Lader M (1987): A comparison of buspirone, diazepam and placebo in patients with chronic anxiety states. J Clin Psychopharmacol 7:148–152.

Olsen RW (1982): Drug interactions at the GABA receptor-ionophore complex. Annu Rev Pharmacol Toxicol 22:245–277.

Patel JB, Malick JB (1982): Pharmacological properties of tracazolate: A new non-benzodiazepine anxiolytic agent. Eur J Pharmacol 78:323–333.

Pecknold JC, Familamiri P, Chang H, Wilson R, Alarcia J, McClure DJ (1985): Buspirone: Anxiolytic? Prog Neuropsychopharmacol Biol Psychiatry 9:639–642.

Pellow S (1985): Can drug effects on anxiety and convulsions be separated? Neurosci Biobehav Rev 9:55–73.

Pellow S, Chopin P, File SE, Briley M (1985a): The validation of open:closed arm entries in an elevated plus-maze as a measure of anxiety in the rat. J Neurosci Methods 14:149–167.

Pellow S, Chopin P, File SE (1985b): Are the anxiogenic effects of yohimbine in the social interaction test mediated at benzodiaze pine receptors? Neurosci Lett 55: 5–9.

Pellow S, File SE (1986a): Anxiolytic and anxiogenic drug effects in exploratory activity in an elevated plus-maze: A novel test of anxiety in the rat. Pharmacol Biochem Behav 24:525–529.

Pellow S, File SE (1986b): Evidence that the β-carboline, ZK 91296, can reduce anxiety in animals at doses well below those causing sedation. Brain Res 363:174–177.

Pellow S, File SE (1986c): The effects of tofisopam, a 3,4-benzodiazepine, in animal models of anxiety, sedation and convulsions. Drug Dev Res 7:61–73.

Pellow S, Johnston AL, File SE (1987): Selective agonists and antagonists for 5-hydroxytryptamine receptor subtypes in the elevated plus-maze in the rat, and interactions with yohimbine and FG 7142. J Pharm Pharmacol 39:917–928.

Peroutka SJ (1985): Selective interaction of novel anxiolytics with 5-hydroxytryptamine $_{1A}$ receptors. Biol Psychiatry 20:971.

Petersen EN, Jensen LF, Honore T, Braestrup C, Kehr W, Stephens DN, Wachtel H, Seidelman D, Schmiechen R (1984): ZK 91296, a partial agonist at benzodiazepine receptors. Psychopharmacology. 83:240–248.

Petersen EN, Jensen LH, Honore T, Braestrup C (1983): Differential pharmacological effects of benzodiazepine receptor inverse agonists. In Biggio G, Costa E (eds): "Benzodiazepine Recognition Site Ligands: Biochemistry and Pharmacology." New York: Raven Press, pp 57–64.

Petersen EN, Paschelke G, Kehr W, Nielsen M, Braestrup C, (1982): Does the reversal of the anticonflict effect of phenobarbital by βCCE and FG 7142 indicate benzodiazepine receptor-mediated anxiogenic properties? Eur J Pharmacol 82:217–221.

Prado de Carvalho L, Greksch G, Chapouthier G, Rossier J (1983): Anxiogenic and non-anxiogenic benzodiazepine antagonists. Nature 301:64–66.

Rowan MJ, Anwyl R (1986): Neurophysiological effects of buspirone and isapirone in the hippocampus: Comparisons with 5- hydroxytryptamine. Eur J Pharmacol 132:93–96.

Saano V, Urtti A (1982): Tofisopam modulates the affinity of benzodiazepine receptors in the rat brain. Pharmacol Biochem Behav 17:367–369.

Schweizer E, Rickels K, Lucki I (1986): Resistance to the antianxiety effect of buspirone in patients with a history of benzodiazepine use. N Engl J med 314:719–720.

Stanton HC, Taylor DP, Riblet LA (1981): Buspirone—An anxioselective drug with dopaminergic action. In Chronister RB, deFrance JF (eds): "The Neurobiology of the Nucleus Accumbens." Brunswick, ME: Haer Institute, pp 316–321.

Stein L, Wise CD, Belluzzi JD (1975): Effects of benzodiazepines on central serotonergic mechanisms. In Garattini S, Mussini E, Randall LO (eds): "Mechanisms of Action of Benzodiazepines." New York: Raven Press, pp 299–326.

Stephens DN, Kehr W (1985): β-Carbolines can enhance or antagonize the effects of punishment in mice. Psychopharmacology 85:143–147.

Stephens DN, Schneider HH (1985): Tolerance to the benzodiazepine diazepam in an animal model of anxiety. Psychopharmacology 87:322–327.

Taylor DP, Eison AS, Eison MS, Riblet LA, Temple DL, Van der Maelen CP (1984): Biochemistry and pharmacology of the anxioselective drug buspirone. Clin Neuropharmacol 7:S476.

Taylor DP, Riblet LA, Stanton HC, Eison AS, Eison MS, Temple DL (1982): Dopamine and antianxiety activity. Pharmacol Biochem Behav 17[Suppl 1]:25–35.

Thatcher Britton K, Rivier J, Vale W, Koob GF (1983): Chlordiazepoxide attenuates CRF effects on conflict test. Soc Neurosci Abstr 9:1122.

Treit D (1985): Evidence that tolerance develops to the anxiolytic effect of diazepam in rats. Pharmacol Biochem Behav 22:383–387.

Tyers MB, Costall B, Domeney A, Jones BJ, Kelley ME, Naylor RJ, Oakley NR (1987): The anxiolytic activities of 5HT$_3$ antagonists in laboratory animals. Neurosci Lett S29:S68.

Tyrer P (1986): Classification of anxiety disorders: a critique of DSM-III. J Affect Disorders 11:99–104.

Tyrer P, Gardner M, Lambourn J, Whitford M (1980): Clinical and pharmacokinetic factors affecting response to phenlzine. Br J Psychiatry 136:359–365.

Vellucci SV, File SE (1979): Chlordiazepoxide loses its anxiolytic action with long-term treatment. Psychopharmacology 62:61–65.

von Frenckell R, Ansseau M, Bonnet D (1986): Evaluation of the sedative properties of PK 8165 (pipequaline), a benzodiazepine partial agonist in normal subjects. Int Clin Psychopharmacol 1:24–35.

Von Voigtlander PF, Straw RN (1985) Alprazolam: review of the pharmacological, pharmacokinetic, and clinical data. Drug Dev Res 6:1–12.

Wheatley D (1982): Buspirone: Multicenter efficacy study. J Clin Psychiatry 43:92–94.

Wood PL, Nair NPV, Lal S, Etienne P (1983): Buspirone: a potential atypical neuroleptic. Life Sci 33:269–273.

Yokoyama N, Ritter B, Neubert AD (1982): 2-Arylpyrazolo4,3-c quinolin-3ones: Novel agonist, partial agonist and antagonist of benzodiazepines. J Med Chem 25:337–339.

Genetics

3
_____

Twin Studies in Panic Disorder

SVENN TORGERSEN, Dr. Philos.

Center for Research in Clinical and Applied Psychology, Department of Psychology, University of Oslo, 0315 Oslo 3, Norway

THE ETIOLOGY OF PANIC DISORDERS

Clinicians engaged in treatment of anxiety disorders have suspected for some time that anxiety problems run in families. Modern diagnostic systems, including the Feighner criteria (Feighner et al., 1972), Research Diagnostic Criteria (RDC) (Spitzer et al., 1978) and DSM III (APA, 1980), structured diagnostic interviews, the Present State Exam (PSE) (Wing et al., 1974), DIS (Robins et al., 1981), and Structured Clinical Interview for Diagnosis (SCID) (Spitzer and Williams, 1984), and refined epidemiological methods have confirmed this. Even more important, however, is the observation that some anxiety disorders seem to be more strongly familial than others. Panic disorder in particular seems to have a high concordance among biologically related family members (Cloninger et al., 1981; Crowe et al., 1980, 1982, 1983; Harris et al., 1983; Noyes et al., 1986). This is discussed further elsewhere in this volume (see Chapter 4).

The question arises of whether the familial transmission is due to shared environmental factors or similarity in the genetic programming. The best way to address this issue is through adoption studies. A higher correlation of anxiety disorders between biological relatives never living together than among adoptive relatives living together would confirm the importance of genetic factors in the development of the disorder. Unfortunately, no adoption study of anxiety disorders has been conducted.

The influence of genetic factors on the development of anxiety disorders can be studied by yet another method; through the study of twins. Because monozygotic (MZ) twins are genetically identical and dizygotic (DZ) twin partners are no more similar genetically than other siblings, a higher concordance among MZ twin partners than among DZ twins would indicate the importance of genetic factors in the development of the disorder. It is erroneously assumed that environmental factors would be similar for DZ and MZ twin partners. This is not true; MZ twins spend much more time together than DZ twins, often share the same friends, and are more often treated as a unit (Torgersen, 1981). It is thus necessary to control for this confounding factor.

It is possible to combine the family and twin method by studying not only the twin partners but also their parents and sibs. This has not been attempted previously with clinical cases, but such a study is now in progress in Norway. This study makes it possible to investigate the mode of inheritance; the interaction between heredity and environment; and the contribution of the genetic, family, and individual variance to the total variance in the frequency and severity of the disorder in the population in question.

A more elegant way to determine the influence of genetic factors on the development of anxiety disorders would be to combine the twin and adoption methods. This is extremely difficult given the rare occurrence of twins who are adopted and raised apart and the relative rarity of the disorder. Such twin pairs would be extremely rare and highly selected. Only three pairs of MZ twins with anxiety traits who were raised apart are described in the literature (Shields, 1962).

Neurobiology of Panic Disorder, Pages 51–58
© 1990 Alan R. Liss, Inc.

A number of twin studies of anxiety disorders have been published. Some have analyzed anxiety disorders as a general group (Shields and Slater, 1966; Torgersen, 1985a); others have focused on specific disorders, e.g., phobias and obsessive compulsive disorders (Carey and Gottesman, 1981; Ihda, 1961; Inouye, 1965; Schepank, 1974; Tienari, 1963; Torgersen, 1979, 1983; Young et al., 1971). However, only a few twin studies have investigated panic reactions or panic disorder specifically (Kendler et al., 1986; Schepank, 1974; Torgersen, 1983). These studies are discussed in this chapter.

Schepank (1974) investigated the partners of 50 twin pairs among whom at least one of the partners had been treated at an outpatient clinic in West Berlin between 1950 and 1970. Twenty-one twin pairs were MZ, 16 same-sex DZ, and 13 opposite-sex DZ. The subjects included 64 adults and 36 children or adolescents. Among these twins, he observed three MZ and four DZ twins with "attacks of free-floating anxiety, death anxiety, or anxiety related to separation from mother or partner." None of their cotwins had the same kind of symptoms. In examining the short case histories of the twin pairs, we observed that three of the twin pairs were children. Furthermore, the case stories indicate that only two probands might have genuine panic disorder, and both were DZ. Both their twin partners had some phobias and obsessive symptoms.

Kendler et al. (1986) analyzed a sample of 3,810 Australian twin pairs who replied to a questionnaire with seven items measuring anxiety and seven items measuring depression. Their overall results indicated that genetic factors seemed to contribute to the replies on all or most of the items. However, of particular interest are replies to two of the items: "Recently, I have been breathless or had a pounding of my heart" and "Recently, for no good reason, I have had feelings of panic." Although the genetic variance of the replies to the other items seemed to be additive, for these two specific items dominant genetic variance seemed to be indicated. Dominant genetic variance means that the genetic effect is nonadditive and a result of two alternative alleles at a locus on the chromosome. A positive answer to these two questions in the Kendler et al.

study (1986) is suggestive of, but certainly does not provide definitive evidence to confirm the diagnosis of panic disorder. With this reservation, it is interesting that Crowe et al. (1981) claimed that panic disorder is transmitted by a single dominant gene. Their arguments stem from a study of four generations of ancestors of probands with panic disorder. They observed that almost all ancestral cases came from the same side of the kindred, either the maternal or the paternal. This observation is an indication of a single dominant gene. However, Carey (1982) has argued that the study of Crowe et al. (1981) is inconclusive. The higher frequency of panic disorder among women speaks against a single dominant gene transmission. Furthermore, Carey's analysis of the observations of Crowe et al. suggests that the findings do not fit what would be expected from a dominant gene model any better than what would be expected with a polygenetic model. He also points out that the Crowe et al. sample is highly selective.

A case report concerning two HLA-identical sib pairs with panic disorder also suggests the potential importance of a single gene model in the transmission of panic disorder (Surman et al., 1983). It is noteworthy that HLA B12 was present in all four individuals with panic disorder. However, because only two sib pairs were studied, it is impossible to reach a definitive conclusion about a genetic link in panic disorder from such a small sample. A recent linkage study of a larger sample, however, seems to indicate that panic disorders might be influenced by a gene on chromosome 16 (Crowe et al., 1988). Only one study has investigated a larger sample of twins with clinical panic disorder diagnosed by DSM III criteria (Torgersen, 1983). Among 318 twin probands, collected in a study of patients from all Norwegian psychiatric institutions, 29 twins turned out to have either panic disorder or agoraphobia with panic attacks. Of the 29 subjects, 13 were MZ twins and 16 were DZ twins.

These two anxiety disorders are grouped together in Table 3–1, as they have been in DSM III-R (APA, 1987). As a comparison, Table 3–1 also shows the results for the other anxiety disorders. Because agoraphobia without panic attacks and obsessive compulsive disorder show some crossover concordance, they are also grouped together along with social phobia. Fi-

TABLE 3–1.
Probandwise Concordance Rates for Various Groups of Anxiety Disorder
(Torgersen, 1983)

Proband diagnosis		Panic disorder or agoraphobia with panic attacks; N (%)	Other phobias or obsessive compulsive disorder; N (%)	Generalized anxiety disorder; N (%)	Any anxiety disorder; N (%)	Total; N (%)
		Cotwin diagnosis				
Panic disorder	MZ	2 (15.4)	0 (0.0)	4 (30.8)	6 (46.2)	13 (100.0)
or agoraphobia with panic	DZ	0 (0.0)	0 (0.0)	4 (25.0)	6 (25.0)	16 (100.0)
Other phobias and	MZ	0 (0.0)	2 (28.6)	1 (14.3)	3 (42.9)	7 (100.0)
obsessive compulsive disorder	DZ	0 (0.0)	0 (0.0)	1 (5.6)	1 (5.6)	17 (100.0)
Generalized	MZ	0 (0.0)	2 (16.7)	0 (0.0)	2 (16.7)	12 (100.0)
anxiety disorder	DZ	0 (10.0)	1 (5.0)	1 (5.0)	4 (20.0)	20 (100.0)

nally, generalized anxiety disorder is described separately from the other anxiety disorders.

Two of 13 MZ pairs are concordant for panic disorder or agoraphobia with panic attacks, compared to none of 16 DZ pairs (Table 3–1). Generalized anxiety disorder is evenly distributed among the cotwins of the probands. In looking at phobias and obsessive compulsive disorders, there is also a fairly high concordance among MZ twin partners and no concordance for the same disorder among the DZ twin partners. Finally, for twins with generalized anxiety disorder, no higher concordance is observed among MZ twins compared to DZ twins. Consequently, the twin study suggests that the development of panic disorder and agoraphobia with panic attacks is influenced by genetic factors. The same conclusion can be reached for other phobias and obsessive compulsive disorder, but these disorders may be transmitted by other genes. The development of generalized anxiety disorder seems uninfluenced by heredity.

The criteria of three panic attacks within a 3 week period for the diagnosis of panic disorder, as stated in the DSM III, is arbitrary and may conceal the true similarity between twin partners. Consequently, we looked at the frequency of anxiety disorder with panic attacks, irrespective of the frequency of attacks, among the cotwins of probands with panic disorder and agoraphobia with panic attacks. Table 3–2 shows that four MZ cotwins (31%) had anxiety disorder with panic attacks compared to none of the DZ cotwins. Among the cotwins of other anxiety disorders, anxiety disorder with panic attacks were almost absent.

It might be argued that the higher concordance in MZ pairs than in DZ pairs could be ascribed to the fact that MZ twin partners spend more time together in childhood, more often share the same friends, and are often treated as a unit. However, it turned out that the childhood similarity in environmental factors was unrelated to concordance rates among the MZ or DZ pairs (Torgersen, 1983). The twin study thus strongly indicates that genetic factors might be involved in the development of panic disorder and agoraphobia with panic attacks. Furthermore, it suggests that anxiety disorders without panic attacks may have a different etiology than anxiety disorders with panic. This viewpoint is shared by Kendler et al. (1986), based on their results mentioned above. Generalized anxiety disorder especially seems to be caused by other factors, and our twin study did not demonstrate any difference between MZ and DZ cotwins in the frequency of these anxiety disorders. It should then be expected that it is easier to demonstrate the influence of environmental factors in the etiology of generalized anxiety disorder than in the anxiety disorders with panic. This was, in

TABLE 3–2.
Anxiety Disorder With Panic Attacks Among Cotwins of Probands With Various Anxiety Disorders

Proband diagnosis		Cotwin diagnosis anxiety disorder with panic attacks; N (%)	Total; N (%)
Panic disorder or	MZ	4 (30.8)	13 (100.0)
agoraphobia with panic	DZ	0 (0.0)	16 (100.0)
Other anxiety	MZ	1 (5.3)	19 (100.0)
disorders	DZ	2 (5.4)	37 (100.0)

fact, what we observed in our twin study (Torgersen, 1986). Whereas twins with panic disorder and agoraphobia with panic attacks in childhood had suffered more often from anxiety than twins with generalized anxiety disorder, the latter had experienced more losses in childhood.

It is important to keep in mind that most of the MZ twin pairs with a proband with panic disorder are discordant. Consequently, environmental factors may be very important in the development of this disorder. The question then arises: What kind of environmental factors are responsible for the observed discordance? An examination of the discordant MZ pairs on a case study basis reveals that the childhood home of twins who later developed panic disorder seemed very safe and reliable to outside observers (Torgersen, 1984). However, to the twins, the family atmosphere was experienced as overcontrolling and strict. This seems to have created in the twins with poorer physical health from birth a more inhibited, passive, less self-assertive personality. In adulthood, a variety of situations triggered the anxiety disorder. Threats to physical security, social status, and independence seem to be among the most frequent precipitating events (see Fig. 3–1).

PANIC DISORDERS AND AFFECTIVE DISORDERS

The discussion about the relationship between anxiety and depression is an old one. Most authors recognize these as separate disorders, but some have claimed that they are different aspects of the same disorder (Lewis, 1934; Mendels et al., 1972). Some have maintained that there is also a mixed disorder, separate from both anxiety and depression (Finlay-Jones and Brown, 1981; Van Valkenburg et al., 1984).

The controversy could be approached with increased precision following the publication of first the DSM III and later the DSM III-R. According to DSM III, major depression is hierarchical above the anxiety disorders. That means that, if both major depression and one or more anxiety disorders exist, the diagnosis of major depression should be applied. If the hierarchy is suspended, a number of patients will have both a major depression and an anxiety disorder. Family studies have shown that the frequency of not only major depression and all anxiety disorders but also alcohol abuse is higher among adult relatives of probands with major depression and panic disorder compared to relatives of probands with major depression without panic disorder (Leckmann et al., 1983). Weissman et al. (1984) observed that children of probands with major depression plus panic disorder had more major depression and anxiety disorders than children of probands with major depression only.

A few twin studies have dealt with the etiology of depression with and without anxiety. Kendler et al. (1987) analyzed the same material from the Australian study discussed earlier (Kendler et al., 1986). By means of a complicated multivariate statistical analysis in which

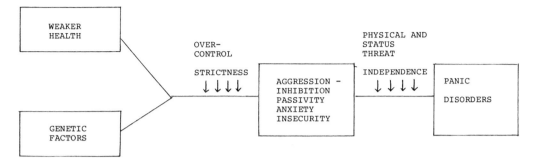

Fig. 3–1. Development of panic disorders.

factors were established by crossover correlations in twin pairs (correlation between symptom x in twin A and symptom y in twin B), they attempted to demonstrate that anxiety symptoms and depressive symptoms had the same genetic origin. Whether the phenotypical expression was anxiety or depression seemed to be due to differentiating environmental factors. However, in their earlier paper (Kendler et al., 1986), they seemed to have demonstrated genetic heterogeneity among their anxiety items, and possibly some environmental family variance among the depressive items. It is, therefore, difficult to understand how the diverse etiologies of the different item could be meaningfully combined in another analysis. As Carey (1987) comments, their calculation method is only one of many ways to calculate genetic and environmental variance, and results are dependent on the statistical method chosen. The study of Kendler et al. demonstrates that important experimentation with different statistical genetic modeling techniques is taking place, and we will need to be patient as these complicated genetic-environmental analyses evolve.

Applying the International Classification System for Diseases (8th edition) (ICD-8), we studied the relationship between anxiety and depression in our twin sample (Torgersen, 1985a). All probands with psychotic symptoms or borderline psychotic conditions were omitted. We observed that there was no difference in concordance among MZ and DZ twin partners in the mixed group of anxiety-depressives. This was also true for the pure anxiety disorders, but not for the pure neurotic depressives. As the concordance for both MZ and DZ

twin partners was high among the pure neurotic depressive and low in the mixed groups, it was hypothesized that traumas in childhood were more important in the etiology of pure neurotic depressives and problems and frustrations in adulthood for the mixed-anxiety-depressions, whereas neither of the two factors was of any importance for the development of pure anxiety disorders. We did observe evidence supportive of these hypotheses (Torgersen, 1985b). Probands with pure neurotic depression had more often lost their parents by death in childhood and had also moved around more. Probands with mixed anxiety disorder had more often never been married.

However, these twin studies have not explicitly dealt with panic disorders among depressives. Recently, we looked at this problem in our sample of depressive twins, diagnosed according to DSM III (Torgersen, 1986). Preliminary results are presented in Table 3–3 and are discussed elsewhere (Torgersen, 1989). As Table 3–3 shows, we observed a much higher concordance both for MZ and DZ twin pairs among twins with major depression plus anxiety disorder with panic attacks compared to twins with major depression without panic. (The anxiety disorders with panic attacks comprise panic disorder, agoraphobia with panic attacks, and generalized anxiety disorder with panic attacks.) The MZ/DZ concordance ratio is also highest in the first group, 3.1 compared to 1.9 among twins with major depression without panic attacks. However, the frequency of anxiety disorders with panic attacks, either concurrent with major depression or not, is not higher among the cotwins of probands with major depression plus panic attacks and nei-

TABLE 3–3.
Major Depression and Anxiety Disorder With and Without Panic Attacks Among Cotwins of Probands With and Without Panic Attacks

Proband diagnosis		Diagnosis of cotwins			
		Major depression; N (%)	Anxiety disorder with panic; N (%)	All anxiety disorders; N (%)	Total; N (%)
Major depression	MZ	5[a] (55.6)	0 (0.0)	0 (0.0)	9 (100.0)
with anxiety disorders with panic attacks	DZ	4[a] (18.2)	1 (4.5)	2 (9.1)	22 (100.0)
Major depression	MZ	5 (20.8)	5 (20.8)	5 (20.8)	24 (100.0)
without anxiety disorders with panic attacks	DZ	4 (10.8)	4 (10.8)	6 (16.2)	37 (100.0)

[a]One is a bipolar disorder.

ther is the frequency of all anxiety disorders. In fact, the frequency is lower.

What does this mean? First, the presence of panic attacks in major depression may indicate a stronger heritability of the affective subtype. Second, major depression with panic attacks does not seem to be a disorder that is etiologically between the anxiety disorders and major depression but rather seems to be a subtype of major depression with a higher threshold of liability according to the multiple threshold theory (Reich et al., 1975) because of stronger genetic loading.

CONCLUSIONS

Twin studies of panic disorders are few, and the number of twin pairs in each study is small. Genetic factors seem to be involved in the development of panic disorders. However, most MZ twin pairs are discordant, pointing to the importance of environmental factors. The kinds of environmental factors that are important is difficult to determine. An examination of MZ pairs discordant for panic disorders suggests that inhibition of aggression and self-assertiveness in childhood, threats to physical security, social status, and seeking independence from parents in adult life may contribute to the development of panic disorders.

Our twin study indicates that panic disorder and agoraphobia with panic attacks may be etiologically related, as is established in DSM III-R. In this revision of DSM III, agoraphobia with panic attacks is subsumed under the panic disorders with the headings of panic disorder

with extensive phobic avoidance and panic disorder with limited phobic avoidance.

On the other hand, agoraphobia without panic attacks, social phobia, and obsessive compulsive disorder may constitute another group of etiologically related anxiety disorders, whereas generalized anxiety disorder seems to differ from other anxiety disorders, with genetic factors having no importance in its development. However, it is conceivable that generalized anxiety disorder with panic attacks is a misclassified panic disorder simply because of the stringent inclusion of the criteria of three panic attacks within a 3 week period.

Concerning the mode of genetic transmission, it is possible that the transmission of panic disorder is controlled by one gene through an autosomal dominant gene, as was suggested by one twin study, some family studies, and a linkage study. It is also possible that a mixed monogenetic-polygenetic model of the transmission of panic disorders is the best explanatory model, perhaps with a specific gene for vulnerability to panic attacks plus a polygenetic inheritance in common with other anxiety disorders and even some affective disorders. In addition, environmental factors may either contribute to the unity or separation between panic disorder and other anxiety disorders, and panic disorders and affective disorders. A test of a genetic-environmental model that takes into consideration all these possibilities may require a large number of twins and relatives and highly sophisticated statistical methods. Panic attacks among patients with major depression imply that the development of the condition is more strongly determined by genetic factors and perhaps also the family environment early in life; the concordance was high both in MZ and DZ twin pairs.

However, most of these statements are mere speculations, because of the relatively small number of twin studies attempted to date. With the heightened interest in twin research over the last few years, it is reasonable to believe that many of these hypotheses will be verified or discarded in the near future.

REFERENCES

APA (1980): "Diagnostic and Statistical Manual of Mental Disorders, 3rd ed." Washington, DC: American Psychiatric Association Press.

APA (1987): "Diagnostic and Statistical Manual of Mental Disorders, 3rd ed., Revised." Washington, DC: American Psychiatric Association Press.

Carey G (1982): Genetic influences on anxiety neuroses and agoraphobia. In Matthew PJ (ed): "The Biology of Anxiety." New York: Bruner/Mazel, pp 37–50.

Carey G (1987): Big genes, little genes, affective disorder, and anxiety: A commentary. Arch Gen Psychiatry 44: 486–491.

Carey G, Gottesman II (1981): Twin and family studies of anxiety, phobic and obsessive disorders. In Klein DF, Rabkin J (eds): "Anxiety: New Research and Changing Concepts." New York: Raven Press, pp 117–136.

Cloninger CR, Martin RI, Clayton P, Guze SB (1981): A blind follow and family study of anxiety neurosis: Preliminary analysis of the St. Louis 500. In Klein DF, Rabkin J (eds): "Anxiety: New Research and Changing Concepts." New York: Raven Press, pp 137–154.

Crowe RR, Gaffney G, Kerber R (1982): Panic attacks in families of patients with mitral valve prolapse. J Affect Disorders 4:121–125.

Crowe RR, Noyes R, Pauls D, Sylman DA (1983): A family study of panic disorder. Arch Gen Psychiatry 40: 1065–1069.

Crowe RR, Noyes R, Wilson AF, Elston RC, Ward LJ (1988): A linkage study of panic disorder. Arch Gen Psychiatry 44:933–937.

Crowe RR, Pauls DS, Kerber RE, Noyes R (1981): Panic disorder and mitral valve prolapse. In Klein DF, Rabkin J (eds): "Anxiety: New Research and Changing Concepts." New York: Raven Press, pp 103–116.

Crowe RR, Pauls DL, Slyman DJ, Noyes R (1980): A familial study of anxiety neurosis: morbidity risk in families of patients with and without mitral valve prolapse. Arch Gen Psychiatry 37:77–79.

Feighner JP, Robsin E, Guze SB, Woodruff RA, Winokur C, Munoz R (1972): Diagnostic criteria for use in psychiatric research. Arch Gen Psychiatry 26:57–63.

Finlay-Jones R, Brown GW (1981): Types of stressful life events and the onset of anxiety and depressive disorders. Psychol Med 11:803–815.

Harris EL, Noyes R, Crowe RR, Chaudry DR (1983): A family study of agoraphobia. Arch Gen Psychiatry 40: 1061–1064.

Ihda S (1961): A study of neurosis by twin method. Psychiatr Neurol Jpn 63:861–892.

Inouye E (1965): Similar and dissimilar manifestations of obsessive-compulsive neurosis in monozygotic twins. Am J Psychiatry 121:1171–1175.

Kendler KS, Heath AC, Martin NG, Eaves LJ (1986): Symptoms of anxiety and depression in a volunteer twin population. The etiologic role of genetic and environmental factors. Arch Gen Psychiatry 43: 213–221.

Kendler KS, Heath AC, Martin NG, Eaves LK (1987): Symptoms of anxiety and symptoms of depression. Same genes, different environments? Arch Gen Psychiatry 44:451–457.

Leckman JF, Weisman MM, Merikangas KR, Pauls DL, Prusoff DA (1983): Panic disorder and major depression: Increased risk of depression, alcoholism, panic and phobic disorders in families of depressive probands with panic disorder. Arch Gen Psychiatry 40:1055–1060.

Lewis AJ (1934): Melancholia, a clinical survey of depressive states. J Ment Sci 80:277–278.

Mendels J, Winstein N, Cochrane C (1972): The relationship between depression and anxiety. Arch Gen Psychiatry 27:649–653.

Noyes R, Crowe RR, Harris EL, Hamro BJ, McChesney CM, Chaudry DR (1986): Relationship between panic disorder and agoraphobia. A family study. Arch Gen Psychiatry 43:227–232.

Reich T, Cloninger CR, Guze SB (1975): The multifactorial model of disease transmission: I. Description of the model and its use in psychiatry. Br J Psychiatry 127:1–10.

Robins LN, Helzer JE, Croughan J, Ratcliff KS (1981): National Institute of Mental Health Diagnostic Interview Schedule. Arch Gen Psychiatry 38:381–392.

Schepank H (1974): "Erb- und Umwelfaktoren bei Neurosen: Tiefenpsychologishe Untersuchungen an 50 Zwillingspaaren." Berlin: Springer-Verlag.

Shields J (1962): "Monozygotic Twins Brought Up Apart and Brought Up Together." London: Oxford University Press.

Shields J, Slater E (1966): La similarite du diagnostic chez les jumeaux et al probleme de la specificite biologique dans les nevroses et les troubles de la personalite. Evol Psychiatrie 31:441–451.

Spitzer RL, Endicott J, Robins E (1978): Research diagnostic criteria, rationality and reliability. Arch Gen Psychiatry 35:773–782.

Spitzer RL, Williams JBW (1984): "Structured Clinical Interview for DSM-III, Axis I (SCID-I)." New York: Biometric Research Department, New York State Psychiatric Institute.

Surman OS, Sheehan DV, Fuller TC, Gallo J (1983): Panic disorder in genotypic HLA identical sibling pairs. Am J Psychiatry 140:237–238.

Tienari P (1963): Psychiatric illnesses in identical twins. Acta Psychiatry Scand Suppl 171:142–185.

Torgersen S (1979): The nature and origin of common phobic fears. Br J Psychiatry 134:343–351.

Torgersen S (1981): Environmental childhood similarity and similarity in adult personality and neurotic development in twin pairs. In Gedda, Parisi P, Nance WE (eds): "Twin Research 3: Part B. Intelligence, Personality, and Development." New York: Alan R. Liss, Inc.

Torgersen S (1983): Genetic factors in anxiety disorder. Arch Gen Psychiatry 40:1085–1089.

Torgersen S (1984): "Twin Pairs Discordant for Affective, Anxiety and Somatoform Disorders: A Study of Environmental Determinants." Oslo: Department of Psychology, University of Oslo.

Torgersen S (1985a): Hereditary differentiation of anxiety and affective neuroses. Br J Psychiatry 146:530–534.

Torgersen S (1985b): Developmental differentiation of anxiety and affective neuroses. Acta Psychiatry Scand 71:304–310.

Torgersen S (1986): Childhood and family characteristics in panic and generalized anxiety disorder. Am J Psychiatry 143:630–632.

Torgersen S (1989): Comorbidity of major depression and anxiety disorders in twin pairs. (Submitted).

Van Valkenburg C, Akiskal HS, Puzantian V, Rosenthal T (1984): Clinical, family history, and naturalistic outcome comparison with panic and major depressive disorders. J Affect Disorders 6:67–82.

Weissman MM, Leckman JF, Merikangas KR, Gammon GD, Prusoff BA (1984): Depression and anxiety disorders in parents and children: results from Yale Family Study. Arch Gen Psychiatry 41:845–852.

Wing JK, Cooper JE, Sartorius N (1974): "The Measurement and Classification of Psychiatric Symptoms: An Introduction Manual for the Present State Examination and CATEGO Programme." London: Cambridge University Press.

Young JPR, Fenton CW, Lader MJ (1971): The inheritance of neurotic trait: A twin study of the Middlesex Hospital Questionnaire. Br J Psychiatry 119:393–398.

4

Molecular Genetics and Panic Disorder: New Approaches to an Old Problem

RAYMOND R. CROWE, MD

Department of Psychiatry, University of Iowa College of Medicine, Iowa City, Iowa 52242

INTRODUCTION

The 1980s have been banner years for genetics. Genes have been located for some of man's most serious and elusive diseases. The discovery of a gene for Huntington's chorea was followed in rapid succession by the identification of genes for cystic fibrosis and Duchenne's muscular dystrophy as well as a host of less publicized diseases, including retinoblastoma, chronic granulomatous disease, and neurofibromatosis (Gusella et al., 1983; Tsui et al., 1985; Monaco et al., 1986; Friend et al., 1986; Royer-Pokora et al., 1986; Barker et al., 1987). Initial doubts about whether this new technology would work with psychiatric disorders have largely been dispelled by the identification of genes for manic-depressive illness and familial Alzheimer's disease (Egeland et al., 1987; Baron et al., 1987; St. George-Hyslop et al., 1987; Tanzi et al., 1987).

These exciting findings raise the question of whether molecular genetics will be important in the study of anxiety disorders. A number of factors suggest that it will. Some of the anxiety disorders are familial, so it is possible to study large families segregating for the disorder. More importantly, rapid advances are being made in our understanding of the basic neuroscience of anxiety. The byproduct of this progress is the cloning of a number of genes with functions relevant to anxiety. This combination of large pedigrees and candidate genes suggests that the molecular genetics of anxiety disorders may be a field ripe for study.

To understand the potential applications of molecular genetics to the anxiety disorders, it will be helpful first to review some of the ways in which it has been successfully applied to other diseases. Second, it will be important to consider the diseases in which breakthroughs have been made to see whether the anxiety disorders fit this pattern. Finally, some of the unique ways in which molecular genetics can be applied to the anxiety disorders will be considered.

APPLYING MOLECULAR GENETICS TO HUMAN DISEASE

The power of the molecular genetic approach lies in the ability to use DNA probes as genetic markers. A probe is a cloned fragment of DNA; a genetic marker is any physical trait that follows Mendel's laws. Thus DNA probes can be used as genetic markers in much the same way as blood groups and HLA types. The technique used for typing with DNA probes to produce restriction fragment length polymorphisms (RFLPs) has been reviewed in a number of publications (Steel, 1984; Gurling, 1985).

Figure 4–1 shows a hypothetical pedigree in which each person has been typed with a DNA probe. It can be seen that each affected person has the "A" and each unaffected person the "B" genotype. This cosegregation of disease with marker within families is referred to as genetic linkage and indicates that the genetic marker lies so close to the disease gene on the chromosome that genetic recombination between the two during meiosis is infrequent. The degree of cosegregation is measured by a statistic called the LOD score, with values of 3.0 or greater confirming linkage and values of

Neurobiology of Panic Disorder, Pages 59–70
© 1990 Alan R. Liss, Inc.

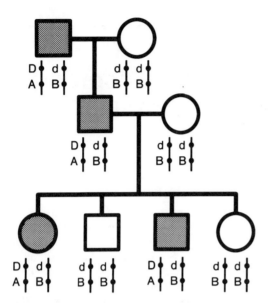

D d   d d
A B   B B

D d   d d
A B   B B

D d   d d   D d   d d
A B   B B   A B   B B

Fig. 4–1. Linkage between a disease locus (D = affected; d = normal) and a marker locus (A,B). The disease gene (D) is dominant, so every person who inherits it develops the disease. Furthermore, the marker alleles, A and B, can be unambiguously genotyped, so each individual can be classified as AA, AB, or BB. The family illustrates cosegregation between disease and the A allele at the marker locus.

−2.0 or less excluding linkage at the marker locus. To take a specific example, a large Amish family segregating for manic-depressive illness was typed with two DNA markers on the short arm of chromosome 11: the insulin gene and the Harvey-ras oncogene. Both genes were found to assort with manic-depressive illness yielding a LOD score of 4.9, confirming a gene for manic-depressive illness on chromosome 11 (Egeland et al., 1987).

The demonstration of linkage identifies the general location of the disease gene, but it does not identify the gene itself; to do this, two strategies have been used. The first is the reverse genetics approach. The term refers to the strategy of proceeding from a linked marker to the disease gene and finally to the protein product of the gene. This is the reverse of the usual procedure of using an amino acid sequence of a protein to identify the gene coding for the protein. The reverse genetics approach can be excruciatingly slow, as evidenced by the fact

that the gene for Huntington's disease has not been located 4 years after the original linkage finding. However, the approach may be paying off in the case of Duchenne's muscular dystrophy and cystic fibrosis (Monaco et al., 1986; Estivill et al., 1987).

The other strategy for identifying disease genes is the candidate gene approach. A candidate gene is a cloned human gene with a function that is relevant to the disease of interest. Returning to the manic-depression story, tyrosine hydroxylase has been found to map to chromosome 11p in the general region of the gene for manic-depressive illness (Craig et al., 1985). Since tyrosine hydroxylase is a major enzyme in the synthetic pathway of norepinephrine, and catecholamines have long been suspected of being involved in manic-depressive illness, tyrosine hydroxylase is a strong candidate gene for manic-depressive illness. If all the affected individuals in the pedigree had a mutant form of the tyrosine hydroxylase gene, then a cause for manic-depressive illness in that family would have been found.

Several other strategies using DNA probes are worth mentioning because of their applicability to anxiety disorders, as discussed below. The first is linkage disequillibrium. This occurs when a disease gene lies so close to a genetic marker that recombination between the two is extremely rare. The result is a strong association between the disease and one form of the marker gene in the population, the mechanism that may underly some of the strong HLA-disease associations. A good example of linkage disequillibrium is the strong association between hyperlipidemia and apolipoprotein gene phenotypes as assessed by DNA markers (Scott et al., 1985).

Finally, DNA probes can be used to search for submicroscopic duplications and deletions of DNA on the chromosome. This is because no DNA will be detected by the probe if the homologous patient DNA is missing (as in deletions), and the radioactive signal will be increased when the amount of homologous DNA is increased (as in duplications).

A number of features characterize the diseases with which we have made progress through these approaches. Obviously, the disease must be genetic, and this was known or strongly suspected with all those cited as ex-

TABLE 4–1.
Two Strategies for Studying Diseases With Genetic Markers

"Candidate gene" strategy (example, amyloid protein)	"Reverse genetics" (example, familial Alzheimer's disease)
Amlyloid protein is extracted from plaques	Familial Alzheimer's disease is mapped to chromosome 21q11–q21
Amino acid sequence is determined	Amloid protein gene is mapped to the same region
Matching oligonucleotide probe is synthesized	Amyloid gene (or a closely linked gene) is a candidate for Alzheimer's disease
Probe detects homologous gene in human DNA	
Human amloid gene is cloned	

amples. It is also clear that the methods are aimed at detecting single genes; therefore, there should be strong evidence that one is dealing with a Mendelian disease, or that families among whom the disease shows Mendelian inheritance can be found. Even though not all cases of manic-depressive illness are familial, the ability to find large pedigrees among whom the transmission is compatible with that of a single gene allowed the disease to be studied with molecular techniques. Another desirable characteristic is genetic homogeneity. The more genetic forms of the illness there are, the more difficult it will be to identify a gene for any one of them. It is not unlikely that some psychiatric disorders have single-locus forms, forms resulting from multifactorial inheritance, and still others from nongenetic causes. One way of increasing the likelihood of a single genetic etiology is by selecting large pedigrees among whom a single gene is likely to be the cause. A clear phenotype is needed for an individual to be designated as "affected" in families being studied. Psychiatric disorders are typically characterized by incomplete penetrance, age and sex effects, and multiple phenotypes. Despite these problems, molecular genetic analysis has identified genes for Huntington's disease, manic-depressive illness, and Alzheimer's disease (Gusella et al., 1983; Egeland et al., 1987; St. George-Hyslop et al., 1987). In fact, Alzheimer's disease provides an instructive example of how molecular genetics has led to some answers in a disorder characterized by many of the above problems (St. George-Hyslop et al., 1987; Goldgaber et al., 1987; Tanzi et al., 1987; Delabar et al., 1987)

(Table 4–1). Although the disease segregates in some families, the majority of cases appear to be sporadic. Moreover, the ability to study Alzheimer's disease in families is complicated by its late onset. Nevertheless, two clues have led to progress. The first is a high rate of Alzheimer-type dementia in older patients with Down's syndrome, suggesting a link with chromosome 21. The second is the deposition of plaques of amyloid protein, which led to the cloning of the gene coding for the amyloid protein. First, DNA markers on chromosome 21 were found to be closely linked to the familial form of Alzheimer's disease. Then, the DNA clone for amyloid protein was found to map to the same region of chromosome 21 as familial Alzheimer's disease. Unfortunately, genetic recombination between the amyloid protein locus and familial Alzheimer's disease have excluded amyloid protein as a candidate gene for Alzheimer's disease. Nevertheless, its close proximity to the Alzheimer's disease locus and the key role of Amyloid protein in Alzheimer's disease make the Amyloid gene an interesting one to study in its own right.

PANIC DISORDER IS A CANDIDATE DISEASE FOR MOLECULAR GENETICS

For genetics research, one needs a clearly defined phenotype and evidence that the transmission follows single locus genetics. Panic disorder comes as close as any psychiatric illness to meeting these criteria. Findings from family and twin studies indicate that the predisposition to panic disorder may be manifest as any of several related anxiety disorders and

TABLE 4–2.
Diagnostic Spectrum of Panic Disorder Based on Family and Twin Findings

Panic disorder	Alcoholism(?)
Agoraphobia	
Panic attacks	Depression(?)

that the familial transmission of this phenotype is consistent with Mendelian genetics.

Defining The Phenotype

Families of panic disorder patients have an aggregation not only of panic disorder but also of several other psychiatric disorders (Table 4–2). Among the anxiety disorders, these include agoraphobia and panic attacks not meeting diagnostic criteria for panic disorder. Conversely, the other anxiety disorders do not appear to aggregate in panic disorder families. Other disorders that have been found in familial aggregation with panic disorder include depression and alcoholism. These findings present serious problems for the genetic study of panic disorder because they indicate that the phenotype is broader than the strict diagnosis of panic disorder, and genetic studies require a clear definition of the affected phenotype.

Agoraphobia is widely considered to be a complication of panic disorder, a view originally proposed by Klein and now adopted by DSM III-R (Klein, 1981; APA, 1987). This view holds that panic attacks are responsible for conditioning the phobic avoidance, and that, once established, the avoidance maintains itself even in the absence of panic attacks. This proposal can be examined by means of family and twin data, since it predicts that each form of the disorder should be found in relatives of index cases with the other form. Indeed, when one looks at the families of agoraphobics, the hypothesis seems to be confirmed. In one study, the rates of panic disorder and agoraphobia were 7.0% and 9.4%, respectively, among relatives of agoraphobics (Noyes et al., 1986). However, the converse was not found. In the same study, the rates of panic disorder and agoraphobia among the relatives of panic disorder patients were 14.9% and 1.7%. Inter-

estingly, the total illness rates (panic disorder plus agoraphobia) in both groups of families were approximately the same, the difference being that the complication of agoraphobia did not develop in the families of the pure panic disorder probands. Nevertheless, these findings do provide support for the hypothesis that agoraphobia and panic disorder are the same illness.

Further evidence comes from twins. Since monozygotic (MZ) twins are genetically identical, discordant MZ twins are a powerful means of studying the variable expressions of disease. As part of a twin study, Torgersen (1983) identified two twin pairs among whom one twin had panic disorder and the other had agoraphobia. Although the small number limits the conclusions, the finding does demonstrate that the same genotype can be expressed as either illness.

Another problem is presented by persons with recurrent panic attacks that fail to meet diagnostic criteria for panic disorder. Both family and twin data indicate that these individuals have a mild form of panic disorder. For instance, we found that 17% of first-degree relatives of panic disorder patients meet DSM III criteria for panic disorder, but an additional 7% have panic attacks that fail to meet criteria because of the infrequency of the attacks or the lack of a sufficient number of criterion symptoms (Crowe et al., 1983). The fact that these borderline cases aggregate in panic disorder but not in control families indicates that they are a form of panic disorder. This conclusion is further supported by Torgersen's (1983) findings of panic attacks (but not panic disorder) in two of thirteen MZ cotwins of index twins with panic disorder.

On the other hand, other anxiety disorders have not been found to aggregate in families with panic disorder and agoraphobia. Specifically, generalized anxiety disorder, obsessive-compulsive disorder, and phobic disorders other than agoraphobia are not increased among relatives or cotwins of panic disorder patients (Crowe et al., 1983).

Anxiety disorders have not been the only disorders found to cluster in families with panic disorder. Leckman et al. (1983) found that families of probands with both depression and panic disorder had an increased incidence of depression, panic disorder, phobia, generalized anxiety disorder, and alcoholism in contrast to the families of probands with depression only. Based on these findings, Leckman et al. proposed a comorbidity for affective and anxiety disorders. In a separate study, depression complicated by panic disorder or agoraphobia in a parent increased the risk for both depression and anxiety disorder in the children (Weissman et al., 1984). Munjack and Moss (1981) found a family history of depression in 38% of agoraphobic families, in 14% of social phobic families, and in 0% of simple phobic families.

Not all studies have supported the comorbidity hypothesis. Our own studies have not identified an increased risk for depression in the families of panic disorder or agoraphobic patients, even when the index patient has a secondary depression (Crowe et al., 1983; Noyes et al., 1986). Likewise, Dealy et al. (1981), studying family histories of panic disorder patients with and without depression, failed to find an increased risk of anxiety disorder, depression, or alcoholism in the first group compared with the second. Another study examined the family histories of four groups of index patients: depression only, depression with panic attacks, panic disorder with secondary depression, and panic disorder only (Van Valkenburg et al., 1984). A higher family history of depression was found in the first two groups and a higher family history of anxiety disorder in the last three. These findings could be interpreted as indicating that depression aggregates only with primary depression in the proband, and anxiety disorder aggregates with panic disorder, whether primary or complicating a depression.

Another disorder identified in the families of panic disorder patients is alcoholism, and there is good agreement in the literature on this finding. Those studies that have not found a statistically significant excess of alcoholism in these families have, nevertheless, found a trend in the expected direction (Cohen et al., 1951; Noyes et al., 1978, 1986, Cloninger et al., 1981; Munjack and Moss, 1981; Crowe et al., 1983).

Taking the diagnostic data on panic disorder together, some tentative conclusions can be drawn regarding which diagnosis the affected phenotype should include. The evidence is strongest for including agoraphobia and limited panic attacks in the spectrum of panic disorder. Conversely, there is no evidence to support the inclusion of other anxiety disorders. The overlap with affective disorders is intriguing, but currently the literature on this issue is divided. Families identified through probands with depression have shown a comorbidity with panic disorder, but the finding has not been replicated in families identified through probands with panic disorder. The present data are not clear enough to consider affective disorder in panic disorder families to be a panic disorder equivalent. The findings with regard to alcoholism are more consistent, but this problem is so common in families of patients with various mental disorders that its specificity to panic disorder should be clarified considerably before considering it a panic disorder equivalent.

Genetic Studies

Panic disorder is the most thoroughly studied anxiety disorder from a genetic standpoint, and the evidence suggests that it is a reasonable candidate for molecular genetic studies. Panic disorder is familial, and large pedigrees among whom it is segregating over several generations are obtainable. Although it is complicated by incomplete penetrance and by age and sex effects, it has a reasonably well defined and penetrant phenotype. Moreover, twin studies are consistent with a genetic etiology, and transmission model studies are consistent with single locus genetics.

Family Studies

The familial findings in panic disorder are based on 12 published family studies spanning over half a century (Oppenheimer and Rothschild, 1918; McInnes, 1937; Wood, 1942; Brown, 1942; Cohen et al., 1951; Wheeler et al., 1948; Noyes et al., 1978, 1986; Cloninger et al., 1981; Crowe et al., 1983; Moran and Andrews, 1985; Hopper et al., 1987) (Table 4–3). Early investigations reported familial clustering of diseases, such as "neurocirculatory asthenia," that correspond closely with panic disorder, although no diagnostic criteria were used. The majority of studies are based on family history obtained from patients, although the studies

TABLE 4–3.
Genetic Findings From Family and Twin Studies

	Range (%)	Median (%)
Families with affected relatives (five studies)	45–67	56
Affected first-degree relatives (12 studies)	6–49	15
Affected second-degree relatives (one study)	9.5	
MZ cotwins (two studies)	31–41	
DZ cotwins (two studies)	0–5	

based on family interviews corroborate the findings. Only the more recent investigations have compared the family rates to those of control groups. Despite these differences, the family study findings are reassuringly consistent.

All the studies that have analyzed the percentage of patients with affected family members have found a high percentage. The actual figures range from 28% to 67%, the median rate being 56%. This figure is fairly close to our own finding of 61% based on family interviews supplemented by family history material for the uninterviewed relatives (Crowe et al., 1983).

Another way of looking at the question of familial aggregation is by calculating the percentage of affected relatives or the age-corrected morbidity risk. Morbidity risks are always higher than simple percentages because they correct for the unaffected relatives who have not passed completely through the age of risk. The range in rates across studies is considerably greater than the small difference that would be expected from the morbidity risk correction. Specifically, the rates have ranged from a low of 6% to a high of 49%, the median being 15%. What is important is that all the rates, with the possible exception of the 6% rate, are higher than expected in the population, and studies with control groups have shown statistically significant differences.

Other features of panic disorder are its age and sex distributions. Family studies are an excellent opportunity for studying sex ratios in that they provide an unselected source of affected persons. The familial findings agree that females are affected two to three times as frequently as males, a finding that agrees well with the recent epidemiological data (Robins et al., 1984). Another point of agreement is the mean age of onset, which is in the mid twenties in both sexes (Crowe et al., 1983; Moran

and Andrews, 1985; Hopper et al., 1987). The mean age was 26 years in our study, with a standard deviation of 11 years (Crowe et al., 1983).

The family findings indicate that panic disorder is familial in a substantial proportion of cases. Nevertheless, since the proportion of affected relatives of either sex does not suggest a simple Mendelian ratio, it cannot be considered a simple Mendelian disease. The deviation from Mendelian ratios could be explained by incomplete penetrance (including age and sex effects), by multifactorial inheritance, or by genetic heterogeneity. The sporadic cases could be explained in one of two ways. They may be familial cases without affected relatives because of small family size and incomplete penetrance. This would be consistent with a hypothesis of genetic homogeneity. On the other hand, the sporadic cases may be a clue that the genetics are more complex than a single locus model.

Twin Studies

Familial aggregation is suggestive of genetic transmission but is not proof of it. Proof of genetic transmission is provided by adoption and twin studies, and since there are no adoption studies of anxiety disorders, one must turn to twins for evidence of a genetic etiology (Table 4–4). Slater and Shields (1967) studied twins with anxiety disorders, a broader concept than the current diagnosis of panic disorder but one that undoubtedly overlaps with it to a considerable degree. Forty-one percent of 17 MZ twins were concordant for anxiety disorders compared with only 4% of 28 dizygotic (DZ) twins. Torgersen's (1983) is the only other study to examine anxiety disorders in twins, and fortunately DSM III diagnoses were used. Thirteen MZ index twins with panic disorder (including agoraphobia with panic attacks) had

TABLE 4–4.
Transmission Model Studies

	Single locus	Polygenic
Ancestral pairs analysis	Supported	Untested
Segregation analysis	Supported	Untested
Sex threshold analysis	Supported	Untested

two cotwins with panic disorder, and another two cotwins had panic attacks. Sixteen DZ twin pairs were studied, and none of the cotwins had panic disorder or panic attacks. Thus four of thirteen MZ and none of sixteen DZ twins had panic attacks. These findings are consistent with a genetic etiology of panic disorder. Moreover, the finding that less than 100% of the MZ cotwins are affected is consistent with the conclusions from family studies that the genetics are more complex than a single locus model. If a single gene is involved, the Torgersen data suggest a penetrance of 30%, close to that predicted by the family data (15% of first-degree relatives affected and 50% at risk equals 30% penetrance).

Transmission Models

If a disease is presumed to be genetic, the mode of inheritance should be sought. Until recently, the inheritance was primarily of academic interest, but this is no longer the case for reasons discussed above. The likelihood that a disease is caused by single locus genetics is now of considerable importance in determining which diseases are the most likely to reward investments in genetic research.

An early model for detecting single locus transmission was based on the theory that a Mendelian disease would be found in ancestral relatives primarily on one side of the family, whereas a multifactorial disease would be found on both sides of the family. Slater (1966) developed a computational model based on pairs of ancestral affected relatives and estimated that, if the number of unilateral pairs exceeded that of bilateral pairs by a ratio of greater than 2:1, a single locus model would be supported. When this model was applied to a group of panic disorder pedigrees, 37 of 41 ancestral pairs were found to be unilateral, the deviation from the expected 2:1 ratio being highly significant and indicative of single locus transmission (Pauls et al., 1979a).

In a subsequent analysis of the same families, a pedigree analysis was used to determine whether the pattern of transmission within the families was consistent with that expected under a Mendelian model (Pauls et al., 1980). Once again, a Mendelian model provided a good fit to the observed data. The analysis estimated a gene frequency of 1.4% (making 2.8% of the population carriers, since each person has two genes at every locus), a 75% penetrance, and a mean age of onset of 25 years.

Since the above analysis failed to account for the pronounced sex ratio characteristic of panic disorder, sex threshold models (single locus and multifactorial) were used to analyze panic disorder families (Crowe et al., 1983). Both models gave a statistically acceptable fit to the observed rates of panic disorder among first-degree relatives. The single locus model predicted a gene frequency of 5%, accounting for a female trait prevalence of 4.5% and a male prevalence of 2.5%.

GENETIC MARKER STUDIES OF PANIC DISORDER

Because of the considerations mentioned above, our group has been examining genetic markers in families segregating for panic disorder (Crowe et al., 1987). These studies were begun before DNA markers were available, and they employed genetic markers based on red cell antigens and protein electrophoresis polymorphisms. Nevertheless, the approach is identical to that employing DNA markers. More recent studies have used DNA clones for candidate genes, an example of which, using a DNA probe for the pro-opiomelanocortin gene, is reviewed here.

Studies Using Linkage Markers

We have studied linkage between panic disorder and 29 genetic markers in 26 pedigrees. One hundred ninety-eight subjects were interviewed and genotyped for the marker systems, and information on another 240 relatives was obtained by family history. Diagnoses of panic disorder with or without agorphobia, and recurrent spontaneous panic attacks were considered to be "affected," and all other diagnoses were considered to be "unaffected."

Linkage was analyzed by the LOD score method (Ott, 1974). A LOD score of at least 3.0

TABLE 4–5.
LOD Scores for Linkage Between Alpha-Haptoglobin (HP) and Properdin Factor B (BF) and Panic Disorder*

	Recombination fraction					
	0.0	0.05	0.10	0.20	0.30	0.40
HP[a]	2.27	2.06	1.79	1.20	0.63	0.20
BF[b]	−2.09	0.37	0.80	0.88	0.60	0.23

[a]Maximum LOD score = 2.27.
[b]Maximum LOD score = 1.04.
*Crowe et al., in press.

is considered to be evidence of linkage, and a LOD score of −2.0 or less excludes linkage to the marker in question. Although none of the markers reached a LOD score of 3.0, two marker systems achieved LOD scores greater than 1.0 (Table 4–5). The largest LOD score was 2.27, and this was obtained at the alpha-haptoglobin locus on chromosome 16q22 at a recombination fraction of 0. The LOD score maximizing at a low recombination fraction indicates that, if panic disorder is linked to alpha-haptoglobin, the marker is relatively close to the disease gene.

The other marker suggestive of linkage was properdin factor B on chromosome 6p21.3, which achieved a LOD score of 1.04 at male and female recombination fractions of 0.27 and 0.10, respectively. In addition, linkage was excluded at 18 of the 29 loci at a recombination fraction of 0, at nine loci at a recombination fraction of 0.05, and at four loci at a recombination fraction of 0.10.

Linkage analysis by the LOD score method assumes that the genetics of the disease are known. It is appropriate for diseases known to be Mendelian with known gene frequencies and dominance relationships. Since none of these can be taken for granted with psychiatric disorders, the LOD score method could lead to erroneous results. Therefore, the data were also analyzed using an identity-by-descent sib-pair method (Haseman and Elston, 1972). This analysis is based on the fact that two sibs can share zero, one, or two alleles identical by descent at a locus in the expected ratio of 1:2:1. However, if both sibs are affected, and the locus is closely linked to the disease, they must share at least one allele (assuming recombination has not occurred). Therefore, the expected 1:2:1 ratio will be distorted in the direction of increased allele sharing between affected pairs

of sibs. These analyses revealed statistically significant evidence of linkage at both the haptoglobin ($P < 0.01$) and properdin factor B ($P < 0.05$) loci.

The data were explored for genetic heterogeneity at the haptoglobin locus. Since nine probands were agoraphobic and 17 had panic disorder without agoraphobia, the LOD scores of these two groups were compared. The nine agoraphobic families contributed a LOD score of 1.51 and the 17 panic disorder families a LOD score of 0.76 (both at recombination fraction 0.0). Nine probands with major depressive disorder (seven secondary to and two independent of the panic disorder) contributed a LOD score of 1.17 and 17 without depression a LOD score of 1.10 (both at recombination fraction 0.0). Finally, the families of six probands with mitral valve prolapse contributed a LOD score of 0.34. In short, linkage at the haptoglobin locus was supported by all the subgroupings we examined.

Although this study failed to confirm linkage between panic disorder and any of the 29 markers tested, it has contributed to the genetic study of panic disorder in several ways. First, two loci have been identified as candidates for linkage to panic disorder. Second, close linkage to another 18 loci could be excluded. These findings allow a better directed approach to linkage, at least for the near future, than would have been the case otherwise. They also demonstrate that panic disorder families can be sufficiently informative to make linkage a feasible approach to the genetics of panic disorder.

Studies With Candidate Gene Probes

An example of a candidate gene of relevance to panic disorder is pro-opiomelanocortin (POMC). POMC codes for a large precursor

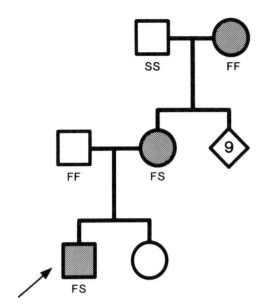

Fig. 4–2. Pedigree showing the transmission of panic disorder (including agoraphobia and limited symptom panic attacks) and a restriction fragment length polymorphism at the pro-opiomelanocortin locus (FF, FS, SS) over three generations. (Adapted from Crowe et al., 1987, with permission of the Elsevier Science Publishers BV, (Biomedical Division), Amsterdam, The Netherlands.)

peptide, which is cleaved to yield beta-lipotropin, beta-endorphin, met-enkephalin, alpha-melanocyte-stimulating hormone (alpha-MSH), and adrenocorticotropic hormone (ACTH), among other peptides (Herbert and Uhler, 1982). Since some panic disorder patients have abnormal dexamethasone suppression tests (Coryell et al., 1985), and since the endorphins and enkephalins may be relevant to abnormal behavior, POMC is a reasonable gene to study in panic disorder.

We studied a clone for the first exon of POMC (p-lambda-P2) in a four-generation family segregating for panic disorder and agoraphobia (Crowe et al., 1987) (Fig. 4–2). The family has been genotyped at the POMC locus as illustrated in Figure 1; F represents the "fast" allele on DNA electrophoresis and S the "slow" allele so that every person can be genotyped as FF, FS, or SS. Figure 4–2 shows that the proband, a 14-year-old boy with panic disorder, inherited the S allele from his mother, a

37-year-old with a 24 year history of panic disorder, since his father is FF. However, his mother inherited her F allele from her affected mother, a 58-year-old with panic disorder, since her father is SS. Therefore, the proband and his affected maternal grandmother share no allele at the POMC locus. Assuming that the father and maternal grandfather are not carriers, and that nonpaternity can be excluded, the POMC gene can be excluded as a cause of panic disorder in this family. This example illustrates the power of the candidate gene approach to exclude a candidate gene when it is not the cause of the disease. The possibilities of nonpaternity and carriers can be dealt with by analyzing additional families and finding further cases of exclusion. This would also minimize the problem of genetic heterogeneity, that a gene could be the cause of the disease in one family but be excluded in another. If the candidate probe was the disease gene, the absence of recombination between disease and probe would result in a high LOD score, with a relatively small number of informative families.

FUTURE PROSPECTS

Finding a disease gene for panic disorder is dependent on two factors; clues to where to look with the reverse genetics strategy and strong candidate genes for the candidate gene strategy. With the anxiety disorders, we may be entering an era when we can make the kind of intuitively guided searches for disease genes that have payed off in other areas of medicine.

It is now generally accepted that a human gene map will become a reality within the near future. A gene map suitible for detecting disease genes through linkage would require a battery of 150–300 marker loci spaced at even intervals along the entire human genome. With a map of this resolution, one can be reasonably sure that linkage would be detected if a disease gene is present and if sufficiently informative families can be collected. Although this is a feasible approach, it is an extremely laborious one. The task can be made considerably easier, however, if one knows where to look. This information can be provided by reports of cytogenetic abnormalities—aneuploidies, translocations, deletions, etc.—that are associated with of the disease of interest. For instance, a family with a chromosome 7/18 translocation associated with symptoms of Tourette's disease was recently reported (Comings et al., 1986), raising the possibility that a gene on chromosome 7 or 18 was inactivated by the translocation, causing the behavioral symptoms. This prompted a report of a patient with a deletion of 18q22.1 with compulsive behavior and panic attacks (Donnai, 1987). Although the patient had hallucinations, unlike Tourette's disease and panic disorder patients, these could be due to other effects of the translocation. Both reports suggest that the 18q22 region is a good candidate for Tourette's disease, and the latter report suggests this region as a candidate for panic disorder as well. Obviously, the association between chromosomal defects and psychiatric symptoms is now of far more than academic interest, and clincans should be encouraged to report all such cases. A seemingly coincidental finding could save years of effort in identifying the location of a disease gene.

Panic disorder presents some of the most promising opportunities to work with candidate gene probes of any of the psychiatric disorders. One of the early theories of panic disorder was based on the observation that panic disorder patients have higher blood lactate levels after exercise than normal persons (Cohen and White, 1950) and that lactate infusions precipitate panic attacks in persons with the disorder (Pitts and McClure, 1967). These findings suggest a link between lactate metabolism and panic disorder. The genes for lactate dehydrogenase A and B have been cloned and would be obvious candidate gene probes with which to study panic disorder.

An even more exciting line of research has evolved from the discovery that the brain contains specific receptors for benzodiazepines (Squires and Braestrup, 1977; Tallman et al., 1980). Receptor agonists, such as the benzodiazepines, decrease anxiety, whereas inverse agonists, such as the beta-carbolines, increase anxiety (Insel et al., 1984). The administration of beta-carbolines to animals produces symptoms compatible with anxiety, and their ingestion by humans results in symptoms of anxiety (Ninan et al., 1982; Dorow et al., 1983).

Recently, an endogenous brain peptide thought to be a ligand for the benzodiazepine receptor was identified (Alho et al., 1985). It antagonizes benzodiazepine receptor binding, and in animals produces symptoms suggesting that it acts as an inverse agonist. These studies suggest that, if the peptide is indeed an endogenous ligand, it probably acts to increase anxiety rather than to relieve it. Thus, genetic mutations resulting in overproduction or increased receptor binding of the peptide could be responsible for anxiety disorders. Now that the gene coding for the peptide has been cloned, it will be possible to test this hypothesis in patients with anxiety disorders (Gray et al., 1986). Furthermore, with the recent cloning of the benzodiazepine receptor protein, it will be possible to test the hypothesis that a genetic defect in the receptor protein structure increases its affinity for its ligand, resulting in pathologically high anxiety levels (Haefely, 1986). Since both hypotheses predict that the candidate gene would be absolutely linked to the disease, their confirmation or exclusion by linkage studies should be straightforward.

REFERENCES

Alho H, Costa E, Ferrero P, Fugimoto M, Cosenza-Murphy D, Guidotti (1985): Diazepam-binding inhibitor: A neuropeptide located in selected neuronal populations of rat brain. Science 229:179–182.

APA (1987): "Diagnostic and Statistical Manual of Mental Disorders, 3rd ed, revised." Washington, DC: APA.

Barker D, Wright E, Nguyen K, Cannon L, Fain P, Goldgar D, Bishop DT, Carey J, Baty B, Kivlin J, Willard H, Waye JS, Greig G, Leinwand L, Nakamura Y, O'Connell P, Leppert M, Lalouel JM, White R, Skolnick M (1987): Gene for Von Recklinghausen neurofibromatosis is in the pericentromeric region of chromosome 17. Science 236:1100–1102.

Baron M, Risch N, Hamburger R, Mandel B, Kushner S, Newman M, Drumer D, Belmaker RH (1987): Genetic linkage between X-chromosome markers and bipolar affective illness. Nature 326:289–292.

Brown FW (1942): Heredity in the psychoneuroses. Proc R Soc Med 35:785–790.

Cloninger CR, Martin RL, Clayton P, Guze SB (1981): A blind follow-up and family study of anxiety neurosis: Preliminary analysis of the St. Louis 500. In Klein DF, Rabkin J (eds): "Anxiety: New Research and Changing Concepts." Raven Press, New York, 1981.

Cohen ME, Badal DW, Kilpatrick A, Reed EW, White PD (1951): The high familial prevalence of neurocirculatory asthenia (anxiety neurosis, effort syndrome). Am J Hum Genet 3:126–158.

Cohen ME, White PD (1950): Life situations, emotions, and neurocirculatory asthenia (anxiety neurosis, neurasthenia, effort syndrome). Proc Assoc Res Nerv Mental Dis 29:832–869.

Comings DE, Comings BG, Diez G, Muhleman D, Okada TA, Sarinana F, Simmer R, Stock D (1986): Evidence the Tourette's syndrome gene is at 18q 22.1. Seventh Int Cong Hum Genet II:620.

Coryell W, Noyes R, Clancy J, Crowe RR, Chaudhry D (1985): Abnormal escape from dexamethasone suppression in agoraphobia and panic attacks. Psychiatry Res 15:301–311.

Craig SP, Buckle VJ, Craig IW, Lamouroux A, Mallet J (1985): Localization of the human tyrosine hydroxylase gene to chromosome 11p15. Cytogenet Cell Genet 40:610.

Crowe RR, Noyes R, Pauls DL, Slymen D (1983): A family study of panic disorder. Arch Gen Psychiatry 40:1065–1069.

Crowe RR, Noyes R, Persico AM (1987): Pro-opiomelanocortin (POMC) gene excluded as a cause of panic disorder in a large family. J Affect Disorders 12:23–27.

Crowe RR, Wilson AF, Elston RC, Noyes R, Ward LI (1987): A linkage study of panic disorder. Arch Gen Psychiatry 44:933–937.

Dealy RS, Ishiki DM, Avery DH, Wilson LG, Dunner DL (1981): Secondary depression in anxiety disorders. Comp Psychiatry 22:612–618.

Delabar JM, Goldgaber D, Lamour Y, Nicole A, Huret JL, De Graouchy J, Brown P, Gajdusek DC, Sinet PM (1987): Beta amyloid gene duplication in Alzheimer's disease and karyotypically normal Down syndrome. Science 235:1390–1392.

Donnai D (1987): Gene location in Tourette syndrome. Lancet i:627.

Dorow R, Horowski R, Paschelke G, Main M, Braestrup C (1983): Severe anxiety induced by FG 7142, a beta-carboline ligand for benzodiazepine receptors. Lancet ii:98–99.

Egeland JA, Gerhard DS, Pauls DL, Sussex JN, Kidd KK, Allen CR, Hostetter AM, Housman DE (1987): Bipolar affective disorders linked to DNA markers on chromosome 11. Nature 325:783–787.

Estivill X, Farrall M, Scambler PJ, Bell GM, Hawley KMF, Lench NJ, Bates GP, Kruyer HC, Frederick PA, Stanier P, Watson EK, Williamson R, Wainwright BJ (1987): A candidate for the cystic fibrosis locus isolated by selection for methylation-free islands. Nature 326:840–845.

Friend SH, Bernards R, Rogel JS, Weinberg RA, Rapaport JM, Albert DM, Dryja TP (1986): A human DNA segment with properties of the gene that predisposes to retinoblastoma and osteosarcoma. Nature 323:643–646.

Goldgaber D, Lerman MI, McBride OW, Saffiotti U, Gajdusek DC (1987): Characterization and chromosomal localization of a cDNA encoding brain amyloid of Alzheimer's disease. Science 235:877–884.

Gray PW, Glaister D, Seeburg PH, Guidotti A, Costa E (1986): Cloning and expression of cDNA for human diazepam binding inhibitor, a natural ligand of an allosteric regulatory site of the gamma-amino-butyric acid type A receptor. Proc Natl Acad Sci USA 83:7547–7551.

Gurling H (1985): Application of molecular biology to

mental illness. Analysis of genomic DNA and brain mRNA. Psychiatr Dev 3:257–273.

Gusella JF, Wexler NS, Conneally PM, Taylor SL, Anderson MA, Tanzi RE, Watkins PC, Ottina K, Wallace MR, Sakaguchi AY, Young AB, Shoulson I, Bonilla E, Martin JB (1983): A polymorphic DNA marker genetically linked to Huntington's disease. Nature 306:234–238.

Haefely WE (1986): The benzodiazepine receptor and its clinical useful ligands. Clin Neuropharmacol 9[Suppl 4]:398–400.

Haseman JK, Elston RC (1972): The investigation of linkage between a quantitative trait and a marker locus. Behav Genet 2:3–19.

Herbert E, Uhler M (1982): Biosynthesis of polyprotein precursors of regulatory peptides. Cell 30:1–2.

Hopper JL, Judd FK, Derrick PL, Burrows GD (1987): A family study of panic disorder. Genet Epidemiol 4:33–41.

Insel TR, Ninan PT, Aloi J, Jimerson DC, Skolnick P, Paul SM (1984): A benzodiazepine receptor-mediated model of anxiety. Arch Gen Psychiatry 41:741–750.

Klein DF (1981): Anxiety reconceptualized. In Klein DF, Rabkin JG (eds): "Anxiety: New Research and Changing Concepts." New York: Raven Press.

Leckman JF, Weissman MN, Merikangas KR, Pauls DL, Prusoff BA (1983): Panic disorder and major depression: Increased risk of depression, alcoholism, panic, and phobic disorders in families of depressed patients with panic disorder. Arch Gen Psychiatry 40:1055–1060.

McInnes RG (1937): Observations on heredity in neurosis. Proc R Soc Med 30:895–904.

Monaco AP, Neve RL, Colletti-Feener C, Bertelson CJ, Kurnit DM, Kunkel LM (1986): Isolation of candidate cDNAs for portions or the Duchenne muscular dystrophy gene. Nature 323:646–650.

Moran C, Andress G (1985): The familial occurrence of agoraphobia. Br J Psychiatry 146:262–267.

Munjack DJ, Moss HB (1981): Affective disorder and alcoholism in families of agoraphobics. Arch Gen Psychiatry 38:869–871.

Ninan PT, Insel TM, Cohen RM, Cook JM, Skolnick P, Paul SM (1982): Benzodiazepine receptor-mediated experimental "anxiety" in primmates. Science 218:1332–1334.

Noyes R, Clancy J, Crowe RR, Slymen D (1978): The familial prevalence of anxiety neurosis. Arch Gen Psychiatry 35:1057–1059.

Noyes R, Crowe RR, Harris EL, Hamra BJ, McChesney CM, Chaudhry DR (1986): Relationship between panic disorder and agoraphobia: A family study. Arch Gen Psychiatry 43:227–232.

Oppenheimer BS, Rothschild MA (1918): The psychoneurotic factor in the irritable heart of soldiers. J Am Med Assoc 70:1919–1922.

Ott J (1974): Estimation of the recombination fraction in human pedigrees: Efficient computation of the liklihood for human linkage studies. Am J Hum Genet 26:588–297.

Pauls DL, Bucher KD, Crowe RR, Noyes R (1980): A genetic study of panic disorder pedigrees. Am J Hum Genet 32:639–644.

Pauls DL, Crowe RR, Noyes R (1979a): Distribution of ancestral secondary cases in anxiety neurosis (panic disorder). J Affect Disorders 1:287–290.

Pauls DL, Noyes R, Crowe RR (1979b): The familial prevalence in second-degree relatives of patients with anxiety neurosis (panic disorder). J Affect Disorders 1:279–285.

Pitts FN, McClure JN (1967): Lactate metabolism in anxiety neurosis. N Engl J Med 277:1329–1336.

Robins LN, Helzer JE, Weissman MN, Orvaschel H, Gruenberg E, Burke JD, Regier DA (1984): Lifetime prevalence of specific psychiatric disorders in three sites. Arch Gen Psychiatry 41:949–958.

Royer-Pokora B, Kunkel LM, Monaco AP, Goff SC, Newburger, PE, Baehner RL, Cole FS, Curnutte JT, Orkan SH (1986): Cloning the gene for an inherited human disorder—chronic granulomatous disease—on the basis of its chromosomal location. Nature 322:32–38.

Scott J, Priestley LM, Knott TJ, Robertson ME, Mann DV, Kostner G, Miller GJ, Miller NE (1985): High-density lipoprotein composition is altered by a common DNA polymorphism adjacent to apoprotein AII gene in man. Lancet 1:771–773.

Slater E (1966): Expectation of abnormality of paternal and maternal sides: A computational model. J Med Genet 3:159–161.

Slater E, Shields J (1967): Genetical aspects of anxiety. In Lader MH (ed): "Studies of Anxiety." Br J Psychiatry, Spec Publ 3, pp 62–71.

Squires RF, Braestrup C (1977): Benzodiazepine receptors in rat brain. Nature 266:732–734.

St. George-Hyslop PH, Tanzi RE, Polinsky RJ, Haines JL, Nee L, Watkins PC, Myers RH, Feldman RG, Pollen D, Drachman D, Growdon J, Bruni A, Foncin JF, Salmon D, Frommelt P, Amaducci L, Sorbi S, Piacentini S, Stewart GD, Hobbs WJ, Conneally PM, Gusella JF (1987): The genetic defect causing familial Alzhei-

mer's disease maps on chromosome 21. Science 235:885–890.

Steel CM (1984): DNA in medicine: The tools, parts I and II. Lancet ii:908–911, 966–968.

Tallman JF, Paul SM, Skolnick P, Gallagher DW (1980): Receptors for the age of anxiety: pharmacology of the benzodiazepines. Science 207:274–281.

Tanzi RE, Gusella JF, Watkins PC, Bruns GAP, St. George-Hyslop PH, Van Kueren ML, Patterson D, Pagan S, Kurnit DM, Neve RL (1987): Amyloid beta protein gene: cDNA, mRNA distribution, and genetic linkage near the Alzhiemer locus. Science 235:880–884.

Torgersen S (1983): Genetic factors in anxiety disorders. Arch Gen Psychiatry 40:1085–1089.

Tsui LC, Buchwald M, Barker D, Braman JC, Knowlton R, Schumm JW, Eiberg H, Mohr J, Kennedy D, Plavsic N, Zsiga M, Markiewicz D, Akots G, Brown V, Helms C, Gravius T, Parker C, Rediker K, Donis-Keller H (1985): Cystic fibrosis locus defined by a genetically linked polymorphic DNA marker. Science 230:1054–1057.

Van Valkenburg CV, Akiskal HS, Puzantian V, Rosenthal T (1984): Anxious depression: Clinical, family history, and naturalistic outcome—comparisons with panic and major depressive disorders. J Affect Disorders 6:67–82.

Weissman MN, Leckman JF, Marikangas KR, Gammon GD, Prusoff BA (1984): Depression and anxiety disorders in parents and children: Results from the Yale Family Study. Arch Gen Psychiatry 41:845–952.

Wheeler ED, White PD, Reed E, Cohen ME (1948): Familial incidence of neurocirculatory asthenia ("anxiety neurosis," "effort syndrome"). J Clin Invest 27:562.

Wood P (1942): Aetiology of DaCosta's syndrome. Br Med J 1:845–851.

5

Origins of Panic Disorder

JEROME KAGAN, PhD, J. STEVEN REZNICK, PhD, NANCY SNIDMAN, PhD,
MAUREEN O. JOHNSON, JANE GIBBONS, MICHELLE GERSTEN, EdD,
JOSEPH BIEDERMAN, MD, AND JERROLD F. ROSENBAUM, MD

Department of Psychology, Harvard University, Cambridge, Massachusetts 02138 (J.K., N.S., M.O.J., J.G.);
Department of Psychology, Yale University, New Haven, Connecticut 06520-7447 (J.S.R.); Child Study Center,
Yale University School of Medicine, New Haven, Connecticut 06510 (M.G.); Department of Psychopharmacology,
Massachusetts General Hospital, Harvard University School of Medicine, Boston, Massachusetts 02114 (J.B., J.F.R.)

INTRODUCTION

Study of the relation between a child's psychological profile and his or her familial environment, which was a popular theme during the period after the Second World War, was guided by both psychoanalytic theory and behavioristic mechanisms. Most psychologists approached the problem with the straightforward environmental assumptions that neurotic patients would reward and punish their children in inconsistent or anomalous ways, fail to establish an affectionate relation with the child, or, as role models, present deviant profiles for their children to observe and to imitate. As a result, the children were expected to develop symptoms directly or as a consequent of conflict and anxiety. Unfortunately, few robust relations emerged from such investigations because most scientists did not actually study the context of socialization but, instead, relied on correlations between psychiatric indices of neurotic symptoms and relatively crude self-report indices of the home environment and parental behavior. Furthermore, as both psychoanalytic and behavioral theory lost a great deal of their attractiveness to academic psychologists during the decade from 1960 to 1970, this kind of inquiry became less appealing to students of human development.

During the subsequent 2 decades, while this category of work in psychology was idling, the hypothesis that genetic factors contributed to mental illness was gaining popularity because of robust associations between particular disorders in parents and distinctive profiles in their children. Two related diagnostic categories cited often as instances of this hypothesis were panic disorder and agoraphobia; these syndromes displayed a pedigree that was absent for most neurotic symptoms (Berg, 1976; Crowe et al., 1983; Gittleman and Klein, 1984; Harris et al., 1983; Marks, 1986; Weissman et al., 1984). Many investigators suggested that adults with panic or agoraphobia, compared with patients diagnosed as having *generalized anxiety*, were more likely to report being anxious and fearful as children (Gittleman-Klein and Klein, 1971; Torgersen, 1983). The children of adult patients with agoraphobia or panic disorder were much more likely to show signs of separation anxiety and school phobia than children of depressive parents but were not more likely to have attention deficit or conduct disorders (Weissman et al., 1984). Additionally, adult agoraphobic women recalled being school phobic themselves (Berg et al., 1974; Berg, 1976). Furthermore, the childhood symptoms of school phobia and adult panic were both alleviated with drugs such as imipramine, whereas the symptoms of generally anxious patients were not alleviated by the same pharmacological treatments (Gelder, 1986; Gittleman-Klein, 1975).

While psychiatrists were probing panic and agoraphobia, a small group of child psychologists, many of whom were unaware of the work on panic disorder, had been studying the developmental history and physiological charac-

Neurobiology of Panic Disorder, Pages 71–87

teristics of extremely shy and fearful children (Bronson, 1970; Daniels and Plomin, 1985; Garcia-Coll et al., 1984). This developmental research suggested that about 10% of white U.S. children were born with a disposition to be extremely irritable as infants; shy and fearful as toddlers; and cautious, quiet, and introverted when they reached school age. Longitudinal studies by Kagan and his colleagues (Kagan et al., 1984; Reznick et al., 1986) revealed that this quality, and its opposite (an outgoing, sociable, bold profile) were among the best preserved personality attributes during the early childhood years. Children selected in the second year of life to be extremely shy or sociable retained their respective profiles through 7.5 years of age, with stability correlations approaching 0.7. In this chapter, we summarize this work in more detail.

INHIBITION TO THE UNFAMILIAR

The empirical record suggests that the temperamental quality defined by an initial tendency to withdraw, to seek a parent, and to inhibit play and vocalization following encounter with unfamiliar people and events persists over the childhood years as part of a coherent network of behavioral and physiological characteristics and has analogues in many mammalian species (Blizard, 1981; Bronson, 1981; Brush et al., 1985; Goldsmith and Gottesman, 1981; Kagan and Moss, 1962; Kagan et al., 1988; McDonald, 1983). The tendency to withdraw from or approach an unfamiliar event emerges as a reliable individual characteristic at about ages 1 year in humans, 2 months in monkeys, and 1 month in cats and dogs. Scott and Fuller (1974) found that variation in reaction to novelty was one of the two most differentiating characteristics among five breeds of dogs, and both Soumi (1984) and Stevenson-Hinde, Stillwell-Barnes, and Zunz (1980) have reported similar variation in laboratory-reared macaque monkeys. This dimension is also central in Jung's theory of psychological types, which made introversion–extraversion the major differentiating characteristic among humans (Jung, 1924). It is also of interest that fearfulness is a highly heritable characteristic in infants under 1 year of age (Goldsmith, 1983; Goldsmith and Gottesman, 1981; Gold-

smith and Campos, 1986), and introversion–extraversion is both the most heritable and also the best preserved personality quality from childhood to the adult years (Floderus-Myrhed et al., 1980; Conley, 1985; Eysenck, 1982; Kagan and Moss, 1962).

Our laboratory has been following two independent groups of white children from intact middle- and working-class families who were selected from large samples when they were either 21 or 31 months of age because they were either consistently shy, timid, and fearful (behaviorally inhibited) or sociable, bold, and fearless (uninhibited) when exposed to unfamiliar rooms, people, and objects. We had to screen over 400 children by telephone and laboratory observation to find groups of approximately 60 inhibited and 60 uninhibited children with equal numbers of boys and girls in each group (see Garcia-Coll et al., 1984; Snidman, 1984; for details).

The children in Cohort 1 were chosen at 21 months of age from a group of 117 who came to our laboratory, where their behavior was video taped and subsequently quantified. The situations were: initial meeting with an unfamiliar examiner in an unfamiliar room, and subsequent encounters with a second unfamiliar room containing toys, an unfamiliar woman displaying three acts with toys that were difficult to remember and to imitate, a third unfamiliar woman, a large metal robot, and finally a brief separation from the mother. Behavioral signs of inhibition were: clinging to or remaining proximal to the mother; fretting or crying, interruption of play, cessation of vocalization, distress after the model's display of the three acts, and reluctance to approach the unfamiliar objects or people. The children who displayed these behaviors consistently across most of the incentives, as well as those who did not, were selected to form groups of 28 extremely inhibited and 30 extremely uninhibited children. These 58 children returned to the laboratory 1 month later to be observed in the same room with the same incentives; the reliability of a continuous index of behavioral inhibition was 0.6.

The original index of inhibited behavior in Cohort 2 at age 31 months was based primarily on behavior with an unfamiliar peer of the same sex and age, with both mothers present,

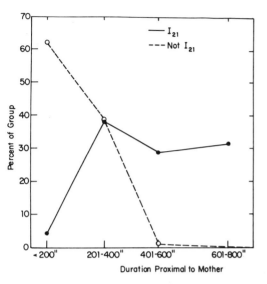

Fig. 5–1. Differences between Cohort 1 inhibited (I) and uninhibited children at 21 months on duration proximal to the mother.

and a brief episode in which the child encountered an unfamiliar woman. The behavioral indexes of inhibition, which were similar to those used with Cohort 1, included long latencies to interact with the unfamiliar child, adult, or toys; withdrawal from the unfamiliar events; and long periods of time proximal to the mother while not playing with an object. Figure 5–1 shows the differences between the two groups in Cohort 1 for duration proximal to the mother across all the episodes and Figure 5–2 the percent of children who displayed crying to separation, remained in physical contact with the mother for more than 10 sec, and fretted or cried to a woman modeling the three acts. Figures 5–3 and 5–4 show the differences between the two groups of Cohort 2 on two of the selection criteria: total time proximal to the mother and latency to approach the unfamiliar peer. Over two-thirds of the children classified as inhibited in Cohorts 1 and 2, but none of the uninhibited children, were proximal to their mother for more than 6.5 min. In Cohort 2, over 80% of the inhibited children but none of the uninhibited children took longer than 10 min to make their first approach to the unfamiliar child.

Each of these sample groups has been seen on several additional occasions. Cohort 1 has

been seen at ages 4 years, 5.5 years, and 7.5 years and Cohort 2 at ages 43 months and 5.5 years, with 15% attrition in each cohort. On the second visit of Cohort 1 at age 4 years and Cohort 2 at age 3.5 years, the primary index of behavioral inhibition was derived from behavior with an unfamiliar child of the same sex and age in a laboratory playroom with both mothers present. At 5.5 years of age, several indexes of inhibition derived from varied situations were aggregated to form a composite index. The separate indexes were based on behavior with 1) an unfamiliar child in a laboratory setting, 2) classmates in a school setting, 3) a female examiner administering tests over a 90 min session, and 4) unfamiliar objects suggestive of risk (a balance beam, a black box with a hole) in an unfamiliar laboratory room.

Preservation of Behavior

The behaviors that characterize inhibited and uninhibited children were moderately preserved from the original to the later assessments. The adjectives "inhibited" and "uninhibited" refer to the original classification at age 21 or 31 months unless otherwise stated (see Table 5–1).

Inhibited behaviors were preserved from the earliest to the latest assessment for both cohorts. In Cohort 1, the correlation between the index of inhibition at 21 months and 5.5 years was 0.52; the comparable correlation for Cohort 2 from 31 months to 5.5 years was 0.55. The preservation of each class of behavior was generalized to the school context. In her doctoral research, Gersten (1986) trained observers who were unaware of the child's classification to code the child's behavior in his or her kindergarten class during the first week of school in September as well as during a day in the spring of the same academic year. The observers noted every 15 sec whether the target child was displaying one or more of a small number of responses. The children in Cohort 1 classified as inhibited at 21 months were more often alone and less often in social interaction with another child or adult ($r = 0.34$, $P < 0.05$).

One of the most sensitive indexes of inhibition in a laboratory situation, especially after 4 or 5 years of age, is a reluctance to talk spontaneously to an examiner during the individual testing session. This relation was robust for

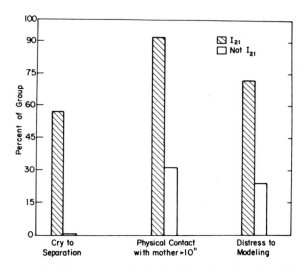

Fig. 5–2. Differences between Cohort 1 inhibited (I) and uninhibited children in separation fear, physical contact with the mother, and distress to modeling.

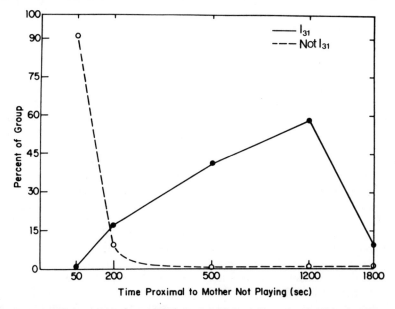

Fig. 5–3. Differences between Cohort 2 inhibited (I) and uninhibited children in time proximal to the mother at 31 months.

Cohort 2 at 5.5 years and for Cohort 1 at both 5.5 and 7.5 years. The two most sensitive variables are latency to utter the first few spontaneous comments to the examiner (i.e., an unprovoked statement and not a reply to an examiner's probe or question) and the total number of spontaneous comments over the entire session. Figures 5–5 and 5–6 show scatter plots of these two conversation variables for the children classified originally as inhibited

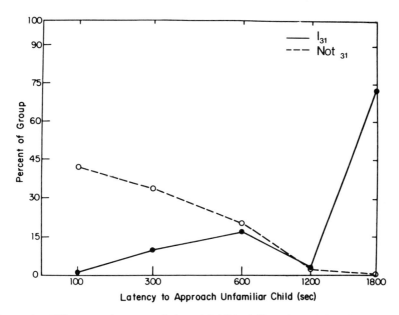

Fig. 5–4. Differences between Cohort 2 inhibited (I) and uninhibited children at 31 months for latency to approach an unfamiliar child.

TABLE 5–1.
Preservation of Inhibited and Uninhibited Behavior Across the Three Assessments in the Two Cohorts (Numbers refer to correlation coefficients)

	Cohort 1				Cohort 2		
Inhibition at	1	2	3	Inhibition at	1	2	3
21 months	—	.51**	.52**	31 months	—	.59**	.55**
4 years	—	—	.67***	43 months	—	—	.45**
5.5 years	—	—	—	5.5 years	—	—	—

**P < 0.01.
***P < 0.001.

or uninhibited in Cohorts 1 and 2. (Note: The correlations among the latencies to the first six comments are over 0.80.) Not one inhibited 5.5-year-old child in Cohort 2, but 14 uninhibited children uttered their second spontaneous comment within 3 min of meeting the examiner and, additionally, made 40 or more comments during the session. By contrast, 13 inhibited but only two uninhibited children had not made their second spontaneous comment after being in the room 10 min and spoke fewer than ten times ($\chi^2 = 21.0$, $P < 0.01$). Among Cohort 1 children at age 7.5 years, 12 uninhibited but only five inhibited children made their sixth spontaneous comment within 5 min and made more than 40 spontaneous com-

ments, whereas 12 inhibited but only 2 uninhibited children took more than 10 min before making their sixth comment and made fewer than 30 spontaneous comments ($\chi^2 = 9.6$, $P < 0.001$).

A sensitive index of inhibition at 7.5 years of age was children's social behavior in a 90 min group play situation consisting of eight or nine unfamiliar children of the same age and sex. The two signs of behavioral inhibition were: infrequent talking to another child and spending a large proportion of the time apart from any other child (defined as greater than arm's length from a peer). These two variables were coded from a combination of a video tape of the entire session and a taped narration of each

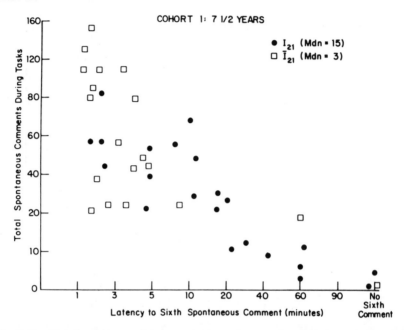

Fig. 5–5. Relation between total spontaneous comments and latency to the sixth spontaneous comment during testing session with Cohort 1 children at age 7.5 years. I, inhibited.

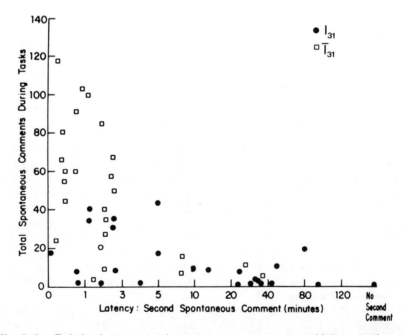

Fig. 5–6. Relation between total spontaneous comments and latency to the second spontaneous comment during testing session with Cohort 2 children at age 5.5 years. I, inhibited.

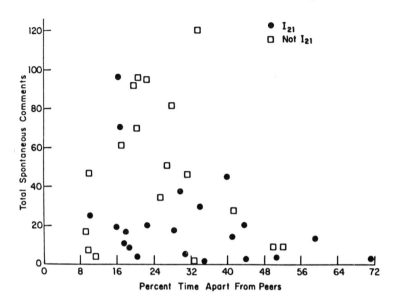

Fig. 5–7. Relation between total spontaneous comments and percent time apart from peers for Cohort 1 children at age 7.5 years. I, inhibited.

child's behavior dictated by a coder who was blind to the child's original behavioral assignment. Figure 5–7 shows the relation between total spontaneous comments and total time in which the child remained apart from any peer in the group play situation for Cohort 1. Ten uninhibited and two inhibited children spoke more than 40 times; 14 inhibited but six uninhibited children spoke fewer than 20 times (χ^2 = 8.4, $P < 0.001$).

There are also more inhibited children who are later than first born—about two-thirds—and more uninhibited children who are first born. This may be due to the fact that first born children are encouraged to be more independent of the mother when the next child arrives. A second possible interpretation assumes that fetal stress is less likely during the first pregnancy than during subsequent pregnancies. A third interpretation is that later born status is associated with a more stressful set of experiences for the small group of infants who are born with a biological disposition to become uncertain to challenge and unfamiliarity. An infant with such a temperamental vulnerability might react with limbic arousal to the mild, but unexpected, intrusions of an older 4-year-old sibling who seizes a toy or pushes the infant from a chair.

Physiological Correlates

We believe that the consistently inhibited children have lower thresholds of excitability in those limbic structures that serve the related psychological states scientists call uncertainty or anxiety. As a result; they are likely to show enhanced activity in the pituitary-adrenal axis, reticular activating system, and sympathetic arm of the autonomic nervous system as well as inhibition of action to unfamiliar events that cannot be assimilated and to threats for which they have no coping response. We now present data revealing a correlation between signs of reactivity in one or more of these systems and behavioral inhibition.

HEART RATE AND VARIABILITY

We measured the child's heart rate and heart rate variability to baseline and cognitive tasks on every assessment, so we can make the firmest statements about these two parameters. Although we use the terms heart rate and heart rate variability in the text, all statistical analyses were performed on the heart period values. Heart rate variability was the average standard deviation of the interbeat intervals for each trial of a particular episode. The mean heart rate and variability for a multitrial episode was the average of the values for the separate trials

TABLE 5–2.
Preservation of Individual Differences in Heart Rate and Variability Across Three Assessments in Two Cohorts (Numbers refer to correlations).

	Cohort 1				Cohort 2		
	21 months	4 years	5.5 years		31 months	43 months	5.5 years
Heart rate							
21 months	—	.23	.15	31 months	—	.53**	.59**
4 years	—	—	.58**	43 months	—	—	.40*
5.5 years	—	—	—	5.5 years	—	—	—
Heart rate variability							
21 months	—	.49**	.39**	31 months	—	.53***	.61***
4 years	—	—	.64***	43 months	—	—	.49**
5.5 years	—	—	—	5.5 years	—	—	—

*$P < 0.05$.
**$P < 0.01$.
***$P < 0.001$.

of that episode. Heart rate and variability were always negatively correlated—high rate with low variability—both under relaxed conditions and under mild cognitive stress (correlations between -0.6 and -0.7). More important, the inhibited children had both higher as well as more stable heart rates than uninhibited children at every age of evaluation, although the differences between the two groups on these two variables were larger during the preschool years than during the assessment at 7.5 years of age. We believe that this is because the stress associated with school led to increased heart rates among some uninhibited children who developed academic problems. In addition, the inhibited children who became more outgoing began to show lower heart rates. At all ages, however, a profile of shy, timid, anxious behavior was associated contemporaneously with a higher heart rate.

Table 5–2 shows the degree of preservation of differences in heart rate and heart rate variability for the two cohorts. Heart rate variability was preserved across all assessments in both cohorts. The preservation of differences in heart rate was significant at all ages for Cohort 2; for Cohort 1 the differences were preserved only from ages 4 to 5.5 years. The magnitudes of preservation for heart rate and variability matched those reported for behavior. Moreover, the consistently inhibited children had the highest heart rates at all ages, and the consistently uninhibited children had the lowest heart rates at all assessments.

It is of interest that the inhibited children with consistently high and stable heart rates had the largest number of fears (e.g., large animals, being left alone in the house, fire, a large body of water). Over half of these children were afraid of monsters in the movies or on television, and one-third had unusual fears or night terrors. One child was afraid of Santa Claus, another of a kidnapper coming to the home, and several of going alone to their bedroom at night. Not one of the uninhibited children had any of these atypical fears; their fears were usually of large dogs or of the dark. Additionally, maternal ratings of the child's shyness with unfamiliar children and fear of going to school were higher among the inhibited children with a high and stable heart rate than among either the inhibited children with a low and variable heart rate or uninhibited children.

Spectral analysis of the heart rate expresses the complex beat-to-beat variation as a power spectrum of the separate rhythms, with peaks at characteristic frequencies. Peaks at low frequencies reflect sympathetic processes, especially blood pressure and temperature regulation. In human subjects, a peak frequency between 0.2 and 0.5 Hz is due primarily to respiration and is mediated by vagal activity. Peaks at lower frequencies are due primarily, but not exclusively, to sympathetic activity. Analysis of the changes in the heart rate power spectrum of the children from Cohort 2 at 43 months of age reveals that more inhibited than uninhibited children shifted to greater power at the lower frequencies from a baseline period prior to cognitive testing to a subsequent baseline after the stress of several difficult cognitive procedures. Moreover, this index of sympathetic activity derived from the spectral analysis at age 43 months predicted inhibited behavior at age 5.5 years ($r = 0.47$, $P < 0.01$).

Pupillary dilation is a second potential index of sympathetic activity, and the inhibited children from both cohorts showed significantly larger pupillary dilation to cognitive tasks than uninhibited children (recall memory for words and digits, a mental comparison of the relative size of objects, and inferring an object from its features). However, the pupil data were not as discriminating of the two groups as heart rate or heart rate variability.

The projections from limbic structures to the skeletal muscles of the larynx and vocal cords also seem to be at a higher level of excitability in inhibited children. Increased tension in these muscles is usually accompanied by a decrease in the variability of the pitch periods of vocal utterances. The increased muscle tension can be due not only to discharge of the nucleus ambiguus but also, indirectly, to sympathetic activity that constricts arterioles serving the muscles of the larynx and vocal folds. Because the vocal cords do not maintain a steady rate as they open and close, the perturbations in the rate at which they open and close is a consequence of many factors, one of which is the tension in the laryngeal muscles (Lieberman, 1961). In her doctoral research, Coster (1986) has found that the inhibited children in Cohort 1 at 5.5 years of age showed less variability in the pitch periods of single word utterances spoken under psychological stress than did uninhibited children.

Because norepinephrine is a primary neurotransmitter of the sympathetic nervous system, a urine sample collected from each child in Cohort 1 at the end of the test battery at age 5.5 years was assayed for norepinephrine and its derivatives using mass fragmentography. The assays yielded values for norepinephrine, normetaephrine, 3-methoxy-4-hydroxyphenylglycol (MHPG), and vanillymandelic acid (VMA). Concentrations of each compound were transformed into moles per gram of creatinine, and an index of total norepinephrine activity was computed. This index reflects primarily peripheral norepinephrine activity. There was a modest correlation between the index of norepinephrine activity at 5.5 years and inhibited behavior at 4 and at 5.5 years ($r = 0.34$ with the index at age 4 years, $r = 0.31$ with the index at age 5.5 years).

To assess activity in the pituitary-adrenal axis, samples of saliva were gathered from both cohorts at 5.5 years of age in the laboratory as well as at home on three mornings before breakfast and, thus, before the stress of the day had begun. These saliva samples were analyzed for unbound cortisol using a modification of the standard radioimmunoassay (RIA) method (Walker, 1984) (see Fig. 5–8). In both groups, the average cortisol level across the three home samples was significantly correlated with the original index of inhibition. Indeed, cortisol levels in Cohort 1 at 5.5 years were more discriminating of the two groups than any other physiological variable. Moreover, inhibited children with high levels of cortisol in both home and laboratory samples, compared with inhibited children with lower cortisol values, were more fearful and had more psychosomatic symptoms (see Levine et al., 1978; Tennes et al., 1977).

AGGREGATE INDEX OF PHYSIOLOGICAL RESPONSIVITY

Although the inhibited children in Cohort 1 showed the peripheral physiological consequences predicted from the hypothesis of lower thresholds of reactivity in the limbic system, only about one-third of the inhibited children showed signs of higher activity in all the target systems, and most of the correlations among the individual variables were low and nonsignificant, with the single exception of a correlation of 0.84 between heart period and heart period variability. The statistical independence of the separate physiological variables is not atypical (see Nesse et al., 1985). To assess the predictive power of an aggregate index of responsivity across the separate indexes, we computed a mean standard score for eight physiological variables quantified on Cohort 1 at 5.5 years of age. The eight variables were: 1) cortisol level in the morning at home, 2) cortisol level in the laboratory, 3) heart period during cognitive tasks, 4) heart period variability during cognitive tasks, 5) pupillary

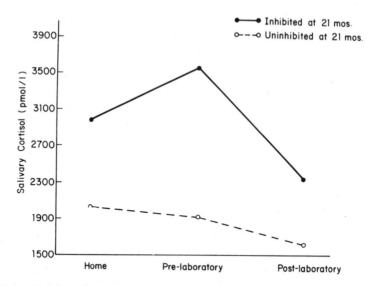

Fig. 5–8.   Cortisol values at age 5.5 years for children classified as inhibited and uninhibited at 21 months.

dilation during cognitive tasks, 6) variability of pitch periods of vocal utterances under cognitive stress, 7) standard deviation of all the fundamental frequency values, and 8) total norepinephrine activity in the laboratory urine sample. We reversed the values for variables 3, 4, 6, and 7 so that a high standard score reflected greater limbic arousal. The correlations between the mean of the eight physiological variables and each of its component scores range from 0.36 to 0.56. The relation between the aggregate of the eight physiological variables and the index of behavioral inhibition at each age for 22 inhibited and 21 uninhibited children was highest with the original index of inhibition at 21 months (r = 0.70, P < 0.001) but was significant at the two later ages (r = 0.66 with the index at age 4 years; r = 0.58 with the index at age 5.5 years). It is of interest that two of the three formerly inhibited children with the lowest physiological indexes had become increasingly less inhibited across the period of study whereas two of the three formerly uninhibited children with the highest indexes had become more inhibited at 5-and-a-half years. Thus, the direction of change in behavior over the 4 years of study is accompanied by the expected level of physiological reactivity at age 5.5 years.

Eye Color and Behavior

It is an odd, but interesting, fact that the incidence of blue eyes is significantly higher among the inhibited children in both longitudinal cohorts, and the frequency of brown eyes is more common among uninhibited children. Furthermore, we have found a significant association between inhibited behavior and blue eyes in three independent studies of children who had not been initially selected for inhibited or uninhibited behavior. In the first unpublished investigation, Reznick and his colleagues discovered that the children who were consistently inhibited in the laboratory at 14, 20, and 32 months of age were more likely to have blue eyes than brown eyes. For her doctoral research, Rosenberg selected infants on eye color (blue vs. brown) and later evaluated them in the laboratory when they were 22 months old. Blue-eyed children had significantly higher scores than brown-eyed children on indexes of behavioral inhibition. Finally, in an earlier study, Rosenberg and Kagan (1987) asked teachers of 133 classrooms from kindergarten to third grade to nominate from among their white pupils the one child who was most timid and shy and the one child who was most sociable and outgoing. More shy children had blue eyes; outgoing children had brown eyes. About 60% of the children in each of the behavioral groups had the expected eye color. The probability of these five independent investigations each yielding the same significant association between eye color and behavioral inhibition is less than one in one million.

Although this association seems inexplicable on the surface, there are at least two possible physiological mechanisms. One explanation appeals to the effects of the pituitary peptide pro-opiomelanocortin (POMC) and its derivatives, especially alpha-melanocyte-stimulating hormone (alpha-MSH), to explain the association between eye color and behavioral inhibition. POMC is the precursor of both alpha-MSH and beta-endorphin (beta-END) (Margules, 1979). The former has several physiological effects, one of which is stimulation of melanin synthesis (Kastin et al., 1971; Pawelek and Korner, 1982). In addition, beta-END alters sensitivity to pain and stress, reduces arterial blood pressure, and decreases vascular sympathetic tone. Because alpha-MSH and beta-END are both derived from POMC, children born with low levels of the precursor might have low levels of alpha-MSH (and hence light pigmentation of the eye) as well as low levels of beta-END (and therefore heightened sensitivity to pain or stress). In addition, alpha-MSH is itself a neuromodulator that can influence human emotion directly. For example, administration of alpha-MSH to humans produces changes in cardiac and vascular processes, patterns of evoked potentials similar to those that accompany limbic arousal, and self-reports of reduced anxiety (Miller et al., 1974; Sandman et al., 1975). This argument, therefore, holds that low levels of alpha-MSH would be associated with both lighter eye color and heightened excitability in the limbic structures.

A second explanation involves the possible effects of cortisol on the brain of the developing embryo and fetus. Meyer (1985) has noted that high levels of cortisol in pregnant rats, which can result from exposure to stress, have significant effects on the embryogenesis of the central nervous system. Placental cortisol inhibits transcription of the POMC gene, thus limiting the synthesis of alpha-MSH and beta-END. Cortisol also stimulates the action of the enzyme dopamine beta-hydroxyalse, which is responsible for the last step in the formation of norepinephrine and enhances the development of adrenergic, rather than cholinergic, neurons in the embryo's autonomic nervous system. Finally, both cortisol and norepinephrine are able to inhibit the production and dispersion of melanin in the melanocytes. Thus an infant born to a mother who produced high levels of cortisol during her pregnancy might be more likely than the average fetus to have light eyes, because of low levels of alpha-MSH, or higher levels of cortisol and norepinephrine. These children would also have more excitable limbic structures because of high levels of central norepinephrine. Although these two hypothetical mechanisms are admittedly speculative, the association between eye color and behavior in white children is unusually robust and invites theoretical attention.

The entire corpus of data, together with reports from behavioral geneticists revealing that qualities relating to social anxiety and introversion are among the most heritable in children and adults, suggests that extreme forms of fearfulness and timidity in children may be under some genetic influence. That conclusion, considered in conjunction with the psychiatric hypothesis of a genetic influence on panic and agoraphobia, suggests the wisdom of studying children living with parents who have panic syndrome to determine whether these children show signs of inhibited behavior. Below we summarize one such investigation.

CHILDREN OF PARENTS WITH PANIC DISORDER

The subjects were 32 white children 4–7 years of age. Eighteen of the children had a parent diagnosed as having or having had panic disorder with or without agoraphobia. The 14 control children had parents diagnosed as having major depressive disorder or parents who were treated for other behavioral problems, such as obesity or tobacco dependence, at the same hospital setting as the parent with panic disorder. The control group included a few children whose sibs had attention deficit disorder and were being treated in an outpatient hospital setting. All the parents were white and were residents of the greater Boston area. Families were asked to participate in this project by research staff who were blind to the presence or absence of any psychiatric difficulties in the children. The parents were evaluated using the NIMH-DIS and the anxiety module of the SCID to confirm the clinical diagnosis and evaluate comorbidity. All diagnostic information was reviewed by the two psychiatrist authors (J.F.R. and J.B.) before the assignment to a diagnostic group. Panic disorder or agoraphobia parents were further stratified into those who also had comorbidity of major depressive disorder. All diagnoses of parents were made independent of any laboratory findings on the children. Each child of a parent in the experimental group was matched for age, sex, socioeconomic status, and ordinal position with a control child whose parent did not have panic or agoraphobia.

Assessments of the Children

The children were assessed in a laboratory setting at Harvard University by a woman who had no knowledge of the parental diagnoses. The rationale for the laboratory protocol described below was based on the desire to obtain an index of the child's behavior with an unfamiliar examiner as well as indexes of heart rate and heart rate variability because of the significant association between inhibited behavior and a high and stable heart rate during mental work. After the child entered the testing room with the mother, electrodes were placed on the child's chest for the recording of heart rate and respiration. The procedure began with a 30 sec quiet period during which the child was asked to sit still followed by a baseline period during which the child sat quietly while an examiner read part of a story accompanied by pictures. Each child was then given five cognitive tests that were mildly stressful. In the first, the child was asked to look carefully at 24 chromatic slides of familiar objects presented one at a time because he or she would be asked to recognize them. Immediately after viewing the 24 slides, the child saw a second group of 24 slides, half of which contained the familiar pictures just seen and half of which were novel. The child was asked to indicate which pictures were new and which were familiar. The child was then asked to remember a set of words in a series of three, four, five, or six words. In the third cognitive

task, the child was shown an object on a stand and requested to explore with the right hand three similar objects behind a curtain that the child could not see. Only one of the three hidden objects was identical to the object that was visible. The child was asked to select the one haptically explored object that was identical to the one to which he or she had visual access. The child was then asked to watch the examiner as she touched a series of xylophone keys in a different spatial pattern and to duplicate the pattern displayed by the examiner. Finally, the child was given a parallel test of recogintion memory using the same procedure as described earlier but with different pictures. Following these cognitive tests, the child was asked to sit quietly while the examiner read a continuation of the earlier story and then was asked just to sit quietly for an additional 30 seconds.

The video tapes of the testing session were coded for a small number of variables: latency to the first, second, and third spontaneous comments made by the child (a spontaneous comment referred to any utterance that was not provoked by an examiner's question); total number of spontaneous comments during the testing session; frequency of smiles, small movements of the fingers, movements of the mouth or lips, and gross body trunk movements. A sample of 12 video tapes randomly selected were coded by a second coder. The reliabilities for the variables ranged from .91 to .97 for these variables.

Profiles of the Two Groups

There were no significant differences between the children from the two groups with respect to smiling or any of the motoricity variables. However, the variables related to spontaneous speech did differentiate the two groups. As was noted in our discussion of the data from the two longitudinal cohorts, the two most sensitive indexes of behavioral inhibition in a laboratory setting for children between 4 and 7 years of age were 1) latency to the first few spontaneous comments and 2) total number of spontaneous comments. The children of the panic patients took significantly longer to utter their first, second, and third spontaneous comments and spoke significantly less often than the control subjects. Correlations among

TABLE 5–3.
Mean Values for the Major Behavioral Variables for Panic Disorder and Control Children

Variable	Child of panic disorder parent	Control children	t	P
Latency to first spontaneous comment	15 min, 40 sec	2 min, 10 sec	3.54	<.01
Total number of spontaneous comments	4.5	23.1	4.04	<.001
Total motoricity (sum of finger, body, facial movements)	1.8	3.0	0.7	ns
Smiles	6.0	9.5	0.8	ns

the latencies to each of the first three comments were very high (average correlation was 0.9), so we shall deal only the latency to the first spontaneous comment (see Table 5–3).

Figure 5–9 illustrates a scatter plot of these two speech variables for all 32 children. Nine of the 14 control children but none of the experimental children had both a latency to the first spontaneous comment under 3 min and eight or more spontaneous comments. By contrast, 13 of the 18 children of parents with panic disorder or agoraphobia, but only one control child, did not speak until 4 min had elapsed and made fewer than seven spontaneous comments ($\chi^2 = 18.4, P < 0.01$). The mean differences between these two groups on these two variables were also significant ($t = 3.54, P < 0.01$ for latency to the first spontaneous comment; $t = 4.04, P < 0.01$ for total spontaneous comments). These results are in close accord with the data gathered on the inhibited and uninhibited children in the longitudinal cohorts, for the former also displayed a long latency to speak spontaneously and uttered very few spontaneous comments.

Heart Rate and Heart Rate Variability

The mean heart rate and variability values were similar for the two groups on all the episodes. Because the data from the longitudinal cohorts had revealed that inhibited behavior was associated with a higher and more stable heart rate, this result was disappointing. However, a large number of inhibited children in our two longitudinal cohorts had displayed an increase in heart rate across the episodes of a cognitive battery, whereas most uninhibited children did not show this acceleration. Therefore, we examined each child's heart rate values across each of the episodes and classified

each protocol as acceleratory if there was 1) a higher mean heart rate on the last three, compared with the first three, episodes and 2) a linear acceleratory trend across the episodes. An uneven or saw-toothed pattern of heart rate was classified as nonaccelerating. Each child's protocol was classified twice, with an agreement of 90%. One child of a panic disorder parent did not have a heart rate record because of technical difficulties. The children of panic disorder parents were more likely than control children to display an acceleratory trend; nine of the 17 (55%) panic children but only four of the 14 (29%) control children showed an acceleratory trend. This difference just missed statistical significance.

However, classification of each child as inhibited or uninhibited, based on the data in Figure 5–9 rather than the parental diagnosis, was significantly related to an acceleratory trend. Ten of the 13 children in the quadrant marked by long latencies (greater than 8 min) and few spontaneous comments (fewer than eight) showed an acceleratory trend, in contrast to three of nine children in the quadrant marked by short latencies (less than 3 min) and many spontaneous comments (greater than eight) ($\chi^2 = 4.0, P < 0.05$). Thus, as with our longitudinal data, behaviorally inhibited children showed an acceleratory trend across the episodes.

The fact that the child's behavior with the examiner was a more robust correlate of an acceleratory trend than the parental diagnosis suggests that the cardiac pattern is indexing the child's level of uncertainty in the situation and is not a defining characteristic of children whose parents have panic disorder. Although there was no difference between panic and control children in the frequency of blue eyes,

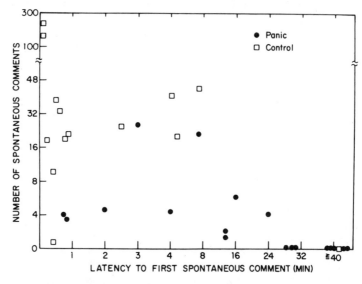

Fig. 5–9. Relation between the number of spontaneous comments and latency to the first spontaneous comment for children of panic parents and controls.

the proportion of blue-eyed children in both groups, 63%, was higher than the expected frequency of 40–45% for white children from the New England area. However, it should be remembered that the control children in this study had sibs or parents with psychological symptoms. Thus the higher proportion of blue eyes among the controls may not be surprising. It is of interest that in only two of the 32 families did the child, sibs, parents, and both sets of grandparents all have blue eyes. In both families, the mother was a panic disorder patient.

DISCUSSION

Children of parents with panic disorder or agoraphobia, with or without depression, were more inhibited behaviorally than control children. Many resembled the 5–7-year-old inhibited children in our two longitudinal cohorts. Although mean heart rate and heart rate variability did not discriminate the two diagnostic groups, the children who were extremely quiet were more likely to show an acceleratory trend over the course of the testing episode, a characteristic also prominent among the inhibited children in our longitudinal studies. This finding is in accord with evidence of greater sympathetic activity in panic patients (e.g., high heart rate and skin conductivity and lower skin temperature; see Freedman et al., 1984).

One possible explanation for the lack of difference between the panic and control children on mean heart rate and heart rate variability is that the former should not be regarded as members of the psychological category we call temperamentally inhibited even though aspects of their phenotype are similar. The children of panic disorder parents who appear inhibited could have acquired their quiet demeanor as a product of socialization and modeling by their anxious parents. One reason for rejecting this interpretation is that one-third of the inhibited children in our two longitudinal cohorts had mothers who were experiencing, or had experienced, panic attacks, some as severe as those of the mothers in the clinical sample.

We believe that the children of the panic disorder parents and the inhibited children in our longitudinal cohorts belong to the same psychological category but that heart rate and heart rate variability need not be consistent signs of this temperamental disposition. Heart rate and variability are monitored, first, by bodily needs and, second, by cognitive effort.

These functions always take precedence over the processes associated with an inhibited temperament. One of the most robust findings in the literature is that a psychological commitment to and investment of effort in a task are associated with a rise and stabilization of heart rate (Kagan and Reznick, 1984). Our longitudinal data indicate that, if a child is not involved in a task, heart rate is often low and variable. In the present sample, there were some children of panic disorder parents who were dramatically more inhibited than any of those in our longitudinal cohorts. A few such children were so frightened they failed to become engaged by the cognitive tasks and had low and variable heart rates. However, almost all the control children became involved in the tasks, and as a result many had a high and stable heart rate.

It is important to ask why the restraint on speech is such a sensitive index of the behavioral quality of inhibition, especially after 4 years of age. Many observers of children have noted that one of the most reliable reactions to an unexpected event that cannot be assimilated, especially an unfamiliar person or context, is to become vocally quiet until assimilation has occurred. The laryngeal muscles, which exert proximal control on oscillations of the vocal cords, are controlled directly by neurons in the motor cortex. Indirect control is maintained by cerebellar relays coursing through the reticular activating system and the basal ganglia. Additionally, sympathetic fibers from the cervical ganglion produce vasoconstriction of capillaries serving the laryngeal muscles and, as a result, increased muscle tone in these muscles. Thus tension in the larynx follows an increase in activity in both the reticular activation system and the sympathetic nervous systems (Stevens and Hirano, 1981). One possible hypothesis is that limbic excitability following encounter with unfamiliar or challenging events leads simultaneously to increased activity in the reticular activating system and sympathetic chain and, as a result, constriction of laryngeal muscles, which, in turn, produces a resistance to phonation. This resistance makes speaking more effortful. A more psychological hypothesis, which ascribes more direct influence to brain processes, suggests that limbic excitability influences the frontal lobe which, in turn, leads to inhibition of speech.

If one moves from immediate to final causes and asks why vocal quieting evolved as a reaction to uncertainty, one possibility is that it would be adaptive in times of danger for the organism to become quiet so as not to reveal its presence. According to Goodall (1986), chimpanzees cease vocalizing to unfamiliar events that might be associated with apprehension. Perhaps the human is biologically prepared to inhibit speech when in an acute state of uncertainty, even though some adults have learned, over the course of development, to control their uncertainty. Some even develop a press of speech. Hence, the relation between inhibition of speech and the state of uncertainty is probably more robust in young children than in adults, even though fear of speaking to strangers or in public is the cardinal symptom of the diagnostic category called "social phobia" (Turner et al., 1986).

In summary, young children born to and living with a parent who has had, or is experiencing, panic or agoraphobia attacks are extremely reluctant to talk to an unfamiliar but friendly examiner. In addition, these children show sympathetic activation to cognitive stress as reflected in an acceleratory heart rate trend across a series of cognitive episodes. These characteristics—timid behavior and heart rate acceleration—also differentiate temperamentally inhibited from uninhibited children of the same age. Although these data are in accordance with the hypothesis of a biologically based disposition to inhibited behavior in the children of panic disorder parents, they are also consistent with the traditional interpretation that emphasizes the role of modeling and social reinforcement. Future work will have to assess the relative contribution of these factors.

If behavioral inhibition is an early precursor for the development of later anxiety disorder, three hypotheses are testable with the sample at hand. First, behavioral inhibition should be more prevalent in young offspring of parents with panic disorder and agoraphobia. This chapter and a previous report (Rosenbaum et al., 1988) contain evidence supporting that hypothesis. Second, in light of the association between child and adult anxiety disorder, behaviorally inhibited children should manifest higher rates of anxiety disorder, and parents of these children, drawn from nonclinically ascertained samples, should also have higher rates of diagnosable anxiety disorder. With respect to the second hypothesis, we have examined the rates of overall psychopathology and anxiety disorders, in particular, in children classified as either inhibited or uninhibited in the sample of children of panic disorder patients and other psychiatric controls as well as in inhibited and uninhibited children from one of our longitudinal cohorts. Rates of disorders were also compared with a group of normal children derived from a general hospital pediatric clinic population. There were higher rates of anxiety disorders in inhibited children compared with uninhibited children and the pediatric control group (Biederman et al., 1988). Thus, by 8 years of age, behavioral inhibition is associated with anxiety disorders in children. Finally, we are examining the rates of diagnosable anxiety disorder in the parents of children from one of the longitudinal cohorts. If risk for anxiety disorders is familial and if behavioral inhibition is a marker of anxiety proneness, parents of young children with behavioral inhibition should have higher rates of anxiety disorders. A preliminary analysis of these data indicates that this is the case, although behavioral inhibition may confer a nonspecific risk for any anxiety disorder.

ACKNOWLEDGMENTS

This research was supported in part by grants from the John D. and Catherine T. MacArthur Foundation and the National Institute of Mental Health (MH 40619).

REFERENCES

Berg I (1976): School phobia in the children of agoraphobic women. Br J Psychiatry 128:86–89.

Berg I, Marks, I, McGuire R, Lipsedge M (1974): School phobia and agoraphobia. Psychol Med 4:428–434.

Biederman J, Rosenbaum FJ, Hirshfeld DR, Gersten M, Meminger SR, Kagan J (1988): Psychiatric correlates of behavioral inhibition in young children of parents with and without psychiatric disorders. Submitted for publication.

Blizard DA (1981): The Maudsley reactive and nonreactive strains. Behav Genet 11:469–489.

Bronson GW (1970): Fear of visual novelty. Dev Psychol 2:33–40.

Bronson WC (1981): "Toddlers' Behaviors With Age Mates. Norwood, NJ: Ablex.

Brush FR, Baron S, Froehlich JC, Ison JR, Pellegrino LJ, Phillips DS, Sakellaris RC, Williams VN (1985): Genetic differences in avoidance learning in Rattus norvegicus. J Comp Psychol 99:60–73.

Conley JJ (1985): Longitudinal stability of personality traits: A multitrait-multimethod-multioccassion analysis. J Personal Social Psychol 49:1266–1282.

Coster W (1986): Aspects of voice and conversation in behaviorally inhibited and uninhibited children. Doctoral dissertation, Harvard University.

Crowe RR, Noyes R, Pauls DL, Slymen D (1983): A family study of panic disorder. Arch Gen Psychiatry 40:1065–1069.

Daniels D, Plomin R (1985): Origins of individual differences in shyness. Dev Psychol 21:118–121.

Eysenck HF (1982): "Personality, Genetics, and Behavior". New York: Praeger.

Floderus-Myrhed B, Pedersen N, Rasmuson I (1980): Assessment of heritability for personality based on a short form of the Eysenck personality inventory. Behav Genet 10:153–162.

Freedman RR, Ianni P, Ettedgui E, Pohl R, Rainey JM (1984): Psychophysiological factors in panic disorder. Psychopathology 17:66–73.

Garcia-Coll C, Kagan J, Reznick JS (1984): Behavioral inhibition in young children. Child Dev 55:1005–1019.

Gelder MG (1986): Panic attack: New approaches to an old problem. Br J Psychiatry 49:346–352.

Gersten M (1986): The contribution of temperament to behavior in natural contexts. Doctoral dissertation, Harvard Graduate School of Education.

Gittelman R, Klein DF (1984): Relationship between separation anxiety in panic and agoraphobic disorders. Psychopathology 17:56–65.

Gittelman-Klein R (1975): Pharmacotherapy and management of pathological separation anxiety. Int J Mental Health 4:255–271.

Gittelman-Klein R, Klein DF (1971): Controlled imipramine treatment of school phobia. Arch Gen Psychiatry 40:1061–1066.

Goldsmith HH (1983): Genetic influences on personality from infancy to adulthood. Child Dev 54:331–355.

Goldsmith HH, Campos JJ (1986): Fundamental issues in the study of early temperament: The Denver twin temperament study. In Lamb MH, Brown A (eds); "Advances in Developmental Psychology." Hillsdale, NJ. Lawrence Erlbaum, pp 261–283.

Goldsmith HH, Gottesman II (1981): Origins of variation in behavioral style. Child Dev 52:91–103.

Goodall J (1986): "The Chimpanzees of Gombe." Cambridge, MA: Harvard University Press.

Harris EC, Noyes R, Crowe RR, Chaudry DR (1983): Family studies of agoraphobia. Arch Gen Psychiatry 40:1061–1066.

Jung CG (1924): "Psychological Types." New York: Harcourt Brace and Company.

Kagan J, Moss HA (1962): "Birth to Maturity." New York: John Wiley and Sons.

Kagan J, Reznick JS (1984): Task involvement and cardiac response in young children. Aust J Psychol 36: 135–147.

Kagan J, Reznick JS, Clarke C, Snidman N, Garcia-Coll C (1984): Behavioral inhibition to the unfamiliar. Child Dev 55:2212–2225.

Kagan J, Reznick JS, Snidman N (1988): Biological bases of childhood shyness. Science 240:167–171.

Kastin AJ, Miller LH, Gonzalez-Barcena D, Hawley WD, Dyster-Aas K, Schally AV, Velasco de Parra ML, Velasco M (1971): Psychophysiologic correlates of MSH activity in man. Physiol Behav 7:893–896.

Levine S, Coe CL, Smotherman WP, Kaplan JN (1978): Prolonged cortisol elevation in the infant squirrel monkey after reunion with mother. Physiol Behav 20: 7–10.

Lieberman P (1961): Perturbations in vocal pitch. J Acoust Soc Am 33:597–603.

Margules DL (1979): Beta-endorphin and endoloxone: Hormones of the autonomic nervous system for the conversion or expenditure of bodily resources and energy in anticipation of famine or feast. Neurosci Biobehav Rev 3:155–162.

Marks IM (1986): Genetics of fear and anxiety disorder. Br J Psychiatry 149:406–418.

McDonald K (1983): Stability of individual differences in behavior in a litter of wolf cubs. J Comp Psychol 97:99–106.

Meyer JS (1985): Biochemical effects of corticosteriods on neural tissues. Physiol Rev 65:946–1020.

Miller LH, Kastin AJ, Sandman CA, Fink M, Van Veen WJ (1974): Polypeptide influences on attention, memory and anxiety in man. Pharmacol Biochem Behav 2:663–668.

Nesse RM, Curtis GC, Thyer BA, McCann DS, Huber-Smith M, Knopf RF (1985): Endocrine and cardiovascular responses during phobic anxiety. Psychosom Med 47:320–332.

Pawelek JM, Korner AM (1982): The biosynthesis of mammalian melanin. Am Sci 70:136–145.

Reznick JS, Kagan J, Snidman N, Gersten M, Baak K, Rosenberg A (1986): Inhibited and uninhibited behavior: A follow-up study. Child Dev 51:660–680.

Rosenbaum JF, Biederman J, Gersten M, Meminger SR, Herman JB, Kagan J, Reznick JS, Snidman N (1988): Behavioral inhibition in children of parents with panic disorder and agoraphobia: A controlled study. Arch Gen Psychiatry 45:463–470.

Rosenberg A, Kagan J (1987): Iris pigmentation and behavioral inhibition. Dev Psychobiol 20:377–392.

Sandman CA, George JM, Nolan JD, Van Riezen H, Kastin AJ (1975): Enhancement of attention in man with ACTH/MSH 4-10. Physiol Behav 15:427–431.

Scott JP, Fuller JL (1974): "Dog Behavior: The Genetic Basis." Chicago: University of Chicago Press (Phoenix Edition). (Originally published 1965.)

Snidman N (1984): Behavioral restraint and the central nervous system. Doctoral dissertation. University of California, Los Angeles.

Stevens KN, Hirano M (eds) (1981): "Vocal Fold Physiology." Tokyo: University of Tokyo Press.

Stevenson-Hinde J, Stillwell-Barnes R, Zunz M (1980): Subjective assessment of rhesus monkeys over four successive years. Primates 21:66–82.

Suomi SJ (1984): The development of affect in rhesus monkeys. In Fox NA, Davidson RJ (eds); "The Psychology of Affective Development." Hillsdale, NJ: Lawrence Erlbaum, pp 119–159.

Tennes K, Downey K, Vernadakis A (1977): Urinary cortisol excretion rates and anxiety in normal one-year-old infants. Psychosom Med 39:178–187.

Torgersen S (1983): Genetic factors in anxiety disorders. Arch Gen Psychiatry 40:1085–1089.

Turner SM, Beidel DC, Dancu CV, Keys DJ (1986): Psychopathology of social phobia and comparison to avoidant personality disorder. J Abnorm Psychol 4: 389–394.

Walker RF (1984): Salivary cortisol determinations in the assessment of adrenal activity. In Ferguson DB (ed); "Steriod Hormones in Saliva." Basel: Karger, pp 33–50.

Weissman MW, Leckman JF, Merikangas KR, Gammon GD, Prusoff BA (1984): Depression and anxiety disorders in parents and children. Arch Gen Psychiatry 41: 845–852.

Postulated Brain Mechanisms for Panic Anxiety

6

Noradrenergic Dysregulation in Panic Disorder

DENNIS S. CHARNEY, MD, SCOTT W. WOODS, MD, LAWRENCE H. PRICE, MD,
WAYNE K. GOODMAN, MD, WILLIAM M. GLAZER, MD, AND
GEORGE R. HENINGER, MD

Clinical Neuroscience Research Unit, Connecticut Mental Health Center, and Department of Psychiatry, Yale
University School of Medicine, New Haven, Connecticut 06508

INTRODUCTION

Abnormal regulation of noradrenergic neuronal function has been hypothesized to be involved in the pathophysiology of diverse disorders, such as panic disorder (PD), generalized anxiety disorder (GAD), major depression, obsessive–compulsive disorder (OCD), and schizophrenia (Charney et al., 1984a; Insel et al., 1984; Redmond, 1979; Siever and Davis, 1985; van Kammen and Antelman, 1984). This chapter reviews the major results of a series of investigations in which we have evaluated noradrenergic function in these disorders by determining the behavioral, biochemical, and cardiovascular responses to challenge doses of the alpha-2-adrenergic receptor antagonist yohimbine and agonist clonidine (Aghajanian, 1978; Cedarbaum and Aghajanian, 1977). Complete and more extensive reports of these individual studies have been published elsewhere (Charney and Heninger, 1986; Charney at al., 1982b, 1987a,c; Price et al., 1986; Sternberg et al., 1982; Glazer et al., 1987; Rasmussen et al., 1987; Heninger et al., 1987).

SUBJECTS AND METHODS

PD Patients

Sixty-eight patients meeting DSM III criteria for agoraphobia with panic attacks (APA) or PD (49 females, mean age 39 ± 2 years; 19 males, mean age 34 ± 3 years) and 20 healthy subjects (11 females, mean age 43 ± 2 years; nine males, mean age 34 ± 3 years) participated in oral yohimbine (20 mg) and placebo challenge tests (Charney et al., 1984a, 1987a). Twenty-six APA or PD patients (24 females, two males, mean age 36 ± 2 years) and 21 healthy subjects (18 females, three males, mean age 32 ± 2 years) participated in iv clonidine (0.15 mg over 5 min) and placebo challenge tests (Charney and Heninger, 1986).

GAD Patients

Twenty patients meeting DSM III criteria for GAD (12 females, mean age 35 ± 7; eight males, mean age 36 ± 6) and 20 healthy subjects (11 females, mean age 43 ± 2 years; nine males, mean age 34 ± 3 years) participated in oral yohimbine (20 mg) and placebo challenge tests (Charney et al., 1987c).

Major Depression Patients

Forty-five patients meeting DSM III criteria for major depression with (N = 25; 18 females, seven males, mean age 46 ± 14 years) or without (N = 20; ten females, ten males, mean age 35 ± 8 years) melancholia and 20 healthy subjects (11 females, nine males, mean age 39 ± 9 years) participated in oral yohimbine (20 mg) and placebo challenge tests (Heninger et al., 1987; Price et al., 1986). Fifteen patients meeting Research Diagnostic Criteria for major depressive episode, endogenous subtype (eight females, mean age 49 ± 13 years; seven males, mean age 42 ± 17 years) and 12 healthy subjects (five females, mean age 40 ± 16 years; seven males, mean age 40 ± 16 years) partici-

Neurobiology of Panic Disorder, Pages 91–105

pated in oral clonidine (5 μg/kg) and placebo challenge tests (Charney et al., 1982b).

OCD Patients

Twelve patients meeting DSM III criteria for OCD (11 females, one male, mean age 39 ± 9 years) and 12 healthy subjects (11 females, one male, mean age 43 ± 7 years) participated in oral yohimbine (20 mg) and placebo challenge tests (Rasmussen et al., 1987).

Schizophrenic Patients

Eighteen schizophrenic patients meeting DSM III criteria for schizophrenia (six females, 12 males, mean age 39.9 ± 14.1 years) and 16 healthy subjects (four females, 12 males, mean age 31 ± 12 years) participated in oral yohimbine (20 mg) and placebo challenge tests (Glazer et al., 1987). Eleven patients meeting DSM III criteria for schizophrenia (six females, five males, mean age 28 ± 10 years) and 11 healthy subjects (five females, six males, mean age 30 ± 7 years) participated in oral clonidine (5 μg/kg) and placebo challenge tests (Sternberg et al., 1982).

Test Day Procedures

Briefly, the patients and healthy subjects arrived at the research unit by 8:30 AM of each test day. Throughout each of the test days, the patients and subjects were supine, with their heads elevated. They stood to use the bathroom and to permit recording of their standing blood pressure and pulse rate. Blood was sampled from an iv cannula in a forearm vein that was kept patent with a normal saline solution. The iv cannula was in place for at least 60 min prior to blood sampling. Blood samples were obtained for plasma-free 3-methoxy-4-hydroxyphenylglycol (MHPG) at 15 and 0.5 min prior to the yohimbine, clonidine, or placebo dose and at 60 (iv clonidine and placebo only), 90 (iv clonidine and placebo only), 120, 180, 210 (oral clonidine and placebo only), and 240 min after the dose. Sitting and standing blood pressure and pulse rate were measured in the usual clinical fashion with a mercury sphygmomanometer at 15 min before and at 30 (iv clonidine and placebo only) 60, 90, 120, 180, and 240 min following the dose.

In each study, behavioral ratings using a visual analog scale to measure the change in anxious feelings were made at 15 min before and at 30 (iv clonidine and placebo only), 60, 90, 120, 180, and 240 min following the dose. The scale was scored in millimeters from the left side of a 100 mm line to a perpendicular mark made by the subject at the point corresponding to the anxiety state at the time. Therefore, the score could range from 0 (not at all) to 100 (most ever).

The PD patients were assessed regarding whether they had a panic attack during each yohimbine test session by a research psychiatrist blind to medication state. This determination was based on direct clinical observation and patient's self-report. Two criteria had to be satisfied. 1) The patient or healthy subject was required to report a crescendo increase in severe subjective anxiety, as reflected by at least a 25 mm rise of the anxious analog rating scale following drug administration, which was accomplished by an increase over baseline of 4 or more of the DSM III symptoms of a panic attack. 2) The patients had to report that the anxiety state experienced was similar to that of a naturally occurring panic attack. A healthy subject was considered to have a panic attack if the first set of criteria was satisfied.

The OCD patients were rated by research nurses, blind to the medication administered, for severity of obsessions and compulsions at 5 min before and 90 min after the dose. Symptoms were assessed for duration, distress, and the ability of the patient to control them during the 90 min before and after yohimbine administration. Global obsession and compulsion severity was rated from 0 (none) to 4 (extreme) on a five-point scale. Assay preparation and quantification of the samples for MHPG were carried out as previously described (Dekirmenjian and Maas, 1974; Maas et al., 1976). (Intra and interassay coefficients of variation were 6 and 11%, respectively.)

Data Analysis

The effects of yohimbine and clonidine in patients and healthy subjects on plasma MHPG, cardiovascular parameters, and ratings of anxiety were initially evaluated using an analysis of variance with repeated measures (ANOVA). A major focus of the data analysis was whether the patient groups reacted differently to the yohimbine and clonidine than healthy subjects. The distinction between groups was manifested primarily in the interaction of group (e.g., patients vs. healthy subjects) and drug (e.g., drug vs. placebo) and time of sampling. The significant interactions were further evaluated with paired and nonpaired t tests to assess how and when the patients differed from healthy subjects in their responses. This was primarily done by substracting the baseline value from the value at each time point on the variable of interest. This resulted in a change score at each time point following placebo or active drug. By subtracting the change following placebo from the change following active drug, an estimate of a net change effect (i.e., drug minus placebo difference) could be obtained. Pearson correlations were calculated to evaluate the relationship among the behavioral, biochemical, and cardiovascular parameters in which significant drug effects were identified. Results are reported as significant when $P < 0.05$ with a two-tailed test.

RESULTS

Yohimbine Challenge

ANXIOGENIC EFFECTS

It was only in the PD patients that yohimbine produced significant effects on the visual analog scale of anxiety. In the healthy subjects and other diagnostic groups, significant drug and time of sampling interaction for the anxious rating on the visual analog scale was not identified, and there were no significant yohimbine-placebo differences at any time point. In the total group of PD patients, a highly significant drug and time of sampling interaction was found for anxious ratings. Following placebo, there was a significant decrease from baseline in anxious ratings at all time points, and after yohimbine there was a significant increase in anxious ratings at 60 (18 ± 4, $P < 0.001$) minutes. The yohimbine-placebo increases were significant for the first four time points for anxious ratings after yohimbine administration.

In the comparison of yohimbine's anxiogenic effects in the patients and in the healthy subjects, a significant interaction of group and drug and time was found for the anxious rating ($F = 6.8$, $P < 0.001$). The yohimbine-placebo increases from baseline were significantly

greater in the patients for anxious ratings at 60, 90, and 120 min. The type of anxiety produced in many of the PD patients appeared to be similar to their naturally occurring panic attacks. Yohimbine produced panic attacks in 37 of the 68 PD patients (54%) and in only one of the 20 healthy subjects (5%) ($P < 0.001$, Fisher exact test).

Although group means on the behavioral ratings were not significant, a subgroup of six schizophrenic patients appeared to develop a dysphoric arousal reaction 60–90 min following yohimbine (data not shown) (see Glazer et al., 1987). Yohimbine had no effect on obsessive and compulsive symptoms in the OCD patients. Figure 6–1 illustrates the yohimbine-placebo increase from baseline at 60 min in the visual analog scale rating of anxious for the healthy subjects and each of the diagnostic groups studied.

PLASMA MHPG

The ANOVA examining the effects of yohimbine on plasma MHPG levels revealed significant drug and time interactions for the healthy subjects and all the diagnostic groups. Significant yohimbine-placebo increases in plasma MHPG were identified in all groups at 120, 180, and 240 min after the dose. The ANOVA comparing the effects of yohimbine on plasma MHPG levels in the patient groups and the healthy subjects revealed nonsignificant group and drug and time interactions, and at no time points were there significant yohimbine-placebo differences between the healthy subjects and patient groups identified except for the GAD patients. In the GAD patients, there was a trend toward a significant interaction between group and drug and time ($F = 2.2$, $P < 0.07$). The yohimbine-placebo differences in plasma MHPG were significantly lower at 120 (0.9 ± 0.7 vs. 0.4 ± 0.5, $P < 0.05$) and 180 (0.9 ± 0.7 vs. 0.4 ± 0.7, $P <. 0.05$) min in the GAD patients compared to the healthy subjects.

The group of PD patients who experienced yohimbine-induced panic attacks had significantly greater increases in plasma MHPG following yohimbine than the healthy subjects or the PD patients who did not experience panic attacks. Significant group and drug and time interactions were observed in the comparison of patients who experienced panic attacks and

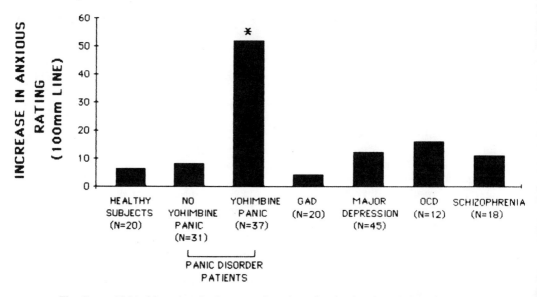

Fig. 6–1. Yohimbine-placebo increase from baseline in visual analog scale rating of anxiety 60 min following the dose. *$P < 0.001$ PD patients reporting yohimbine-induced panic attacks vs. healthy subjects; Student's t test (two-tailed).

the patients who did not (F = 7.2, $P < 0.001$) and the healthy subjects (F = 3.3, $P < 0.05$). Significant yohimbine-placebo differences were identified between the patients who experienced panic attacks and the PD patients who did not and the healthy subjects at 120, 180, and 240 min.

There was a significant positive correlation between the yohimbine-placebo peak increase in anxious ratings and in plasma-free MHPG in the PD patients ($r = 0.37$, $P < 0.003$) but not in the healthy subjects or the other diagnostic groups. Figure 6–2 illustrates the yohimbine-placebo increase from baseline at 120 min in plasma MHPG for the healthy subjects and each of the diagnostic groups.

CARDIOVASCULAR EFFECTS OF YOHIMBINE

In the healthy subjects (N = 20) significant drug and time interactions for sitting systolic, standing systolic, and standing diastolic blood pressures were observed. The yohimbine-placebo differences showed significant mean increases from baseline ranging from 5 to 7 mm Hg in sitting systolic blood pressure at 60, 120, and 180 min and in standing systolic blood pressure at 60, 90, and 180 min after the dose.

Yohimbine had greater effects on blood pressure in the PD patients than in the healthy subjects. Significant drug and time interactions were found for sitting and standing diastolic and systolic blood pressures. Yohimbine-placebo differences indicated significant mean increases from baseline in sitting and standing systolic blood pressures ranging from 6 to 14 mm Hg at all five time points following the dose. The ANOVA comparing the effects of yohimbine on blood pressure in the patients and healthy subjects revealed a group and drug and time interaction for sitting systolic blood pressure (F = 2.7, $P < 0.05$). Yohimbine-placebo differences were significantly greater in the patients for sitting systolic blood pressure at 60 (15 ± 2 vs. 5 ± 2, $P < 0.001$) and 90 min (15 ± 2 vs. 6 ± 3, $P < 0.05$). The patients who reported yohimbine-induced panic attacks had a slightly greater effect on blood pressure compared to the patients who did not.

Yohimbine produced consistent increases in both sitting and standing systolic and diastolic blood pressure in the depressed patients. Significant drug and time interactions were observed for all four of the blood pressure measurements. In the comparison to the healthy subjects, there were no significant group and drug and time effects for any of the four blood

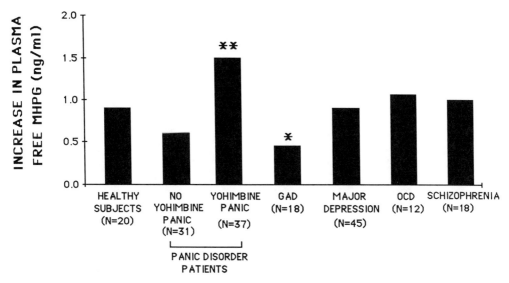

Fig. 6–2. Yohimbine-placebo increase from baseline in plasma-free MHPG 120 min following the dose. *$P < 0.05$ GAD patients vs. healthy subjects; Student's t test (two-tailed). **$P <$ 0.001 PD patients reporting yohimbine-induced panic attacks vs. healthy subjects; Student's t test (two-tailed).

pressure measurements. The effect of yohimbine on blood pressure, however, did appear to be somewhat greater in the depressed patients. For example, the yohimbine-placebo increase in sitting systolic blood pressure was significantly greater in the depressed patients at 60 (10 ± 2 vs. 5 ± 2, $P < 0.01$) and 90 (12 ± 2 vs. 6 ± 3, $P < 0.01$) min.

Significant drug and time interactions were observed for sitting systolic, standing systolic, and standing diastolic blood pressure in the GAD patients. There was not a significant group and drug and time interaction for any of the blood pressures, and at no time were the yohimbine-placebo increases in blood pressure significantly different between the GAD patients and healthy subjects.

In the OCD patients the only significant drug and time of sampling interaction occurred for standing systolic blood pressure. This, however, may be due to the small number of patients studied. Standing systolic blood pressure increased at 60 (13 ± 15, $P < 0.01$) and 90 (13 ± 14, $P < 0.01$) min after yohimbine administration. The comparison of the OCD patients and healthy subjects revealed a significant group and drug and time interaction for standing systolic blood pressure ($F = 2.6$, $P <$

0.05). There was a trend toward a greater increase in standing systolic blood pressure in the patients at 60 (16 ± 17 vs. 4 ± 12, $P = 0.07$) and 90 (13 ± 17 vs. 2 ± 11, $P = 0.09$) min.

The ANOVA for the schizophrenic patients revealed significant drug and time interactions for all four of the blood pressure measurements. The comparison of the effects of yohimbine on blood pressure between the healthy subjects and the schizophrenic patients revealed a group and drug and time interaction for sitting systolic blood pressure that tended toward significance ($F = 2.2$, $P = 0.06$). The increase in sitting systolic blood pressure following yohimbine in comparison to placebo tended to be significantly greater at 90 min in the patients. Figure 6–3 illustrates the yohimbine-placebo increase in sitting systolic blood pressure at 90 min in the healthy subjects and each of the diagnostic groups.

Clonidine Challenge

PLASMA MHPG

Intravenous clonidine produced modest decreases in plasma MHPG in healthy subjects. There was a significant drug and time interaction, and clonidine significantly decreased plasma MHPG levels at 60, 180, and 240 min

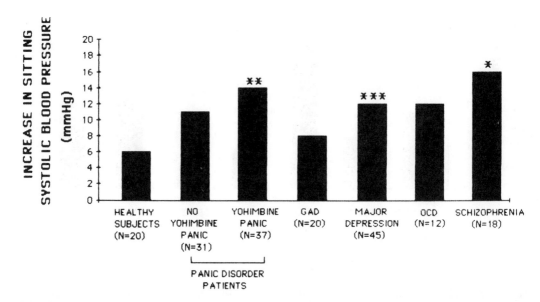

Fig. 6–3. Yohimbine-placebo increase from baseline in sitting systolic blood pressure 90 min following the dose. *P < 0.01 Schizophrenic patients vs. healthy subjects; Student's *t* test (two-tailed). **P < 0.05 PD patients reporting yohimbine-induced panic attacks vs. healthy subjects; Student's *t* test (two-tailed). ***P < 0.01 Depressed patients vs. healthy subjects; Student's *t* test (two-tailed).

after the dose compared to placebo. In the PD patients, clonidine produced greater decreases in plasma MHPG. As in the healthy subjects, there was a significant drug and time interaction, and, in comparison to placebo, clonidine significantly decreased plasma MHPG levels at all time points following drug administration. The ANOVA comparing the effects of clonidine on plasma MHPG in PD patients and healthy subjects revealed a significant interaction between group and drug and time (F = 4.7, P < 0.05). The clonidine-placebo decrease in plasma MHPG was significantly greater in the patients at 120 (−0.2 ± 0.1 vs. −0.7 ± 0.1, P < 0.05) and 240 (−0.4 ± 0.1 vs. −0.8 ± 0.1, P < 0.05) min after the dose.

The study of the effects of oral clonidine on plasma MHPG in depressed patients and healthy subjects revealed significant drug and time interactions, reflecting the ability of clonidine to lower plasma MHPG. The comparison of the two groups revealed a nonsignificant group and drug and time interaction. Of interest, after the administration of placebo, the increase in plasma MHPG levels in the healthy subjects was greater than the small de-

crease observed in the patients. In addition, the decrease in plasma MHPG levels in the patients after clonidine administration was significantly greater than the response to clonidine in the healthy subjects. However, clonidine-placebo decrease in plasma MHPG levels (mean of values at 180, 210, and 240 min) was 0.6 ng/ml in the healthy subjects and 0.8 ng/ml in the patients, a nonsignificant difference.

In the study of schizophrenic patients, there was a highly significant interaction of group and drug and time interaction (F = 13.9, P < 0.001) suggesting a different response of patients and healthy subjects to placebo and clonidine. Similar to the observation in the study of depressed patients, following placebo there was a significant increase in plasma MHPG levels in the healthy subjects, which was significantly different from the small decrease observed in the patients. In addition, there was a decrease in the healthy subjects following active clonidine that approached significance (P < 0.08), whereas the patients had no significant change in plasma MHPG following clonidine. The clonidine-placebo dif-

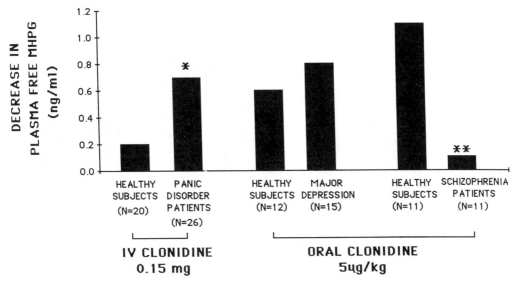

Fig. 6–4. Clonidine-placebo decrease from baseline in plasma free MHPG 120 min after the iv clonidine dose and the mean of values 180, 210, and 240 min after the oral clonidine dose. *$P < 0.05$ PD patients vs. healthy subjects; Student's *t* test (two-tailed). **$P < 0.001$ Schizophrenic patients vs. healthy subjects; Student's *t* test (two-tailed).

ference (mean of values at 180, 210, and 240 min) was significantly greater in the healthy subjects compared to the schizophrenic patients (-1.1 ± 0.8 vs. -0.1 ± 0.4, $P < 0.001$). Figure 6–4 illustrates the clonidine-placebo decreases in plasma MHPG in the healthy subjects and PD, depressed, and schizophrenic patients.

BLOOD PRESSURE

Intravenous clonidine robustly decreased blood pressure in healthy subjects. The ANOVA revealed highly significant drug and time interactions for all four blood pressure measurements. Clonidine, in comparison to placebo, produced significant mean decreases in sitting and standing systolic blood pressure at all time points measured, ranging from 11 to 18 mm Hg. Mean sitting and standing diastolic blood pressure was significantly decreased at almost all time points measured, with decreases ranging from 6 to 11 mm Hg.

In the patients, the iv clonidine produced significant decreases in blood pressure with significant drug and time interactions on all four measures. Clonidine, in comparison to placebo, produced significant mean decreases in sitting and standing systolic and diastolic pressures at all time points measured ranging from 8 to 22 mm Hg.

The comparison of the effect of iv clonidine on blood pressure between the two groups revealed a significant group and drug and time interaction for sitting diastolic ($F = 4.6$, $P < 0.05$) and standing diastolic ($F = 10.9$, $P < 0.01$) blood pressure and a trend toward a significant interaction for sitting systolic blood pressure ($F = 3.5$, $P < 0.07$). The decrease in sitting and standing diastolic blood pressure, respectively, following clonidine in comparison to placebo was significantly greater in the patients at 60 (-13 ± 2 vs. -7 ± 2, $P < 0.05$; -16 ± 2 vs. -8 ± 2, $P < 0.01$) and 90 (-11 ± 2 vs. -4 ± 3, $P < 0.05$; -15 ± 2 vs. -6 ± 2, $P < 0.01$) min after the dose. In addition, the decrease in standing diastolic blood pressure was larger at 30 (-16 ± 2 vs. -11 ± 2, $P < 0.05$) and 240 (-13 ± 2 vs. -7 ± 2, $P < 0.05$) min in the patients.

Oral clonidine produced significant decreases in both systolic and diastolic blood pressures in the healthy subjects and patients with major depression. However, the ANOVAs of the blood pressure data indicated no significant group and drug and time interaction

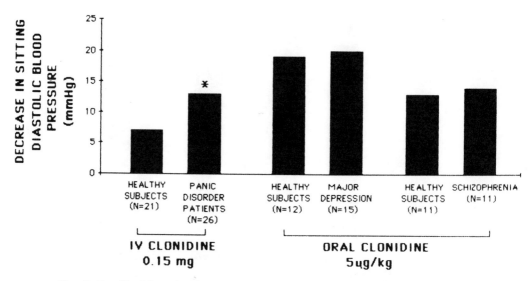

Fig. 6–5. Clonidine-placebo decrease from baseline in sitting diastolic blood pressure 120 min after the iv and oral clonidine doses. *$P < 0.05$ PD patients vs. healthy subjects; Student's t test (two-tailed).

for systolic or diastolic blood pressures, and at no time point was the clonidine-placebo decreases in blood pressure significantly different between the healthy subjects and depressed patients. Similarly, in the schizophrenia study, clonidine produced significant decreases in systolic and diastolic blood pressure in both the patient and healthy subject groups. The ANOVA of the blood pressure data demonstrated no significant group and drug and time interactions, and the magnitude of the clonidine-induced decreases in blood pressure was not different between the two groups at any time point. Figure 6–5 illustrates the clonidine-placebo decreases in sitting diastolic blood pressure in the healthy subjects and PD, depressed, and schizophrenic patients.

DISCUSSION

The strongest findings to emerge from this series of investigations of the effects of yohimbine and clonidine were among the PD patients. The enhanced responses to both yohimbine and clonidine suggest that the pathophysiology of PD may be related in some patients to abnormal regulation of the noradrenergic neuronal system. The increased anxiogenic, plasma MHPG, and cardiovascular re-

sponses to yohimbine in a subgroup of PD patients are supportive of the hypothesis relating anxiety development to noradrenergic neuronal hyperactivity.

Noradrenergic Hyperactivity Hypothesis of Anxiety

The noradrenergic hyperactivity hypothesis of anxiety, development of which has been extensively reviewed elsewhere, is based on preclinical, neuroanatomic, neurophysiologic, pharmacologic, and behavioral investigations (Charney et al., 1984a, 1987a; Jacobs, 1986; Jacobs et al., 1987; Redmond, 1979). These studies provide a basis for relating abnormally high levels of noradrenergic neuronal activity to the behavioral expression of anxiety and fear and the somatic symptoms and cardiovascular alterations that accompany severe anxiety states.

A variety of clinical investigations have provided preliminary support for this hypothesis. Increased levels of urine and plasma norepinephrine and epinephrine and their metabolites have been reported for healthy subjects following emotional stress (Breggin, 1964; Buchsbaum et al., 1981; Lader, 1974). The symptoms associated with withdrawal syndromes of opiate abstinence and abrupt tricyclic antidepressant discontinuation include the symptoms of anxiety and have been associated with increases in the norepinephrine metabolite MHPG in plasma (Charney et al., 1982c, 1984b). In depressed patients, a significant positive correlation has been identified between rated anxiety and cereprospinal fluid (CSF) levels of norepinephrine and MHPG (Post et al., 1978; Redmond et al., 1986) and changes in state of anxiety and urinary MHPG levels (Sweeney et al., 1978). Patients meeting concurrent diagnostic criteria for major depression and PD have been shown to have elevations of urinary MHPG excretion in comparison to patients with major depression only (Garvey et al., 1987). Yohimbine and piperoxane, drugs that increase brain norepinephrine turnover by antagonizing alpha-2-adrenergic autoreceptors, have been shown to produce anxiety states in healthy subjects and, in the case of yohimbine, increased plasma MHPG levels (Charney et al., 1982a; Holmberg and Gershon, 1961; Soffer, 1954).

Relatively few studies have been designed to investigate noradrenergic function in patients with anxiety disorders defined by specific diagnostic criteria. Plasma epinephrine and norepinephrine have been reported to be elevated in patients meeting DSM II criteria for anxiety neurosis and DSM III criteria for PD (Cameron et al., 1984; Wyatt et al., 1971). The effects of iv adrenaline, norepinephrine, epinephrine, and the beta-adrenergic receptor agonist isoproterenol have also been studied in patients with anxiety syndromes, but these studies are difficult to interpret because these agents fail to penetrate the brain (Harbedo and Owman, 1980; MacKenzie et al., 1976; Minneman, 1983).

Effects of Yohimbine in PD

In the reported investigation, yohimbine produced panic attacks in approximately 54% of the patients, and the symptoms reported were similar to their naturally occurring attacks. There is considerable preclinical evidence that this anxiogenic property of yohimbine is mediated via its ability to increase noradrenergic activity by antagonizing the alpha-2-adrenoceptor (Charney et al., 1984a; Goldberg and Robertson, 1983; Pellow et al., 1985; Redmond, 1979). The finding that pa-

tients who experienced yohimbine-induced panic attacks had significantly higher baseline MHPG levels (see Charney et al., 1987a) and greater plasma-free MHPG rises following yohimbine than either the healthy subjects or the patients who did not experience panic attacks supports the hypothesis developed from preclinical studies that relate increased presynaptic brain noradrenergic activity to the development of panic anxiety. Also supportive of this hypothesis was the observation of a significant correlation between the yohimbine-induced increase in plasma MHPG and anxiety.

The complex fashion in which the brain noradrenergic system is regulated suggests that dysfunction at many sites may result in the abnormally increased presynaptic neuronal function observed in the patients who experienced panic attacks. For example, noradrenergic neurons, such as those of the locus ceruleus, are regulated not only by the alpha-2-adrenoceptor but also by other neuronal systems, including benzodiazepine receptors, endogenous opiates, serotonin, acetylcholine, gamma-aminobutyric acid (GABA), epinephrine, CRF, and substance P (Andrade and Aghajanian, 1982, 1985; Bird and Kuhar, 1977; Cedarbaum and Aghajanian, 1976; Foote et al., 1983; Grant et al., 1980, 1984; Guyenet and Aghajanian, 1977, 1979; Segal, 1979; Starke et al., 1975). Abnormal regulation of noradrenergic systems by one or a number of these systems could account for the enhanced ability of yohimbine to raise plasma MHPG levels. Reduced alpha-2-adrenoceptor sensitivity, increased activity of excitatory inputs (e.g., CRF, cholinergic, or substance P), or decreased activity of inhibitory inputs (e.g., opiate, GABA, serotonin, epinephrine) may result in greater increases in noradrenergic neuronal impulse flow, norepinephrine release, and consequently increased norepinephrine turnover by yohimbine.

The mechanism responsible for the excessive anxiety produced by yohimbine in the patients may depend on the increased stimulation of alpha-1- and beta-adrenergic postsynaptic receptors by norepinephrine in a variety of brain regions and the peripheral nervous system. It is possible that the direct blockade of the postsynaptic alpha-2-adrenoceptor by yohimbine also relates to yohimbine's anxiogenic properties (Charney et al., 1984a; Foote et al., 1983; Moore and Bloom, 1979; Unnerstall et al., 1984).

These findings have led to a conceptual model relating episodically increased presynaptic noradrenergic neuronal function to the development of both spontaneous and phobic stimulus-induced panic attacks. Spontaneous attacks may result from the inability of the alpha-2-adrenoceptor and other neuronal inputs properly to regulate normal fluctuations in noradrenergic neuronal activity that may occur in response to mild, nonnoxious stimuli of many kinds (Foote et al., 1980, 1983). The phobic stimulus-induced panic attacks may result from increased norepinephrine neuronal activity and norepinephrine release that occurs following stress (Glavin, 1985). Under normal conditions, increased norepinephrine release would feed back to decrease neuronal activity by stimulating the inhibitory alpha-2-adrenoceptor. However, this mechanism could be impaired in patients with decreased activity of this receptor, thereby producing a prolonged state of noradrenergic hyperactivity and panic anxiety.

The effects of yohimbine on blood pressure provide a less specific index of noradrenergic function than the MHPG response. The ability of yohimbine to increase blood pressure may be due to either pre- or postsynaptic effects or the relative balance between the two. There is considerable preclinical data that norepinephrine has stimulatory effects on blood pressure. On the other hand, there is also evidence that postsynaptic alpha-2-adrenoceptors have inhibitory actions on blood pressure regulation and cortisol secretion (Bousquet and Schwartz, 1983; Kobinger, 1984; Kubo and Yoshimi, 1981; Tung et al., 1983). The ability of yohimbine to produce greater increases in blood pressure in the PD patients may be due to increased norepinephrine release by yohimbine, causing increased blood pressure. However, this explanation is not supported by the lack of correlation among changes in blood pressure and MHPG levels. It is also not consistent with the observation that, in comparison to healthy subjects, significantly greater yohimbine-placebo increases in blood pressure were also seen in the patients who did not ex-

perience yohimbine-induced panic attacks and who did not have increased yohimbine-induced rises in MHPG. An alternative hypothesis is that the enhanced blood pressure of yohimbine in the patients is due to a subsensitivity of postsynaptic alpha-2-adrenoceptors or the regulation of these receptors by other neuronal systems.

Abnormal Regulation of Noradrenergic Activity in PD

The abnormal responses to clonidine in the PD patients were, in general, opposite those caused by yohimbine. Interpretation of the combined results of these investigations must be made with caution, because they were conducted with separate patient populations. It is possible that the abnormalities in noradrenergic function observed are identifying distinct neurobiological subgroups of patients and not a regulatory disturbance common to most patients with PD. Additional studies with both drugs should be conducted in the same population of patients.

The increased and decreased norepinephrine turnover that followed yohimbine and clonidine administration, respectively, in the patients with PD raises the possibility that the noradrenergic system is markedly dysregulated such that the gain of the system is augmented. Inputs that act either to increase or to decrease noradrenergic activity are both amplified. Interpretations of the greater clonidine-induced decrease in plasma MHPG levels in PD patients include increased functional sensitivity of the alpha-2-adrenoceptor, decreased activity of excitatory inputs, and increased activity of inhibitory inputs. However, these mechanisms are inconsistent with the findings that yohimbine produces larger increases in plasma MHPG levels in patients with frequent panic attacks. As was discussed above, reduced rather than increased alpha-2-adrenoceptor functional sensitivity, increased rather than decreased excitatory inputs, and decreased rather than increased inhibitory inputs are consistent with the observed yohimbine effects in PD patients. Therefore, if individual patients are found to have abnormal clonidine and yohimbine MHPG responses, the results of these investigations using yohimbine and clonidine to assess the regulation of noradrenergic activity are difficult to interpret simply in terms of abnormalities in the alpha-2-adrenoceptor or regulatory inputs to the noradrenergic neuronal system.

Abnormal regulation of noradrenergic activity in PD patients may be related to abnormalities in the coupling of alpha-2-adrenoceptor to effector systems located intracellularly that mediate the biological actions produced by receptor activation or antagonism. Activation of the alpha-2-adrenoceptor produces a hyperpolarization of noradrenergic neurons through an increase in potassium conductance (Aghajanian, 1984; Aghajanian and Vander Maelen, 1982; Andrade and Aghajanian, 1984). This results in an inhibition of intracellular adenylate cyclase, a decrease in the levels of the second messenger cyclic adenosine monophosphate (cAMP) (Andrade and Aghajanian, 1985; Kahn et al., 1982; Lefkowitz et al., 1984; Rouot et al., 1980), and consequently a reduction in cAMP-dependent protein phosphorylation (Nestler and Greengard, 1984). Abnormalities in the receptor-effector coupling mechanisms have recently been identified in other disease states, including changes in thyroid or adrenal status, pseudohypoparathyroidism (Lefkowitz et al., 1984), and possibly anorexia nervosa and bulimia (Heufelder et al., 1985). For example, the defect in pseudohypoparathyroidism is due not to an alteration in the beta-receptor but rather to a genetic deficiency of the regulatory protein (Farfel et al., 1980; Heinsimer et al., 1980; Levine et al., 1980).

Similar to the clonidine- and yohimbine-induced changes in plasma MHPG levels, the greater clonidine-induced decreases in blood pressure in a subgroup of PD patients contrasts with the previous finding that yohimbine produced greater increases in blood pressure. As with the regulation of norepinephrine turnover, it is possible that the site of this dysfunction is not the alpha-2-adrenoceptor but is rather at the level of the receptor-effector coupling mechanisms.

Investigations are now needed to elucidate the specific mechanisms that mediate an abnormal regulation of noradrenergic function in PD. Future studies should be designed to evaluate the possible abnormalities in regulatory inputs to noradrenergic neurons, receptor-effector coupling mechanisms, and intracellular

effector systems (Charney and Heninger, 1986; Heufelder et al., 1985; Kafka and Paul, 1986; Lefkowitz et al., 1984; Nestler and Greengard, 1984).

Effects of Yohimbine and Clonidine in Other Psychiatric Disorders

The potentiated responses to clonidine and yohimbine contrast with many of the effects of these drugs in patients with GAD, major depression, OCD, and schizophrenia. The responses to yohimbine in the GAD patients were particularly distinguished from those of the PD patients. These observations support the distinction made between these two disorders. Understanding the relevance of the reduced magnitude of the yohimbine-induced increase in MHPG in the GAD patients will require further investigation.

The lack of clear differences between depressed patients and healthy subjects in the yohimbine-induced increases in plasma MHPG and the clonidine-induced decreases in plasma MHPG as well as the lack of behavioral responses to yohimbine in the depressed patients suggest that the alpha-2-adrenoceptor may not be markedly abnormal in major depression. The comparison of PD patients and the depressed patients clearly reveal that the PD patients are more responsive to yohimbine in terms of their behavioral and MHPG responses. The groups were similar in regard to the cardiovascular effects of yohimbine. A previous study by Siever et al. (1984) using iv clonidine showed that the clonidine-induced decreases in plasma MHPG and heart rate were reduced in depressed patients compared to healthy subjects. These findings suggest a subsensitive rather than a supersensitive alpha-2-adrenoceptor, which has been most frequently hypothesized, and are opposite to the findings in PD patients.

It should be noted that there is considerable clinical data suggesting that postsynaptic alpha-2-adrenoceptors are subsensitive in the depressed patients. The growth hormone response to clonidine is dependent on postsynaptic alpha-2-adrenoceptors, and the growth hormone response to clonidine has repeatedly been shown to be blunted in depression (Siever et al., 1982; Unnerstall et al., 1984). The specificity of this response for major depression, however, remains in question because a blunted growth hormone response to clonidine has also been observed in PD and OCD patients (Charney and Heninger, 1986; Siever, et al., 1983).

The overall behavioral response of OCD patients to oral yohimbine was similar to that of healthy subjects, and no consistent effects on obsessive–compulsive symptoms were observed. In addition, the normal MHPG response to yohimbine in OCD patients suggests that this disorder does not involve abnormal alpha-2-adrenoceptor regulation of noradrenergic activity. It is likely that other neuronal systems, such as the serotonin and dopamine systems, are involved more in the pathophysiology of OCD.

A subgroup of schizophrenic patients appeared to respond differently to yohimbine than healthy subjects. Six patients were noticeably activated about 60 min after the yohimbine dose. However, this subgroup did not demonstrate significantly increased MHPG or blood pressure responses to yohimbine compared to the other patients or healthy subjects. The total schizophrenic group had a trend toward significantly greater increases in blood pressure and MHPG levels following yohimbine compared to the healthy subjects. These findings are consistent with the observations of schizophrenic patients following clonidine administration. The absence of a clonidine-induced decrease in plasma MHPG in the schizophrenic patients supports the hypothesis that some schiozophrenic patients have decreased functioning of presynaptic alpha-2-adrenoceptors. The results of the clonidine and yohimbine studies in schizophrenia must be considered in the context of previous studies of noradrenergic function in schizophrenia. A critical review of such studies is beyond the scope of this report, but it is of interest to note that several investigators have reported increased norepinephrine levels in postmortem brain, CSF, and plasma of drug-free schizophrenic patients (van Kammen and Antelman, 1984). The clinical relevance of the observation that a subgroup of schizophrenics with abnormally increased noradrenergic function may exist needs investigation. For example, clonidine treatment may be a particularly effective therapeutic approach in such patients (Freedman et al., 1982).

In summary, the findings of the series of investigations reported above suggests that abnormal regulation of brain noradrenergic activity may have greater etiological significance in panic disorders than in other psychiatric syndromes. However, the site and specific pathophysiological mechanism underlying this dysfunction remains to be established. Recent methodological advances have brought the study of noradrenergic function to the molecular level as well as to the living brain in vivo. Future studies should focus on positron emission tomography brain imaging following administration of noradrenergic system probes, evaluation of receptor-effector coupling mechanisms, and genetic encoding of noradrenergic neuronal function.

ACKNOWLEDGMENTS

These studies were supported in part by Public Health Service grants MH-25642, MH-36229, MH-38007, MH-30929, and MH-40140 and by the State of Connecticut. M. Fasula, B. Aiken, D. Mordowanec, R. Fleischmann, R. Terwilliger, R. Reynolds, S. Giddings, R. Sturwald, C. Hill, L. Quadrino, and E. Testa of the Ribicoff Research Facilities provided expert technical assistance.

REFERENCES

Aghajanian GK (1978): Tolerance of locus coeruleus neurons to morphine and suppression of withdrawal response by clonidine. Nature 276:186–188.

Aghajanian GK (1984): The physiology of central α- and β-adrenoceptors. In Usdin E, Carlsson A, Dahlström A, Engel J (eds): "Catecholamines, Part B: Neuropharmacology and Central Nervous System—Theoretical Aspects." New York: Alan R. Liss, Inc., pp 85–92.

Aghajanian GK, Vander Maelen CP (1982): α_2-Adrenoceptor-mediated hyperpolarization of locus coeruleus neurons: Intracellular studies in vivo. Science 215:1394–1396.

Andrade R, Aghajanian GK (1982): Single cell activity in the noradrenergic A-5 region: Responses to drugs and peripheral manipulations of blood pressure. Brain Res 242:125–135.

Andrade R, Aghajanian GK (1984): Locus coeruleus activity in vitro: Intrinsic regulation by a calcium-dependent potassium conductance but not α_2-adrenoceptors. J Neurosci 4:161–170.

Andrade R, Aghajanian GK (1985): Opiate- and α_2-adrenoceptor-induced hyperpolarizations of locus ceruleus neurons in brain slices: Reversal by cyclic adenosine 3':5'-monophosphate analogues. J Neurosci 5:2359–2364.

Bird SJ, Kuhar MJ (1977): Iontophoretic application of opiates to the locus coeruleus. Brain Res 122:523–533.

Bousquet P, Schwartz J (1983): Commentary: Alpha-adrenergic drugs: Pharmacological tools for the study of the central vasomotor control. Biochem Pharmacol 32:1459–1465.

Breggin PR (1964): The psychophysiology of anxiety: With a review of literature concerning adrenaline. J Nervous Mental Dis 109:558–568.

Buchsbaum MS, Muscettola G, Goodwin FK (1981): Urinary MHPG, stress response, personality factors and somatosensory evoked potentials in normal subjects and patients with major affective disorders. Neuropsychobiology 7:212–220.

Cameron OG, Smith CB, Hollingsworth PJ, Nesse RM, Curtis GC (1984): Platelet α_2-adrenergic receptor binding and plasma catecholamines: Before and during imipramine treatment in patients with panic anxiety. Arch Gen Psychiatry 41:1144–1148.

Cedarbaum JM, Aghajanian GK (1976): Noradrenergic neurons of the locus coeruleus: Inhibition by epinephrine and activation by the alpha-antagonist piperoxane. Brain Res 112:413–419.

Cedarbaum JM, Aghajanian GK (1977): Catecholamine receptors on locus coeruleus neurons: Pharmacological characterization. Eur J Pharmacol 44:375–385.

Charney DS, Heninger GR, Sternberg DE (1982a): Assessment of alpha-2 adrenergic autoreceptor function in humans: Effects of oral yohimbine. Life Sci 30:2033–2041.

Charney DS, Heninger GR, Sternberg DE, Hafstad KM, Giddings S, Landis DH (1982b): Adrenergic receptor sensitivity in depression: Effects of clonidine in depressed patients and healthy subjects. Arch Gen Psychiatry 39:290–294.

Charney DS, Heninger GR, Sternberg DE, Landis DH (1982c): Abrupt discontinuation of tricyclic antidepressant drugs: Evidence for noradrenergic hyperactivity. Br J Psychiatry 141:377–386.

Charney DS, Heninger GR, Breier A (1984a): Noradrenergic function in panic anxiety: Effects of yohimbine in healthy subjects and patients with agoraphobia and panic disorder. Arch Gen Psychiatry 41:751–763.

Charney DS, Heninger GR (1986): Abnormal regulation of noradrenergic function in panic disorders: Effects of clonidine in healthy subjects and patients with agoraphobia and panic disorder. Arch Gen Psychiatry 43:1042–1054.

Charney DS, Redmond DE Jr, Galloway MP, Kleber HD, Heninger GR, Murberg M, Roth RH (1984b): Naltrexone precipitated opiate withdrawal in methadone addicted human subjects: Evidence for noradrenergic hyperactivity. Life Sci 35:1263–1272.

Charney DS, Woods SW, Goodman WK, Heninger GR (1987a): Neurobiological mechanisms of panic anxiety: Biochemical and behavioral correlates of yohimbine-induced panic attacks. Am J Psychiatry 144:1030–1036.

Charney DS, Woods SW, Heninger GR (1989): Noradren-

ergic function in Generalized Anxiety Disorder. Effects of yohimbine in healthy subjects and patients with generalized anxiety disorder. Psych Res 27:173–182.

Dekirmenjian H, Maas JW (1974): MHPG in plasma. Clin Chim Acta 52:203–208.

Farfel Z, Brickman AS, Kaslow HR, Brothers VM, Bourne HR (1980): Defect of receptor-cyclase coupling protein in pseudohypoparathyroidism. N Engl J Med 303:237–242.

Foote SL, Aston-Jones G, Bloom FE (1980): Impulse activity of locus coeruleus neurons in awake rats and monkeys is a function of sensory stimulation and arousal. Proc Natl Acad Sci USA 77:3033–3037.

Foote SL, Bloom FE, Aston-Jones G (1983): Nucleus locus coeruleus: New evidence of anatomical and physiological specificity. Physiol Rev 63:844–914.

Freedman R, Kirch D, Bell J, Adler L, Pecevich M, Pachtman E, Denver P (1982): Clonidine treatment of schizophrenia. Acta Psychiatrica Scand 65:35–45.

Garvey MJ, Tollefson GD, Orsulak PJ (1987): Elevations of urinary MHPG in depressed patients with panic attacks. Psychiatry Res 20:183–188.

Glavin GB (1985): Stress and brain noradrenaline: A review. Neurosci Biobehav Rev 9:233–243.

Glazer WM, Charney DS, Heninger GR (1987): Noradrenergic function in schizophrenia. Arch Gen Psychiatry 44:898–904.

Goldberg MR, Robertson D (1983): Yohimbine: A pharmacological probe for study of the α_2-adrenoreceptor. Pharmacol Rev 35:143–180.

Grant SJ, Huang YH, Redmond DE Jr (1980): Benzodiazepines attenuate single unit activity in the locus coeruleus. Life Sci 27:2231–2236.

Grant SJ, Mayor R, Redmond DE Jr (1984): Effects of alprazolam, a novel triozolobenzodiazepine, on locus coeruleus unit activity. Soc Neurosci Abstr 10:952.

Guyenet PG, Aghajanian GK (1977): Excitation of neurons in the nucleus locus coeruleus by substance P and related peptides. Brain Res 136:178–184.

Guyenet PG, Aghajanian GK (1979): ACh, substance P and met-enkephalin in the locus coeruleus: Pharmacological evidence for independent sites of action. Eur J Pharmacol 53:319–328.

Harbedo JE, Owman C (1980): Barrier mechanisms for neurotransmitter monoamines and their precursors at the blood-brain interface. Ann Neurol 8:1–11.

Heinsimer JA, Davies AO, Downs RW (1980): Impaired formation of β-adrenergic receptor-nucleotide regulatory protein in erythrocytes from patients with pseudohypoparathyroidism. Biochem Biophys Res Commun 94:1319–1324.

Heninger GR, Charney DS, Price LH (1988): Alpha-2-adrenergic receptor sensitivity in depression: The plasma MHPG, behavioral, and cardiovascular responses to yohimbine. 45:718–726.

Heufelder A, Warnhoff M, Pirke KM (1985): Platelet β_2-adrenoceptor and adenylate cyclase in patients with anorexia nervosa and bulimia. J Clin Endocrinol Metab 61:1053–1060.

Holmberg G, Gershon S (1961): Autonomic and psychi-

104 Charney et al.

atric effects of yohimbine hydrochloride. Psychopharmacology 2:93–106.

Insel TR, Mueller EA, Gillin JC, Seiver LJ, Murphy DL (1984): Biological markers in obsessive-compulsive and affective disorders. J Psychiatr Res 4:407–423.

Jacobs BL (1986): Single unit activity of locus coeruleus neurons in behaving animals. Prog Neurobiol 27:183–194.

Jacobs BL, Abercrombie ED, Morilak DA, Fornal CA (1987): Brain norepinephrine and stress: Single unit studies of locus coeruleus neurons in behaving animals. IV Int Symp Proc Catecholamines Stress (in press).

Kafka MS, Paul SM (1986): Platelet α_2-adrenergic receptors in depression. Arch Gen Psychiatry 43:91–95.

Kahn DJ, Mitrius JC, U'Prichard DC (1982): Alpha$_2$-adrenergic receptors in neuroblastoma X glioma hybrid cells: Characterization with agonist and antagonist radioligands and relationship to adenylate cyclase. Mol Pharmacol 21:17–26.

Kobinger W (1984): α-adrenoceptors in cardiovascular regulation. In Ziegler MG, Lake CR (eds): "Norepinephrine." Baltimore: Williams & Willkins, pp 307–326.

Kubo T, Yoshimi M (1981): Pharmacological characterization of the α-adrenoceptors responsible for a decrease of blood pressure in the nucleus tractus solitarii of the rat. Arch Pharmacol 317:120–125.

Lader M (1974): The peripheral and central role of the catecholamines in the mechanism of anxiety. Int Pharmacopsychiatry 9:125–137.

Lefkowitz RJ, Caron MG, Stiles GL (1984): Mechanisms of membrane-receptor regulation: Biochemical, physiological, and clinical insights derived from studies of the adrenergic receptors. N Engl J Med 310:1570–1579.

Levine MA, Downs RW Jr, Singer M, Marx SJ, Aurbach GD, Spiegel AM (1980): Deficient activity of guanine nucleotide regulatory protein in erythrocytes from patients with pseudohypoparathyroidism. Biochem Biophys Res Commun 94:1319–1324.

Maas JW, Hattox SE, Roth RH (1976): The determination of a brain arteriovenous difference for 3-methoxy-4-hydroxyphenylethyleneglycol (MHPG). Brain Res 118:167–174.

MacKenzie ET, McCulloch J, O'Keane M, Pickard JD, Harper AM (1976): Cerebral circulation and norepinephrine: Relevance of the blood-brain barrier. Am J Physiol 231:483–488.

Minneman KP (1983): Peripheral catecholamine administration does not alter cerebral β-adrenergic receptor density. Brain Res 264:328–331.

Moore RY, Bloom FE (1979): Central catecholamine neuron systems: Anatomy and physiology of the norepinephrine and epinephrine systems. Annu Rev Neurosci 2:113–168.

Nestler EJ, Greengard P (1984): "Protein Phosphorylation in the Nervous System." New York: John Wiley & Sons Inc.

Pellow S, Chopin P, File SE (1985): Are the anxiogenic effects of yohimbine mediated by its action at benzodiazepine receptors? Neurosci Lett 55:5–9.

Post RM, Lake CR, Jimerson DC, Bunny WE, Wood JH,

Ziegler MG, Goodwin FK (1978): CSF norepinephrine in affective illness. Am J Psychiatry 135:907–912.

Price LH, Charney DS, Rubin AL, Heninger GR (1986): Alpha-2 adrenergic receptor function in depression: The cortisol response to yohimbine. Arch Gen Psychiatry 43:849–858.

Rasmussen SA, Goodman WK, Woods SW, Heninger GR, Charney DS (1987): Effects of yohimbine in Obsessive-Compulsive Disorder. Psychopharmacology 93:308–313.

Redmond DE Jr (1979): New and old evidence for the involvement of a brain norepinephrine system in anxiety. In Fann WE (ed): "The Phenomenology and Treatment of Anxiety." New York: Spectrum Press, pp 153–203.

Redmond DE Jr, Katz MM, Maas JW, Swann A, Casper R, Davis JM (1986): Cerebrospinal fluid amine metabolites: Relationships with behavioral measurements in depressed, manic, and healthy control subjects. Arch Gen Psychiatry 43:938–948.

Rouot BR, U'Prichard DC, Snyder SH (1980): Multiple alpha-2 noradrenergic receptor sites in rat brain: Selective regulation of high affinity [^{3}H]clonidine binding by guanine nucleotides and divalent cations. J Neurochem 34:374–384.

Segal M (1979): Serotonergic innervation of the locus coeruleus from the dorsal raphe and its action on responses to noxious stimuli. J Physiol 286:401–415.

Siever LJ, Davis KL (1985): Overview: toward a dysregulation hypothesis of depression. Am J Psychiatry 142:1017–1031.

Siever LJ, Insel TR, Jimerson DC, Lake CR, Uhde TW, Aloi J, Murphy DL (1983): Growth hormone response to clonidine in obsessive-compulsive patients. Br J Psychiatry 142:184–187.

Siever LJ, Uhde TW, Jimerson DC (1984): Differential inhibitory noradrenergic responses to clonidine in 25 depressed patients and 24 normal control subjects. Am J Psychiatry 141:733–741.

Siever LJ, Uhde TW, Silberman EK, Jimerson DC, Aloi JA, Post RM, Murphy DL (1982): The growth hormone response to clonidine as a probe of noradrenergic receptor responsiveness in affective disorder patients and controls. Psychiatr Res 6:171–183.

Soffer A (1954): Regatine and benadine in the diagnoses of pheochromocytoma. Med Clin North Am 38:375–384.

Starke K, Borowski E, Endo T (1975): Preferential blockade of presynaptic α-adrenoceptors by yohimbine. Eur J Pharmacol 34:385–388.

Sternberg DE, Charney DS, Heninger GR, Leckman JF, Hafstad KM, Landis DH (1982): Impaired presynaptic regulation of norepinephrine in schizophrenia: Effects of clonidine in schizophrenic patients and normal controls. Arch Gen Psychiatry 39:285–289.

Sweeney DR, Maas JW, Heninger GR (1978): State anxiety and urinary MHPG. Arch Gen Psychiatry 35:1418–1423.

Tung CS, Onuora CO, Robertson D, Goldberg MR (1983): Hypertensive effect of yohimbine following selective injection into the nucleus tractus solitarii of normotensive rats. Brain Res 277:193–195.

Unnerstall JR, Kopajtic TA, Kuhar MJ (1984): Distribution of α_2 agonist binding sites in the rat and human central nervous system: Analysis of some functional, anatomic correlates of the pharmacologic effects of clonidine and related adrenergic agents. Brain Res Rev 7:69–101.

van Kammen DP, Antelman S (1984): Minireview. Im-

paired noradrenergic transmission in schizophrenia? Life Sci 34:1403–1413.

Wyatt RJ, Portnoy B, Kupfer DJ, Snyder F, Engelman K (1971): Resting catecholamine concentrations in patients with depression and anxiety. Arch Gen Psychiatry 24:65–70.

7

Isoproterenol-Induced Panic: A Beta-Adrenergic Model of Panic Anxiety

ROBERT POHL, MD, **VIKRAM YERAGANI,** MD, **RICHARD BALON,** MD, **AURELIO ORTIZ,** MD, PhD, AND **ASAF ALEEM,** MD

Department of Psychiatry, Wayne State University, Detroit, Michigan 48207 (R.P., V.Y., R.B., A.O., A.A.); Lafayette Clinic, Detroit, Michigan 48207 (R.P., V.Y., R.B., A.O.); Veterans Administration Hospital, Allen Park, Michigan 48101 (A.A.)

INTRODUCTION

Catecholamines have long been implicated in the pathophysiology of anxiety. Cannon (1915) demonstrated early in this century that the intense behavioral displays associated with fear and rage in cats were associated with tachycardia, pupillary dilatation, piloerection, and decreased visceral activity. These symptoms were associated with release of epinephrine from the adrenals and could be reproduced by the intravenous administration of epinephrine. In man, epinephrine has been reported to reproduce the symptoms of "irritable heart," a syndromic diagnosis used by cardiologists of that era to describe a heterogeneous group of patients with functional cardiac symptoms and anxiety (Wearn and Sturgis, 1919). Subcutaneous injections of epinephrine have been reported to produce "cold" anxiety in many individuals, "as if" they felt afraid. However, it was noted at the same time that some patients experienced intense emotional states that were characterized by anxiety, crying, sobbing, and sighing. Individuals with this "second-degree" reaction were predisposed by hyperthyroidism, emotional instability, psychoneurosis, or excitement (Maranon, 1924).

Epinephrine injections provoked anxiety attacks in patients with a history of an anxiety disorder but did not provoke attacks in subjects with other psychiatric disorders (Lindemann, 1935; Lindemann and Finesinger, 1938). Norepinephrine has also been reported to induce anxiety attacks in panic disorder patients (Pyke and Greenberg, 1986).

Plasma epinephrine is released from the adrenal medulla, plasma norepinephrine from sympathetic nerve endings. Plasma norepinephrine levels are usually too low to be physiologically significant (Kopin, 1984). Although catecholamine release, especially epinephrine release, is associated with acute anxiety, catecholamines can be released under a variety of mundane circumstances. These include postural changes, anticipation of exertion, mental concentration, public speaking, coffee ingestion, and smoking. Stress increases catecholamine output in normal people (Levi, 1972), but catecholamine levels in generalized anxiety disorder patients and controls are similar (Mathew et al., 1982). These findings suggest that catecholamine levels per se have no casual relationship to anxiety as an illness and that the sensitivity of anxiety patients to catecholamines (Lindemann and Finesinger, 1938) may reflect a psychological or physiological sensitivity that is characteristic of the illness.

The relationship of epinephrine, a mixed alpha- and beta-adrenergic agonist, to anxiety suggests that the beta-receptor may play a role. In addition, the symptoms of a panic attack, namely, heart palpitations, shortness of breath,

Neurobiology of Panic Disorder, Pages 107–120

chest discomfort, choking, and tremulousness, point to the beta-adrenergic system. Isoproterenol, a sympathomimetic amine that acts almost exclusively on beta-receptors, can be used to study the response of anxiety disorder patients to beta-receptor stimulation. Frohlich et al. (1969) found that nine of fourteen patients with a history of anxiety symptoms developed intense anxiety states ("hysterical outbursts") during infusions of 2–3 µg/min isoproterenol, a dosage that did not affect normal subjects. Easton and Sherman (1976) found that 0.5–2.6 µg/min isoproterenol produced anxiety states in five subjects with a history of panic attacks. In both studies, the anxiety states quickly subsided after iv injections of 10 mg propranolol and 2–5 mg propranolol, respectively. Schmidt and Elizabeth (1982) also reported that patients with DSM III diagnosed panic disorder reporting to an emergency room experienced panic attacks and tachycardia during isoproterenol infusions.

Previous reports from this laboratory have suggested that isoproterenol provokes panic attacks more often in panic disorder patients than in control subjects and that isoproterenol and lactate attacks resembled spontaneously occurring panic attacks equally often (Rainey et al., 1984a,b). This chapter reviews recent findings with isoproterenol as a provocative agent for inducing panic attacks in the laboratory. In addition, we attempt to relate a beta-receptor model of anxiety to other provocative infusions and to the pharmacotherapy of anxiety disorders.

ISOPROTERENOL INFUSIONS

Methods

Subjects were between 18 and 58 years of age and had taken no psychotropic medication from 2 weeks before the first infusion until after the infusion series was completed. All panic disorder patients met Research Diagnostic Criteria (RDC) (Spitzer et al., 1978) for panic disorder. Patients with bulimia and posttraumatic stress disorder met DSM III criteria for those disorders. All patients were actively symptomatic, and panic disorder patients averaged at least one panic attack weekly. The 45 control subjects had no personal history of panic disorder and no psychiatric history. All subjects were healthy, and all gave informed consent.

Isoproterenol was administered as part of a study of the effects of dextrose, isoproterenol, and sodium lactate infusions. Each infusion was administered through a 21-gauge butterfly needle placed in an arm vein. Infusions were administered double-blind, in random order, and at intervals of at least 1 week. Infusions were preceded by a 10 min slow drip of 5% dextrose in sterile water (D5W). Sodium lactate was administered as a 1 M solution. The isoproterenol infusion solution consisted of 20 µg isoproterenol in D5W. During the infusion, the flow rate was adjusted by gravity feed to deliver 6 ml/kg over 20 min.

Patients were rated just prior to the start of the infusion and then every 2 min during the infusion with a panic description scale (PDS). This 21-item scale (Rainey et al., 1984a) includes all the RDC criteria for panic. Patients rate each item on a five-point scale, as not present, mild, moderate, severe, or very severe. Only 18 of the 21 items are included in the scoring; two items ("paralyzed" and "going blind") are not RDC symptoms of anxiety, and another ("feeling generally nervous") was used to help the rating investigator evaluate the patient's overall anxiety level.

RDC criteria were used to identify panic attacks during the infusions, with each symptom counted only if it increased from baseline values. To meet criteria for panic, patients had to develop at least four symptoms or have an increase in the severity of symptoms present just prior to the infusion. An increase in subjective apprehension or fear was also required, and the anxiety had to be of at least moderate intensity. Infusions were stopped as soon as it was established that the patient met criteria for a panic attack. Panic disorder subjects who panicked were then asked to rate the similarity and severity of their panic attacks relative to their usual attacks. The severity rating was identical to the severity rating used for items in the PDS. For similarity, patients were asked to respond with not similar, somewhat similar, moderately similar, very similar, or identical.

Isoproterenol was administered at a fixed rate (1 µg/min) that did not take into account differences in weight. To account for differences in weight, isoproterenol dosage is fre-

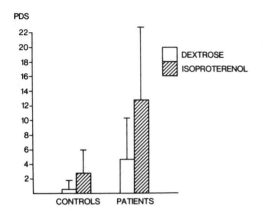

Fig. 7–1. Comparison of all controls (n = 42) and patients (n = 80) who gave complete data for the panic description scale (PDS). Each bar represents the difference between the peak score and the preinfusion baseline score (delta PDS) for either dextrose or isoproterenol infusions.

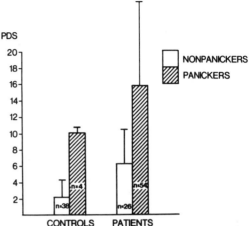

Fig. 7–2. Comparison of subjects who panic during isoproterenol infusions with those who do not. Each bar represents the difference between the peak score and the preinfusion baseline score (delta PDS) for isoproterenol infusions.

quently reported as the amount of isoproterenol administered per minute per kilogram. Variance in rates of administration per kilogram between subjects was largely the result of differences in subject weight; there was a high correlation between weight and the rate of isoproterenol administration per kilogram (r = 0.831, P < 0.01).

Isoproterenol Infusions in Panic Disorder Patients and Controls

PATIENTS VS. CONTROLS

Eighty-six panic disorder patients and 45 controls were infused with isoproterenol; there was no significant difference in either age or rate of isoproterenol administered per kilogram between these two groups (Pohl et al., 1988b). Sixty-six percent of the panic disorder patients panicked, compared to 9% of the controls, a significant difference (X^2 = 36.8, P < 0.001). The response of 80 patients and 42 controls with complete panic description scale (PDS) data can be seen in Figure 7–1. The *increase* in the PDS over baseline, or delta PDS, in patients as a group is more than four times the delta PDS in controls. This difference occurred in spite of the shorter duration of infusions in the panic disorder group (mean 12.9 min) compared to controls (mean 18.9 min). Panic disorder patients had shorter infusions

because the infusion was stopped when a panic attack occurred.

There was also a moderate increase in anxiety with dextrose infusions, although the delta PDS with isoproterenol was much greater (Fig. 7–1). This finding suggests that separate placebo infusions are a useful control condition for research in this group of patients.

PANICKERS VS. NONPANICKERS

The response of patients who panicked with isoproterenol can be compared to the patients who did not in Figure 7–2. Nonpanickers all received a full 20 min infusion; the panickers received an infusion that was on average less than half as long. The panic attacks experienced by patients were moderately intense. The mean delta PDS score was 15.9; this score was in addition to the baseline mean of 6.2 on the PDS. A subject who began the infusion without anxiety symptoms, and who developed eight symptoms during the infusion, would have to rate them all as moderate in intensity to achieve a PDS delta score of 16.

Patients were also asked to rate the global similarity and severity of the attacks to those of their usual episodes. The mean similarity rating for isoproterenol attacks was between "moderately" and "very much" like previous episodes. The attacks were rated on average as moderately severe. However, patients may have perceived the attacks as less severe because of the laboratory setting, which included the presence of physicians and nurses. Some patients spontaneously volunteered that they would have been much more anxious if the episode had occurred while they were alone.

PANIC ATTACKS IN CONTROLS

Normal controls have been known occasionally to experience panic attacks during lactate infusions (Ehlers et al., 1986; Fink et al., 1969; Kelly et al., 1971; Pitts and McClure, 1967). Four controls panicked with isoproterenol; none of the controls panicked with dextrose. The control attacks were somewhat less severe than the attacks experienced by patients (Fig. 7–2), possibly because the control attacks were a novel experience and easier to define because of the relative absence of baseline anxiety. The isoproterenol attacks in controls appeared qualitatively similar to those that occurred in patients. The most frequent symptoms during the attacks were feeling frightened or afraid, nervousness, heart pounding, chest pain or tightness, and feeling choked or smothered. Three of the four controls who panicked with isoproterenol also panicked with lactate, and seven patients panicked with lactate alone (Balon et al., 1988a,b).

EFFECTS OF SEX AND DOSE

Seventy-eight percent of the 50 female and 50% of the 36 male patients panicked, a significant difference between sexes (Pohl et al., 1988b). However, females weighed less than males and so had a higher rate of isoproterenol administration per kilogram. When 23 males were weight matched to 23 females, there was no longer any difference between sexes in either dosage per kilogram or in panic attack frequency.

The rate of isoproterenol administration per kilogram appeared to affect the frequency of panic (Pohl et al., 1988b). When the patients were split into low-, moderate-, and high-dosage groups, the group with the lowest dosage (8.2 ± 1.8 ng/min/kg) had a 55% rate of panic. Those with the highest dosage (18.5 ± 3.2 ng/min/kg) panicked 79% of the time, a rate well within the range usually achieved by sodium lactate infusions.

POSTTREATMENT REINFUSIONS OF ISOPROTERENOL

A second series of infusions after successful treatment with tricyclic antidepressants was also performed double-blind at intervals of at least 1 week in ten subjects. Reinfusions were randomly assigned a second time rather than given in the pretreatment sequence, since both the investigators and the patients were aware of the effects of each infusion from the pretreatment series.

The posttreatment rate of panic was similar to that experienced by controls. Seven of the ten patients had isoproterenol panic attacks before treatment, whereas only one had an attack after treatment (Pohl et al., 1985). This difference occurred even though the mean duration of infusions given after treatment was more than twice the duration before treatment.

PANIC ATTACKS ASSOCIATED WITH DEXTROSE INFUSIONS

Fourteen of the 86 panic disorder patients panicked during dextrose infusions, significantly fewer than the 57 who panicked with isoproterenol ($Z = 6.56$, $P < 0.01$). The dextrose attacks were of interest because they appeared to be "naturally" occurring episodes that were either spontaneous or related to the anxiogenic effects of the experimental setting. These "naturally" occurring episodes could then be compared to isoproterenol-associated episodes.

Nine patients experienced both isoproterenol and dextrose panic attacks, allowing for a within subject comparison. The mean PDS ratings for these patients just prior to the infusion and at the peak of their attack are shown in Figure 7–3. There is no significant difference between dextrose and isoproterenol either prior to the attack or at the peak of the PDS rating. Patients showed robust increases in anxiety ratings for both types of attack.

These nine patients were also asked to rate the similarity and severity of their laboratory attacks in comparison to their usual attacks. As can be seen in Figure 7–4, there is no significant difference between dextrose and isoproterenol attacks with these ratings. There was no trend for dextrose attacks to be rated as more similar to the patient's usual attack; isoproterenol attacks were, if anything, judged to

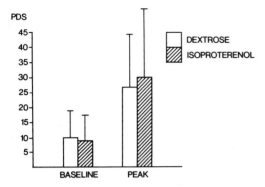

Fig. 7–3. Comparison of panic attacks that occur during isoproterenol infusions with those that occur during dextrose infusions in nine subjects who had both types of attack. Both baseline and peak panic description scales are represented.

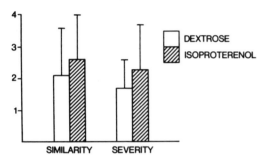

Fig. 7–4. Comparison of panic attacks that occur during isoproterenol infusions with those that occur during dextrose infusions in nine subjects who had both types of attack. Ratings of both the similarity and severity of the attacks are represented.

be closer to the patients' usual attacks, and there was a tendency for isoproterenol attacks to be rated as more severe.

PLASMA 3-METHOXY-4-HYDROXYPHYLGLCOL (MHPG) LEVELS

Plasma levels of MHPG were obtained from ten of the panic disorder patients and nine of the controls (Pohl et al., 1987) in an attempt to detect any increase in central sympathetic outflow associated with either the diagnosis of panic disorder or with isoproterenol-provoked panic attacks. Plasma MHPG levels in patients were not elevated at baseline, during isoproterenol infusions, at the point of panic, or up to

20 min after the onset of panic. In fact, MHPG levels were slightly higher in controls than in patients for almost all comparisons, and this held true even when only the control nonpanickers were compared to patient panickers. MHPG levels were also not elevated in all subjects who panicked compared to all those who did not. Although there were some significant correlations between MHPG levels and anxiety ratings, these correlations were infrequent and could be explained by chance alone. Identical findings were also obtained for lactate infusions in the same subjects.

In drawing conclusions from these MHPG results, it is important to realize that the time sequence for an increase in central noradrenergic activity to be reflected in the periphery is not known, and it may take hours. However, it does appear that at rest there is no increase in MHPG in panic disorder patients, suggesting that there is no resting increase in noradrenergic tone.

Isoproterenol Infusions in Bulimics

Bulimia is an eating disorder characterized by recurrent episodes of binge eating that is viewed by the patient as abnormal and is usually followed by vomiting, fasting, or laxative or diuretic abuse. Like panic disorder patients, patients with bulimia respond well to both tricyclic and monoamine oxidase inhibitor antidepressants (Pohl et al., 1982; Pope et al., 1983; Walsh et al., 1984). Abraham and Beaumont (1982) have reported that bulimic patients often complain of anxiety and tension before a binge, and that 80% describe symptoms of autonomic arousal, such as palpitations, tremulousness, and sweating, all common symptoms of panic attacks. In a survey of 275 patients with bulimia, feeling "tense, anxious" was the most common reason given for binging (Mitchell et al., 1985).

These similarities prompted us to consider a possible relationship between bulimia and panic disorder. In our study of 13 bulimic subjects, seven had actively symptomatic panic attacks (Pohl et al., 1986c). Nine of the 13 bulimics were infused with isoproterenol; three of these patients panicked. Eight patients also received lactate; four of these patients panicked. Only one attack occurred during placebo infusions. All the lactate panickers had a history of panic, whereas two of the three isoproterenol panickers had no such history.

These results suggest that there may be a large subset of bulimic patients with coexisting panic attacks. Although bulimics had fewer lactate-induced panic attacks than panic disorder patients, the lactate response of bulimics with a history of panic disorder resembled that of panic disorder patients. Bulimics may also be sensitive to the panic-provoking effects of isoproterenol, but this sensitivity did not depend on a history of panic attacks.

Isoproterenol Infusions in Posttraumatic Stress Disorder Patients

Posttraumatic Stress Disorder (PTSD) and panic disorder appear to be closely related. Over 50% of PTSD patients experience panic attacks (Mellman and Davis, 1985; Sierles et al., 1983), and in clinical studies flashbacks and panic attacks appear to be closely related phenomena (Mellman and Davis, 1985). Like panic attacks, flashbacks and nightmares can be suppressed by the use of imipramine and phenelzine (Burstein, 1984; Hogben and Cornfield, 1981; Levenson et al., 1982). In a family study of the relatives of PTSD patients, 22% of the first-degree relatives suffered from an anxiety disorder (Davidson et al., 1985).

To investigate the relationship between panic disorder and PTSD, we administered both lactate and isoproterenol infusions to seven Vietnam veterans with PTSD (Rainey et al., 1987). All the patients had flashbacks with lactate infusions; six of them also had panic attacks. With isoproterenol, two patients experienced flashbacks and panic attacks. These findings suggest that both sodium lactate and, to a lesser degree, isoproterenol can induce flashbacks and panic attacks in PTSD patients. The involvement of beta-receptors in this disorder is also suggested by a study by Kolb (1984) in which 12 PTSD patients treated with propranolol experienced a significant decrease in startle responses, nightmares, hyperalertness, and explosiveness. Further studies to examine beta-adrenergic function in PTSD patients are warranted.

BETA-RECEPTOR STUDIES

In the studies discussed above, panic disorder patients were more sensitive than normal controls to the anxiogenic effects of isoproterenol. One possible explanation for this phenomenon would be an increased sensitivity of beta-receptors. For this reason, studies of beta-receptor function in anxiety disorder patients are of interest. The studies of peripheral beta-adrenergic function in anxiety disorder patients are conflicting, but much of the evidence points to a decreased sensitivity or number of beta-receptors.

An indirect measure of the affinity of isoproterenol for chronotropic beta-receptors has been made by plotting the relationship between heart rate response and isoproterenol dosage. With this technique, affinity for beta-receptors was higher in patients with "neurocirculatory asthenia" than in normal individuals or in patients with borderline hypertension or hyperthyroidism (Hirakawa et al., 1981; Ito et al., 1983; Tonai et al., 1978). The dosages used in these studies ranged up to 3 μg of isoproterenol administered iv over 1 min. This dosage was not associated with any increase in circulating epinephrine or norepinephrine, suggesting that the heart rate response was a direct effect of the exogenously administered isoproterenol.

The diagnostic criteria for neurocirculatory asthenia were the presence of at least sighing respiration, anterior chest discomfort, and easy fatigability; other criteria included vegetative nerve disorder and a psychosomatic background (Ito, personal communication). It seems likely to us that there would be an overlap between this group of patients and panic disorder patients.

We have examined the heart rate data for 46 panic disorder patients and 29 controls given continuous infusions of isoproterenol using the methods described above (Pohl et al., 1986a). Heart rates were obtained at baseline and at 2 min intervals during the infusion. Patients had higher baseline heart rates than controls (82 vs. 75), but the overall difference in heart rates was insignificant. Isoproterenol rapidly and similarly increased heart rate for both groups. There was also no difference between isoproterenol panickers and nonpanickers. However, the continuous infusion design is not as useful as bolus infusions for determining chronotropic sensitivity to isoproterenol.

Other studies suggest that panic disorder patients have decreased sensitivity to peripheral beta-receptor stimulation. In a study designed to test the hypothesis that panic disorder patients had increased beta-adrenergic sensitivity, Nesse et al. (1984) measured heart rate during a series of logarithimically increasing iv bolus doses of isoproterenol hydrochloride. Although the mean baseline heart rate for panic patients was 25.5 beats faster than in controls, the heart rate response to isoproterenol in patients was less than in controls. For example, the mean dosage required to raise the heart rate 25 beats per minute was 2.75 μg for patients but 0.91 μg for controls. Heart rate response appeared to be independent of baseline heart rate. These findings suggest that the responsiveness of chronotropic beta-receptors is decreased in panic disorder. Bolus infusions of isoproterenol did not provoke panic attacks.

The panic disorder patients in the above study also showed a small increase in norepinephrine levels and substantially higher resting levels of epinephrine than controls, suggesting that panic disorder patients have down-regulated beta-receptors as the result of increased adrenergic function. Catecholamines are known to modulate the activity of their receptors. For example, frog erythrocytes exposed to isoproterenol developed a decreased number of beta-adrenoceptors and a decrease in adenylate cyclase responsiveness (Mickey et al., 1975; Mukherjee et al., 1976). Agonist-induced changes in receptor sensitivity can be large. Treatment with the beta-adrenergic agonists ephedrine and terbutaline resulted in at least a 50% decrease in lymphocyte beta-receptors after 8 days of administration in normal human volunteers (Aarons et al., 1983).

There is direct evidence that the responsiveness of beta-receptors is decreased in anxiety disorder. In 14 patients with incapacitating anxiety, the lymphocytic cyclic adenosine monophosphate (cAMP) response to the beta-agonist isoproterenol was significantly lower than in controls (Lima and Turner, 1983). This decrease is not specific for anxiety disorders because decreased isoproterenol-induced lymphocytic cAMP has also been a finding in depressed and manic patients (Extein et al., 1979).

Although it appears from receptor studies that beta-receptors are less responsive in panic disorder patients, there are some caveats. First, the studies measure peripheral, not central, nervous system beta-receptor function. Second, beta-receptor function appears to be a dynamic activity and may conceivably change rapidly in patients who experience panic attacks. Third, there is evidence that beta-receptor regulation can vary in different tissues in response to the same stimulus. Davies and Lefkowitz (1980) have found that cortisone acetate administered to normal volunteers induced an acute rise in granulocyte beta-adrenoceptor density and adenylate cyclase activity but an acute fall in lymphocyte beta-adrenoceptor density. This "differential regulation" of a single receptor subtype in response to the same stimulus suggests that changes in white blood cell or chronotropic beta-receptors may not reflect the status of beta-receptors in other tissues even when the receptors are known to be of the same subtype.

RELATIONSHIP TO TREATMENT MODELS

Beta-Blockers

If anxiety states are mediated through beta-receptors, one would predict that the administration of beta-blocking drugs would be an effective treatment. The effect of beta-blockers on anxiety states has been reviewed by a number of authors (Noyes et al., 1981; Noyes, 1982; Pitts and Allen, 1979); a complete review will not be included here. Most of the controlled studies are limited by study populations that do not discriminate between panic and generalized anxiety. In addition, most studies use modest dosages for relatively brief periods of 1–3 weeks.

The results of these studies have been mixed. Of ten placebo-controlled studies reviewed by Noyes (1982), six studies found a beta-blocker to be superior to placebo for the treatment of anxiety disorder. Beta-blockers often appear to have an affect on somatic anxiety but little or no affect on psychological symptoms. For example, Granville-Grossman and Turner (1966), in a double-blind, 2 week, cross-over comparison of placebo and 80 mg/day of propranolol in 15 anxiety neurotics, found that only autonomically mediated symptoms were significantly improved. In a 1 week, double-blind, cross-over study of 12 chronically anxious patients, daily dosages of 120–360 mg propranolol produced improvement that was equal to 6–18 mg diazepam and better than placebo in patients with predominantly somatic anxiety but inferior to diazepam and no better than placebo for patients with predominantly psychic symptoms, (Tyrer and Lader, 1974).

Only one study has tested the efficacy of beta-blockers in DSM III defined agoraphobia with panic attacks and panic disorder. Noyes et al. (1984) studied 21 patients; one of these only met criteria for generalized anxiety disorder. In this study, a median dosage of 240 mg propranolol was compared to a median daily dose of 30 mg diazepam. Each drug was given for 2 weeks in a double-blind, cross-over design. Propranolol was inferior to diazepam on all measures, and appeared to have no influence on the number of attacks or their severity. In addition, patients who reported predominantly somatic symptoms were no more likely to improve on propranolol than were patients with predominantly psychic symptoms.

The finding that beta-blockers have little therapeutic effect on psychic anxiety is not consistent across all studies. A number of controlled studies show that beta-blockers do have an effect on psychological symptoms (Becker, 1975; Burrows et al., 1976; Johnson et al., 1976; Tyrer and Lader, 1973). In a controlled study with propranolol, Kathol et al. (1980) found that a high dosage of 160 mg daily produced a significant reduction of psychological symptoms. Given the available data to date, it appears that beta-blockers may reduce psychic anxiety if the dosage is high enough, but the effect on some of the somatic symptoms of anxiety is more prominent (Noyes et al., 1981). Overall, the clinical efficacy of beta-blockers seems to be modest, especially when compared to other treatments.

It is not clear whether the efficacy of beta-blocking drugs can be used as a litmus test for a beta-adrenergic model. The sensitivity of beta-receptors may change in response to beta-blockade. In seven patients with incapacitating anxiety treated with 80 mg propranolol twice per day, there was a significant increase in the response of lymphocytic cAMP to isoproterenol (Lima and Turner, 1983). In their study of propranolol in patients with panic attacks, Noyes et al. (1984) noted that six patients who showed some improvement during the first week of propranolol treatment showed no improvement the second week, suggesting that tolerance developed to the therapeutic effects of propranolol. Adaptive changes in response to beta-blockade may dictate that tests of the beta-receptor model study only the acute effects of beta-blockers. Treatment studies of the clinical efficacy of beta-blockers can address this problem with frequent clinical ratings and an analysis of the time course of any improvement. Ambulatory monitoring might also be useful for assessing the time course of any improvement from beta-blockers; panic attacks are accompanied by substantial increases in heart rate during naturally occurring panic attacks (Freedman et al., 1985).

Antidepressants

Tricyclic antidepressants prevent panic attacks, and their efficacy in panic disorder patients in a number of controlled studies has been reviewed (Pohl et al., 1982). Tricyclic antidepressants down-regulate beta-adrenoceptors (Sulser and Mobley, 1981; U'Prichard and Enna, 1979), decreasing beta-adrenergic-induced increases in cAMP (Wolfe et al., 1978). This is not an acute effect but appears to be an adaptive response to chronically increased noradrenergic stimulation. The time course of the effects of tricyclic antidepressants is consistent with a noradrenergic, beta-receptor mediated hypothesis of anxiety. Some panic disorder patients are very sensitive to imipramine and initially develop insomnia, jitteriness, irritability, and increased anxiety (Pohl et al., 1986b, 1988a; Zitrin et al., 1978); therapeutic effects occur later, when compensatory down-regulation of beta-receptors would be expected to occur.

Zimelidine, a second-generation antidepressant that has been withdrawn from the market, appears to be effective for phobic anxiety (Evans and Moore, 1981). Chronic zimelidine administration significantly reduced the density of beta-adrenoceptors in rat cerebral tissue (Ross et al., 1981) and reduced isoproterenol induced cAMP (Schoffelmeer et al., 1984).

On the other hand, bupropion is an effective antidepressant (Fabre and McLendon, 1978; Stern and Marto-Truax, 1980) but lacks anti-panic effects. In a study of 12 panic disorder patients placed on bupropion for 35 days, not a single patient improved (Sheehan et al., 1983). All patients subsequently responded to either phenelzine or imipramine. The effect of bupropion on the beta-adrenergic system is less clear. Bupropion has been reported not to produce desensitization of beta-receptors (Bryant et al., 1983; Maxwell et al., 1981), but other investigators report that bupropion decreased binding of dihydroalprenolol in cerebral cortical homogenates (Sellinger-Barnette et al., 1980).

Other Drugs

Alprazolam, a benzodiazepine, is effective for the treatment of panic disorder in double-blind, placebo-controlled studies (Chouinard et al., 1982; Sheehan et al., 1984). In normal rats, alprazolam did not alter the density of cerebral cortex beta-adrenoceptors but did partially block the increase in receptors induced by chronic iv infusion of reserpine (Sethy and Hodges, 1982). These results suggest that the effect of alprazolam in panic disorder might be mediated in part by an effect on beta-receptors.

The beta-adrenergic model does not explain the fact that lithium carbonate (Rosenblatt et al., 1979) down-regulates beta-receptors but is not known to exert anxiolytic effects. This treatment however has not been systematically investigated for the treatment of panic disorder; it would be interesting to test the efficacy of lithium in this population.

RELATIONSHIP TO OTHER MODELS
Provocative Drugs
SODIUM LACTATE

Sodium lactate is a well established model for the laboratory induction of panic attacks (Bonn et al., 1971; Fink et al., 1969; Liebowitz et al., 1984; Pitts and McClure, 1967; Pohl et al., 1985). To test the hypothesis that lactate-induced panic acts on hyperresponsive beta-receptors, Gorman et al. (1983) administered propranolol before giving sodium lactate to six panic disorder patients who had previously

experienced lactate-induced panic. Each patient received an iv infusion of propranolol hydrochloride (0.2 mg/kg) over 30 min just before reinfusion with 10 ml/kg of 0.5 M racemic lactate over 20 min. The dosage of propranolol given had previously been shown to achieve complete peripheral beta-blockade (Jose and Taylor, 1969). Propranolol failed to block panic attacks or to increase the dosage of sodium lactate required to produce a panic attack. Moreover, propranolol did not blunt lactate-induced increases in heart rate or anxiety ratings on the Acute Panic Inventory.

The failure of propranolol to block lactate-induced panic implies that beta-receptors are not crucial for lactate-induced panic, assuming that lactate itself does not affect the ability of propranolol to block beta-receptors. However, Scebat et al. (1978) have reported that the effects of propranolol on heart rate and cardiac index in dogs can be reversed by small dosages of sodium lactate. Similar results were obtained in human volunteers given the beta-blocker pindolol. The reversal of cardiac beta-blockade occurred with doses of sodium lactate that are much smaller than that used to induce panic. These findings suggest that it is difficult to determine whether lactate-induced panic is mediated by beta-receptors.

YOHIMBINE

Yohimbine is an alpha-2 antagonist that can produce anxiety in psychiatric patients and normal volunteers (Holmberg and Gershon, 1961). In panic disorder patients, the drug produced significantly greater anxiety, palpitations, hot and cold flashes, restlessness, tremors, and piloerection than in normal controls (Charney et al., 1984b). Yohimbine increases plasma norepinephrine in a variety of species, including man (Ginsberg and Robertson, 1983), and increases norepinephrine turnover as measured by increases in MHPG. In man, this effect is more pronounced in patients with frequent panic attacks (Charney et al., 1984a).

The effect of beta-blockade on yohimbine-induced anxiety is not known. Beta-blockers do attenuate enhancement of yohimbine toxicity in mice (Quinton, 1963). Yohimbine has not been given to panic disorder patients before and after treatment with tricyclic antidepressants. It has been well established that yohimbine-induced excitation and toxicity in rats is enhanced by tricyclic antidepressants (Ginsberg and Robertson, 1983) and tricyclic antidepressants enhance the autonomic symptoms of yohimbine in humans (Holmberg and Gershon, 1961). These results suggest that panic disorder patients on tricyclic antidepressants may be more rather than less sensitive to a reinfusion of yohimbine. The validity of both the isoproterenol and the lactate models has been supported by the finding that isoproterenol (Pohl et al., 1985) and lactate-induced anxiety attacks (Liebowitz et al., 1984) do not occur or are attenuated in panic disorder patients after treatment with tricyclic antidepressants.

CAFFEINE

Panic disorder patients report that caffeine produces more anxiety and sleep problems than is found in normal controls (Boulenger et al., 1984), and panic disorder patients experience severe anxiety or panic attacks when given dosages of caffeine not associated with anxiety in normal subjects (Boulenger et al., 1986). In another study, 10 mg/kg caffeine produced significantly greater increases in subject-rated anxiety, nervousness, fear, nausea, palpitations, restlessness, and tremors in panic disorder patients compared to normal controls. Fifteen of 21 panic disorder patients reported that the effects of caffeine were similar to those experienced during panic attacks (Charney et al., 1985).

Caffeine increases levels of plasma epinephrine and norepinephrine in human subjects (Robertson et al., 1978, 1981) and can therefore be expected to stimulate beta-receptors. The effect of caffeine on epinephrine appears to be especially pronounced, suggesting that caffeine may promote the release of catecholamines from the adrenal medulla. However, caffeine is known to affect benzodiazepine and adenosine receptors (Boulenger et al., 1982; Marangos et al., 1979; Snyder and Sklar, 1984) and these receptors could be reasonably expected to affect anxiety. Unlike yohimbine, caffeine appears to produce anxiety symptoms in normal volunteers (Charney et al., 1984a) and panic-like symptoms in panic disorder patients (Charney et al., 1985), without affecting norepinephrine turnover as measured by plasma MHPG.

The Noradrenergic Model of Anxiety

LOCUS CERULEUS (LC)

The LC contains the majority of the norepinephrine-containing neurons in the brain. There is a large body of evidence that suggests that the LC is involved in the expression of anxiety; this evidence has been extensively reviewed by Redmond (1979). Stimulation of the LC in monkeys results in fear-like behavior, and the effects of yohimbine are consistent with a noradrenergic, LC hypothesis. Several anxiolytic drugs decrease LC firing.

Norepinephrine-containing efferent axons from the LC affect postsynaptic beta-receptors that are widely distributed throughout the cerebrum, limbic system, cerebellum, and spinal cord (see Grant and Redmond, 1981, for review). The density of beta-receptors is especially great in the limbic forebrain, hippocampus, and cerebral cortex (Alexander et al., 1975). Connections to postsynaptic beta-adrenoceptors appear to be essential for LC-mediated anxiety; the behavioral effects of LC stimulation in monkeys is almost completely blocked by the beta-blocker propranolol (Huang et al., 1977).

The noradrenergic hypothesis therefore predicts that the administration of a pure beta-adrenergic agonist would produce anxiety in man (Redmond, 1979). In our studies, the anxiety induced by isoproterenol is much more intense in patients than in controls, suggesting that patients may have abnormally sensitive or abnormally regulated beta-receptors rather than increased LC activity. An abnormally sensitive beta-receptor would result in an accentuated response to LC stimulation, and a decrease in LC firing would help to adjust for receptor sensitivity. However, there is an interaction between the LC and its postsynaptic receptors, and abnormally sensitive beta-receptors could conceivably be the result of a disturbance in LC function. Noradrenergic projections from the LC have a significant effect on the sensitivity of beta-adrenoceptors in the frontal cortex, hippocampus, and cerebellum and possibly the amygdala, septum, and thalamus (U'Prichard et al., 1980).

Blood–Brain Barrier

The LC is highly vascularized, and may not have an effective blood–brain barrier. In monkeys, there is a direct apposition of blood vessels to perikarya and dendrites of monoaminergic neurons (Felten and Crutcher, 1979). However, the anxiogenic effects of LC stimulation, or of beta-agonist administration, would presumably be related to postsynaptic effects elsewhere in the brain.

Surprisingly, little is known of the central nervous system effects of catecholamines. Although catecholamines do not appear to readily cross the blood–brain barrier, they appear to have some central nervous system effects. For example, although only modest amounts of tritiated epinephrine crosses the blood–brain barrier into the hypothalamus of cats (Weil-Malherbe et al., 1959), there is indirect evidence that it can penetrate sufficiently to exert some central effects (Rothballer et al., 1959). In addition, small iv doses of epinephrine produced repeatable electroencephalogram (EEG) activation and behavioral arousal in naturally sleeping cats with permanently implanted cortical electrodes (Rothballer et al., 1959). Isoproterenol has similar central nervous system effects, suggesting that physiologically active amounts of the drug can cross the blood–brain barrier. Intravenous infusions of isoproterenol result in EEG changes in curarized animals (Goldstein and Munoz, 1961). Electrocortical and behavioral arousal can also be obtained with intravenously administered isoproterenol given to kittens 4 weeks of age or older (Marley and Key, 1963).

CONCLUSIONS

Although catecholamines have been implicated in the pathogenesis of human anxiety since close to the turn of the century, the role of the beta-adrenergic system is just beginning to be investigated. The sensitivity of panic disorder patients to isoproterenol suggests that panic symptoms are mediated by beta-receptors. Panic disorder patients exposed to continuous infusions of isoproterenol experience panic attacks that are qualitatively similar to their usual attacks; these episodes include central as well as peripheral symptoms of anxiety.

However, as with most provocative models, it is difficult to separate the psychological effects of peripheral symptomatology (heart pounding for isoproterenol, tingling and vibratory sensations for sodium lactate) from direct physiological effects on biological systems that control anxiety.

Circumstantial evidence points towards a direct effect on biological systems, rather than a psychological effect mediated by peripheral symptoms. Patients have a decreased sensitivity to the anxiogenic effect of infusions after pharmacological treatment, and control subjects who have never before panicked occasionally panic with these provocative infusions. In addition, the model is consistent with the observed symptomatology in these patients, with the noradrenergic model, and with known effects of drugs that are effective for panic disorder.

The increased sensitivity of panic disorder patients to beta-agonists does not necessarily implicate the beta-receptor itself. Other receptor systems may also be involved or may interact with the beta-adrenergic system. An eventual understanding of isoproterenol-induced panic attacks may depend on a greater understanding of both receptor function and receptor regulation.

REFERENCES

Aarons RD, Nies AS, Gerber JG, Molinoff PB (1983): Decreased beta-adrenergic receptor density on human lymphocytes after chronic treatment with agonists. J Pharmacol Exp Ther 224:1–6.

Abraham SF, Beumont PJV (1982): How patients describe bulimia or binge eating. Psychol Med 12:625–635.

Alexander RW, Davis JN, Lefkowitz RJ (1975): Direct identification and characterisation of beta-adrenergic receptors in rat brain. Nature 258:437–440.

Balon R, Pohl R, Yeragani VK, Rainey JM Jr, Berchou R (1988a): Follow-up of controls with lactate and isoproterenol induced panic attacks. Am J Psychiatry 145:238–241.

Balon R, Pohl R, Yeragani VK, Rainey JM, Weinberg P (1988b): Lactate- and isoproterenol-induced panic attacks in panic disorder patients and controls. Psychiatr Res 23:153–160.

Becker AL (1975): Oxprenolol and propranolol in anxiety states: A double-blind comparative study. S Afr Med J 50:627–629.

Bonn JA, Harrison J, Rees WL (1971): Lactate-induced anxiety: Therapeutic applications. Br J Psychiatry 119:468–471.

Boulenger JP, Bierer LM, Uhde TW (1986): Anxiogenic effects of caffeine in normal controls and patients with panic disorder. In Shagass C, Josiassen RC, Bridger WH, Weiss KJ, Stoff D, Simpson GM (eds): "Biological Psychiatry 1985: Proceedings of the IVth World Congress of Biological Psychiatry." New York: Elsevier Science Publishing Co. Inc., pp 454–456.

Boulenger JP, Patel J, Marangos PJ (1982): Effects of caffeine and theophylline on adenosine and benzodiazepine receptors in human brain. Neurosci Lett 30: 161–166.

Boulenger JP, Uhde TW, Wolff EA III, Post RM (1984): Increased sensitivity to caffeine in patients with panic disorders: Preliminary evidence. Arch Gen Psychiatry 41:1067–1071.

Bryant SG, Guernsey BG, Ingrim NB (1983): Review of bupropion. Clin Pharmacol 2:525–537.

Burrows GD, Davies B, Fail L, Poynton C, Stevenson H (1976): A placebo controlled trial of diazepam and oxprenolol for Anxiety. Psychopharmacology 50:177–179.

Burstein A (1984): Treatment of post-traumatic stress disorder with imipramine. Psychosomatics 25:681–687.

Cannon WB (1915): "Bodily Changes in Pain, Fear and Rage. New York: Appleton.

Charney DS, Galloway MP, Heninger GR (1984a): The effects of caffeine on plasma MHPG, subjective anxiety, autonomic symptoms and blood pressure in healthy humans. Life Sciences 35:135–144.

Charney DS, Heninger GR, Breier A (1984b): Noradrenergic function in panic anxiety: Effects of yohimbine in healthy subjects and patients with agoraphobia and panic disorder. Arch Gen Psychiatry 41:751–763.

Charney DS, Heninger GR, Jatlow PI (1985): Increased anxiogenic effects of caffeine in panic disorders. Arch Gen Psychiatry 42:233–243.

Chouinard G, Annable L, Fontaine R, Solyom L (1982): Alprazolam in the treatment of generalized anxiety and panic disorders: A double-blind placebo-controlled study. Psychopharmacology 77:229–233.

Davidson J, Swartz M, Storck M Krishnan RR, Hammett E (1985): A diagnostic and family study of post-traumatic stress disorder. Am J Psychiatry 142:90–93.

Davies AO, Lefkowitz RJ (1980): Corticosteroid-induced differential regulation of beta-adrenergic receptors in circulating human polymorphonuclear leukocytes and mononuclear leukocytes. J Clin Endocrinol Metab 51:599–605.

Easton JD, Sherman DG (1976): Somatic anxiety attacks and propranolol. Arch Neurol 33:689–691.

Ehlers A, Margraf J, Roth WT, Taylor CB, Maddock RJ, Sheik J, Kopell ML, McClenahan KL, Gossard D, Blowers GH, Agras WS, Kopell BS (1986): Lactate infusions and panic attacks: Do patients and controls respond differently? Psychiatry Res 17:295–308.

Evans L, Moore G (1981): The treatment of phobic anxiety by zimelidine. Acta Psychiatr Scand 63[Suppl 290]:342–345.

Extein I, Tallman J, Smith CC, Goodwin FK (1979): Changes in lymphocytic beta-adrenergic receptors in depression and mania. Psychiatry Res 1:191–197.

Fabre LF, McLendon DM (1978): Double-blind placebo-controlled study of bupropion hydrochloride (Wellbatrin) in the treatment of depressed inpatients. Curr Ther Res 23:393–402.

Felton DL, Crutcher KA (1979): Neuronal-vascular relationships in the raphe nuclei, locus ceruleus, and substantia nigra in primates. Am J Anat 155:467–482.

Fink M, Taylor MA, Volavka J (1969): Anxiety precipitated by lactate. N Engl J Med 281:1129.

Freedman RR, Ianni P, Ettedgui E, Puthezhath N (1985): Ambulatory monitoring of panic disorder. Arch Gen Psychiatry 42:244–248.

Frohlich ED, Tarazi RC, Dustan HP (1969): Hyperdynamic beta-adrenergic circulatory state. Arch Intern Med 123:1–7.

Ginsberg MR, Robertson D (1983): Yohimbine: A Pharmacological probe for study of the alpha-2 adrenoreceptor. Pharmacol Rev 351:143–180.

Goldstein L, Munoz C (1961): Influence of adrenergic stimulant and blocking drugs on cerebral and electrical activity in curarized animals. J Pharmacol Exp Ther 132:345–353.

Gorman JM, Levy GF, Liebowitz MR, McGrath P, Appleby IL, Dillon DJ, Davies SO, Klein DF (1983): Effect of acute beta-adrenergic blockade on lactate-induced panic. Arch Gen Psychiatry 40:1079–1082.

Grant SJ, Redmond DE Jr (1981): The neuroanatomy and pharmacology of the nucleus locus ceruleus. In Lal H, Fielding S (eds): "Pharmacology of Clonidine." New York: Alan R. Liss, Inc., pp 5–27.

Granville-Grossman KL, Turner P (1966): The effect of propranolol on anxiety. Lancet i:788–790.

Hirakawa S, Ito H, Tonai N, Kamubara K, Minatoguchi S, Dsamura M (1981): Estimated affinity of the chronotropic beta-adrenergic receptor of human heart, with special reference to the hyperthyroidism. Paper presented at the Third International Study Group of Research in Cardiac Metabolism, Nagoya, Japan, November 6, 1981.

Hogben GL, Cornfield RB (1981): Treatment of war neurosis with phenelzine. Arch Gen Psychiatry 38:440–445.

Holmberg G, Gershon S (1961): Autonomic and psychic effects of yohimbine hydrochloride. Psychopharmacologia 2:93–106.

Huang YH, Maas JW, Redmond DE Jr (1977): Evidence for noradrenergic specificity of behavioral effects of electrical stimulation of the nucleus locus ceruleus. Soc Neurosci Abstr 3:251.

Ito H, Tonai N, Hirakawa S (1983): Estimated affinity of isoproterenol to cardiac chronotropic beta-receptor and of phenylephrine to vasoconstrictive alpha-receptor of the systemic resistance vessels in human borderline hypertension. Jpn Circ J 47:240–255.

Johnson S, Singh B, Leeman M (1976): Controlled evaluation of the beta-adrenoceptor blocking drug oxprenolol in anxiety. Med J Aust 1:909–912.

Jose DG, Taylor RR (1969): Autonomic blockade by propranolol and atropine to study intrinsic myocardial function. J Clin Invest 48:2009–2031.

Kathol RG, Noyes R Jr, Slymen DJ, Crowe RR, Clancy J, Kerber RE (1980): Propranolol in chronic anxiety disorders: A controlled study. Arch Gen Psychiatry 37: 1361–1365.

Kelly D, Mitchell-Heggs N, Sherman D (1971): Anxiety and the effects of sodium lactate assessed clinically and physiologically. Br J Psychiatry 119:129–141.

Kolb LC (1984): The post-traumatic stress disorders of combat: A subgroup with a conditioned emotional response. Military Med 149:237–243.

Kopin IJ (1984): Avenues of investigation for the role of catecholamines in anxiety. Psychopathology 17 [Suppl 1]:83–97.

Levenson H, Lanman R, Rankin M, (1982): Traumatic war neurosis and phenelzine. Arch Gen Psychiatry 39:1345.

Levi L (1972): Stress and distress in response to psychosocial stimuli. Acta Med Scand 528[Suppl]:1–157.

Liebowitz MR, Fyer AJ, Gorman JM, Dillon D, Appleby IL, Levy G, Anderson S, Levitt M, Palij M, Davies SO, Klein DF (1984): Lactate provocation of panic attacks: I. Clinical and behavioral findings. Arch Gen Psychiatry 41:764–770.

Lima DR, Turner P (1983): Propranolol increases reduced beta-receptor function in severely anxious patients. Lancet 2:1505.

Lindemann E (1935): The psychopathological effect of drugs affecting the vegetative system. Am J Psychiatry 91:983–1008.

Lindemann E, Finesinger J (1938). The effect of adrenalin and mecholyl in states of anxiety in psychoneurotic patients. Am J Psychiatry 95:353–370.

Marangos PJ, Paul SM, Parma AM, Goodwin FK, Syapin P, Skolnick P (1979): Purinergic inhibition to diazepam binding to rat brain (in vitro). Life Sci 24:851–858.

Maranon G (1924): Contribution a l'etude de l'action emotive de l'adrenaline. Rev Fr Endocrinol 2:301–325

Marley E, Key BJ (1963): Maturation of the electrocorticogram and behaviour in the kitten and guinea-pig and the effect of some sympathomimetic amines. Electroenceph Clin Neurophysiol 15:620–636.

Mathew RJ, Ho BT, Francis DJ, Taylor DL, Weinman ML (1982): Catecholamines and anxiety. Acta Psychiatr Scand 65:142–147.

Maxwell RA, Mehta NB, Tucker WE Jr, Schroeder DH, Stern WC (1981): Bupropion. In Goldberg ME (ed): "Pharmacological and biochemical properties of drug substances. Vol 3." Washington, DC: American Pharmaceutical Association Academy of Pharmaceutical Sciences.

Mellman TA, David GC (1985): Combat-related flashbacks in post-traumatic stress disorder: Phenomenology and similarity to panic attacks. J Clin Psychiatry 46:379–384.

Mickey J, Tate R, Lefkowitz J (1975): Subsensitivity of adenylate cyclase and decreased beta-adrenergic receptor binding after chronic exposure to (-) isoproterenol in vitro. J Biol Chem 250:5727–5729.

Mitchell JE, Hatsukami D, Eckert ED, Pyle RL (1985): Characteristics of 275 patients with bulimia. Am J Psychiatry 142:482–485.

Mukherjee C, Caron MB, Lefkowitz RJ (1976): Regulation of adenylate cyclase coupled beta-adrenergic receptors by beta-adrenergic catecholamines. Endocrinology 99:347–357.

Nesse RM, Cameron OG, Curtis GC, McCann DS, Huber-Smith MJ (1984): Adrenergic function in patients with panic anxiety. Arch Gen Psychiatry 41:771–776.

Noyes R Jr (1982): Beta-blocking drugs and anxiety. Psychosomatics 23:155–170.

Noyes R Jr, Anderson DJ, Clancy J, Crowe RR, Slymen DJ, Ghoneim MM, Hinrichs JV (1984): Diazepam and propranolol in panic disorder and agoraphobia. Arch Gen Psychiatry 41:287–292.

Noyes R Jr, Kathol R, Clancy J, Crowe DR (1981): Antianxiety effects of propranolol: A Review of Clinical Studies. In Klein DF, Rabkin J (eds): "Anxiety: New Research and Changing Concepts." New York: Raven Press, pp 81–93.

Pitts FN Jr, Allen R (1979): Beta-adrenergic Blocking Agents in the Treatment of Anxiety. In Fann WE, Karacan I, Porkorny AD, Williams RL (eds): "Phenomenology and Treatment of Anxiety," Jamaica, NY: Spectrum Publications, Inc., pp 337–361.

Pitts FN Jr, McClure JN Jr (1967): Lactate metabolism in anxiety neurosis. N Engl J Med 277:1328–1336.

Pohl R, Berchou R, Rainey JM (1982): Tricyclic antidepressants and monoamine oxidase inhibitors in the treatment of agoraphobia. J Clin Psychopharmacol 2: 399–407.

Pohl R, Ettedgui E, Bridges M, Lycaki H, Jimerson D, Kopin I, Rainey JM (1987): Plasma MHPG levels in lactate and isoproterenol anxiety states. Biol Psychiatry 22:1127–1136.

Pohl R, Ortiz A, Lycaki H, Yeragani V, Weinberg P, Rainey JM (1986a): Heart rate during isoproterenol-induced panic attacks. Abstracts of the 41st Annual Convention and Scientific Program, Society of Biological Psychiatry, May 7–11, Washington, DC, p 144.

Pohl R, Rainey J, Ortiz A, Balon R, Singh H, Berchou R (1985): Isoproterenol anxiety states. Psychopharmacol Bull 21:424–427.

Pohl R, Yeragani VK, Balon R, Lycaki H (1988a): The jitteriness syndrome in panic disorder patients treated with antidepressants. J Clin Psychiatry 49:100–104.

Pohl R, Yeragani VK, Balon R, Rainey JM, Lycaki H, Ortiz A, Berchou R, Weinberg P (1988b): Isoproterenol-induced panic attacks. Biol Psychiatry 24:891–902.

Pohl R, Yeragani VK, Ortiz A, Rainey JM Jr, Gershon S (1986b): Response of tricyclic-induced jitteriness to a phenothiazine in two patients. J Clin Psychiatry 47: 427.

Pohl R, Yeragani V, Rainey J, Balon R, Ortiz A, Berchou R, Lycaki H, Weinberg P (1986c): Isoproterenol and lactate infusions in bulimics with and without panic anxiety. Abstracts of the 15th Collegium Internationale Neuro-Psychopharmacologicum Congress, San Juan, December 14–17, p 187.

Pope HG Jr, Hudson JI, Jonas JM, Yurgelon-Todd D (1983): Bulimia treated with imipramine: A placebo-controlled, double-blind study. Am J Psychiatry 140: 554–558.

Pyke RE, Greenberg HS (1986): Norepinephrine challenges in panic patients. J Clin Psychopharmacol 6: 279–285.

Quinton RM (1963): The increase in the toxicity of yohimbine induced by imipramine and other drugs in mice. Br J Pharmacol 21:51–66.

Rainey JM Jr, Aleem A, Ortiz A, Yeragani V, Pohl R, Berchou R (1987): A laboratory procedure for the induction of flashbacks. Amer J Psychiatry 144:1317–1319.

Rainey JM, Ettedgui E, Pohl R, Balon R, Weinberg P, Yelonek S, Berchou R (1984a): The beta receptor: Isoproterenol anxiety states. Psychopathology 17[Suppl 3]:40–51.

Rainey JM, Pohl R, Williams M, Knitter E, Freedman R, Ettedgui E (1984b): A comparison of lactate and isoproterenol anxiety states. Psychopathology 17[Suppl 1]:74–82.

Redmond DE Jr (1979): New and old evidence for the involvement of a brain norepinephrine system in anxiety. In Fann WE, Karacan I, Pokorny AD, Williams RL (eds); "Phenomenology and Treatment of Anxiety." New York: Spectrum Press, pp 153–203.

Robertson D, Frolick JC, Carr RK, Watson JT, Hollingfield JW, Shand DG, Oates JA (1978): Effects of caffeine on plasma renin activity, catecholamines and blood pressure. N Engl J Med 298:181–185.

Robertson D, Wade D, Workman R, Woosley RL, Oates JA (1981): Tolerance to the humoral and hemodynamic effects of caffeine in man. J Clin Invest 67:1111–1117.

Rosenblatt JE, Pert CB, Tallman JF, Pert A, Bunney WE Jr (1979): The effect of imipramine and lithium on alpha- and beta-receptor binding in rat brain. Brain 160:186–191.

Ross SB, Hall H, Renyi AL, Westerlund D (1981): Effects of zimelidine on serotoninergic and noradrenergic neurons after repeated administration in the rat. Psychopharmacology 72:219–225.

Rothballer AB (1959): The effects of catecholamines on the central nervous system. Pharmacol Rev 11:494–547.

Scebat A, Castan RR, Chiche J, Fernandez F, Gerbaux A (1978): Action d'une perfusion de lactate de soude sur les effets hemodynamiques de beta-bloquants. Arch Mal Coeur 71:306–313.

Schmidt HS, Elizabeth JI (1982): Mitral valve prolapse: Relationship to panic attacks/anxiety disorders and beta-adrenergic hypersensitivity. Paper presented at the 37th Annual Meeting of the Society of Biological Psychiatry, Toronto, May 7.

Schoffelmeer AN, Hoorneman EM, Sminia P, Mulder AH (1984): Presynaptic alpha 2- and postsynaptic beta-adrenoreceptor sensitivity in slices of rat neocortex after chronic treatment with various antidepressant drugs. Neuropharmacology 23:115–119.

Sellinger-Barnette MM, Mendels J, Frazer A (1980): The effect of psychoactive drugs on beta-adrenergic receptor binding sites in rat brain. Neuropharmacology 19:447–454.

Sethy VH, Hodges DH (1982): Role of beta-adrenergic receptors in the antidepressant activity of alprazolam. Res Commun Chem Pathol Pharmacol 36:329–332.

Sheehan DV, Coleman JH, Greenblatt DJ, Jones KJ, Levine PH, Orsulak PJ, Peterson M, Schildkraut JJ, Uzogara E, Watkins D (1984): Some biochemical correlates of panic attacks with agoraphobia and their response to a new treatment. J Clin Psychopharmacol 4:66–75.

Sheehan DV, Davidson J, Manschreck T, Van Wyck Fleet J (1983): Lack of efficacy of a new antidepressant (bupropion) in the treatment of panic disorder with phobias. J Clin Psychopharmacol 3:28–31.

Sierles FS, Chan JJ, McFarland RE, Taylor MA (1983): Post-traumatic stress disorder and concurrent psychiatric illness: A preliminary report. Am J Psychiatry 140:1177–1179.

Snyder SH, Sklar P (1984): Behavior and molecular actions of caffeine: Focus on adenosine. J Psychiatr Res 18:91–106.

Spitzer R, Endicott J, Robins E (1978): "Research Diagnostic Criteria (RDC) for a Selected Group of Functional Disorders, 3rd ed." New York: New York State Psychiatric Institute.

Stern WC, Harto-Truax N (1980): Two multicenter studies of the antidepressant effects of bupropion HCl versus placebo. Psychopharmacol Bull 16:43–46.

Sulser F, Mobley PL (1981): Regulation of central noradrenergic receptor function: New vistas on the mode of action of antidepressant treatments. In: Usdin E, Bunney WB, Davis JM (eds): "Neuroreceptors: Basic Clinical Aspects." New York: John Wiley and Sons Inc., pp 55–83.

Tonai N, Ito H, Arakawa M, Aso T, Mori M, Hirakawa S (1978): "Affinity" of the chronotropic receptors for the intravenous isoproterenol, with emphasis on the peculiarity of patients with neurocirculatory asthenia. Paper presented at the Eighth World Congress of Cardiology, Tokyo, Japan, September 17, 1978.

Tyrer PJ, Lader MH (1973): Effects of beta-adrenergic blockade with sotalol in chronic anxiety. Clin Pharmacol Ther 14:418–426.

Tyrer PJ, Lader MH (1974): Response to propranolol and diazepam in somatic and psychic anxiety. Br Med J 2:14–16.

U'Prichard DC, Enna SJ (1979): In vitro modulation of CNS beta-receptor number by antidepressants and beta-agonists. Eur J Pharmacol 59:297–301.

U'Prichard DC, Reisine TD, Mason ST, Fibiger HC, Yamamura HI (1980): Modulation of rat brain alpha- and beta-adrenergic receptor populations by lesion of the dorsal noradrenergic bundle. Brain Res 187:143–154.

Walsh BT, Stewart JW, Roose SP, Gladis M, Glassman AH (1984): Treatment of bulimia with phenelzine: A double-blind, placebo-controlled study. Arch Gen Psychiatry 41:1105–1109.

Wearn J, Sturgis C (1919): Studies on epinephrine: Effects of the injection of epinephrine in soldiers with "irritable heart." Arch Intern Med 24:247–268.

Weil-Malherbe N, Axelrod J, Tomchick R (1959): Blood-brain barrier for adrenaline. Science 129:1226–1227.

Wolfe BB, Harden TK, Sporn JR, Molinoff PB (1978): Presynaptic modulation of beta-adrenergic receptors in rat cerebral cortex after treatment with antidepressants. J Pharmacol Exp Ther 207:446–457.

Zitrin CM, Klein DF, Woerner GR (1978): Behavior therapy, supportive psychotherapy, imipramine and phobias. Arch Gen Psychiatry 35:307–316.

8

Serotonin Abnormalities in Panic Disorder

J.C. PECKNOLD, MD

Douglas Hospital, Verdun, Quebec, Canada H4H 1R3

INTRODUCTION

Serotonin (5-HT) has been thought to be involved in affective disorders for several decades. New pharmacological, receptor, behavioral, epidemiological, and neuroendocrine studies suggest that 5-HT plays a role in the anxiety disorders. One hypothesis is that increased anxiety results from an increased activity in central 5-HT-ergic neurons. This chapter reviews support for this hypothesis from animal pharmacological studies and lesion studies and from reduction of 5-HT and enhancement of 5-HT function, as well as evidence that benzodiazepines reduce 5-HT turnover. Buspirone, a nonbenzodiazepine anxiolytic, has also been found selectively to decrease 5-HT activation and to increase that of norepinephrine and dopamine. The other hypothesis is that there is a 5-HT-ergic deficiency in anxiety, particularly in panic disorder. This chapter reviews the evidence for this hypothesis deriving from the efficacy of 5-HT agonists in panic disorder as well as some findings with 5-HT probes and reviews the hypothesis of 5-HT involvement in lactate infusions. The role of 5-HT in the affective disorders, the link between depression and anxiety, and 5-HT involvement in anxiety disorders such as obsessive–compulsive disorder are considered.

THE LINK BETWEEN ANXIETY AND DEPRESSIVE DISORDERS

The Mixture of Anxiety and Depression

According to Lehmann (1983), anxiety and depression are closely associated dysphoric af-

fects. Almost every depressed patient is anxious: However, not all anxious patients are depressed. Dealy et al. (1981) found that, among a group of patients with anxiety neurosis, significantly more of the patients who had a history of major depression had a history of panic attacks. Many patients with panic disorder and agoraphobia have had symptoms of depression or a depressive episode at some time in their lives. A number of studies have identified a temporal sequence between occurrence of panic disorder and depression (Raskin et al., 1974; Bowen and Kohut, 1979; Munjack and Moss, 1981; Leckman et al., 1983; 1984; Cloninger et al., 1981; Breier et al., 1984, 1985, 1986). In the recent cross-national collaborative study of over 500 patients, 29% had a major depressive episode (secondary depression) at some time after the panic disorder began (Lesser et al., 1988). Van Valkenburg et al. (1984) used panic attacks as a clinical marker for anxious depression and noted that patients with both syndromes, depression and panic attacks, seem quite similar clinically and in treatment response to the anxious depressive patients described by Overall et al. (1966) and by Paykel (1972). Fawcett and Kravits (1983) note that, among 200 patients with RDC-defined major depression, 21% had a history of panic attacks and 62% had moderate psychic anxiety. Severe psychic anxiety was found in 38%.

Leckman et al. (1983) reported that major depression plus panic disorder in probands was associated with a marked increase in risk to relatives for a number of psychiatric disorders. Relatives were more than twice as likely to have major depression, panic disorder, phobia,

Neurobiology of Panic Disorder, Pages 121–142
© 1990 Alan R. Liss, Inc.

or alcoholism than the relatives of probands with major depression without any anxiety disorder. The authors argued for a partially shared diathesis between panic disorder and some cases of major depression. They also stated that metabolic differences may exist that could distinguish patients with depression and panic disorder from depressed patients without an anxiety disorder. Breier, Charney, and Heninger (1985) summarized the evidence and found support for a hypothesis of a common underlying vulnerability for panic disorder and depression. Price et al. (1987) were unable to find evidence for either a major locus or a polygenic mode of inheritance in a group of probands with major depression with panic or in a subset with early onset of primary major depression.

5-HT in Affective Disorder

Certain tricyclic antidepressants enhance transmission through 5-HT synapses by blocking the reuptake of 5-HT (Carlsson et al., 1969). Several of the newer, more specific 5-HT uptake inhibitors have antidepressant activity; these include zimeldine (Claghorn et al., 1983; Heel et al., 1982, Pecknold et al., 1985b), citalopram (Bjerkenstedt et al., 1984; Hattel et al., 1983), fluvoxamine (Amin et al., 1984), fluoxetine (Lentrelhan et al., 1984), and indalpine (Sechter et al., 1984). Willner's (1985) review has shown that many antidepressant treatments potentiate presynaptic 5-HT function and that these effects persist during chronic treatment. Most antidepressant treatments, including those that are potent receptor antagonists when given acutely, enhance postsynaptic receptor function on chronic administration. The overall picture is one of enhanced transmission at the 5-HT synapse. This conclusion is consistent with the original indoleamine hypothesis of depression but not with the hypersensitive 5-HT receptor theory. Sulser (1987) notes that both norepinephrine and 5-HT are required for the process of down-regulation of central beta-adrenoceptor systems by antidepressants and has suggested a 5-HT–norepinephrine link hypothesis of affective disorders. This hypothesis holds that the linked aminergic receptor systems function as an amplification/adaptational system of vital functions. Any impairment of the norepineph-

rine information flow that results in a lack of adaptation would lead to pathophysiological symptoms, for example, a depressed mood.

In summary, it seems clear that 5-HT-ergic mechanisms are involved in affective disorder. It is also evident that there is a clear link in some patients and families between panic disorder and depressive illness. Two platelet probes of 5-HT function, imipramine-binding and 5-HT uptake have been used in affective disorder. The importance of investigating 5-HT probes in platelets, which may have relevance to both depressive disorder and panic disorder, is discussed below.

Obsessive–Compulsive Disorder and Generalized Anxiety Disorder

Obsessive–compulsive disorder has been found to occur frequently in patients with agoraphobia and panic (Klein, 1964; Marks and Herset, 1970; Gelder et al., 1967; Deutsch, 1982). Cloninger et al. (1981) reported that 22% of patients with panic disorder developed obsessions and compulsions, and Breier et al. (1986) reported this occurrence in 17% of patients.

5-HT-ergic involvement in obsessive–compulsive disorder has been postulated because of the beneficial effect of L-tryptophan (Yaryura-Tobias and Bhagavan, 1977) and of clomipramine, a tricyclic antidepressant that blocks 5-HT reuptake (Thoren et al., 1980a,b; Ananth et al., 1980; Volavka et al., 1985; Zohar and Insel, 1987). In two studies, the plasma level of clomipramine but not that of desmethylclomipramine was correlated significantly with the reduction of obsessive–compulsive but not depressive symptoms (Stern et al., 1980; Insel et al., 1983). In a third study, clinical improvement was correlated significantly with a reduction in the cerebrospinal fluid (CSF) 5-HT metabolite 5-hydroxyindoleacetic acid (5-HIAA) (Thoren et al., 1980a,b). Other antidepressants, such as nortriptyline (Thoren et al., 1980a,b), amitriptyline (Ananth et al., 1981), and clorgyline (Insel et al., 1983), had no impact on obsessional symptoms. In the treatment of childhood obsessive–compulsive disorder (Flament et al., 1987), clomipramine was more effective than placebo. Clinical improvement during drug treatment was closely correlated with pretreatment platelet 5-HT concentration and monoamine oxidase activity as well as with the decrease in both measures during clomipramine administration. The authors suggest that the effects of clomipramine on 5-HT uptake may be essential to the antiobsessional action.

The specificity of clomipramine effect on amine uptake has been questioned, because the metabolite desmethylclomipramine, which represents the major form of the drug in plasma (Traskman et al., 1979; Vandel et al., 1982), has potent inhibitory effects on norepinephrine uptake (Ross and Renyi, 1977). However, this metabolite shares with the parent compound both a strong effect on 5-HT reuptake in vitro (Linnoila et al., 1982) and a high affinity for the putative 5-HT transporter, the imipramine binding site on platelets (Paul et al., 1980b).

Zimeldine (Kahn et al., 1984; Prasad, 1984) has also been reported to be effective for obsessive-compulsive illness. However, Insel et al. (1985) were unable to find an increased antiobsessional effect for zimeldine in comparison with desipramine. They also found that platelet [^{3}H]-imipramine binding and 5-HT uptake were not significantly different between the obsessive-compulsive disorder patients and a control group. However, the level of the metabolite 5-HIAA in CSF was significantly higher in a small cohort of obsessional patients compared to healthy volunteers, possibly reflecting increased brain 5-HT turnover. In this study, nonresponders to zimeldine or desipramine improved significantly during a subsequent double-blind trial of clomipramine. Other 5-HT-ergic agents, such as fluoxetine (Fontaine and Chouinard, 1985; Turner et al., 1985) and fluvoxamine (Goodman et al., 1986; Perse et al., 1987) have also been reported to be effective antiobsessionals. Zohar et al. (1987) found that metachlorophenylpiperazine (MCCP), a 5-HT agonist exacerbated obsessive–compulsive symptoms. This finding would be consistent with the negative correlation between clinical improvement and 5-HIAA changes in CSF and with adaptive down-regulation of postsynaptic 5-HT receptors after long-term treatment with chlomipramine, zimeldine, and fluoxetine.

Generalized anxiety disorder has been diagnosed frequently in patients before, during, and after the onset of panic attacks and agoraphobia (Marks, 1970; Snaith, 1968; Roberts, 1964; Buglass et al., 1977; Thorpe and Burns, 1983). Breier et al. (1986) report that 80% of their patients with panic disorder and agoraphobia had at least one episode of generalized anxiety disorder, 30% had an episode that occurred prior to and overlapped with the onset of panic attacks, and 60% had onset of generalized anxiety concomitant with panic disorder and agoraphobia.

The role of 5-HT-ergic mechanisms in generalized anxiety disorder is currently unclear. Ritanserin, a selective 5-HT$_2$ antagonist, has been reported to be effective compared to benzodiazepine and placebo (Ceulemans et al., 1985). An open trial of 5-hydroxytryptophan (Kahn and Westenberg, 1985) was effective in the treatment of generalized anxiety. Buspirone, a nonbenzodiazepine, has been proved to have clinical anxiolytic potency equal to that of diazepam and superior to that of placebo in patients with generalized anxiety disorder (Feighner et al., 1982; Wheatley, 1982; Rickels et al., 1982; Pecknold et al., 1985a) and equal to that of clorazepate (Cohn et al., 1986). Buspirone exerts a differential effect on monoaminergic neuronal activites, suppressing 5-HT-ergic activity and enhancing dopaminergic and noradrenergic cell firing. Buspirone, like the benzodiazepines, inhibits the firing of 5-HT-ergic cells in the dorsal raphe but, unlike the benzodiazepines, moderately enhances the firing of noradrenergic neurons (Eison and Temple, 1986). Buspirone exerts its effects on the 5-HT system through interaction with the recently identified 5-HT$_{1A}$ receptor located on cell bodies of ascending 5-HT neurons originating in the raphe nuclei (Temple and Yocca, 1986). Findings of 5-HT connections to obsessive–compulsive disorder and generalized anxiety disorder indicate that this neurotransmitter is involved in panic disorder, given the comorbidity with the other two anxiety disorders.

PHARMACOLOGICAL DATA LINKING 5-HT AND ANXIETY DISORDERS

Several lines of pharmacological, behavioral, and biochemical evidence recently reviewed by Iversen (1984) involve 5-HT-ergic neurons in the control of anxiety. There is also evidence that the anxiolytic action of benzodiazepines is mediated through a reduction in central 5-HT neurotransmission (Gardner, 1985). However, some data concerning 5-HT antagonists have called into question 5-HT activity in models of anxiety following manipulations of the function of central 5-HT pathways (Commissaris et al., 1981; Gardner, 1985; Kilts et al., 1981; Petersen and Lassen, 1981; Johnston and File, 1986).

Lesion Studies

Lesions of 5-HT-ergic pathways produce anxiolytic profiles in conflict paradigms (Geller and Seifter, 1960; Iverson, 1983; Estes and Skinner, 1941) in some studies (Pelham et al., 1975; Tye et al., 1979; Thiebot et al., 1984) but not in others (Thiebot et al., 1982; Commissaris, et al., 1981). Abundant data, however, indicate that a reduction or a blockade of 5-HT transmission specifically evokes, as do benzodiazepines, response suppression in punishment paradigms (Geller and Blum, 1970; Graeff and Schoendfeld, 1970; Robichaud and Sledge, 1969; Sepinwall and Cook, 1980; Stein et al., 1975, 1977; Thiebot et al., 1983; Tye et al., 1977).

Reduction of 5-HT Function

The 5-HT synthesis inhibitor parachlorophenylalanine (PCPA) produces anxiolytic effects in several animal tests, including conflict procedures and social interaction. Multiple investigators (File and Hyde, 1977; Geller and Blum, 1970; Robichaud and Sledge, 1969; Stevens and Fechter, 1969; Tenne, 1967; Stein et al., 1973) have demonstrated the reverse of the anxiolytic effects of PCPA by administration of the 5-HT precursor 5-hydroxytryptophan. However, other studies have found the effects of PCPA on punished responding to be weak, transient, and inconsistent (Blakey and Parker, 1973; Cook and Sepinwall, 1975).

Enhancement of 5-HT Function

Electric stimulation of the median raphe causes a behavioral inhibition resembling fear responses to threatening events (Graeff and Filho, 1978). Microiontophoretic injections of 5-HT into the dorsal raphe were found to release punished responding (Thiebot et al., 1982). Because such injections may depress

the firing rate of dorsal raphe neurons, through an action on autoreceptors, the results appeared to support the hypothesis that decreased 5-HT activity results in attenuation of behavioral inhibition.

Interpretation Problems With 5-HT Agonists and Antagonists

The net effect of these agents will depend on the nature and degree of their effect on 5-HT receptors at different sites, e.g., $5\text{-HT}_1/5\text{-HT}_2$ postsynaptic receptors, autoreceptors, and 5-HT receptors on the nerve terminals of neurons releasing or modulating the release of other neurotransmitters (Gardner, 1985). In summary, a major problem in interpretation of behavioral effects is that activation of different synaptic 5-HT receptors may lead to different, even opposing, functional effects (Gardner, 1985; Goodwin and Green, 1985; Green et al., 1984). The relative contributions to any given behavior of different pathways with degrees of involvement of different postsynaptic receptors are poorly understood. Having stated this, however, it appears that the balance of animal pharmacological evidence, including lesion studies, reduction of 5-HT function, and enhancement of 5-HT function, suggests that decreased 5-HT-ergic transmission produces an anxiolytic profile.

BIOCHEMICAL AND BEHAVIORAL EVIDENCE IMPLICATING 5-HT SYSTEMS IN THE ANXIOLYTIC ACTION OF BENZODIAZEPINE AND NONBENZODIAZEPINE ANXIOLYTICS

Benzodiazepines have been reported to decrease 5-HT turnover (Corrodi et al., 1971; Haefely et al., 1981; Pratt et al., 1985; Saner and Pletscher, 1979), to slow down the firing rate of 5-HT neurons (Laurent et al., 1983; Pratt et al., 1979; Trulson et al., 1982) and to reduce 5-HT released from nerve endings (Soubrie et al., 1983). Benzodiazepines applied to the raphe nuclei, the main origin of ascending 5-HT neurons, or microinjections of either GABA mimetics or 5-HT itself into the raphe dorsalis, elicit various effects that mimic those of peripherally administered benzodiazepines. These treatments enhance locomotor activity (Sainati and Lorens, 1983) and facilitate feeding behavior (Przewlocka et al., 1979); also, they released suppressed behavior in a conditioned conflict paradigm, an effect that is prevented by the destruction of 5-HT raphe neurons (Thiebot et al., 1982). Increased brain concentrations of L-tryptophan, the precursor of 5-HT, have been reported following benzodiazepine administration (Pratt et al., 1979; Valzelli et al., 1980), possibly resulting from increased uptake of L-tryptophan (Hockel et al., 1979). Several studies have found that benzodiazepines increase brain 5-HT concentrations, probably by decreasing 5-HT turnover (Chase et al., 1970; Lidbrink et al., 1973; Pratt et al., 1979).

Both acute and, particularly, chronic diazepam administration elevated synaptosomal 5-HT, suggesting that the release of 5-HT was reduced (Rastogi et al., 1978; Cook and Sepinwall, 1975; File and Vellucci, 1978). Wise et al. (1972) reported a reduction of 5-HT turnover after both acute and chronic oxazepam treatment, but a reduction in norepinephrine turnover only after acute treatment, and suggested that the anxiolytic effects of the benzodiazepines were due to reduction of 5-HT turnover, whereas their sedative effects, to which tolerance rapidly develops with chronic treatment, were due to reduction in norepinephrine turnover.

In summary, under certain experimental conditions, although not all (Thiebot, 1986), a reduction of 5-HT transmission undoubtedly mimics the effects of benzodiazepines. Two nonbenzodiazepine anxiolytics, buspirone and ritanserin, have been found to be clinically effective in several trials. Buspirone decreases 5-HT selectively and ritanserin is a selective 5-HT$_2$ antagonist with no partial agonist properties.

PSYCHOPHARMACOLOGICAL STUDIES IN PANIC DISORDERS AND PHOBIAS

Several studies of agoraphobia have reported the superiority of imipramine to chlorpromazine (Klein, 1964), to placebo (Zitrin et al., 1980, 1983; Sheehan et al., 1980), and to chlordiazepoxide (McNair and Kahn, 1981). Marks et al. (1983) found no superiority of imipramine over placebo in the treatment of agoraphobic patients; however, all the patients in that study received concomitant behavior therapy.

Mavissakalian et al. (1983, 1984) have proposed that the efficacy of imipramine in agoraphobia may be due predominantly to the 5-HT-ergic action of the drug. In a study of 15 agoraphobic patients who received imipramine, the plasma imipramine level, but not that of desipramine, correlated significantly with improvement, especially of the phobia in agoraphobic patients. It was suggested that the parent drug, imipramine, is essentially 5-HT-ergic, whereas the active N-desmethyl metabolite desipramine is mostly adrenergic (Maas, 1975; Ross and Renyi, 1975; Riblet et al., 1979); thus the antiphobic effect of imipramine may be mediated through the 5-HT system.

Kahn and Westenberg (1985) used L-5-hydroxytryptophan (5-HTP) in an open study and found that panic attacks ceased in the seven patients who had experienced them and that there was significant improvement in nine of the ten patients. 5-HTP, the immediate precursor of 5-HT, stimulates 5-HT synthesis (Van Praag and Westenberg, 1980). Both tryptophan and 5-HTP increase CSF 5-HIAA after transport blockade by probenecid (Van Praag, 1983), and this indicates an increase in CNS 5-HT metabolism (Korf and Van Praag, 1971; Mignot et al., 1985). Tryptophan, however, does not increase catecholamine activity, whereas 5-HTP, thought to result in increased catecholaminergic formation (Van Praag, 1984), increases CSF concentrations of the major catecholamine metabolites as well (Van Praag, 1986). Therefore, it appears that, although 5-HTP acts predominantly on 5-HT-ergic function, it also has important catecholaminergic effects.

Clomipramine appeared in initial uncontrolled studies to be effective in the treatment of phobic states (Colgan, 1975; Marshall, 1971, 1977; Waxman, 1975; Wooton and Bailey, 1975, 1977; Carey et al., 1975). A large uncontrolled multicenter study (Beaumont, 1977) found clomipramine, at a dose of 100 mg or less, to be highly effective in the treatment of 765 patients with phobic anxiety. Improvement was noted in 70–80%, and over 50% of patients were symptom-free. By the end of the trial, 51% of patients were symptom-free of general anxiety and 47% of situational anxiety; 55% were free of the physiological accompaniments of phobia, and 63% were free of avoidance behavior.

Karabanow (1977), in a placebo-controlled study, investigated the effect of clomipramine on depressed patients with obsessive–compulsive and phobic symptoms and found clomipramine significantly more effective after only 2 weeks of treatment. A comparison between clomipramine and diazepam in phobic and obsessive states (Waxman, 1977) showed that patients suffering the panic-like general anxiety related to illness and death responded better to clomipramine. Among a small sample of purely phobic cases, Escobar and Landbloom (1976) found that clomipramine tended to produce a greater improvement than placebo. Kahn et al. (1986) found clomipramine to be more effective than placebo in a controlled study of panic disorder and agoraphobia.

Allsopp et al. (1984) found in a study of 33 agoraphobic or social phobic patients that clomipramine was significantly superior to diazepam in improving and in maintaining improvement in situational anxiety, interference in life-style, accompanied travel distance, and total score on an agoraphobia inventory. Diazepam showed the greatest improvement by week 6, with some deterioration subsequently, whereas the clomipramine group continued to improve to the end of the trial at week 8. Thirty-three percent of the patients at the end of the study were taking less than 50 mg of clomipramine, and 65% were taking 75 mg or less. These control studies show the effectiveness of clomipramine in terms of situational anxiety and phobic anxiety as well as measures of phobia; unfortunately, specific panic attack measures were not employed.

In an uncontrolled study of clomipramine, Gloger et al. (1981) treated 20 panic disorder patients or patients with agoraphobia and panic attacks, as defined by DSM III criteria. They found that, after 8 weeks of treatment, 75% of the patients were asymptomatic and 90% of the patients had only mild infrequent panic attacks as well as moderate improvement of agoraphobic fears. Forty-five percent of the patients responded at dosages less than or equal to 50 mg/day, as opposed to the recommended dosage for imipramine of 150–225 mg/day (Klein, 1964).

Pecknold et al. (1982) treated 40 patients, 24 agoraphobics and 16 social phobics, with clomipramine and either 8 g of tryptophan or placebo. Statistical improvement was found for all groups on the Psychiatric Questionnaire of Phobic Neurosis. On the Hamilton Depression Scale, the agoraphobic and the social phobic patients on placebo showed significant improvement, and, on the Brief Psychiatric Rating Scale, only the social phobics on tryptophan did not improve. The presence of depression in these groups did not affect outcome. Both the Zung Anxiety Scale and the Social Adjustment Scale showed improvement in all subjects. Panic attacks, which were found in all the agoraphobic patients and in 80% of the social phobic patients, responded to treatment within a 3 week period. After 8 weeks of treatment, the tryptophan and the placebo were withdrawn although the clomipramine was maintained at the existing dosage. Nine patients who were on tryptophan and clomipramine regressed on withdrawal of tryptophan. These included six agoraphobic and three social phobic patients.

Tryptophan, a 5-HT precursor, increases the production of 5-HT in 5-HT neurons. However, at high doses, tryptophan interferes with the entrance of tyrosine into the CNS, decreasing the synthesis rate of catecholamines (Wertman et al., 1981). Hence, although the desmethyl metabolites of clomipramine result in considerable reuptake blocking of norepinephrine (Traskman et al., 1979), it appears that combined clomipramine and tryptophan would act predominantly on 5-HT-ergic pathways. The finding that patients on clomipramine alone, as well as those on combined clomipramine and tryptophan, improved significantly implies a role for both norepinephrine and 5-HT in the therapeutic process. The finding that certain patients relapsed after the withdrawal of tryptophan suggests that there is a subgroup of phobic disorder patients who are sensitive to changes in 5-HT.

Zimeldine is a selective inhibitor of 5-HT uptake, with little effect on norepinephrine uptake (Ross et al., 1980). Its principal metabolite norzimeldine is an even more potent 5-HT uptake blocker (Siwers et al., 1977). Koczkas et al. (1981) carried out a pilot study of zimeldine at a dose of 200–300 mg/day with 13 patients with phobic neurosis. After 6 weeks of treatment, six patients dropped out of the study because they were not appreciably improved, but seven patients showed definite improvement and completed a treatment course of at least 12 weeks. Significant relief of anxiety symptoms, particularly somatic anxiety, was noted. It was also noted that after treatment all the patients returned to work. Two of these patients had previously been treated with phenelzine. Three patients in the nonresponder group were subsequently treated with phenelzine and showed improvement. Evans and Moore (1980) carried out a pilot open study of zimeldine in seven patients diagnosed as suffering from phobic anxiety. One patient dropped out of the study. Of the remaining six patients, all but one improved.

Evans et al. (1986) carried out a controlled 6 week study comparing zimeldine and imipramine with placebo after a 2 week placebo washout in 44 patients with agoraphobia and panic attacks. The authors found that imipramine was not therapeutically superior to placebo on any of the rating scales. Zimeldine was superior to imipramine on the Fear Survey Schedule, the Hamilton Depression Scale, the Hamilton Anxiety Scale, and the Gurley Phobic Scale (total score and agoraphobia subscore). Zimeldine was also superior to placebo on the Fear Survey Schedule.

Trazodone was compared with alprazolam and imipramine by Charney et al. (1986) in 74 patients with a panic disorder in an active treatment period of 8 weeks after a 3 week placebo washout. Both imipramine and alprazolam were highly effective in reducing symptoms of generalized anxiety, frequency of panic attacks, and phobic avoidance. Alprazolam demonstrated therapeutic properties within the first week, whereas the imipramine apparently was not efficacious until the fourth week of treatment. Relative to imipramine and alprazolam, trazodone was not an effective treatment for panic disorder. Only 17 trazodone-treated patients completed at least 4 weeks of treatment, and only two patients were considered good or complete responders. The remaining 25 patients of the 27 were judged to be nonresponders. However, they subsequently responded to treatment with alprazolam or to imipramine or phenelzine. During the treatment period, a relatively low dosage of trazodone (150–200 mg/day) was used in most patients. This is considerably below recommended levels for depression. Trazodone has been shown in animal studies to inhibit the reuptake of 5-HT (Wielosz et al., 1977; Massotti et al., 1976; Riblet et al., 1979), to cause beta-receptor subsensitivity (Maggi et al., 1980), and to induce significant changes in 5-HT_2 receptor binding, with only a slight effect on alpha-2-adrenoceptors (Enna and Kendall, 1981). Trazodone seems to increase the concentration of intrasynaptic norepinephrine by blocking presynaptic alpha-adrenoceptors rather than by blocking norepinephrine transport (Maggi et al., 1980; Riblet et al., 1979). Trazodone also produces a beta-adrenoceptor subsensitivity after chronic administration (Clements-Jewrey, 1978; Maggi et al., 1980). Perhaps the effect of trazodone on 5-HT metabolism is dose-dependent, that it is an antagonist at low doses and an agonist at high doses (Baran et al., 1979). This may explain the lack of effect on panic disorder in the study of Charney et al. (1986), particularly insofar as Mavissakalian et al. (1987) found trazodone at a dosage of 300 mg/day to be effective in an open study of a small sample of panic disorder patients.

The monoamine oxidase inhibitors (MAOI), especially phenelzine, have proved effective in the treatment of phobic anxiety in uncontrolled studies (Kelly et al., 1977; King, 1962; Sargant, 1962; West, 1959) and controlled studies (Lipsedge et al., 1973; Solyom et al., 1973; Tyrer et al., 1973). Phenelzine pretreatment was found to prevent panic attacks from lactate infusions (Kelly et al., 1971). Phenelzine was also found to be superior to imipramine as well as to placebo (Sheehan et al., 1980). The MAOIs appear to increase brain 5-HT much more patently than other monoamines (Modigh and Svensson, 1972); hence the efficacy of the MAOIs in panic disorder may relate to their 5-HT-ergic activity.

In summary, clomipramine and zimeldine, which appear to exert a principal effect on 5-HT-ergic transmission, with a secondary effect on noradrenergic transmission, have strong antipanic effects. The effectiveness of the more traditional antipanic agents, imipramine and phenelzine, may also be mediated through their effect on 5-HT activity.

ROLE OF 5-HT IN LACTATE
AND CO$_2$ INHALATION

Lactate Infusion

Pitts and McClure (1967) reported that sodium lactate infusion regularly produced panic attacks in patients with panic disorders but rarely in controls. This was subsequently confirmed by other groups (Bonn et al., 1971; Fink et al., 1970; Kelley et al., 1971; Appelby et al., 1981; Rifkin et al., 1981; Liebowitz et al., 1984, 1986; Rainey et al., 1984). Fyer et al. (1985) propose that lactate vulnerability may be a trait characteristic of panic disorder. There are several hypotheses for the mechanism of action of lactate in the induction of panic attacks. These include sensitivity of panic patients to beta-adrenergic agonists (Pitts and Allen, 1979), peripheral catecholamine release with central noradrenergic stimulation (Redmond, 1979), endogenous opioid dysregulation (Klein, 1981), central CO$_2$ hypersensitivity (Liebowitz et al., 1985; Gorman et al., 1984), chemoreceptor hypersensitivity (Carr and Sheehan, 1984), and alteration of the ratio of nicotinamide adenosine dinucleotide to the reduced form (Liebowitz et al., 1986). Liebowitz et al. (1986) recently reviewed some experiments and noted that neither depression of ionized calcium nor induction of metabolic alkalosis is sufficient to cause a panic attack during a lactate infusion.

The locus ceruleus and its projections may play a part in panic attacks (Redmond, 1979). Clonidine, an alpha-adrenoceptor agonist that decreases noradrenergic function, is essentially a locus ceruleus inhibitor, which has been reported to block panic attacks transiently (Hoehn-Saric et al., 1981; Liebowitz et al., 1981). Yohimbine is an alpha-2-adrenoceptor antagonist that is reported to have an anxiogenic effect and even to trigger panic attacks in 50% of patients with panic disorder (Charney et al., 1984a, 1987). Charney and Heninger (1986a) report on the basis of their work with clonidine and yohimbine that a subgroup of patients with panic disorder exhibits abnormal plasma MHPG, blood pressures, and growth hormone and sedative responses to clonidine and that this subgroup exhibits marked abnormalities in the regulation of noradrenergic function rather than a simple deficiency or excess. However, clonidine may not be specific for adrenergic systems and may involve other neurotransmitters (Liebowitz et al., 1986). It has been shown that the activity in 5-HT synapses is an important determinant for the magnitude of the growth hormone responses to clonidine (Soderpalm et al., 1987).

Lingjaerde (1985) has hypothesized that 5-HT reuptake stimulation may be involved in lactate-induced panic attacks. It seems that lactate produces a marked increase of 5-HT uptake (Lingjaerde, 1971) and acts at a hypothetical activating site associated with the 5-HT transport carrier complex, by increasing the effectiveness of chloride ion required in 5-HT transport through platelet membrane (Lingjaerde, 1977). Since active transport of 5-HT through the plasma membranes is similar in platelets and neurons (Sneddon, 1973), lactate may stimulate serotonin uptake in 5-HT-ergic neurons. Hence a more rapid inactivation of synaptic cleft 5-HT would reduce the activity of 5-HT transmission. Lingjaerde (1985) suggests a second, less direct stimulation of neuronal 5-HT reuptake by lactate, namely, by lower intracerebral pH. The central acidosis produced by lactate (Gorman et al., 1984) results in an increase of 5-HT uptake rate (Lingjaerde, 1977). By either of these methods, a reduction in 5-HT-ergic transmission would reduce the 5-HT inhibitory system (Gray, 1982) acting on the locus ceruleus (Charney et al., 1984a) and might thereby trigger a panic attack.

The interaction between 5-HT-ergic and noradrenergic systems may be relevant to the manifestation of anxiety (Hoehn-Saric, 1982). In monkeys, the locus ceruleus contains 5-HT-ergic as well as noradrenergic cells. Also, the raphe 5-HT nuclei receive input from noradrenergic neurons, and the locus ceruleus receives innervation from the raphe (Mason and Fibiger, 1979; Hoehn-Saric, 1982; Iversen, 1984). Gray (1982) describes a behavioral inhibition system that consists anatomically of the septohippocampal system and summarizes evidence supporting the involvement of 5-HT-ergic input to the septohippocampal system from the raphe nuclei and noradrenergic input from the locus ceruleus. The 5-HT-ergic input may promote behavioral inhibition, whereas the noradrenergic input seems to influence the arousal and attentional functions of behavioral inhibition systems (Gray, 1982).

CO$_2$ Inhalation

Gorman et al. (1984) observed that aspiration of 5% CO$_2$ produces panic attacks in vulnerable patients with a frequency comparable to that of lactate. Elevated cerebral CO$_2$ is a locus ceruleus stimulant (Elam et al., 1987), is hypothesized to lead to central chemoreceptor hypersensitivity (Carr and Sheehan, 1984), and has been proposed as a common mechanism for the panic-inducing effect of both lactate and CO$_2$ (Liebowitz et al., 1985; Gorman et al., 1984). Also, as was mentioned by Lingjaerde (1985), elevated cerebral CO$_2$ lowers the cerebral pH, which in turn increases the cerebral 5-HT reuptake ratio (Lingjaerde, 1977).

In summary, the induction of panic attacks by CO$_2$ inhalation and lactate infusion may to be linked to the locus ceruleus. Although there is more evidence for noradrenergic involvement, 5-HT inhibition of the locus ceruleus may also be implicated.

5-HT PROBES IN PANIC DISORDER

Intravenous L-Tryptophan Effect on Prolactin Secretion

Heninger et al. (1984) have reported that an infusion of tryptophan with concurrent measurement of serum prolactin is blunted in patients with major depression in comparison with normal subjects. In another study, the same group (Charney et al., 1984a,b) reported that amitriptyline and desipramine significantly increased the prolactin rise induced by tryptophan in comparison with a preceding placebo.

Charney and Heninger (1986b) determined prolactin levels before, during, and after a 20 min infusion of 7 g tryptophan in 23 drug-free patients who met DSM III criteria for agoraphobia with panic attacks or panic disorder and in 21 age- and sex-matched healthy subjects. Seven of the patient group also met the criteria for concurrent major depression. In nine of the patients, the tryptophan infusion was repeated during alprazolam treatment. The alprazolam mean dosage was 3.8 mg/day (range of 2–6 mg/day), and mean duration of treatment was 9.9 weeks (range 8–16 weeks). The authors found that tryptophan induced significant increases in serum prolactin values both in the healthy subjects and in the panic disorder patients. There were no significant differences between the two groups. The seven patients with concurrent panic disorder and major depression were not significantly different from the rest of the panic group in their prolactin response. In the nine patients who went on to alprazolam therapy, the prolactin response to the tryptophan infusion was no different during alprazolam treatment than during the placebo phase despite clinical improvement with this relatively low dosage of alprazolam. The authors suggest that 5-HT function may be normal in panic disorder and, furthermore, that the antipanic mechanism of action of alprazolam may be unrelated to effects on 5-HT activity.

[³H]Imipramine Binding and 5-HT Uptake Binding Sites

The high-affinity binding site for [³H]-imipramine is present in membranes prepared from various regions of the brain of several species, including man (Langer et al., 1981, 1982; Raisman et al., 1979a,b, 1980) and on platelet membranes (Briley et al., 1979; Langer et al., 1980b). This binding site possesses most of the characteristics of a recognition site for a pharmacological receptor (Langer and Briley, 1981). It is inhibited with high affinity by tricyclic antidepressants and by nontricyclic inhibitors of neuronal 5-HT uptake (Langer et al., 1984a,b). The only neurotransmitter known to inhibit [³H]-imipramine binding is 5-HT (Raisman et al., 1980). The association of [³H]-imipramine binding with the transporter for the 5-HT uptake mechanism in serotogenic nerve endings has been established (Brunello et al., 1982; Gross et al., 1981; Langer et al., 1980a; Sette et al., 1981). It is likely that [³H]-imipramine binding labels a physiologically relevant site that modulates 5-HT uptake (Langer et al., 1983) rather than a simple tricyclic recognition site. In platelets, competitive interaction between 5-HT and imipramine for the same sites has been proposed (Talvanheimo and Rudnick, 1980), as has a noncompetitive or mixed-type interaction (Lingjaerde, 1979). Wennogle and Meyerson (1985) note that there is no evidence for cooperative interaction at the imipramine recognition site in platelets. Possibly 5-HT can modulate the dissociation of [^{3}H]-imipramine on platelet membranes, indicating binding of these ligands (imipramine and 5-HT) to different but allosterically coupled sites (Langer et al., 1983; Wennogle and Meyerson, 1983). In the brain, the [^{3}H]-imipramine binding sites and the recognition site for 5-HT reuptake are independent but are allosterically coupled (Sette et al., 1983). Thus the imipramine binding site is distinct from, and allosterically coupled to, the 5-HT uptake site (Wennogle and Meyersen, 1985; Briley et al., 1981; Barbaccia et al., 1983b). Each tricyclic binding site may be associated with two adjacent 5-HT transport sites (Rudnick et al., 1983). Endogenous modulators or autocoids (Barbaccia et al., 1983a; Angel and Paul, 1984) would provide fine control of the velocity of the 5-HT transporter and thus regulate the availability of free 5-HT. A potent inhibitor of [^{3}H]-imipramine binding, 5-methoxytryptaline, also inhibits [^{3}H]-5-HT uptake and may be a candidate for this autocoid (Langer et al., 1984a).

Imipramine Binding

A reduction in the number of binding sites for the tricyclic antidepressant imipramine on platelets appears to be a potential peripheral biochemical marker of depression (Briley et al., 1980a,b; Paul et al., 1981; Asarch et al., 1981; Langer et al., 1981; Suranyi-Cadotte et al., 1982). These [^{3}H]-imipramine binding sites may be associated but not identical with the uptake of 5-HT in the brain (Langer et al., 1980b; Palkovits, 1981; Barbaccia et al., 1983a) and platelets (Paul et al., 1980a, Rehavi et al., 1981; Wood et al., 1983; Suranyi-Cadotte et al., 1985b). Platelet [^{3}H]-imipramine binding could be a useful model to investigate abnormalities of CNS 5-HT-ergic function. Reduced platelet [^{3}H]-imipramine binding has been reported in depressed patients but not in patients with other disorders thought potentially to involve altered 5-HT-ergic function, such as schizophrenia (Wood et al., 1983), schizoaffective disorder (Suranyi-Cadotte et al., 1983), alcoholism (Athee et al., 1981), arterial hypertension (Kamal et al., 1984a,b), Alzheimer's disease, and Parkinson's disease (Suranyi-Cadotte et al., 1985a).

Studies in Panic Disorder

We studied 43 patients with panic disorder and agoraphobia (Pecknold et al., 1987). These patients with panic disorder included those who never had a depressive episode (56%) (according to DSM III criteria for major depressive disorder) and those who met concurrent DSM III criteria for both panic disorder and major depressive disorder at presentation (16%). There were also patients with panic disorder who had had DSM III-defined major depression in the past (44%). The panic disorder patients were compared to patients who met criteria for major depression (research diagnostic criteria of Feighner et al, 1972) who also met criteria (Winokur, 1983) for primary pure familial depression.

Figure 8–1 illustrates mean platelet [^{3}H]-imipramine binding variables in healthy volunteers and patients with primary major depression and panic disorder. The affinity (Kd, nM) of [^{3}H]-imipramine for its binding site on platelet membranes of depressed and panic disorder patients was not significantly different from that of normals. As is shown in Figure 8–1, the number (Bmax ± SD; fmoles/mg protein) of [^{3}H]-imipramine binding sites on platelets of depressed patients was significantly lower than for normal subjects. Furthermore, patients with primary major depression had Bmax values that were also significantly reduced compared to panic disorder patients. In the panic group, the mean density of [^{3}H]-imipramine binding sites was not significantly different from healthy volunteers. These data alone are suggestive of a distinct difference between panic disorder and primary depressive disorder. The distinction between the two disorders is further reflected by the finding of Bmax values similar to those of controls, even in those panic disorder patients who presented with concurrent panic disorder and major depression as well as those with panic disorder and a history of major depression. In panic disorder patients who presented with concurrent depressive disorder, severity of depression, as indicated by Hamilton Depression Rating scores, did not correlate significantly with either Bmax ($r = -0.19$, $P = 0.35$ ns) or Kd ($r = 0.02$, $P = 0.48$, ns) values.

Our study demonstrated that a reduction in number of high-affinity platelet [^{3}H]-imip-

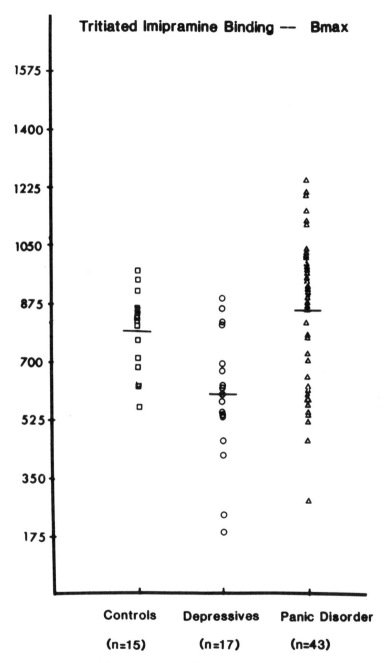

Fig. 8–1.   Platelet tritiated imipramine binding (Bmax) for depressed (n = 17) and panic disorder patients (n = 43) compared to normal controls (n = 15). Horizontal line (——) indicated mean value within each group.

ramine binding sites may distinguish patients with primary major depression from panic disorder subjects. In depressed patients, the num-ber (Bmax) of [3H]-imipramine binding sites was significantly lower than in normal subjects, as has been reported previously (Briley et al., 1980a; Paul et al., 1981; Asarch et al., 1981; Suranyi-Cadotte et al., 1982). In contrast, panic disorder patients had Bmax values that were not significantly different from those of normal volunteers. The apparently normal Bmax values in panic disorder patients observed here are in agreement with an earlier report by Roy-Byrne and Uhde (1985), who found similar [^{3}H]-imipramine binding variables in nondepressed panic disorder and normal subjects, but are at variance with the findings of Lewis et al. (1985), who found a decreased Bmax in agoraphobic patients. In our study, normal Bmax values were observed even in those panic disorder patients who had concurrent major depression or a history of major depression. This finding further supports the distinction between primary major depression and panic disorder and suggests that the presence of secondary depression is not sufficient to alter the characteristics of [^{3}H]-imipramine binding sites. The reduction in the density of platelet [^{3}H]-imipramine binding sites may, therefore, be a selective peripheral marker of primary depressive disorder.

5-HT Uptake

5-HT uptake refers to the transport of 5-hydroxytryptamine through the platelet plasma membrane. After having penetrated the platelet membrane, most 5-HT is stored in the dense granules, but the rate-limiting step in the overall uptake process is the passage through the plasma membrane (Lingjaerde, 1977).

There are reports of reduced 5-HT uptake in depression (Coppen et al., 1978; Ehsanullah, 1980; Hallstrom et al., 1976; Pare et al., 1974; Rausch et al., 1982; Ross et al., 1980; Tuomisto and Tukiainen, 1976; Tuomisto et al., 1979), mostly endogenous unipolar or bipolar depression. It appears to be the maximal uptake rate (Vmax) that is reduced, whereas the apparent affinity constant (Km) is unchanged (Coppen et al., 1978; Meltzer et al., 1981; Tuomisto and Tukiainen, 1976; Tuomisto et al., 1979).

Studies in Panic Disorder Patients

We studied 5-HT uptake in 47 patients with panic disorder, 17 patients with primary major depression, and 15 normal volunteers (Pecknold et al., 1988). Panic disorder patients fulfilled DSM III criteria. Ninety-four percent of these patients had no concurrent major depression (DSM III criteria) and 6% did have. Seventy-two percent had had no previous depressive episode, and 28% had had a previous major depression according to DSM III criteria that developed subsequent to the first onset of the panic disorder. Panic disorder patients had a diagnosis of agoraphobia (89%) or limited phobic avoidance (11%).

All depressed patients met research diagnostic criteria for major depressive disorder (Feighner et al., 1972) and the criteria (Winokur, 1983) for primary pure familial depression and had Hamilton Depression Rating scores equal to or greater than 20. The maximum rate of uptake of 5-HT into platelets (Vmax) was found to be significantly lower in both the depressed and panic disorders groups than in the control group (F = 5.46, df = 2, 76, P < 0.006; see Fig. 8–2) (Neuman-Keuls).

Because the Vmax of platelet 5-HT uptake has been reported to be reduced in depression, we assessed the effect of present or a history of depression in panic disorder patients. Interestingly, panic disorder patients with current and/or past episodes of major depression had values actually slightly higher than the mean Vmax value of the panic patients without history of major depression (Fig. 8–2).

There was no significant correlation between Vmax and Hamilton Depression, Hamilton Anxiety, or Panic Scale scores in the panic disorder group. However, in the panic disorder group, there was a significant positive low-order correlation between Vmax and the last measure of the Sheehan-Gelder Phobia Scale (r = 0.24, P < 0.05), indicating that the panic disorder patients with higher Vmax values experience more avoidance.

Our results demonstrate that, compared to normal subjects, patients with panic disorder and familial depression have similar significant decreases in platelet 5-HT uptake. The reduction in the maximum rate of uptake (Vmax) for 5-HT in platelets of depressed patients observed here is in agreement with previous studies (Coppen et al., 1978; Tuomisto and Tukiainen, 1976; Meltzer et al., 1981; Wood et al., 1983). Our finding of a reduced Vmax in patients with panic disorder is at variance with the findings of Norman et al. (1986), who found higher Vmax values in their 45 panic disorder

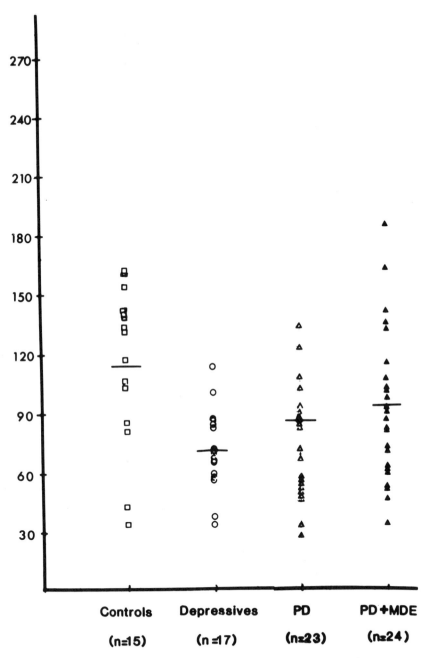

Fig. 8–2.   Platelet serotonin uptake (Vmax) for depressed (n = 17); panic disorder (PD, n = 23) and panic disorder patients with major depressive episode (MDE n = 24) compared to normal controls (n = 15). Horizontal line (——) indicates mean value within each group.

patients than in 21 normal controls. The authors correlate their finding with the observation by Evans et al. (1985) of lowered plasma 5-HT levels in panic patients, suggesting that both findings are a consequence of increased mitochondrial platelet MAO activity observed in panic patients (Yu et al., 1983). However, several reports support the hypothesis that low 5-HT levels are at least partially attributed to reduced platelet 5-HT uptake (Tuomisto and Tukiainen, 1976; Meltzer et al., 1981; Kaplan and Mann, 1982). Other mechanisms that may explain a reduced 5-HT content include an increased intracellular conjugation or degradation, a defect of storage in intracellular dense granules, and an increased release of the amine from platelets (Le Quan-Bui et al., 1984).

The 5-HT uptake and imipramine binding data were analyzed together (Pecknold and Suranyi-Cadotte, 1986). Those panic disorder patients were selected who had low 5-HT Vmax values, comparable to those of depressive patients (range 50–90), and also the patients who had an imipramine binding Bmax comparable to that of the depressive group (range 395–700). There were eight panic disorder patients in this group; we will call them the "panic-depressive subgroup." This group was not significantly different from the controls, depressives, or other panic disorder group regarding sex. The depressive group was significantly older than the remaining three groups. Examining the 5-HT Vmax with analysis of covariance controlling for age, we found that the control group had a significantly higher score than the panic-depressive subgroup and depressive groups. When looking at the imipramine binding Bmax, also on analysis of covariance, both the panic-depressive subgroup and the depressed groups had Bmax scores significantly lower than control and panic disorder groups.

In comparing the panic-depressive subgroup with the rest of the panic patients, there were no significant differences in terms of sex, history of the previous depression, or presence of a current secondary depression. Also the total Hamilton Anxiety score, the total Hamilton Depression score, and the Panic Attack total score failed to differentiate the panic-depressive subgroup from the panic group. There was, however, a significant difference between the two panic groups on rapid eye movement (REM) sleep latency. The panic-depressive subgroup included a greater proportion of patients with an early REM sleep latency than did the panic disorder group as a whole.

In summary, we have demonstrated that a reduction in the number of high-affinity platelet [^{3}H]-imipramine binding sites (Bmax) may distinguish patients with primary major familial depression from panic disorder patients. This finding indicates that, for the panic disorder group, we cannot demonstrate a shared diathesis with pure familial depressive illness.

We have also demonstrated that for the panic disorder group, as a whole, and for the major familial depression group there is a similar and significant decrease in platelet 5-HT uptake below normal levels. This suggests the possibility of a 5-HT mechanism in panic disorder.

Finally, it appears that a very small group of patients, 17% of our group, may have a shared diathesis with depression. The prediction of pathophysiological and therapeutic outcome for this patient group are important subjects for future study.

CONCLUSIONS

The phenomenological and epidemiological linkage of anxiety and depressive disorders suggests a similar implication of both the noradrenergic and 5-HT-ergic systems. Support for 5-HT-ergic involvement is found in several lines of pharmacological and behavioral evidence in animal studies. Interpretation of this data is difficult because the correspondence of animal behaviors to generalized anxiety and to panic disorder in human beings is not clear. Furthermore, the activation of different synaptic 5-HT receptors may lead to different and even opposing functional effects. Nevertheless, overwhelming evidence links 5-HT-ergic mechanisms to various phenomena of anxiety. The anatomical and physiological hypotheses of Gray (1982) propose that the 5-HT-ergic system may be an inhibitory behavioral system impinging on the locus ceruleus and indeed on the septohippocampal system. Lingjaerde's (1985) hypothesis is that 5-HT reuptake is stimulated by lactate. This produces a central reduction in 5-HT-ergic transmission, which reduces the 5-HT-inhibiting system acting on the locus ceruleus. The result of the reduction of the inhibition system contributes to the triggering of a panic attack. The postulated deficit of 5-HT has been observed in our studies of platelet 5-HT uptake in patients with panic disorder.

Psychopharmacological studies show that

antipanic agents such as phenelzine and imipramine may act through a 5-HT-ergic mechanism. The more potent or more selective 5-HT agonists such as clomipramine and zimeldine produce an even greater therapeutic improvement and do so at lower therapeutic dosages. All these agents given subchronically either increase the responsiveness of postsynaptic 5-HT receptors or decrease the sensitivity of 5-HT autoreceptors. In either case, they facilitate 5-HT-ergic neurotransmission and augment the inhibitory 5-HT-ergic behavioral system, which reduces the likelihood of a panic attack. The precise interaction of 5-HT-ergic and noradrenergic mechanisms in panic disorder is not yet clear, and the interrelationships of general anxiety reactions and of depression also have to be clarified.

REFERENCES

Allsopp LF, Cooper GL, Poole PH (1984): Clomipramine and diazepam in the treatment of agoraphobia and social phobias in general practice. Curr Med Res Opinion 9:64–70.

Amin MM, Ananth JV, Coleman BS, Darcourt G, Farkas T, Goldstein B, Lapierre YD, Paykel E, Wakelin JS (1984): Fluvoxamine: antidepressant effects confirmed in a placebo-controlled study. Clin Neuropharmacol 7[Suppl 1]:580–581.

Ananth J, Pecknold JC, Van der Steen N, Engelsmann F (1980): Double blind comparative study of clomipramine and amitriptyline in obsessive neurosis. Prog. Neuropsychopharmacol Biol Psychiatry 5:257–264.

Angel I, Paul SN (1984): Inhibition of synaptosomal 5[^{3}H]-hydroxytryptamine uptake by endogenous factor(s) in human blood. FEBS Lett 171:280–284.

Appelby I, Klein D, Sachar E, Levitt M (1981): Biochemical indices of lactate-induced panic: A preliminary report. In Klein DF, Rabkin J (eds): "Anxiety: New Research and Changing Concepts." New York: Raven Press.

Asarch KB, Shih JC, Kubesar A (1981): Decreased 3H-imipramine binding in depressed males and females. Commun Psychopharmacol 4:425–432.

Athee L, Briley M, Raisman R, Lebrec D, Langer SZ (1981): Reduced uptake of serotonin but unchanged 3H-imipramine binding in the platelets of cirrhotic patients. Life Sci 29:2323–2329.

Baran L, Maj J, Rogo'z Z, et al. (1979): On the central antiserotonin action of trazodone. Pol J Pharmacol Pharm 31:25–33.

Barbaccia ML, Brunello N, Chuang DM, Costa E (1983b): On the mode of action of imipramine: Relationship between serotonergic axon terminal function and down-regulation of beta adrenergic receptors. Neuropharmacology 22:373–383.

Barbaccia ML, Gandolfi O, Chuang DM, Costa E (1983a): Modulation of neuronal serotonin uptake by a puta-

tive endogenous ligand of imipramine recognition sites. Proc Natl Acad Sci USA 80:5134–5138.

Beaumont G (1977): A large open multicentre trial of clomipramine (anafranil) in the management ofphobic disorders. J Int Med Res 5[Suppl 5]:116–123.

Bjerkenstedt L, Edman G, Flyckt L, Sedvall G, Wiesel F (1984): Clinical and biochemical effects of citalopram in depressed patients. Clinical Psychopharmacol 7[Suppl 1]:874–875.

Blakey TA, Parker LF (1973): effects of parachlorophenylalanine on experimentally induced conflict behaviour. Pharmacol Biochem Behav 1:600–613.

Bonn J, Harrison J, Rees W (1971): Lactate-induced anxiety: therapeutic application. Br J Psychiatry 119:468.

Bowen RC, Kohut J (1979): The relationship between agoraphobia and primary affective disorders. Can J Psychiatry 24:317–321.

Breier MS, Charney DS, Heninger GR (1984): Major depression in patients with agoraphobia and panic disorder. Arch Gen Psychiatry 41:1129–1135.

Breier A, Charney DS, Heninger GR (1985): The diagnostic validity of anxiety disorders and their relationship to depressive illness. Am J Psychiatry 142:787–797.

Breier A, Charney DS, Heninger GR (1986): Agoraphobia with panic attacks: Development, diagnostic stability, and course of illness. Arch Gen Psychiatry 43:1029–1036.

Briley MS, Raisman R, Langer SZ (1979): Human platelets possess high-affinity binding sites for ^{3}H-imipramine. Eur J Pharmacol 58:347–348.

Briley MS, Langer SZ, Raisman R, Sechter D, Zarifian E (1980a): Tritiated imipramine binding sites are decreased in platelets of untreated depressed patients. Science 209:303–305.

Briley MS, Raisman R, Sechter D, Zarifian E, Langer SZ (1980b): ^{3}H-Imipramine binding in human platelets: A new biochemical parameter in depression. Neuropharmacology 19:1209–1210.

Briley MS, Langer SZ, Sette M (1981): Allosteric interaction between the 3H-imipramine binding and the serotonin uptake mechanism. Br J Pharmacol 74:817–818.

Brunello M, Chuang D, Costa E (1982): Different synaptic localizations of mianserin and imipramine binding sites. Science 215:1112–1115.

Buglass D, Clarke J, Henderson AS, Kreitman N, Presley AS (1977): A study of agoraphobic housewives. Psychol Med 7:73–86.

Carey MS, Hawkinson R, Kornhaber A, Wellish CS (1975): The use of clomipramine in phobic patients: preliminary research report. Curr Ther Res 17:107–110.

Carlsson A, Corrodi H, Fuxe K, Hokfelt T (1969): Effect of antidepressant drugs on the depletion on intraneuronal brain 5-hydroxytryptamine stores caused by 4-methyl-alpha-ethyl-metatyramine. Eur J Pharmacol 5:357–366.

Carr D, Sheehan D (1984): Panic anxiety: A new biological model. J Clin Psychiatry 45:323–330.

Ceulemans DLS, Hoppenbrouwers M-LJA, Gelders YG, Reyntjens (1985): The influence of ritanserin, a serotonin antagonist, in anxiety disorders: A double-blind placebo controlled study verus lorazepam. Pharmacopsychiatry 18:303–305.

Charney DS, Heninger GR (1986a): Abnormal regulation of noradrenergic function in panic disorders. Effects of clonidine in healthy subjects and patients with agoraphobia and panic disorders. Arch Gen Psychiatry 43:1042–1054.

Charney DS, Heninger GR (1986b): Serotonin function in panic disorders: The effect of intravenous tryptophan in healthy subjects and patients with panic disorders before and during alprazolam treatment. Arch Gen Psychiatry 43:1059–1065.

Charney DS, Heninger GR, Breier A (1984a): Noradrenergic function in panic anxiety: Effects of yohimbine in healthy subjects and patients with agoraphobia and panic disorder. Arch Gen Psychiatry 41:751–763.

Charney DS, Heninger GR, Sternberg DE (1984b): Serotonin function and mechanism of action of antidepressant treatments: Effects of amitriptaline and desipramine. Arch Gen Psychiatry 41:359–365.

Charney DS, Woods SW, Goodman WK, Heninger GR (1987): Neurobiological mechanisms of panic anxiety: biochemical and behavioural correlates of yohimbine-induced panic attacks. Am J Psychiatry 144:1030–1036.

Charney DS, Woods SW, Goodman WK, Rifkin B, Kinch M, Aiken B, Quadrino CM, Heninger GR (1986): Drug treatment of panic disorders: The comparative efficacy of imipramine, alprazolam, and trazodone. J Clin Psychiatry 47:580–586.

Chase TN, Katz RI, Kopin IJ (1970): Effect of diazepam on fate of intracisternally injected serotonin C-14. Neuropharmacology 9:103–108.

Claghorn J, Gershon S, Goldstein BJ, Behrnetz S, Bush DF, Huitfeldt B (1983): A double-blind evaluation of zimeldine in comparison to placebo and amitriptyline in patients with major depressive disorder. Prog Neuropsychopharmacol 7:367–382.

Cleland WW (1967): The statistical analysis of enzyme kinetic dats. Adv Enzymol 29:1–32.

Clements-Jewrey S (1978): The development of cortical beta-adrenoceptor subsensitivity in the rat by chronic treatment with trazodone, doxepin, and mianserine. Neuropharmacology 17:779–781.

Cloninger CR, Martin RL, Clayton R, et al. (1981): A blind follow-up and family study of anxiety neurosis: Preliminary analyses of the St. Louis 500. In Klein DF, Raskin J (eds): "Anxiety: New Research and Changing Concepts." New York: Raven Press, pp 137–168.

Cohn B, Wilcox CS, Melzer HY (1986): Neuroendocrine effects of buspirone in patients with generalized anxiety disorder. Am J Med 80[Suppl 3B]:36–40.

Colgan A (1975): A pilot study of anafranil in the treatment of phobic states. Scottish Med J 20:55–70.

Commissaris RL, Lyness WH, Rech RH (1981): The effects of d-lysergic acid diethylamide (LSD), 2,5-dimethoxy-4-methylamphetamine (DOM), pentobarbital, and methaqualone on punished responding in control and 5,7-dihydroxytryptamine-treated rats. Pharmacol Biochem Behav 14:617–623.

Cook L, Sepinwall J (1975): Behaviour analysis of the effects of mechanisms of action of benzodiazepines. In

Costa E, Greengard P (eds): "Mechanism of Action of Benzodiazepines." New York: Raven Press, pp 1–28.

Coppen A, Swade C, Wood K (1978): Platelet 5-hydroxytryptamine accumulation in depressive illness. Clin Chim Acta 87:165–168.

Corrodi HK, Fuxe P, Lidbrink P, Olson L (1971): Minor tranquillizers, stress and central catecholamine neurons. Brain Res 29:1–16.

Dealy RS, Ishiki DM, Avery DH, Wilson LG, Dumes DL (1981): Secondary depression in anxiety disorders. Comp Psychiatry 22:612–618.

Den Boer JA, Westenberg HGM, Kamerbeek WOJ, Verhoeven WMA, Kahn RS (1987): Effect of serotonin uptake inhibitors in anxiety disorders: A double-blind comparison of clomipramine and fluvoxamine. Int Clin Psychopharmacol 2:21–32.

Deutsch H (1982): The genesis of agoraphobia. Int J Psychoanal 10:51–69.

Ehsanullah RSB (1980): Uptake of 5-hydroxytryptamine and dopamine into platelets from depressed patients and normal subjects—Influence of clomipramine, desmethylclomipramine and maprotiline. Postgrad Med J [Suppl 1]:31–35.

Eison AS, Tample DL (1986): Buspirone: review of its pharmacology and current perspectives on its mechanism of action. Am J Med 80[Suppl 3B]:1–9.

Elam M, Yoa J, Thoren P (1981): Hypercapnia and hypoxia: Chemoreceptor mediated control of locus ceruleus neurones and splanchnic, sympathetic nerves. Brain Res 222:373–381.

Enna SJ, Kendall DA (1981): Interaction of antidepressants with brain neurotransmitter receptors. J Clin Psychopharmacol 1:12–65.

Escobar J, Landbloom P (1976): Treatment of phobic neurosis with clomipramine: a controlled clinical trial. Curr Ther Res 20:680–685.

Estes WK, Skinner BF (1941): Some quantitative properties of anxiety. J Exp Psychol 29:390–400.

Evans L, Best J, Moore G, et al. (1980): Zimelidine—A serotonin uptake blocker in the treatment of phobic anxiety. Prog Neuropsychopharmacol 4:75–79.

Evans L, Kenardy J, Schneider P, Hoey H (1986): Effect of a selective serotonin uptake inhibitor in agoraphobia with panic attacks. Acta Psychiatr Scand 73:49–53.

Evans L, Moore G (1981): The treatment of phobic anxiety by zimeldine. Acta Psych Scand 63[Suppl 290]:342–345.

Evans L, Schneider P, Ross-Lee, et al. (1985): Plasma serotonin levels in agoraphobia. Am J Psychiatry 142:267.

Fawcett J, Kravits HM (1983): Anxiety syndromes and their relationship to depressive illness. J Clin Psychiatry 44:8–11.

Feighner JP, Merideth CH, Henrickson GA (1982): A double-blind comparison of buspirone and diazepam in outpatients with generalized anxiety disorder. J Clin Psychiatry 43:12, 103–107.

Feighner JP, Robins E, Guze SB, et al. (1972): Diagnostic criteria for use in psychiatric research. Arch Gen Psychiatry 26:57–63.

File SE, Hyde JRG (1977): The effects of p-chlorophenylalanine and ethanolamine-0-sulphate in an animal test of anxiety. J Pharmacol 29:735–738.

File SE, Vellucci SV (1978): Studies on the role of ACTH and of 5-HT in anxiety, using an animal model. J Pharm Pharmacol 30:105–110.

Fink M, Taylor MA, Volavka J (1970): Anxiety precipitated by lactate (letter). N Engl J Med 281:1129.

Flament MF, Rapoport JL, Murphy DL, Lake CR, Berg CJ (1987): Biochemical changes during clomipramine treatment of childhood obsessive-compulsive disorder. Arch Gen Psychiatry 44:219–225.

Fontaine R, Chouinard G (1985): Antiobsessive effect of fluoxetine. Am J Psychiatry 142:989.

Fyer AJ, Liebowitz MR, Gorman JM, Davies SO, Klein DF (1985): Lactate vulnerability of remitted panic patients. Psychiatry Res 14:143.

Gardner CR (1985): Pharmacological studies of the role of serotonin in animal models of anxiety. In Green AR (ed): "Neuropharmacology of Serotonin." New York: Oxford University Press, pp 281–325.

Gardner CR (1986): Recent developments in 5-HT-related pharmacology of animal models of anxiety. Pharmacol Biochem Behav 24:1479–1485.

Gelder MG, Marks IM, Wolff HH (1967): Desensitization and psychotherapy in the treatment of phobic states: A controlled enquiry. Br J Psychiatry 113:53–73.

Geller I, Blum K (1970): The effects of 5-HTP on parachlorophenylalanine (pCPA) attenuation of "conflict" behaviour in the rat. Eur J Pharmacol 9:319–324.

Geller I, Seifter J (1960): The effects of meprobamate, barbiturates, d-amphetamine, and promaxine on experimentally induced conflict in the rat. Psychopharmacologia 1:482–492.

Gloger S, Grunhaus L, Birmacher B, Troudart T (1981): Treatment of spontaneous panic attacks with clomipramine. Am J Psychiatry 138:1215–1217.

Goodman WK, Price LH, Rasmussen SA, Charney DS, Woods SN, Heninger GRL (1986): Evidence for abnormal serotonergic function in obsessive-compulsive disorder. Abstract 317.6. Abstracts of the 16th Annual Meeting of the Society for Neuroscience, Washington, DC, Nov 9–14, 1986.

Goodwin GM, Green AR (1985): A behavioural and biochemical study in mice and rats of putative selective agonists and antagonists for 5-HT, and 5-HT$_2$ receptors. Br J Pharmacol 84:743–753.

Gorman JM, Askanazi J, Liebowitz MR, et al. (1984): Response to hyperventilation in a group of patients with panic disorder. Am J Psychiatry 141:857–861.

Gorman JM, Liebowitz MR, Fyer AJ, Goetz D, Campeas RB, Fyer MR, Davies SO, Ulein DF (1987): An open trial of fluoxetine in the treatment of panic attacks. J Clin Psychopharmacol 7:329–332.

Graeff FG, Filho NGS (1978): Behavioural inhibition induced by electrical stimulation of the median raphe nucleus of the rat. Physiol Behav 21:477–484.

Graeff FG, Schoenfeld RI (1970): Tryptamine mechanisms in punished and nonpunished behaviour. J Pharmacol Exp Ther 173:277–283.

Gray JA (1982): The neuropsychology of anxiety: An inquiry into the functions of the septo-hippocampal system. New York: Oxford University Press.

Green AR, Guy AP, Gardner CR (1984): The behavioural effects of RU24969, a suggested 5-HT1 receptor agonist in rodents and the effect on the behaviour of treatments with antidepressants. Neuropharmacology 23:655–661.

Gross G, Gothert M, Ender H-C, Schumann H-J (1981): ^{3}H-imipramine binding sites in the rat brain: selective localization on serotoninergic neurons. Naunyn-Schmiedebergs Arch Pharmacol 317:310–314.

Haefely WL, Pieri L, Polc P, Schaffner R (1981): General pharmacology and neuropharmacology of benzodiazepine derivatives. In Hoffmerster F, Stille G (eds): "Handbook of Experimental Pharmacology. Vol 55, Part II." Berlin: Springer-Verlag, pp 13–262.

Hallstrom COS, Linford Rees W, Pare CMB, Trenchard A, Turner P (1976): Platelet uptake of 5-hydroxytryptamine and dopamine in depression. Postgrad Med J 52[Suppl 3]:40–44.

Heel RC, Morley PA, Brogden RN, Carmine AA, Speight TM, Avery GS (1982): Zimeldine: a review of its pharmacological properties and therapeutic efficacy in depressive illness. Drugs 24:169–206.

Heninger GR, Charney DS, Sternberg DE (1984): Serotonergic function in depression: Prolactin response to intravenous tryptophan in depressed patients and healthy subjects. Arch Gen Psychiatry 41:398–404.

Hockel SHJ, Muller WE, Wollert U (1979): Diazepam increases L-tryptophan intake into various regions of the rat brain. Res Commun Psychol Psychiatry Behav 4:467–475.

Hoehn-Saric R (1982): Neurotransmitters in anxiety. Arch Gen Psychiatry 39:735–742.

Hoehn-Saric R, Merchant AF, Keyser ML, et al. (1981): Effects of clonidine on anxiety disorders. Arch Gen Psychiatry 38:1278–1282.

Hytell J, Overo KF, Arnt J (1984): Biochemical effects and drug levels in rats after long-term treatment with the specific 5-HT uptake inhibitor citalopram. Psychopharmacology 83:20–27.

Insel TR, Mueller EA, Alterman I, Linnoila M, Murphy DL (1985): Obsessive-compulsive disorder and serotonin: Is there a connection? Biol Psychiatry 20:1174–1188.

Insel TR, Murphy DL, Cohen RM, Alterman I, Kilts C, Linnoila M (1983): Obsessive-compulsive disorder: A double-blind trial of clomipramine and clorgyline. Arch Gen Psychiatry 40:605–612.

Iversen SD (1983): Animal models of anxiety. In Trimble M (ed): "Benzodiazepines Divided: A Multidisciplinary Review." New York: Wiley, pp 87–97.

Iversen SD (1984): 5-HT and anxiety. Neuropharmacology 23:1553–1560.

Johnston AL, File SE (1986): 5-HT and anxiety: Promises and pitfalls. Pharmacol Biochem Behav 24:1467–1470.

Kahn RS, Westenberg HGM (1985): L-5-hydroxytryptophan in the treatment of anxiety disorders. J Affect Disorders 8:197–200.

Kahn RS, Westernberg HGM, Jolles J (1984): Zimeldine treatment of obsessive-compulsive disorder. Acta Psychiatr Scand 69:259–261.

Kahn RS, Westenberg HGM, Verhoeven WMA, Gisperde Wied CC (1987): Effect of a serotonin precursor and uptake inhibitor in anxiety disorders; a double-blind comparison of 5-HTP, clomipramine, and placebo. Int Clin Psychopharmacol 2:33–45.

Kamal LA, Le Quan-Bui KH, Meyer P (1984): Decreased uptake of 3H-serotonin and endogenous content of serotonin in blood platelets in hypertensive patients. Hypertension 6:568–573.

Kamal LA, Raisman R, Meyer P, et al. (1984): Reduced V-MAX of ^{3}H-serotonin uptake but unchanged ^{3}H-imipramine binding in the platelets of untreated hypertensive subjects. Life Sci 34:2083–2088.

Kaplan RD, Mann JJ (1982): Altered platelet serotonin uptake kinetics in schizophrenia and depression. Life Sci 31:583–586.

Karabanow O (1977): Double-blind controlled study in phobias and obsessions. J Int Med Res 5[Suppl 5]:42–48.

Kelly D, Mitchell-Heggs N, Sherman D (1971): Anxiety and the effects of sodium lactate assessed clinically and psychologically. Br J Psychiatry 119:129–141.

Kilts CD, Commissaris RL, Rech RH (1981): Comparison of anticonflict drug effects in three experimental animal models of anxiety. Psychopharmacology 74:290–296.

King A. (1981): Phenalzine treatment of Roth's calamity syndrome. Med J Aust 1:879–883.

Klein DF (1964): The delineation of two drug-responsive anxiety syndromes. Psychopharmacology 5:397–408.

Klein DF (1981): Anxiety reconceptualized. In Klein DF, Rabkin JG (eds): "Anxiety, New Research and Changing Concepts." New York: Raven Press.

Koczkas S, Holberg G, Wedin L (1981): A pilot study of the effect of the 5HT-uptake inhibitor, zimeldine, on phobic anxiety. Acta Psychiatr Scand 63[Suppl 290]:328–341.

Korf J, Van Praag HM (1971): Amine metabolism in the human brain: Further evaluation of the probenecid test. Brain Res 35:221–230.

Langer SZ, Briley M (1981): High affinity 3H-imipramine binding: a new biological tool for studies in depression. Trends Neurosci 4:28–31.

Langer SZ, Javoy-Agid F, Raisman R, Briley M, Agid Y (1981): Distribution of high-affinity binding sites for imipramine in human brain. J Neurochem 37:267–271.

Langer SZ, Lee CR, Segonzac A, Tateishi T, Schormaher H, Wimblod B (1984a): Possible endocrine role of the pineal gland for 6-methoxy-tetrahydrobetacarboline, a putative endogenous neuromodulation for the ^{3}H-imipramine recognition site. Eur J Pharmacol 102:379–380.

Langer SZ, Moret C, Raisman R, Dubocovitch ML, Briley MS (1980a): High affinity ^{3}H-imipramine binding in rat hypothalamus is associated with the uptake of serotonin but not norepinephrine. Life Sci 210:1133–1135.

Langer SZ, Raisman R, Briley M (1980b): Stereoselective inhibition of ^{3}H-imipramine binding by antidepressant drugs and their derivatives. Eur J Pharmacol 64:89–90.

Langer SZ, Raisman R, Sechter D, Gay C, Loo H, Zarifian

E (1984b): ^{3}H-Imipramine and ^{4}H-desipramine binding sites in depression. In Usdin E, Asberg M, Bertilsson L, Sjoqvist F (eds): "Frontiers in Biochemical and Pharmacological Research in Depression." New York: Raven Press, pp 113–126.

Langer SZ, Sette M, Raisman R (1983): Association of [3H]-imipramine binding with serotonin uptake and of [3H]-desipramine binding with noradrenaline uptake: potential research tools in depression. In Gram L, Usdin E, Dahl S, Kragh-Sorensen P, Sjoqvist F, Morselli PL (eds): "Clinical Pharmacology in Psychiatry: Bridging the Experimental Therapeutic Gap." London: Macmillan Press Ltd., pp 339–348.

Langer SZ, Zarifian E, Briley M, Raisman R, Sechter D (1982): High-affinity 3H-imipramine binding: A new biological marker in depression. Pharmacopsychiatr Neuropsychopharmacol 15:3–10.

Laurent JP, Margold M, Hunkel V, Haefely W (1983): Reduction by two benzodiazepines and pentobarbitone of the multiunit activity in substantia nigra, hippocampus, nucleus locus coeruleus, and dorsal raphe nucleus of "encephale isole" rats. Neuropharmacology 22:501–512.

Leckman JF, Weissman MM, Merikangas KR, et al. (1983): Panic disorder increases risk of major depression, alcoholism, panic, and phobic disorders in affective ill families. Arch Gen Psychiatry 40:1055–1060.

Leckman JF, Weissman MM, Prusoff BA, et al. (1984): Subtypes of depression. Family study perspective. Arch Gen Psychiatry 41:833–838.

Lehmann HE (1983): The clinician's view of anxiety and depression. J Clin Psychiatry 44:3–7.

Lemberger L, Bergstrom R, Aronoff G, Farid N, Wolen R (1984): Specific serotonin uptake blockers: Clinical pharmacology and antidepressant action. Clin Neuropharmacol 7[Suppl 1]:324–325.

Le Quan-Bui KH, Plaisant O, LeBoyer M, et al. (1984): Reduced platelet serotonin in depression. Psychiatry Res 13:129–139.

Lesser IM, Rubin RT, Pecknold JC, Rifkin A, Swinson RP, Ballenger JC, Burrows GD, Dupont RL, Noyes R (1988): Secondary depression in panic disorder and agoraphobia. I. Frequency, severity, and relationship to panic and phobic depression. Arch Gen Psychiatry. 45:437–443.

Lewis DA, Noyes R Jr, Coryell W, Clancy J (1985): Tritiated imipramine binding to platelets is decreased in patients with agoraphobia. Psychiatry Res 16:1–9.

Lidbrink PH, Corrodi H, Fuxe K, Olson L (1973): The effects of benzodiazepines, meprobamate, and barbiturates on central monoamine neurons. In Garattini S, Mussini E, Randall LO (eds): "The Benzodiazepines." New York: Raven Press, pp 203–224.

Liebowitz MR, Fyer AJ, McGrath P, et al. (1981): Clonidine treatment of panic disorder. Psychopharmacol Bull 17:122–123.

Liebowitz MR, Fyer AJ, Gorman JM, et al. (1984): Lactate provocation of panic attacks, I: Clinical and behavioural findings. Arch Gen Psychiatry 41:764–770.

Liebowitz MR, Gorman JM, Fyer AJ, et al. (1985): Lactate provocation of panic attacks, II: Biochemical and physiological findings. Arch Gen Psychiatry 42:709–719.

Liebowitz MR, Gorman JM, Fyer A, Dillon D, Levitt M,

Klein DF (1986): Possible mechanisms for lactate's induction of panic. Am J Psychiatry 143:495–502.

Lingjaerde O (1971): Uptake of serotonin in blood platelets in vitro. III: Effects of acetate and other monocarboxylic acids. Acta Physiol Scand 83:309–318.

Lingjaerde O (1977): Platelet uptake and storage of serotonin. In Essman WB (ed): "Serotonin in Health and Disease, Vol IV." New York: Spectrum Publications, pp 139–199.

Lingjaerde O (1979): Inhibitory effect of chlorimipramine and related drugs on serotonin uptake in platelets: more complicated than previously thought. Psychopharmacology 61:245–249.

Lingjaerde O (1985): Lactate-induced panic attacks: possible involvement of serotonin reuptake stimulation. Acta Psychiatry Scand 72:206–208.

Linnoila M, Insel T, Kitts C, Potter WZ, Murphy DL (1982): Plasma steady-state concentrations of hydroxylated metabolites of clomipramine. Clin Pharmacol Ther 32:208–211.

Lipsedge J S, Hattoff J, Huggins P et al. (1973): The management of severe agoraphobia: A comparison of Iproniazid and systemic desensitization. Psychopharmacolgica 32:67—80.

Maas JW (1975): Biogenic amines and depression. Arch Gen Psychiatry 32:1357–1361.

Maggi A, U'Prichard DC, Enna SJ (1980): Differential effects of antidepressant treatment on brain monoaminergic receptors. Eur J Pharmacol 61:91–98.

Malmgren R (1981): Methodological aspects of studies on the 5-HT uptake mechanism in normal platelets. Acta pharmac, tox 49:277–284.

Marks IM (1970): Agoraphobic syndrome (phobic anxiety state). Arch Gen Psychiatry 23:538–553.

Marks IM, Herst E (1970): The open door: A survey of agoraphobics in Britain. Soc Psychiatry 1:16–24.

Marks IM, Gray S, Cohen D, et al. (1983): Imipramine and brief therapist-aided exposure in agoraphobics having self-exposure homework. Arch Gen Psychiatry 40:153–162.

Marshall WK (1971): Treatment of obsessional illness and phobic anxiety states with clomipramine. Br J Psychiatry 199:467.

Marshall WK (1977): Clinical experience in the treatment of phobic disorders. J Int Med Res 5[Suppl 5]:65.

Mason ST, Fibiger HC (1979): Anxiety: The locus coeruleus disconnection. Life Sci 25:2141–2147.

Massotti M, Scotti De Carolis A, Longo VG (1976): Effects of trazodone on behaviour and brain amine content of mice. Curr Ther Res 19:133–139.

Mavissakalian M, Michelson L, Dealy RS (1983): Pharmacological treatment of agoraphobia: imipramine versus imipramine with programmed practice. Br J Psychiatry 143:348–355.

Mavissakalian M, Perez J (1985): Imipramine in the treatment of agoraphobia: Dose-response relationships. Am J Psychiatry 142:1032–1036.

Mavissakalian M, Perez J, Bowler K, Dealy R (1987): Trazodone in the treatment of panic disorder and agoraphobia with panic attacks. Am J Psychiatry 144:785–787.

Mavissakalian M, Perez JM, Michelson L (1984): The relationship of plasma imipramine and N-desmethylimipramine to improvement in agoraphobia. J Clin Psychopharmacol 4:36–40.

McNair DM, Kahn RJ (1981): Imipramine compared with a benzodiazepine for agoraphobia. In Klein DF, Rabkin J (eds): "Anxiety: New Research and Changing Concepts." New York: Raven Press.

Mellman TA, Uhde TW (1987): Obsessive compulsive symptoms in panic disorder. Am J Psychiatry 144:1573–1576.

Meltzer HY, Ramesh CA, Arora RC, Baber R, Tricou BJ (1981): Serotonin uptake in blood platelets of psychiatric patients. Arch Gen Psychiatry 38:1322–1326.

Mignot E, Serrano H, Laude D, Elghozi JL, Dedek J, Scatton B (1985): Measurement of 5-HIAA levels in ventricular CSF (by LCEC) and in striatum (by in vivo voltametry) during pharmacological modifications of serotonin metabolism in the rat. J Neural Transmiss 62:117–124.

Modigh K, Svensson T H (1972): On the role of central nervous system catecholamines and 5-hydroxytryptamine in the nialamide-induced behavioral syndrome. Br J Pharm 46:32–45.

Munjack DC, Moss HB (1981): Affective disorder and alcoholism in families of agoraphobics. Arch Gen Psychiatry 38:869–871.

Norman TR, Judd FK, Gregory M, et al (1986): Platelet serotonin uptake in panic disorder. J Affect Disord 11:69–72.

Overall JE, Hollister L, Johnson M, et al. (1966): Nosology of depression and differential response to drugs. J Am Med Assoc 195:946–948.

Palkovitcs M, Raisman R, Briley MS, Langer SZ (1981): Regional distribution of ^{3}H-imipramine binding in rat brain. Brain Res 210:493–498.

Pare CMB, Trenchard A, Turner P (1974): 5-Hydroxytryptamine in depression. Adv Biochem Psychopharmacol 11:275–279.

Paul SM, Rehavi M, Hulihan B, Skolnick P, Goodwin FK (1980a): A rapid and sensitive radioreceptor assay for tertiary amine tricyclic antidepressants. Commun Psychopharmacol 4:487–494.

Paul SM, Rehavi M, Skolnick KP, Ballenger JC, Goodwin K (1981): Depressed patients have decreased binding of tritiated imipramine to platelet serotonin transporter. Arch Gen Psychiatry 38:1315–1317.

Paul SM, Rehavi M, Skolnick KP, Goodwin FK (1980b): Demonstration of specific "high affinity" binding sites for [^{3}H]imipramine on human platelets. Life Sci 26:953–959.

Paykel ES (1972): Depressive typologies and response to amitriptyline. Br J Psychiatry 120:147–156.

Pecknold JC, McClure DJ, Appeltauer L, Allan T, Wrzesinki L (1982): Does tryptophan potentiate clomipramine in the treatment of agoraphobic and social phobic patients? Br J Psychiatry 140:484–490.

Pecknold JC, Chang H, Fleury D, Koszychi D, Quirion R, Nair NPV, Suranyi-Cadotte BE (1987): Platelet imipramine binding in patients with panic disorder and major familial depression. J Psychiatry Res 21:319–326.

Pecknold JC, Familamiri R, Chang H, Wilson R, Alarcia

J, McClure DJ (1985a): Buspirone: Anxiolytic. Prog Neuropsychopharmacol Biol Psychiatry 9:639–642.

Pecknold JC, McClure DJ, Chang H (1985b): Zimeldine: comparative study in depression. Curr Ther Res 38: 808–816.

Pecknold JC, Suranyi-Cadotte BE (1986): Panic disorder and depression: 5HT and imipramine binding studies. Clin Neuropharmacol 9(4):46–48.

Pecknold JC, Suranyi-Cadotte BE, Chang H, Nair NPV (1988): Serotonin uptake in panic disorder and agoraphobia. Neuropsychopharmacology 1:173–176.

Pelham RW, Osterberg AC, Thibault L, Tanikella (1975): Interactions between plasma corticosterone and anxiolytic drugs of conflict behaviour in rats. Paper presented at 4th Int Cong Soc Psychoneuroendocrinol, Aspen, Colorado.

Perse TL, Greist JH, Jefferson JW, Rosenfeld R, Dar R (1987): Fluvoxamine treatment of obsessive compulsive disorder. Am J Psychiatry 144:1543–1548.

Petersen EN, Lassen JB (1981): A water lick conflict paradigm using drug experienced rats. Psychopharmacology 75:236–239.

Pitts FN, Allen RE (1979): Biochemical induction of anxiety. In Fann WE, Karacan I, Pokorny AD, et al. (eds): "Phenomenology and Treatment of Anxiety." New York: Spectrum Publications.

Pitts FN, McClure JN (1967): Lactate metabolism in anxiety neurosis. N Engl J Med 277:1328–1336.

Prasad A (1984): A double blind study of imipramine versus zimeldine in treatment of obsessive-compulsive neurosis. Pharmacopsychiatria 17:61–62.

Pratt J, Jenner P, Marsden CD (1985): Comparison of the effects of benzodiazepines and other anticonvulsant drugs on synthesis and utilization of 5-HT in mouse brain. Neuropharmacology 24:59–68.

Pratt J, Jenner P, Reynolds EH, Marsden CD (1979): Clonazepam induces decreased serotonin activity in mouse brain. Neuropharmacology 18:791–799.

Price RA, Kidd KK, Weissman MM (1987): Early onset (under age 30 years) and panic disorder as markers for etiologic homogeneity in major depression. Arch Gen Psychiatry 44:434–440.

Przewlocka B, Stala L, Scheel-Kruger J (1979): Evidence that GABA in the nucleus dorsalis raphe induces stimulation of locomotor activity and eating behaviour. Life Sci 25:937–946.

Rainey JM, Pohl RB, Williams M, et al. (1984): A comparison of lactate and isoproterenol anxiety states. Psychopathology 17:74–82.

Raisman R, Briley M, Langer SZ (1979a): High-affinity ^{3}H-imipramine binding in rat cerebral cortex. Eur J Pharmacol 54:307–308.

Raisman R, Briley M, Langer SZ (1979b): Specific tricyclic antidepressant binding sites in rat brain. Nature 281:148–150.

Raisman R, Briley M, Langer SZ (1980): Specific tricyclic antidepressant binding sites in rat brain characterized by high affinity 3H-imipramine binding. Eur J Pharmacol 61:373–380.

Raskin A, Schulterbrandt JG, Reatig N, Crook TH, Odle D (1974): Depression subtypes and response to phenelzine, diazepam, and a placebo. Arch Gen Psychiatry 30:66–75.

Rastogi RB, Lapierre YD, Singhal RL (1978): Synaptosomal uptake of norepinephrine and 5-hydroxytryptamine and synthesis of catecholamines during benzodiazepine treatment. Can J Physiol Pharmacol 56:777–784.

Rausch JL, Shah NS, Burch EA, Donald AG (1982): Platelet serotonin uptake in depressed patients: Circadian effect. Biol Psychiatry 17:121–123.

Redmond DE (1979): New and old evidence for the involvement of a brain norepinephrine system in anxiety. In Fann WE, Karacan I, Pokorny AD, et al. (eds): "Phenomenology and Treatment of Anxiety." New York: Spectrum Publications.

Rehavi M, Ittah Y, Rick KC, Skolnick KP, Goodwin FK, Paul SM (1981): 2-Nitroimipramine: A selective irreversible inhibitor of [^{3}H]serotonin uptake and [^{3}H]imipramine binding in platelets. Biochem Biophys Res Commun 99:954–959.

Riblet LA, Gatewood CF, Mayol RF (1979): Comparative effects of trazedone and tricyclic antidepressants on uptake of selected neurotransmitters by isolated rat brain synaptosomes. Psychopharmacology 63:99–101.

Rickels K, Weisman K, Norstad N, Singer M, Stoltz D, Brown A, Danton J (1982): Buspirone and diazepam in anxiety: a controlled study. J Clin Psychiatry 43:12, 81–86.

Rifkin A, Klein DF, Dillon D, Levitt M (1981): Blockade by imipramine or desipramine of panic induced by sodium lactate. Am J Psychiatry 138:676.

Roberts AH (1964): Housebound housewives: A follow-up study of a phobic anxiety state. Br J Psychiatry 110:191–197.

Robichaud RC, Sledge KL (1969): The effects of p-chlorophenylalanine on experimentally induced conflict in the rat. Life Sci 8:965–969.

Ross, SB, Aperia B, Beck-Friis J, Jansa S, Wetterberg L, Aberg A (1980): Inhibition of 5-hydroxytryptamine uptake in human platelets by antidepressant agents in vivo. Psychopharmacology 67:1–7.

Ross SB, Renyi AL (1975): Tricyclic antidepressant agents. 1. Comparison of the inhibition of the uptake of ^{3}H-noradrenaline and ^{14}C-5-hydroxytryptamine in slices and crude synaptosome preparations of the midbrain-hypothalamus region of the rat brain. Acta Pharmacol Toxicol 36:382–394.

Ross SB, Renyi AL (1977): Inhibition of the neuronal uptake of 5-hydroxytryptamine and noradrenalin in rat brain by (Z) and (E)-3-(4-bromophenyl)-N,N-dimethyl-3-(3-pyridyl)allylamines and their secondary analogues. Neuropharmacology 16:57–63.

Rotman Z, Zemishlany Z, Munitz H, Wijsenbeek H (1982): The active uptake of serotonin by platelets of schizophrenic patients and their families: Possibility of a genetic marker. Psychopharmacology 77:171–174.

Roy-Byrne PP, Uhde TW (1985): Panic disorder and major depression: biological relationships. Psychopharmac Bull 21:551–554.

Rudnick G, Talvenheimo J, Fishkes H, Nelson PJ (1983): Imipramine binding and serotonin uptake in blood platelets of depressed patients: Trait markers of affective illness? Sodium ion requirements for serotonin transport and imipramine binding. Psychopharmacol Bull 19:545–549.

Sainati SM, Lorens SA (1983): Intra-raphe benzodiazepines enhance rat locomotor activity: interactions with GABA. Pharmacol Biochem Behav 18:407–414.

Saner A, Pletscher A (1979): Effects of diazepam on cerebral 5-hydroxytryptamine synthesis. Eur J Pharmacol 55:315–318.

Sargant W. (1962): The treatment of anxiety states and atypical depressions by the MAOI drugs. J Neuropsychiatry 3 (Suppl 1) 96–103.

Sechter D, Poirier MF, Loo H (1984): Clinical studies with 5-hydroxytryptamine binding sites in synaptic membranes from rat brain after long-term administration of tricyclic antidepressants. Eur J Pharmacol 58: 75–83.

Sepinwall J, Cook K (1980): Mechanism of action of the benzodiazepines—Behavioural aspect. Fed Proc 39: 3024–3031.

Sette M, Briley MS, Langer SZ (1983): Complex inhibition of [³H]imipramine binding by serotonin and non-tricyclic serotonin uptake blockers. J Neurochem 40: 622–628.

Sette M, Raisman R, Briley M, Langer SZ (1981): Localization of tricyclic antidepressant binding sites on serotonin nerve terminals in rat hypothalamus. J Neurochem 37:40–42.

Sheehan DV, Ballenger J, Jacobsen G (1980): Treatment of endogenous anxiety with phobic, hysterical, and hypochondriacal symptoms. Arch Gen Psychiatry 37: 51–59.

Siwers B, Ringberger V, Tuck JR, Sjoqvist F (1977): Initial clinical trial based on a biochemical methodology of zimeldine (a serotonin uptake inhibitor) in depressed patients. Clin Pharmacol Ther 21:194–200.

Snaith RP (1968): A clinical investigation of phobia. Br J Psychiatry 114:673–697.

Sneddon JM (1973): Blood platelets as a model for monoamine containing neurones. In Kerkut GA, Phillis JW (eds): "Progress in Neurobiology, Vol I, part 2." New York: Pergamon Press, pp 153–198.

Soderpalm B, Andersson L, Carlsson M, Modigh K, Eriksson E (1987): Serotonergic influence on the growth hormone response to Clonidine in rat. J Neuroltransm 69:105–114.

Solyom L, Heseltine G F D, McClure D J, et al. (1973): Behaviour therapy versus drug therapy in the drug treatment of phobic neurosis. Can Psychiatr Assoc J 18:25–31.

Soubrie P, Blas C, Feron A, Glowinski J (1983): Chlordiazepoxide reduces in vivo serotonin release in the basal ganglia of "encephale isole", but not of anaesthetized cats: evidence for a dorsal raphe site of action. J Pharmacol Exp Ther 226:526–532.

Stein L, Belluzzi JD, Wise CD (1975): Effects of benzodiazepines on central serotonergic mechanisms. In Costa E, Greengard P (eds): "Mechanism of Action of Benzodiazepines." New York: Raven Press, pp 29–44.

Stein L, Belluzzi JD, Wise CD (1977): Benzodiazepines: behavioural and neurochemical mechanisms. Am J Psychiatry 134:665–669.

Stein L, Wise CD, Berger BD (1973): Antianxiety action of benzodiazepines: decrease in activity of serotonin neurons in the punishment systems. In Garattini S, Mussini E, Randall LO (eds): "The Benzodiazepines." New York: Raven Press, pp 299–326.

Stern RS, Marks IM, Wright J, Luscombe DK (1980): Clomipramine: plasma levels, side effects, and outcome in obsessive-compulsive neurosis. Postgrad Med J 56: 134–139.

Stevens DA, Fechter LD (1969): The effects of p-chlorophenylalanine, a depletor of brain serotonin, on behaviour. II. Retardation of passive avoidance learning. Life Sci 8:379–385.

Sulser F (1987): Serotonin-norepinephrine receptor interactions in the brain: implications for the pharmacology and pathophysiology of affective disorders. J Clin Psychiatry 48:12–18.

Suranyi-Cadotte BE, Gautier S, Lafaille F, Deflors S, Dam TV, Nair NPV, Quirion R (1985a): Platelet ³H-imipramine binding distinguishes depression from Alzheimer dementia. Life Sci 37:2305–2311.

Suranyi-Cadotte BE, Quirion R, Nair NPV, Lafaille F, Schwartz A (1985b): Imipramine treatment differentially affects platelet ³H-imipramine binding and serotonin uptake in depressed patients. Life Sci 36:795–799.

Suranyi-Cadotte BE, Wood PL, Nair NPV, Schwartz G (1982): Normalization of [³H]-imipramine binding in depressed patients during remission. Eur J Pharmacol 85:357–358.

Suranyi-Cadotte BE, Wood PL, Schwartz G, Nair NPV (1983): Altered platelet ³H-imipramine binding in schizoaffective and depressive disorders. Biol Psychiatry 18:923–927.

Talvenheimo J, Rudnick G (1980): Solubilization of the platelet plasma membrane serotonin transporter in an active form. J Biol Chem 255:8606–8611.

Temple DL, Yocca FD (1986): Current perspectives on the mechanism of action of buspirone. Abstract p 154. Abstracts of the 15th CINP Meeting, San Juan, Puerto Rico, Dec. 14–17, 1986.

Tennen SS (1967): The effects of p-chlorophenylalanine, a serotonin depletor, on avoidance acquisition, pain sensitivity, and related behaviour in the rat. Psychopharmacologia 10:204–219.

Thiebot MH (1986): Are serotonergic neurones involved in the control of anxiety and in the anxiolytic activity of benzodiazepines? Pharmacol Biochem Behav 24: 1471–1477.

Thiebot MH, Hamon M, Soubrie P (1982): Attenuation of induced anxiety in rats by chlordiazepoxide: role of raphe dorsalis benzodiazepine binding sites and serotonergic neurones. Neuroscience 7:2287–2294.

Thiebot MH, Hamon M, Soubrie P (1983): The involvement of nigral serotonin innervation in the control of punishment-induced behavioural inhibition in rats. Pharmacol Biochem Behav 19:225–229.

Thiebot MH, Hamon M, Soubrie P (1984): Serotonergic neurones and anxiety-related behaviour in rats. In Zarifian E, Trimble MR (eds): "Psychopharmacology of the Limbic System." New York: Wiley, pp 164–173.

Thoren P, Asberg M, Bertilsson L, Mellstrom B, Sjoqvist F, Traskman L (1980a): Clomipramine treatment of obsessive-compulsive disorder. II. Biochemical aspects. Arch Gen Psychiatry 37:1289–1294.

Thoren P, Asberg M, Cronholm B, Jornestedt L, Traskman L (1980b): Clomipramine treatment of obsessive-compulsive disorder: A controlled clinical trial. Arch Gen Psychiatry 37:1281–1285.

Thorpe GL, Burns LE (1983): "The Agoraphobic Syndrome." New York: Wiley.

Torgersen S (1983): Genetic factors in anxiety disorders. Arch Gen Psychiatry 40:1085–1089.

Traskman L, Asberg M, Bertilsson L (1979): Plasma levels of chlorimipramine and its desmethyl metabolite during treatment of depression. Clin Pharmacol Ther 26:600–669.

Trulson ME, Preussler DW, Howell GA, Frederickson CJ (1982): Raphe unit activity in freely moving cats: Effects of benzodiazepines. Neuropharmacology 21:1050–1082.

Tuomisto J, Tukiainen E (1976): Depressed uptake of 5-hydroxytryptamine in blood platelets from depressed patients. Nature 262:596–598.

Tuomisto J, Tukiainen E, Ahlfors UG (1979): Decreased uptake of 5-hydroxytryptamine in blood platelets from depressed patients with endogenous depression. Psychopharmacology 65:141–147.

Turner SM, Jacob RG, Beidel DC, Himmelhoch J (1985): Fluoxetine treatment of obsessive-compulsive disorder. J Clin Psychopharmacol 5:207–212.

Tye NC, Everitt BJ, Iversen SD (1977): 5-Hydroxytryptamine and punishment. Nature 268:741–743.

Tye NC, Iversen SD, Green AR (1979): The effects of benzodiazepines and serotonergic manipulations on punished responding. Neuropharmacology 18:689–695.

Tyrer P, Candy J, Kelly D A (1973): A study of the clinical effects of Phenelzine and placebo in the treatment of phobic anxiety. Psychopharmacologia 32:237–254.

Valzelli L, Bernasconi S, Coene, Petkov VV (1980): Effect of different psychoactive drugs of serum and brain tryptophan levels. Neuropsychobiology 6:224–229.

Vandel B, Vandel S, Jounet JM (1982): Relationship between the plasma concentration of clomipramine and desmethylclomipramine in depressive patients and the clinical response. Eur J Clin Pharmacol 22:15–20.

Van Praag HM (1983): In search of the action mechanism of antidepressants, 5-HTP tyrosine mixtures in depression. Neuropharmacology 22:433–440.

Van Praag HM (1984): Studies in the mechanism of action of serotonin precursors in depression. Psychopharmacol Bull 20:599–602.

Van Praag HM (1986): Serotonin precursors with and without tyrosine in the treatment of depression. In Chogass C, Josias R, Bridger W, Weiss K, Shoff D, Simpson J (eds): "Biological Psychiatry." New York: Elsevier.

Van Praag HM, Westenberg HGM (1983): The treatment of depressions with L-5-hydroxytryptophan. In Van Praag HM, Merdlewicz J (eds): "Treatment of Depression with Monoamine Precursors." Karger, Basel, pp 94–128.

Van Valkenburg C, Akiskal HS, Puzantian V, et al. (1984): Anxious depression, clinical family history and naturalistic outcome—Comparison with panic and major depressive disorders. J Affect Disorders 6:67–82.

Volavka J, Neziroglu F, Yaryura-Tobias JA (1985): Clomipramine and imipramine in obsessive-compulsive disorder. Psychiatry Res 14:83–91.

Waxman D (1975): An investigation into the use of anafranil in phobic and obsessional disorders. Scottish Med J 20:1–61.

Waxman D (1977): A clinical trial of clomipramine and diazepam in the treatment of phobic and obsessional illness. J Int Med Res 5[Suppl 5]:99–110.

Wennogle LP, Meyerson L (1983): Serotonin modulates the dissociation of [³H]imipramine from human platelets recognition sites. Eur J Pharmacol 86:303–307.

Wennogle LP, Meyerson LR (1985): Serotonin uptake inhibitors differentially modulate high affinity imipramine dissociation in human platelet membranes. Life Sci 36:1541–1550.

West E D, Dally P J (1959): Effects of Iproniazid in depressive syndromes. Br Med J 1:1491.

Wheatley D (1982): Buspirone: multicenter efficacy study. J Clin Psychiatry 43:12, 92–94.

Wielosz M, Dall'olio A, DeGaetano G, et al. (1977): Effect of two nontricyclic antidepressant drugs on [¹⁴C]5-hydroxytryptamine uptake by rat platelets. J Pharm Pharmacol 29:546–549.

Willner P (1985): Antidepressants and serotonergic neurotransmission: An integrative review. Psychopharmacology 85:387–404.

Winokur G (1983): Unipolar depression: Is it divisible into autonomous subtypes? Arch Gen Psychiatry 36:47–52.

Wise CD, Berger BD, Stein L (1972): Benzodiazepines: anxiety-reducing activity by reduction of serotonin turnover in the brain. Science 177:180–183.

Wood PL, Suranyi-Cadotte BE, Nair NPV, LaFaille F, Schwartz G (1983): Lack of association between [³H]imipramine binding sites and uptake of serotonin in control, depressed and schizophrenic patients. Neuropharmacology 22:1211–1214.

Wooton LW, Bailey RI (1975): Experiences with clomipramine (anafranil) in the treatment of the phobic anxiety states in general practice. J Int Med Res 3[Suppl 1]:101.

Wooton LW, Bailey RI (1977): The management of phobic disorders in general practice. J Int Med Res 5[Suppl 5]:124–125.

Wurtman R J, Hefti F, Melamed E (1981): Precursor control of neurotransmitter synthesis. Pharmacol Rev 32:315–335.

Yaryura-Tobias JS, Bhagavan HN (1977): L-tryptophan in obsessive–compulsive disorders. Am J Psychiatry 134:1298–1299.

Yu P, Bowen RG, Davis BA, Boulton AA (1983): A study of the catabolism of trace amines in mentally disordered individuals with particular reference to agoraphobic patients with panic attacks. Prog Neuropsychopharmacol Biol Psychiatry 7:611–615.

Zitrin CM, Klein DF, Woerner MG (1980): Treatment of agoraphobia with group exposure in vivo and imipramine. Arch Gen Psychiatry 37:63–72.

Zohar J, Insel TR (1987): Obsessive-compulsive disorder: psychobiological approaches to diagnosis, treatment, and pathophysiology. Biol Psychiatry 22:667–687.

Zohar J, Mueller EA, Insel TR, Zohar-Kadouch RC, Murphy DL (1987): Serotonin responsivity in obsessive-compulsive disorder. Arch Gen Psychiatry 44:946–951.

9

Tribulin and Stress: Clinical Studies on a New Neurochemical System

VIVETTE GLOVER, PhD, AND M. SANDLER, MD

Department of Chemical Pathology, Queen Charlotte's Maternity Hospital, London W6 OXG, England

INTRODUCTION

There is good evidence, outlined below, for the existence of an endogenous monoamine oxidase inhibitor (MAOI)/central benzodiazepine (BZ) receptor binding inhibitor (or inhibitors), which we have called "tribulin" (Sandler, 1982). There is also good evidence that tribulin is released during periods of stress or anxiety, including panic attacks. This research is still at an early stage, and the functional importance of tribulin is not yet clear. Increased output of an endogenous MAOI during stress, to conserve catecholamines and delay their further metabolism, would make physiological sense. Were it to act at BZ receptors as an inverse agonist, as do some of the beta-carbolines (Dorow et al., 1983; Insel et al., 1984), it may well be responsible for generating sensations of anxiety or panic. However, at this stage of our knowledge, it is also possible that it is a byproduct of the metabolism of other more functionally important compounds.

Tribulin differs from the peptide endogenous MAOIs (Becker et al., 1983; Giambalvo, 1984) and from some of the putative endogenous BZ receptor ligands (e.g. Guidotti et al., 1983) reported in the literature in being a nonpeptide, small molecule. Obviously, there may well be several different endogenous factors that act to control each system.

PURIFICATION AND PROPERTIES OF TRIBULIN

Tribulin has now been completely purified from normal human urine (Elsworth et al., 1986; also, unpublished observations) using a sequence of organic solvent extractions and high-performance liquid chromatography (HPLC) columns, taking peaks for MAO inhibition. It is a low-molecular-weight, very slightly basic compound, which is soluble in water and in ethyl acetate but not in heptane. It would thus be expected to cross cell membranes quite easily. Its IC50 with MAO in the standard assay procedure is about 10 μM and for the central BZ receptor (using clonazepam) about 120 μM. This purified compound is much less active against the peripheral BZ receptor (unpublished observations). Our previous characterization of tribulin was with impure preparations (Clow et al., 1983; Elsworth et al., 1986; Glover et al., 1980) and the work should be repeated with the pure compound. However, these earlier studies suggested that it acts reversibly against MAO, is roughly equipotent against MAO-A and -B, and competes with tyramine. It also seemed to compete with clonazepam at the central BZ receptor and showed no gamma-aminobutyric acid (GABA) shift. It did not inhibit benzylamine oxidase, or spiperone binding to dopamine receptors, and thus does not appear to be a general enzyme or receptor poison.

The structure of tribulin is currently being determined by mass spectrometry, and it is

Neurobiology of Panic Disorder, Pages 143–152
© 1990 Alan R. Liss, Inc.

now known to be an indole derivative.* It is possible that, in the near future, a gas chromatographic-mass spectrometric assay will be available.

ASSAY METHODS

Tribulin has been determined by measuring its inhibition of MAO and inhibition of BZ binding to corresponding receptors. These assays have now been standardized for urine and tissue extracts, as described in detail below. In the earlier studies, several different methods were used, so that the actual percentages of inhibition obtained are not comparable with figures obtained later. The earlier clinical investigations were performed measuring MAO inhibition only, and this was also the case in some later experiments, when only limited material was available. In all studies in which both inhibitory activities have been measured, there was a significant correlation between them, supporting the concept that the factor whose production is raised in stress or anxiety has both properties. In no clinical study was either activity significantly related to the initial urinary volume or creatinine content. For tissue distribution studies, displacement of the central BZ ligand clonazepam was used; for clinical studies, the less specific flunitrazepam was the ligand.

Determination of MAO and BZ Receptor Binding Inhibitory Activities in Human Urine

Urine samples were collected in bottles well washed with water and stored at −20°C. Both inhibitory activities appear stable in urine for periods of at least 1 year. All urine samples were diluted with water to a constant concentration of 600 μg creatinine in 2 ml, acidified to pH 1 with M HCl, and extracted into 2 vol redistilled ethyl acetate. The organic phase was reduced to dryness under nitrogen.

For estimation of MAO inhibitory activity, samples were reconstituted to their original volume in 100 mM sodium phosphate buffer, pH 7.4; 100 μl aliquots were then added to 100 μl of 100 mM sodium phosphate buffer, pH 7.4, together with 20 μl of 1% (w/v) rat liver

*Note added in proof: Since this chapter went to press we have identified the major urinary MAO inhibitory component as isatin (indole-2,3-dione). (Glover et al., 1988.)

homogenate in 10 mM sodium phosphate buffer, pH 7.4, and 20 μl [14C]tyramine (specific activity, 50 mCi/mmol; Radiochemical Centre, Amersham, England), diluted with unlabelled material to give a final concentration of 83 μM. The mixture was incubated for 30 min at 37°C, and a standard MAO assay procedure was then followed (Glover et al., 1982).

For estimation of BZ receptor binding inhibition, the dried samples were reconstituted to one-sixth their original volume in 25 mM sodium phosphate buffer, pH 7.1, and 100 μl aliquots were added to 500 μl of five times washed rat whole-brain homogenate (0.5%, w/v), 300 μl of 25 mM sodium phosphate buffer, pH 7.1, and 100 μl of [3H]flunitrazepam (specific activity of 92 Ci/mmol, final concentration 2 nM; Radiochemical Centre). The reaction mixture was incubated at 0°C for 30 min and then rapidly filtered under vacuum. Filters were washed twice with 5 ml cold 25 mM sodium phosphate buffer, pH 7.1, and then suspended in 8 ml of Instagel. Specific binding was determined by incorporation of 3 μM diazepam. Controls with water instead of urine throughout the procedure were included for both assays.

Determination of MAO and BZ Receptor Binding Inhibitory Activities in Rat Tissue

For duplicate assays of both MAO and BZ binding inhibition, tissues from six rats were pooled, weighed, and homogenized (20–50% w/v) with an Ultraturrax homogenizer in cold 2 M HCl and centrifuged (0–4°C for 10 min at 12,500g). Supernatants were transferred to 30 ml glass tubes and extracted into 2 vol of redistilled ethyl acetate. After centrifugation (10 min at 2,500g), the organic layers were carefully removed, divided into two aliquots, and dried under nitrogen. Controls, containing the same volumes of 2 M HCl as those used for tissue homogenization, were also extracted into ethyl acetate and carried through the whole procedure.

For measurement of MAO inhibitory activity, residues were taken up in 250 μl of 100 mM phosphate buffer, pH 7.4. Aliquots (100 μl) were incubated with 20 μl of MAO preparation (1% w/v homogenates of rat liver) and 10 μl of [14C]tyramine, specific activity 50 mCi/mmol, diluted with unlabelled tyramine to

TABLE 9–1.
Distribution of Endogenous MAO and BZ Inhibitory Activities (MAO I and BZ I) in Rat Tissues*

Tissue	MAO I (units/g)	BZ I (units/g)
Superior cervical ganglion	383 ± 75	169 ± 49
Vas deferens	7.8 ± 1.3	14.4 ± 5.5
Heart	4.5 ± 0.6	1.4 ± 0.1
Cerebellum	3.1 ± 0.3	1.1 ± 0.3
Spleen	1.7 ± 0.1	0.9 ± 0.4
Cerebrum	1.9 ± 0.2	0.7 ± 0.2
Liver	1.2 ± 0.1	0.4 ± 0.1
Kidney	1.2 ± 0.1	0.4 ± 0.1
Lung	0.4 ± 0.1	0.3 ± 0.1
Adrenal	Undetectable	Undetectable

*Results are means ± SEM of four experiments. A unit is arbitrarily defined as that amount of material producing 25% of inhibition in each test assay system. (Reproduced from Armando et al., 1986, with permission of the publisher.)

TABLE 9–2.
Urinary Output of Endogenous MAO and BZ Inhibitory Activities (MAO I and BZ I) (mean ± SEM) From Rats Subjected to 2 hr of Cold-Restraint Stress†

	n	MAOI	BZI
Controlss	11	27.2 ± 4.0	18.0 ± 3.5
Stress	9	49.3 ± 4.2**	31.1 ± 3.6*

*$P < 0.05$, **$P < 0.01$ vs. controls (two-tailed Student's t test). Correlation MAO I/BZ I, $r = 0.87$, $P < 0.001$.

†Reproduced from Glover et al., 1984a, with permission of Gordon and Breach, Science Publishers S.A.

give a final concentration in the incubation mixture of 83 μM. A standard MAO assay was then carried out (Glover et al., 1982). For measurement of BZ binding inhibition, a procedure was followed similar to that for human urine, as described above, but on a smaller scale. The samples were taken up in 250 μl of 25 mM phosphate buffer, pH 7.1, and 100 μl aliquots were incorporated into an assay system to determine inhibition of [³H]clonazepam (specific activity 43.5 Ci/mmol, Hoffman-LaRoche, Nutley, NJ; final concentration in the incubation mixture 1 nM) binding to rat brain membranes (0.5% w/v homogenate) in a final volume of 255 μl.

Blanks for both assays were obtained using 100 μl of buffer instead of tissue or control extracts. Controls inhibited both reactions by about 10–15%. The potency of each sample was calculated as percentage inhibition compared with the activity of its respective control. For a single assay of either activity, it is possible to use tissues from an individual animal.

ANIMAL STUDIES

Distribution of Tribulin in Rat Tissues

The distribution of the two inhibitory activities in rat tissues has been found to be highly correlated. (Table 9–1) (Armando et al., 1986). Highest levels were present in the superior cervical ganglion. Similarly high levels have also been noted in the pineal (I. Armando, V. Glover, M. Sandler, and G. Oxenkrug, unpublished observations). Higher activities were present in vas deferens than in heart or brain, and no activity was detectable in the adrenal gland.

The quite disparate levels in different organs show that the effects do not stem from some general tissue component. This distribution also makes it unlikely that we are dealing with a nonspecific dietary factor. The distribution points to a possible regulatory role for tribulin in certain catecholamine systems, in that the superior cervical ganglia, pineal, and vas deferens are rich in norepinephrine. However, the distribution of both activities shows some marked differences from that of catecholamines: The adrenal gland, in particular, the richest source in the body of both epinephrine and norepinephrine and, indeed, of other stress-related hormones, had no detectable level of either inhibitory activity; in the brain, too, higher inhibitory activity was present in cerebellum than in cerebrum, the reverse of the distribution of catecholamines.

Stress Causes Increased Production of Rat Tribulin

Cold-restraint stress brought about an increased output of inhibitory activities in rat urine (Table 9–2) (Glover et al., 1984a). Prior administration of BZ drugs significantly re-

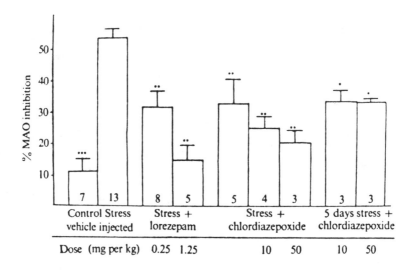

Fig. 9–1. Effect of cold stress on endogenous MAOI with and without various benzodiazepine (BZ) dosage schedules compared with control animals. Values are means ± SEM. No. of animals is given at the base of each bar. ***$P <$ 0.001 compared with vehicle-injected stressed group (two-tailed Student's t test). **$P <$ 0.01, different from vehicle-injected stressed group (Neuman-Keul's test) ($P < 0.05$). The data from the stressed group were subjected to analysis of variance and showed a significant drug effect (F = 8.76, d.f. = 7.35; $P < 0.0001$). (Reprinted from Glover et al., 1981, with permission of *Nature*, ©1981 Macmillan Magazines Ltd.)

duced the output (Fig. 9–1) (Glover et al., 1981). Armando et al. (1988) reported similarly that cold-restraint stress causes an increase of both activities in rat heart and kidney, although not in the other tissues listed in Table 9–1. This finding was not paralleled by an increase in epinephrine or norepinephrine in heart or kidney: In fact, concentration of norepinephrine in heart decreased significantly following stress.

We have recently noted that cold-restraint stress can increase MAO inhibitory activity in rat brain also (Table 9–3) (S.K. Bhattacharya, V. Glover, M. Sandler, I. McIntyre, and G. Oxenkrug, in preparation). The effects were similar in young and old rats. Restraint alone caused a somewhat smaller increase. The fact that tribulin seems to increase in some tissues but not in others during stress suggests a certain specificity of function and not, for example, merely a nonspecific change in production of material from gut flora.

Pharmacological Manipulation of Rat Tribulin

The administration of both pentylenetetrazole, which produces an anxiety model in animals, and (−)−ephedrine, a sympathomimetic that can provoke feelings of fear or anxiety, gave rise to a significant increase in rat brain MAO inhibitory activity (Table 9–4). BZ binding inhibition was not measured in this experiment (S.K. Bhattacharya, A. Clow, V. Glover, M. Sandler, in preparation). The effects of the former were countered by prior administration of diazepam and of the latter by propranolol, although neither drug had any significant effect alone. Ethanol brought about a significant decrease in urinary MAOI output in a different rat experiment. Loading with tryptamine, tryptophan, or methanol had no significant effect (Armando et al., 1983).

These results support the hypothesis that high tribulin output is linked with different conditions of stress or anxiety and can be

TABLE 9–3.
Effect of 2 hr of Stress on Endogenous MAOI in Rat Brain†

	n	Mean ± SEM % inhibition MAO	different from controls
Controls	5	24.9 ± 1.6	
Immobilisation stress	5	34.8 ± 3.2	$P<0.05$
Cold-immobilization stress	5	42.2 ± 1.2	$P<0.001$

†Reproduced from Bhattacharya et al., in preparation.

TABLE 9–4.
Effect of Drugs on Endogenous MAOI Level in Rat Brain
(Mean ± SEM)†

Dose (mg/kg)	Drug	n	Percent MAO inhibition	Different from control
	Control	18	26.8 ± 2.3	
20	Pentylenetetrazole	12	44.9 ± 2.4	$P<0.001$
2.5	Diazepam	9	24.9 ± 2.2	N.S
	Pentylenetetrazole			
	+ diazepam	6	23.3 ± 4.8	N.S
20	Ephedrine	6	38.1 ± 3.0	$P<0.001$
5	Propranolol	6	27.0 ± 1.7	N.S
	Propranolol			
	+ ephedrine	6	24.5 ± 1.4	N.S

†Reproduced from Bhattacharya et al., in preparation.

counteracted by tranquilizers such as diazepam or ethanol. They do not, however, pinpoint the mechanism.

Tribulin in Other Species

An endogenously generated MAOI, extractable into ethyl acetate, has been found in urine from cattle, goat, sheep, and pig. The MAOI from pig's urine was shown to be competitive with tyramine, to be increased by some forms of stress, and to be reduced by anesthesia (Sharman et al., 1987).

Possible Effects of Tribulin In Vivo

All the measurements of change in tribulin level would be of greater significance if backed by evidence that the two inhibitory activities are functionally effective in vivo. Biggio et al. (1984) reported that handling stress in naive animals reduces GABA binding to brain membranes, an effect they ascribed to the release of an endogenous BZ inverse agonist. Several groups have found that stress causes a reduction in MAO activity as measured in homogenates ex vivo. Welch and Welch (1970) as-

cribed some of their findings on the effects of stress on monoamine levels to the effect of a reversible MAOI. Maura and Vaccari (1975) showed that a combined stress of flashing lights, sounds, and cage oscillations causes a significant decrease in rat brain MAO activity. The recovery was faster than protein turnover, so the authors ascribed the effect to a reversible MAO inhibitor. Boucher et al. (1986) found that cold stress causes a decrease in brown fat MAO activity. Armando et al. (1987) also found that cold restraint stress causes a significant decrease in heart and kidney MAO activity, although the activity of the enzyme in other tissues was unchanged.

A different approach to the determination of whether tribulin has an effect in vivo is to see whether it competes with other drugs (Green, 1984). We have recently used this approach with the irreversible MAO-inhibiting drug phenelzine (A. Clow, V. Glover, G. Oxenkrug, M. McIntyre, and M. Sandler, in preparation). Phenelzine, in fact, administered to stressed rats, caused significantly less inhibition of brain MAO ex vivo than in unstressed con-

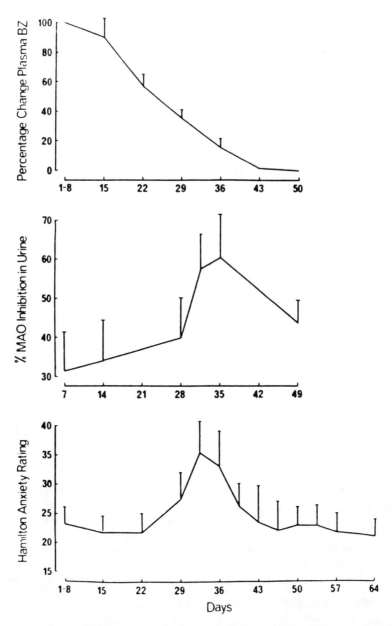

Fig. 9–2. Benzodiazepine withdrawal: mean (±SEM) percentage changes in plasma benzodiazepine receptor binding activity plotted against time: days 1–14, full dose; days 15 to 28, half dose; medication stopped on day 28. Mean-percentage (±SEM) inhibition of MAO in differ- ent 24 hr samples. Mean scores (±SEM) of Hamilton Anxiety Ratings plotted against the same time scale. (Reprinted from Petursson et al., 1982, with permission of the Royal College of Psychiatrists.)

trols. This finding would be compatible with a protective action of a raised level of reversible endogenous MAOI partially masking the en- zyme and protecting it from the action of phenelzine, although other mechanisms could also operate.

TABLE 9–5.
Output of MAO I, BZ I, VMA, and HVA (μmoles/mmol Creatinine $\pm$ SEM) in the Urine of Panic-Susceptible Patients Following Lactate or Saline Infusion and in Normal Subjects Following Lactate Infusion*

	n	MAO I			BZ I		
		Before	After	P	Before	After	P
All subjects given lactate	22	24.1 ± 2.2	29.3 ± 2.2	<0.001	26.6 ± 2.3	31.6 ± 2.9	<0.02
Patients given lactate	14	23.8 ± 3.6	29.3 ± 2.9	<0.01	28.8 ± 3.1	35.2 ± 3.8	<0.05
Normals given lactate	8	24.5 ± 2.2	28.6 ± 3.4	NS	22.8 ± 2.8	25.2 ± 3.8	NS
Patients given saline	5	30.6 ± 3.7	28.3 ± 4.1	NS	41.4 ± 5.7	41.6 ± 5.2	NS

	n	VMA			HVA		
		Before	After	P	Before	After	P
All subjects given lactate	21	3.08 ± 0.10	1.71 ± 0.09	<0.001	2.76 ± 0.22	2.26 ± 0.16	<0.005
Patients given lactate	14	2.18 ± 0.11	1.84 ± 0.12	<0.05	2.54 ± 0.18	2.16 ± 0.14	<0.05
Normals given lactate	8	1.89 ± 0.19	1.47 ± 0.12	<0.05	3.13 ± 0.52	2.43 ± 0.36	<0.05
Patients given saline	5	1.76 ± 0.24	1.80 ± 0.12	NS	2.78 ± 0.45	2.92 ± 0.23	NS

*Comparison of percentage inhibition, before and after infusion, using Student's paired t test. (Reproduced from Clow et al., 1988, with permission of the Royal College of Psychiatrists.)

CLINICAL STUDIES

Tribulin in Anxiety and Panic

Tribulin output in human urine has been found to be raised in generalized anxiety disorder (Clow et al., 1984; A. Clow, V. Glover, M. Sandler, and J. Tiller, in preparation), in lactate-induced panic attacks (Clow et al., 1988), and during BZ withdrawal (Petursson et al., 1982). Figure 9–2 shows that mean output of endogenous MAOI paralleled mean rise in Hamilton Anxiety Rating in a group of patients showing a characteristic withdrawal reaction following cessation of long-term BZ treatment. This result complements that in the rat (Fig. 9–1), in which output was increased following cold-restraint stress but was reduced by BZ pretreatment.

Lactate infusion brought about an increased urinary output of tribulin, both inhibitory activities being measured in this study (Table 9–5) (Clow et al., 1988). Urine samples were collected from the same individual before and after lactate or saline infusion and diluted to constant creatinine concentration before assay, and the changes in individual output were compared. Lactate infusion caused increases in tribulin levels (MAO and BZ inhibitory activities) both in panic patients (Diagnosed by DSM III criteria), all of whom who experienced an attack, and in controls, who did not have a

panic attack. However, in the controls, these increases failed to reach statistical significance. Larger subject numbers would be needed to determine whether lactate is responsible for an increased output in all subjects. Saline infusion did not result in increased output in either group. There was no significant difference in baseline values between panic patients and controls. Thus it was the "within-subject" changes that were significant.

One interesting finding in this study was that lactate infusion was responsible for a significant *decrease* in urinary output of 4-hydroxy-3-methoxymandelic acid (VMA) and homovanillic acid (HVA) in both patients and controls (Table 9–5). This observation complements the finding of Carr et al. (1986), who noted that plasma norepinephrine concentrations increased, whereas those of its metabolite, 4-hydroxy-3-methoxyphenylglycol (HMPG), decreased after lactate infusion in both panic patients and controls. These results show that changes in metabolite level may not necessarily parallel those in the parent catecholamines. An in vivo MAO inhibitory action of tribulin could be one possible cause.

We have also found mean urinary tribulin levels (both inhibitory activities being measured) to be significantly raised in drug-free patients with generalized anxiety disorder (Ta-

TABLE 9–6.
Hamilton Anxiety Rating (HAM-A) and Urinary Output of Endogenous MAO and BZ Inhibitory Activites in Patients With Generalized Anxiety Disorder (GAD) Before (A) and After (B) Treatment and Controls (Means ± SEM)†

	n	HAM-A	MAO I	BZ I
Controls	19	1.7 ± 0.1	14.4 ± 0.3	18.7 ± 0.3
GAD A	38	20.5 ± 0.9**	19.8 ± 0.9**	23.8 ± 1.3*
GAD B	38	5.1 ± 1.0	21.1 ± 1.3**	22.7 ± 1.1*

*P < 0.02,

**P < 0.001 vs. controls (two-tailed Students' t test). Correlation MAO I/BZ I in GAD patients A, r = 0.54, P < 0.0001.

†Reproduced from Clow et al., 1988, with permission of Springer-Verlag, Heidelberg.

TABLE 9–7.
Psychiatric Diagnosis and Urinary MAO Inhibition in Samples From Various Diagnostic Categories (Mean ± SEM)†

Group	n	MAO I
Controls	28	27.1 ± 1.9
All patients	50	28.3 ± 2.2
Schizophrenia, total	10	18.9 ± 3.5
Acute	4	24.0 ± 5.9
Chronic	6	15.5 ± 4.4*
Depression	19	25.1 ± 3.9
Mania	3	33.7 ± 3.4
Alcoholism postwithdrawal	9	40.4 ± 4.4**
Other	9	31.7 ± 5.1

*P <0.02, **P<0.01 vs. controls (two-tailed Student's t test).

†Reproduced from Petursson et al., 1981, with permission of Elsevier Science Publishers BV (Biomedical Division.)

ble 9–6) compared to age- and sex-matched controls (A. Clow, V. Glover, M. Sandler, and J. Tiller, in preparation). There was a significant correlation (r = 0.39, P < 0.01) between MAO inhibitory level and Hamilton Anxiety Rating within the patient group before treatment. When patient and control values were combined for analysis, there was a significant correlation between Hamilton Anxiety score and each inhibitory activity (both r = 0.60, P < 0.001) in the whole group. These patients were treated by nondrug, relaxation therapy. After 6 weeks, their anxiety score was reduced, but there was no effect on tribulin output (Table 9–6). In fact, a significant correlation between output of the two inhibitory activities re-

TABLE 9–8.
Relationship Between Urinary MAO Inhibition and Acute Symptoms/Hyperkinesia (group 1) and Chronic Symptoms/Bradykinesia (group 2) (Mean ± SEM)†

Group	n	MAO I
1) Agitated depression, mania, acute schizophrenia, postwithdrawal alcoholism	20	34.3 ± 3.0
2) Retarded depression, chronic schizophrenia	21	21.2 ± 3.4*

*P < 0.02 vs. Group 1 (two-tailed Student's t test).

†Reproduced from Petursson et al., 1981, with permission of Elsevier Science Publishers BV (Biomedical Division.)

TABLE 9–9.
Summary of Clinical Studies

Tribulin raised in	Tribulin normal in
Lactate- induced panic attacks (Clow et al., 1988)	Essential tremor (unpublished observations)
Generalized anxiety disorder (Clow et al., 1984)	Pregnancy (unpublished observations)
Benzodiazepine withdrawal (Petursson et al., 1982)	Post-traumatic stress disorder (between attacks) (unpublished observations)
Alcohol withdrawal (Petursson et al., 1981, Bhattacharya et al., 1982) Epilepsy (Clow et al., 1987)	Parkinson's disease (unpublished observations)

mained on the two occasions (MAO r = 0.55, P < 0.0001; BZ r = 0.65, P < 0.0001), showing that, in these patients, tribulin output values remained fairly stable with time in the different individuals.

Other Human Studies

The pattern of tribulin output in a normal population has not yet been well characterized. There is evidence that it can be increased by exercise: Output of both inhibitory activities was raised in normal children after strenuous exercise on a treadmill (Armando et al., 1984). We also have preliminary data that tribulin output is significantly higher in females than in males and that it is increased with age (unpublished data). Tribulin output has not yet been studied adequately in depressive illness. In a preliminary screen of urine samples from 50 psychiatric inpatients, depressive patients appeared to show values similar to those of controls (Table 9–7) (Petursson et al., 1981). The group with the highest output in this study was postwithdrawal alcoholics. Chronic schizophrenics had low output and the three manic patients relatively high output values. Output in patients with hyperkinetic clinical features (agitated depression, mania, acute schizophrenia, postwithdrawal alcoholics) was about 50% higher and significantly greater than in those with bradykinesia (retarded depression, chronic schizophrenia) (Table 9–8). The finding of raised MAOI output in postwithdrawal alcoholics, including those who were drug-free, was confirmed in a subsequent study (Bhattacharya et al., 1982). In this investigation, it was also shown that 0.5 g of oral L-dopa reduced the raised output in the alcoholics to control levels.

In a screen of neurological patients, the group as a whole was also found to have significantly raised output of both inhibitory activities compared with controls (Clow et al., 1987), with a highly significant degree of correlation between them of 0.48 (P < 0.001). In a recent study, we have found that epileptics and neurological patients suffering pain had particularly high levels. Parkinson's disease patients did not (unpublished observations). A summary of the clinical results is given in Table 9–9.

Tribulin also appears to be present in plasma

(Glover et al., 1984b), at about one-twentieth the level in urine. However, no systematic clinical studies have yet been performed.

DISCUSSION

Tribulin output or tissue concentration appears to be raised in a variety of different conditions, all related to stress, agitation, or anxiety. The finding is clearly specific not to a single diagnostic condition but rather to a symptom cluster (see Tables 9–8, 9–9) or possibly to some component of these different disorders. BZ treatment is useful in a range of conditions, with considerable overlap with those in which tribulin has been implicated (see Table 9–9). It is thus not unlikely that this range of disorders also shares some disturbances in pathology. Whether the increase in tribulin is part of the cause or part of the effect and whether it will have any diagnostic value or implication for drug treatment are questions to be answered in the future.

REFERENCES

Armando I, Barontini M, Levin G, Simsolo R, Glover V, Sandler M (1984): Exercise increases endogenous urinary monoamine oxidase-benzodiazepine receptor ligand inhibitory activity in normal children. J Autonom Nervous System 11:95–100.

Armando I, Glover V, Sandler M (1986): Distribution of endogenous benzodiazepine receptor ligand-monoamine oxidase inhibitory activity (tribulin) in tissues. Life Sci 38:2063–2067.

Armando I, Glover V, Sandler M, File SE (1983): Output of endogenous monoamine oxidase inhibitor: Effect of ethanol, tryptamine and tryptophan. J Neural Transmiss 56:85–90.

Armando I, Levin G, Barontini M (1988): Stress increases endogenous benzodiazepine receptor ligand-monoamine oxidase inhibitory activity (tribulin) in rat tissues. J Neural Transmiss 71:29–37.

Becker RE, Giambalvo C, Fox RA, Macho M (1983): Endogenous inhibitors of monoamine oxidase present in human cerebrospinal fluid. Science 221:476–478.

Bhattacharya SK, Glover V, Sandler M, Clow A, Topham A, Bernadt M, Murray R (1982): Raised endogenous monoamine oxidase inhibitor output in postwithdrawal alcoholics: Effects of L-dopa and ethanol. Biol Psychiatry 17:829–836.

Biggio G, Concas A, Serra M, Salis M, Corda MG, Nurchi V, Crisponi C, Gessa GL (1984): Stress and β-carbolines decrease the density of low affinity GABA binding sites, an effect reversed by diazepam. Brain Res 305:13–18.

Boucher T, Strolin Benedetti M, Jamin C (1986): Amine oxidase activities of interscapular brown adipose tissue of cold-exposed rat. Pharmacol Toxicol 60 [Suppl 1]:7.

Carr DB, Sheehan DV, Surman OS, Coleman JH, Greenblatt DJ, Heninger GR, Jones KH, Levine PH, Watkins WD (1986): Neuroendocrine correlates of lactate-induced anxiety and their response to chronic alprazolam therapy. Am J Psychiatry 143:483–494.

Clow A, Glover V, Armando I, Sandler M (1983): New endogenous benzodiazepine receptor ligand in human urine: Identity with endogenous MAO inhibitor? Life Sci 33:735–741.

Clow A, Glover V, Elsworth JD, Tiller JWG, Sandler M (1984): Increased tribulin output in general anxiety disorder. J Pharm Pharmacol 36:61W.

Clow A, Glover V, Sandler M, Elwes R, Reynolds EH (1987): Tribulin output in neurological disorders. Br J Clin Pharmacol 24:403–404.

Clow A, Glover V, Weg W, Walker PL, Sheehan DV, Carr DB, Sandler M (1988): Urinary catecholamine metabolite and tribulin output during lactate infusion. Br J Psychiatry 152:122–126.

Dorow R, Horowski R, Paschelke G, Amin M (1983): Severe anxiety induced by FG 7142, a β-carboline ligand for benzodiazepine receptors. Lancet ii:98–99.

Elsworth JD, Dewar D, Glover G, Goodwin BL, Clow A, Sandler M (1986): Purification and characterization of tribulin, an endogenous inhibitor of monoamine oxidase and of benzodiazepine receptor binding. J Neural Transmiss 67:45–56.

Giambalvo CT (1984): Purification of endogenous modulators of monoamine oxidase from plasma. Biochem Pharmacol 33:3929–3932.

Glover V, Bhattacharya SK, Sandler M, File SE (1981): Benzodiazepines reduce stress-augmented increase in rat urine monoamine oxidase inhibitor. Nature 292:347–349.

Glover V, Clow A, Elsworth J, Armando I, Sandler M (1984a): Increased output of endogenous monoamine oxidase inhibitor in stress: A link with the benzodiazepine system? In Usdin E, Kvetnansky R, Axelrod J (eds): "Stress. The Role of Catecholamines and Other Neurotransmitters, Vol 1." New York: Gordon and Breach Science Publishers, pp 457–465.

Glover V, Halket JM, Watkins PJ, Clow A, Goodwin BL, Sandler M (1988): Isatin: identity with the purified endogenous monoamine oxidase inhibitor tribulin. J Neurochem 51:656–659.

Glover V, Liebowitz J, Armando I, Sandler M (1982): β-Carbolines as selective monoamine oxidase inhibitors: In vivo implications. J Neural Transmiss 54:209–218.

Glover V, Reveley MA, Sandler M (1980): A monoamine oxidase inhibitor in human urine. Biochem Pharmacol 29:467–470.

Glover V, Segarajasinghe CE, Clow A, Elsworth JD, Sandler M (1984b): Endogenous monoamine oxidase inhibitors in rat brain and human plasma. J Pharm Pharmacol 36:12W.

Green AL (1984): Assessment of the potency of reversible MAO inhibitors in vivo. In Tipton KF, Dostert P, Strolin Benedetti M (eds): "Monoamine Oxidase and Disease: Prospects for Therapy With Reversible Inhibitors." London: Academic Press, pp 73–81.

Guidotti A, Forchetti CM, Corda MG, Konkel D, Bennett CD, Costa E (1983): Isolation, characterization, and purification to homogeneity of an endogenous polypeptide with agonistic action on benzodiazepine receptors. Proc Natl Acad Sci USA 80:3531–3535.

Insel TR, Ninan PT, Aloi J, Jimerson DC, Skolnick P, Paul SM (1984): A benzodiazepine receptor-mediated model of anxiety. Arch Gen Psychiatry 41:741–750.

Maura G, Vaccari A (1975): Relationships between age of submission to environmental stress and monoamine oxidase activity in rats. Experientia 31:191–193.

Petursson H, Bhattacharya SK, Glover V, Sandler M, Lader MH (1982): Urinary monoamine oxidase inhibitor and benzodiazepine withdrawal. Br J Psychiatry 140:7–10.

Petursson H, Reveley MA, Glover V, Sandler M (1981): Urinary MAO inhibitor in psychiatric illness. Psychiatry Res 5:335–340.

Sandler M (1982): The emergence of tribulin. Trends Pharmac Sci 3:471–472.

Sharman DF, Stephens DB, Cohen G, Holzbauer M (1987): Variations in the monoamine oxidase-inhibitory activity ("tribulin?") in pig's urine. J Neural Transmiss 69:229–242.

Welch BL, Welch AS (1970): Control of brain catecholamines and serotonin during acute stress after d-amphetamine by natural inhibition of monoamine oxidase: An hypothesis. In Costa E, Garattini S (eds): "Amphetamines and Related Compounds." New York: Raven Press, pp 415–445.

Challenge Strategies

10

Potential Mechanisms for Sodium Lactate's Induction of Panic

DIANA P. SANDBERG, MD, AND MICHAEL R. LIEBOWITZ, MD

New York State Psychiatric Institute and Department of Psychiatry, College of Physicians and Surgeons, Columbia University, New York, New York 10032

INTRODUCTION

For centuries physicians observed the condition known as neurocirculatory asthenia. In the 1950s, Cohen and White noted that a sample of 61 young male neurasthenics had higher blood lactate levels than normals during exercise. The findings were replicated by Holmgren and Strom (1959), Jones and Mellersh (1946), and Linko (1950). In 1967 Pitts and Mc-Clure published the famous experiment that demonstrated in a double-blind design that the infusion of intravenous (iv) sodium lactate induced panic anxiety in 13 of 14 patients with anxiety attacks and two of ten controls, while infusion of a comparable amount of hypertonic glucose solution did not cause panic in either group. Since that time investigators around the world have been replicating the result and attempting to understand the mechanism of panic induction (Bonn et al., 1971; Ehlers et al., 1986; Fink et al., 1969; Freedman et al., 1984; Kelly et al., 1971; Knott et al., 1981; Liebowitz et al., 1984a; Rainey et al., 1984b; Sheehan et al., 1984). In this chapter, we first describe the procedure and present results from our own laboratory. Each hypothesized mechanism is then discussed in the light of testing performed thus far and further warranted investigations.

SODIUM LACTATE INFUSION

Subjects in our facility are diagnosed by SADS-LA, meeting DSM III criteria for panic

disorder or agoraphobia with panic attacks. They are excluded on the basis of current major depression, inability to be medication free for 2 weeks, current alcohol or drug abuse, or concurrent medical illnesses that increase the risk of infusion. Normal controls are excluded if a semistructured interview reveals any Axis I illness or if there is an anxiety disorder in any first-degree relative.

Following medical screening, subjects are scheduled for infusions. The day before infusion, subjects in the sample analyzed here came to the laboratory to meet the staff and to become acclimated to the equipment and setting. We now do this the same day in the 90 min prior to iv insertion. Subjects must abstain from caffeine, alcohol, and cigarettes for 12 hr and fast after midnight before the procedure. Upon arrival on infusion day, equipment is placed to measure respiratory rate and depth, electrocardiogram (EKG), electroencephalogram (EEG), blood pressure (BP), skin temperature, and skin conductance. A baseline rating and a usual panic attack rating is obtained on the 17 item Acute Panic Inventory (API), an instrument designed to detect individual symptoms of panic attacks (Dillon et al., 1987). Subjects are asked to lie down, and an indwelling iv catheter is inserted into each antecubital fossa, one for infusion and one for blood sampling.

A slow iv of 5% dextrose in water or, more recently, normal saline is administered for 30 min to test the response to placebo and to allow biological reactions to the venipunctures to abate. After 2 min of rapid saline infusion, the single-blind switch to 0.5 molar DL-

Neurobiology of Panic Disorder, Pages 155–172

sodium lactate is made. The lactate is administered at body temperature over 20 min or until the point of panic, at which time the infusion is stopped. Total dose for complete infusion is 10 ml/kg body weight. The patient is blind to whether he or she is receiving sugar or salt water or lactate at any given time. The research psychiatrist is now blind to diagnosis and patient or normal control status, although our earlier data include nonblind infusions. The psychiatrist is blind to heart rate and blood pressure as well. The API, along with anxiety and apprehension self-ratings on a scale of 0–10, is administered repeatedly during both the saline and lactate phases. Patients are encouraged to verbalize any physical or emotional sensations experienced. A psychiatrist, a psychologist, and a laboratory technician sit by the bedside throughout the procedure.

The call of panic versus no panic is by the physician's judgement. We require a crescendo of both subjective fear and somatic symptoms typical of panic attacks according to DSM III criteria. Physical symptoms without fear or physiologic reactions to lactate, such as vibrations and the urge to urinate, are not rated as panic attacks. Any lactate infusion that runs over 22 min is considered invalid and dropped from the analysis, since we have found prolongation of infusion will nullify the panicogenic effect. The infusion is stopped immediately if the patient has a panic attack.

Blood is drawn at baseline and repeatedly for pH, pCO_2, HCO_3, epinephrine, norepinephrine, lactate, pyruvate, ionized calcium, phosphate, prolactin, and cortisol measurements. A complete set of blood work is always obtained at the point of panic.

OUTCOME

Among our sample of 43 patients and 20 normal controls, 31 (72%) of patients and 0 controls were judged to panic by nonblind research psychiatrists (Liebowitz et al., 1984a). There were no differences between the panic rates for uncomplicated panic disorder and agoraphobia with panic attacks. The mean time to panic was 12.3 min. Dose of metabolically active L-lactate does not appear important; a small sample of individuals given 0.5 M L-lactate had no dif-

ference in panic rate or time to panic from those given 0.5 M racemic DL-lactate (A. Fyer, unpublished data). We measured the amount of lactate remaining in the bottle for lactate panickers to see if they were infused more rapidly than nonpanickers; the rates of infusion were virtually identical. Presence or absence of mitral valve prolapse had no effect on outcome (Gorman et al., 1981). Our rates for lactate panic are lower than found in many other studies; our stringent criteria for panic increase the specificity but lower the sensitivity.

PHYSIOLOGIC RESPONSE IN PATIENTS AND CONTROLS

Table 10–1 summarizes the biological data for each variable in panickers, nonpanickers, and normals every 5 min during DL-sodium lactate infusion. Because some patients did not panic during lactate infusion, we divided the study sample into three groups: patients who panicked with lactate, patients who did not panic with lactate, and normal controls, none of whom panicked with lactate. The analyses were complicated by the fact that infusions were terminated at the point of panic, and therefore total lactate dose varied. To permit comparisons that controlled for the amount of lactate received, panickers were divided into four groups: those who panicked between 2.5 and 7.5 min, 7.5 and 12.5 min, 12.5 and 17.5 min, and 17.5 and 22.5 min. Biochemical and physiological measurements in these four groups made at the actual point of panic were compared with the 5, 10, 15, and 20 min values, respectively, for the no panic and control groups.

During lactate infusion, patients and controls alike develop combined metabolic and respiratory alkalosis and high prolactin levels. Neither group shows changes in cortisol or adrenocorticotropic hormone (ACTH) (Levin et al. 1987). Patients have higher baseline heart rates and signs of chronic hyperventilation, including low pCO_2, low HCO_3, low PO_4, and normal pH, than controls, regardless of whether they go on to panic with lactate. Low baseline PO_4 does seem to predict panic with lactate (Gorman et al., 1986). During the infusion, panicking and nonpanicking patients alike develop higher lactate and pyruvate levels and greater ionized calcium and pH changes than do normal controls. There are no differences in these variables between panicking and nonpanicking patients.

Those who panic with lactate regularly show signs of acute hyperventilation (hyperventilation-induced hypocapnea), decreased HCO_3, and a sudden increase in heart rate. No consistent differences were found in lactate levels, epinephrine levels, pH, calcium, inorganic phosphate, or systolic blood pressure during infusion, though many patients had high baseline epinephrine levels. Elevation of plasma norepinephrine was present in 5 min and 20 min panickers only, and diastolic blood pressure elevations were present in 15 and 20 min panickers only.

The heart rate changes have been more finely analyzed by Gorman et al. (1987). They have derived a formula, called the heart rate index (HRI), that reflects the abrupt rise in heart rate that is superimposed on the baseline tachycardia in patients immediately preceding the onset of a lactate-induced panic attack. They have further shown that the tachycardia is not secondary to an increase in vagal tone, since the vagally controlled respiratory variation in heart rate remains intact during lactate panic. The tachycardia is not prevented by acute beta-blockade with iv propanolol, suggesting it is mediated through another system.

It is difficult to compare our results with those from other centers because of different test conditions. Criteria for panic may also differ among centers. Diagnostic uncertainty, especially in earlier studies, may have led to inclusion of generalized anxiety disorder, simple phobia, social phobia, and others as well as panic disorder and agoraphobia with panic attacks (see Table 10–2 for a summary of lactate studies). Carr et al. (1986) performed lactate infusions under conditions similar to ours and replicated our biochemical findings, especially the lack of peripheral catecholamine surge, the flat cortisol curve, and the nonspecific prolactin rise. They also measured growth hormone (GH) and luteinizing hormone (LH) and discovered a dissociation; LH was flat in patients and controls, but GH rose markedly in panicking and nonpanicking patients while remaining flat in controls. Beta-endorphin activity fell slightly in both patients and controls.

Lapierre and Knott (1984) made careful psychophysiological measures to reflect the state of central, autonomic, and somatic nervous systems during sodium lactate infusion for panickers and nonpanickers. Subjects were 23 patients with DSM III panic disorder and 16 patients with DSM III generalized anxiety disorder. Design was double blind 5% dextrose in water followed by 0.5 M DL-sodium lactate versus 0.5 M DL-sodium lactate followed by 5% dextrose in water. Measurements were made of tonic EEG, averaged evoked potentials, reaction time, vertical electro-oculographic activity, tonic electromyographic activity, and tonic heart rate. They observed that 6 of 23 panic disorder patients panicked with lactate, and 2 of 16 generalized anxiety disorder patients panicked. There were no baseline differences, except that panic patients had lower levels of subjective anxiety than did generalized anxiety patients. No significant difference in any baseline levels distinguished panickers from nonpanickers. For nonpanickers, there were no significant differences in any electrophysiologic variable during infusion. Panickers had significantly higher blink frequency, EMG tension, and heart rate.

VALIDITY OF LACTATE-INDUCED PANIC AS A MODEL FOR NATURALLY OCCURRING ATTACKS

The first test of a valid model is whether it is able to discern patients from controls and whether it is specific to the diagnosis of panic disorder or agoraphobia with panic attacks (Liebowitz et al., 1987). In our laboratory the rate of lactate-induced panic in panic patients is approximately 75% if the doctor is not blind to diagnosis and 60% if the doctor is blind. Zero out of 20 normal controls had a panic attack. A small study of lactate infusions in obsessive–compulsive disorder by Gorman et al. (1985b) showed that one of seven panicked. Liebowitz et al. (1985a) infused 16 social phobics without spontaneous panic attacks and only 1 of 16 panicked. Preliminary data from Lindy et al. (personal communication, 1987) shows that patients with bulimia are not significantly more vulnerable to lactate-induced panic than are normal controls. Depressed patients with a history of panic attacks panic at rates similar to panic disorder patients during lactate infusion, while those without panic

TABLE 10–1.
Physiological and Biochemical Measurements During Lactate Infusion of 43 Panic Patients and 20 Control Subjects*

Variable	Infusion time (minutes)	Control subjects			Reaction of patient to lactate infusion					
					No panic			Panic (at the point of panic)		
		No.	Mean	SD	No.	Mean	SD	No.	Mean	SD
Heart rate (beats/min)	0	14	62.79	10.80	8	74.06	10.33	8	96.75	21.78
	5	14	66.29	12.09	8	84.00	13.56	9	112.67	17.01
	10	14	75.64	14.41	8	89.81	11.44	6	126.50	16.01
	15	14	83.78	12.58	8	95.81	10.44	7	115.50	21.69
	20	14	89.68	12.76	8	100.69	9.83			
Blood pressure (mm Hg) systolic	0	13	108.31	12.08	8	112.75	11.41	7	109.71	14.53
	5	13	114.08	13.64	8	117.75	13.16	9	123.11	19.70
	10	13	120.46	13.98	8	120.50	14.92	7	129.43	18.25
	15	13	123.00	13.38	8	124.25	14.64	8	134.25	10.28
	20	13	122.92	14.09	8	120.00	14.42			
Blood pressure (mm Hg) diastolic	0	12	69.33	7.10	8	70.75	8.81	7	69.43	9.07
	5	12	70.17	6.35	8	73.00	9.26	9	74.56	11.91
	10	12	71.33	7.69	8	70.73	5.65	6	84.33	6.98
	15	12	69.67	10.01	8	70.00	8.07	8	84.00	9.44
	20	12	69.33	7.92	8	68.75	8.00			
L-lactate (mg/dl)	0	14	8.10	2.05	11	7.03	1.06	6	20.57	6.06
	5	14	17.46	4.00	11	20.89	6.56	8	38.06	9.90
	10	14	27.74	6.26	11	32.68	6.84	7	37.55	6.13
	15	14	34.94	8.47	11	42.56	8.29	8	46.83	9.11
	20	14	43.52	7.63	11	49.74	6.43			
Pyruvate (mg/dl)	0	14	0.68	0.14	11	0.63	0.13	6	1.04	0.06
	5	14	0.89	0.21	11	1.02	0.23	8	1.95	0.54
	10	14	1.38	0.29	11	1.66	0.24	5	2.14	0.38
	15	14	1.64	0.33	11	2.08	0.32	8	2.27	0.41
	20	14	2.02	0.34	11	2.60	0.35			
Calcium (mmol/liter)	0	3	1.08	0.09	4	1.06	0.08	1	0.95	0
	5	3	1.02	0.12	4	0.98	0.11	1	1.10	0
	10	3	0.99	0.13	4	0.90	0.13	4	0.90	0.10
	15	3	0.96	0.15	4	0.85	0.11	4	0.92	0.14
	20	3	0.91	0.13	4	0.83	0.08			
Phosphate (mg/dl)	0	8	2.72	0.61	7	2.45	0.25	6	2.12	0.91
	5	8	2.55	0.51	7	2.29	0.31	5	2.07	0.38
	10	8	2.44	0.49	7	2.18	0.23	5	1.81	0.84
	15	8	2.39	0.51	7	2.03	0.32	7	1.90	0.46
	20	8	2.25	0.47	7	1.92	0.36			

(continued)

Physiological and Biochemical Measurements During Lactate Infusion (continued)

Variable	Infusion time (minutes)	Control subjects			Reaction of patient to lactate infusion					
					No panic			Panic (at the point of panic)		
		No.	Mean	SD	No.	Mean	SD	No.	Mean	SD
Epinephrine (pg/ml)	0	12	55.33	35.57	11	72.18	61.91			
	5	12	53.67	37.07	11	80.64	114.03	7	135.57	138.24
	10	12	63.67	34.40	11	75.27	79.81	8	146.00	101.25
	15	12	68.50	46.67	11	68.25	86.25	6	145.17	105.86
	20	12	70.92	45.10	11	73.18	74.18	8	121.37	105.85
Norepinephrine (pg/ml)	0	13	236.69	108.18	11	248.64	86.62			
	5	13	218.92	113.52	11	254.00	104.70	7	135.57	138.24
	10	13	246.61	132.65	11	272.64	128.48	8	146.00	101.25
	15	13	226.31	134.18	11	279.91	131.13	6	311.67	155.79
	20	13	220.08	135.94	11	250.91	137.36	8	410.00	249.71
Cortisol (μ/dl)	0	17	11.10	4.56	12	11.41	7.38			
	5	0	—	—	0	—	—	7	9.57	3.43
	10	17	9.29	3.78	12	9.58	6.43	6	11.28	4.07
	15	0	—	—	0	—	—	6	12.60	4.30
	20	17	8.99	3.74	12	9.42	6.23	8	15.91	11.12
Prolactin (ng/ml) Men	0	10	6.63	2.70	4	6.08	1.66			
	10	10	6.19	1.95	4	5.93	2.38	2	12.30	0.99
	20	10	7.62	2.67	4	9.28	2.99	5	10.50	4.74
Women	0	7	13.36	4.50	8	15.06	7.03			
	10	7	12.73	3.66	8	18.11	8.03	5	18.10	0.99
	20	7	17.13	7.41	8	26.24	12.30	3	18.10	6.13
PCO₂ (mm HG)	0	12	43.42	4.27	9	39.11	4.73			
	5	12	42.67	4.12	9	37.89	5.75	6	33.17	10.66
	10	12	42.83	—	9	36.67	6.14	5	31.60	2.79
	15	12	41.53	4.50	9	35.89	6.07	5	33.20	6.69
	20	12	41.00	3.81	9	34.89	5.73	6	34.33	5.82
pH	0	14	7.38		10	7.39				
	5	14	7.39		10	7.44		6	7.45	
	10	14	7.42		10	7.47		5	7.49	
	15	14	7.45		10	7.50		5	7.50	
	20	14	7.47		10	7.52		7	7.54	
Bicarbonate (mmol/liter)	0	12	24.95	1.91	9	22.80	2.36			
	5	12	25.13	1.69	9	24.65	1.40	6	22.07	3.62
	10	12	26.95	1.75	9	25.45	1.66	5	23.56	2.04
	15	12	27.61	2.60	9	26.22	1.91	5	25.24	3.21
	20	12	28.75	1.62	9	26.90	2.70	6	27.81	4.81

*Number of subjects varies because measurement of some variables was started after the study began. (Reproduced from *Archives of General Psychiatry*, 1985. 42:709–719. ©1985, American Medical Association.)

TABLE 10–2.
Comparison of Lactate Studies*

Source	Study samples	Technique	Findings
Pitts and McClure (1967)	14 anxiety neurotics with panic attacks, 10 normal controls	0.5 M sodium (DL) lactate, 10 ml/kg over 20 min; parallel infusions with lactate plus calcium and glucose in saline controls; infusion not stopped for panic; double-blind	93% patients panicked with lactate; 7% panicked with lactate plus calcium; none panicked with glucose in saline; 20% controls panicked with lactate; mean time to panic, 1–2 min after starting lactate; marked after-effects in 10 patients
Fink et al. (1969)	5 anxiety patients, 4 normal controls	Same as Pitts and McClure (1967)	100% patients panicked with lactate; 25% controls became anxious with lactate; patients had less intense and briefer anxiety reactions with lactate plus calcium and none with glucose in saline; mean time for panic, 8–12 min
Kelly et al. (1971)	20 anxiety neurotics with panic attacks, 10 normal controls	0.5 M sodium (DL) lactate, 10 ml/kg over 20 min following saline infusion; single-blind; infusion stopped if patient panicked; reinfused 8 patients after MAOI therapy	80% of patients panicked with lactate; 10% of controls panicked with lactate; 10% of patients panicked with saline; mean time to panic, 12 min; 5 MAOI responders had fewer symptoms on reinfusion; 3 nonresponders did not
Bonn et al. (1971)	Sample 1: 24 anxiety neurotics with panic attacks, 9 normal controls	1.0 M sodium (DL) lactate, 5 ml/kg given over 20 min; saline control; blindness not specified	80% of first 20 patients panicked with lactate; reaction of controls not given; no panic attacks with saline; mean time to panic, 14 min
	Sample 2: 23 anxiety neurotics	Twice-weekly lactate infusion for 3 week	Overall anxiety diminished with repeated provocations
Lapierre et al. (1984)	23 patients with DSM III panic disorder, 16 patients with DSM III generalized anxiety disorder	0.5 M sodium (DL) lactate, 10 ml/kg over 20 min after 5% dextrose in water infusion; double-blind	6 of 23 with panic disorder panicked; 2 of 16 with generalized anxiety disorder panicked
Liebowitz et al. (1984a)	43 patients with DSM III panic disorder or agoraphobia with panic, 20 normal controls	0.5 M sodium (DL) lactate over 20 min after 5% dextrose in water or normal saline; infusion stopped if patient panicked; single-blind	72% patients panicked; 0% controls panicked; mean time to panic, 12.3 min

(continued)

TABLE 10–2.
Comparison of Lactate Studies* *(continued)*

Source	Study samples	Technique	Findings
Freedman et al. (1984)	8 patients with DSM III panic disorder, 9 normal controls	1.0 M sodium (DL) lactate 6 ml/kg over 20 min; infusion stopped if panic; double-blind	7 of 8 patients panicked with lactate; 3 of 9 controls panicked with lactate; 3 of 8 patients panicked with placebo; 0 of 9 controls panicked with placebo
Ehlers et al. (1986)	10 patients with panic disorder or agoraphobia with panic, 10 normal controls	1.0 M sodium (DL) lactate over 20 min after 0.5 normal saline; infusion stopped if panic; single-blind	Incidence of panic not given; patients more anxious at baseline; no difference between patients' and normal controls; symptom changes during infusion
Carr et al. (1986)	25 patients with panic disorder of agoraphobia, 10 normal controls	0.5 M sodium (DL) lactate or placebo at 10 ml/kg over 20 min; infusion stopped if panic; double-blind; reinfused after alprazolam	90% of patients anxious, 0% controls anxious with lactate; no anxiety in patients or controls on placebo; alprazolam blocked lactate-induced anxiety
Arbab et al. (1971)	6 normal subjects	1.0 M sodium (DL) lactate, 5 ml/kg over 20 min following pretreatment with iv propranolol hydrochloride (10 mg) or saline; blindness not specified	No effect of propranolol on response to lactate; incidence of lactate panic not given
Grosz and Farmer (1972)	10 normal subjects	Parallel infusion of 0.5 M sodium (DL) lactate, 0.5 M sodium bicarbonate, 0.555 M glucose in 0.15 M sodium chloride; all infused at 8 ml/kg over 30 min; double-blind	Incidence of panic not given; similar symptoms with lactate and bicarbonate

*MAOI, monoamine oxidase inhibitor; iv, intravenous.

history are immune to lactate (McGrath et al., 1985). Infrequent panickers also appear to be lactate vulnerable, but they may panic at a lower rate than do frequent panickers.

Another validity test is whether the lactate-induced attacks resemble the patients' spontaneous attacks. Table 10–3 compares patient ratings of their usual attacks and of their lactate-induced attack using the 17 item API (Liebowitz et al., 1984a). Both measures were made on infusion day. Generally, the spontaneous and lactate-induced panics are similar.

The items "twitching" and "urinary urgency" probably reflect nonspecific effects of lactate infusion rather than anxiety. The API change scores during the infusion also correlate highly with the ratings of panic or no panic by the research psychiatrist, who is blind to both heart rate and panic history (Dillon et al., 1987). The in vivo ambulatory heart rate data show that the rise in heart rate seen during lactate panic (Liebowitz et al., 1985b) also occurs during natural attacks. Taylor et al. (1986) found a heart rate increase of at least 20 beats/

TABLE 10–3.
Symptoms of Usual Versus Lactate-Induced Panic Attacks[†]

API Variable	Usual, Mean (SD) (N = 31)	Lactate, Mean (SD) (N = 31)	Comparison*
Feeling faint	1.19 (1.11)	0.87 (1.23)	NS
Fear of dying	1.23 (1.28)	0.58 (1.12)	t (30) = 2.77, $P \leq 0.02$
Fearfulness	2.36 (0.87)	2.36 (1.02)	NS
Palpitations	1.97 (1.11)	1.97 (1.11)	NS
Difficulty in breathing, rapid breathing	1.97 (1.11)	2.00 (1.16)	NS
Urgency to urinate	0.48 (0.96)	1.07 (1.37)	t (30) = 2.68, $P \leq 0.02$
Urgency to defecate	0.23 (0.56)	0.10 (0.40)	NS
Dizziness	1.94 (1.12)	1.74 (1.29)	NS
Confusion	1.94 (1.18)	1.36 (1.36)	t (30) = 0.38, $P \leq 0.03$
Sense of unreality	0.97 (1.17)	0.42 (0.89)	t (30) = 2.78, $P \leq 0.007$
Detachment from body	0.87 (1.12)	0.61 (1.00)	NS
Difficulty concentrating	2.36 (1.02)	1.74 (1.29)	t (30) = 2.03, $P \leq 0.02$
Sweating	1.84 (1.07)	1.07 (1.24)	t (30) = 3.03, $P \leq 0.007$
Difficulty speaking	1.55 (1.21)	1.58 (1.41)	NS
Difficulty doing a job	2.48 (0.63)	2.71 (0.82)	NS
Twitching	1.45 (1.12)	2.29 (1.01)	t (30) = 3.24, $P \leq 0.003$
Nausea, vomiting	0.90 (1.14)	0.77 (1.28)	NS
Overall score	25.73 (7.90)	23.24 (9.42)	NS

[†]API, Acute Panic Inventory. Ratings: 0, none; 1, mild; 2, moderate; and 3, severe. (Reproduced from *Archives of General Psychiatry*, 1984. 41:764–770. ©1984, American Medical Association).
*Bonferroni correction, significant $P \leq 0.003$.

min in 19 of 33 panic attacks; the intensity of panic correlated with the likelihood of heart rate increase. Freedman et al. (1985) found evidence of abrupt heart rate increases in seven of eight naturally occurring panic attacks. Naturally occurring panic attacks vary widely in symptomatology. It is possible that the increase in heart rate occurs only in patients with cardiorespiratory symptoms during attacks and that those with attacks consisting mainly of dizziness and depersonalization do not become tachycardic. To answer this question, a combination of detailed symptom ratings (by API, for example) and ambulatory monitoring in a heterogeneous group of panickers will be required.

A third successful test supporting the validity of the lactate model is that chornic administration of antipanic drugs such as monoamine oxidase inhibitors (MAOI) (Kelly et al., 1971), tricyclics (Fyer et al., 1985; Rifkin et al., 1981), and alprazolam (Liebowitz et al., 1986a; Sheehan et al., 1984) all block lactate-induced anxiety in patients previously lactate-vulnerable and now clinically well on medication.

Kelly et al. reinfused five MAO responders and three MAO nonresponders; only the nonresponders became panicky again. Fyer et al. (1985) reinfused 13 patients well on tricyclics, and none panicked. Liebowitz et al. (1986a) reinfused nine patients well on alprazolam, and only two of nine panicked. There is preliminary evidence that medication-free, remitted panic patients remain lactate-vulnerable and that lactate vulnerability may be a trait marker (Fyer et al., 1985). Medications that are not antipanic drugs, such as diazepam and propanolol, do not block lactate-induced panic attacks when administered acutely, although diazepam does increase the time to panic (Liebowitz, unpublished data). Acute blockade with clonidine, an antipanic medication of equivocal efficacy, also delays time to panic but does not block the lactate panic response (Liebowitz, unpublished data). Acute blockade with imipramine would be useful in understanding the mechanisms of both induction and blockade of panic. To the degree that lactate-induced panic is a valid model for naturally occurring panic attacks, understanding the mechanism may provide insights into the pathophysiology of the illness.

MECHANISMS FOR LACTATE'S INDUCTION OF PANIC

The mechanism by which sodium lactate induces panic attacks in patients with panic disorder remains unclear. Much discussion and research has been directed toward this important question, and many hypotheses have been generated and tested. Here we first list the known possibilities and then discuss them individually (Table 10–4).

A. Alteration of peripheral biochemistry

    1. Hypocalcemia

    2. Hypoglycemia

    3. Peripheral catecholamine release or altered beta-adrenergic sensitivity

    4. Alkalosis

B. Alteration of central biochemistry

    1. Central noradrenergic (alpha) stimulation or endogenous opioid or 5-HT dysregulation

    2. Hyperventilation, carbon dioxide sensitivity, or chemoreceptor hypersensitivity

    3. Alteration of $NAD^+/NADH$ ratio

    4. Nonspecific stress that frightens persons conditioned to view physical symptoms with alarm

Hypocalcemia

Sodium lactate clearly lowers serum ionized calcium; perhaps lactate binds to ionized calcium at the excitable membrane surface and thereby lowers both serum calcium and the threshold for firing. Pitts and McClure (1967) hypothesized that hypocalcemia was the mechanism of lactate-induced panic and reported that the addition of calcium to the lactate solution attenuated and often prevented the anxiety response. Grosz and Farmer (1972) criticized that work, stating that the lactate doses used were not high enough to induce hypocalcemia. However, Fink et al. (1969) replicated the calcium chloride blockade of lactate panicogenesis in five anxiety neurotics. Pitts and Allen (1979) tested the hypocalcemia hypothesis by infusing panic patients with the calcium chelator EDTA. Hypocalcemia suffi-

cient to induce tetany occurred, but none of the patients panicked. Fyer et al. (1984) showed that sodium lactate infusions in 22 patients who panicked, 11 patients who did not panic, and 6 normal controls produced significantly decreased serum ionized calcium in all groups. No association was found between the rate or magnitude of decrease in ionized calcium and the occurrence of a panic attack during the infusion. These data suggest calcium supplementation may compensate for some other panicogenic effect of lactate, but further study of the issue is needed.

Hypoglycemia

Hypoglycemia results in a rapid increase in epinephrine secretion and presumably produces the concomitant anxiety symptoms. Patients with panic attacks are often told by physicians that they have hypoglycemia. Gorman et al. (1984c) measured blood glucose levels serially during sodium lactate infusion in 10 patients with panic disorder or agoraphobia. All were fasting for 8 hr prior to the procedure, and all had a panic attack during the lactate infusion. The lowest blood sugar obtained at the point of panic was 81 mg/dl. The mean drop in blood sugar level during the infusion was 3.1 ± 3.0 mg/dl. Therefore sodium lactate-induced panics seem unrelated to hypoglycemia. Gorman et al. (1984b) also measured insulin levels at the point of panic during the same ten infusions to determine whether hyperinsulinism balanced by epinephrine-enhanced gluconeogenesis was related to panic. Insulin levels were all normal.

Uhde et al. (1984) performed glucose tolerance tests in patients with panic disorder and found no correlation with blood glucose and panic, even in those who became hypoglycemic during the test. Rapid induction of hypoglycemia through insulin administration to anxiety patients also fails to elicit panic, suggesting that hypoglycemia is not a major factor in panic disorder.

Peripheral Catecholamine Release and/or Altered Beta-Receptor Sensitivity

As discussed above, no consistent changes in plasma epinephrine were found to be associated with lactate-induced panic. This is in contrast to performance anxiety, in which

TABLE 10–4.
Pontential Mechanisms for Lactate's Induction of Panic

Mechanism	EVIDENCE	
	For	Against
Hypocalcemia	1. Adding calcium to lactate prevents panic	1. EDTA is not panicogenic 2. Serum-ionized calcium is the same in infusion panickers, nonpanickers, and controls
Hypoglycemia	1. Symptoms of hypoglycemia resemble panic attacks	1. Normal glucose levels during infusion 2. Normal insulin levels during infusion 3. Normal glucose tolerance tests 4. Normal insulin tolerance test
Alkalosis	1. Patients are chronic hyperventilators 2. Lactate induces alkalosis 3. Sodium bicarbonate infusion makes normals anxious	1. Acute hyperventilation is not panicogenic 2. Alkalosis does not precede symptom onset
Beta-receptor hypersenstivity or peripheral catechol release	1. Isoproteronal induces panic when given by iv drip	1. There is evidence of beta-receptor down-regulation, including high serum epinephrine and blunted heart rate response to isoproterenol 2. Beta-blockade does not prevent lactate-induced panic or tachycardia 3. Epinephrine does not rise during lactate induced panic
Central noradrenergic, serotonergic, or opioid dysregulation	1. Clonidine treats panic disorder 2. Patients are hypersensitive to HR and and BP decrease with clonidine infusion 3. Yohimbine causes anxiety in patients 4. Tricyclics block serotonin reuptake and are effective antipanic drugs 5. Serum MHPG levels are elevated in panic disorder	1. Naloxone in moderate doses does not cause panic or alter lactate panic 2. Clonidine pretreatment does not prevent lactate panic 3. Tryptophan infusions do not differ in patients and controls
Carbon dioxide or chemoceptor sensitivity	1. CO_2 inhalation induces panic 2. Lactate is metabolized to CO_2 3. Patients show signs of chronic hyperventilation 4. Breathing retraining may treat panic attacks	1. $[^{14}C]$ labeled lactate does not appear to metabolize to $[^{14}C]O_2$.
NAD^+/NADH ratio alteration	1. Passive rise in lactate causes increased acidosis, which increases chemoceptor firing	1. 30-fold change in lactate/pyruvate ratio does not change the redox state of the cell
Cognitive	1. Evidence of cognitive instructions changing affective reaction during lactate infusion in normals and CO_2 inhalation in panic disorder.	1. Other nonspecific stressors do not make patients panicky 2. Lactate can cause panic in sleeping patients 3. Antipanic drugs alone block lactate panic

there are definite acute rises in plasma epinephrine during public speaking, and patients respond therapeutically to beta-blockers (Dimsdale and Moss, 1980; Levin et al., unpublished data; Neftel et al., 1982). Plasma norepinephrine and blood pressure were higher in panickers at some points in the infusion, but these differences were not consistent. The norepinephrine increases may be a result of panic rather than a cause, because peripheral norepinephrine is merely leakage from sympathetic synapses. Nevertheless, many patients did have higher baseline epinephrine values than controls on infusion day (Liebowitz et al., 1985a), and there is evidence that both alpha-2- and beta-adrenoceptors may be down-regulated (hyposensitive) in panic disorder.

To measure beta-receptor function, Lima and Turner (1983) studied lymphocyte cyclic adenosine monophosphate (cAMP) response to isoprenaline in anxious patients and normals. They looked at baseline response and at response after treatment with either 160 mg propanolol per day or 30 mg diazepam per day. Baseline cAMP response to isoprenaline stimulation was significantly lower in patients than in controls. After 4 weeks of propanolol treatment there was a significant increase in cAMP response, but no change in response after 4 weeks of diazepam treatment. This evidence of beta-receptor down-regulation in anxiety patients was also found by the same investigators in hypertensive patients. Nesse et al. (1984) infused eight patients with panic disorder and six normal controls with a series of up to seven logarithmically increasing bolus iv doses of isoproterenol over a 4 hr period. These patients and controls underwent periods of standing up and isometric exercise as well. Six other patients underwent supine saline infusions alone. The investigators found that patients had markedly elevated resting heart rate, plasma epinephrine, and growth hormone. Plasma norepinephrine levels were mildly elevated in patients. There was no anxiety response to isoproterenol. Heart rate response to isoproterenol was decreased in panic disorder patients, suggesting beta-receptor hyposensitivity resulting from chronically increased adrenergic functioning.

Some investigators have also evaluated the possibility of beta-receptor hypersensitivity.

Lindemann and Finesinger (1938) infused 20 "neurotics" with epinephrine and found that the subgroup with worry, derpession, and with "overwhelming attacks of distress" panicked with epinephrine, while the group with more discrete phobias and fears were immune to epinephrine but were made more anxious by the cholinergic agonist mecholyl. There were no controls. Frohlich et al. (1969) found that anxious hypertensives become more anxious than nonanxious hypertensives and normals during infusion of the beta-agonist isoproterenol. It is not clear what anxiety disorder the patients had. Rainey et al. (1984a) infused lactate, 5% dextrose in water, and isoproterenol into 11 panic disorder patients and 10 normal controls. The infusions were randomly sequential and double-blind. Eight of 11 panic patients and 2 of 10 controls had a panic attack by RDC criteria during the isoproterenol infusion compared with 10 of 11 patients and 3 of 10 controls with sodium lactate. Four of 11 patients also panicked with 5% dextrose. Patients rated the anxiety during isoproterenol infusion as milder than during sodium lactate, but described both experiences as being very similar to their spontaneous attacks. These experiments could reflect beta-receptor hypersensitivity (see Chapter 7, this volume).

Gorman et al. (1983) took six subjects with panic disorder who had panic attacks with sodium lactate and repeated the lactate infusions after administering iv propanolol to produce acute beta-adrenergic blockade. In all cases, propanolol pretreatment failed to prevent panic attacks, tachycardia, and increased systolic BP during lactate infusion. It also failed to lower baseline anxiety ratings on the day of infusion, although it did lower baseline heart rate. In contrast, Easton and Sherman (1976) found that in six patients, all of whom panicked with isoproterenol, the isoproterenol panic was blocked by propanolol. Therefore, some central regulating system must be activated and overrides the peripheral beta-blockade during lactate administration.

There is also work investigating the role of alpha-stimulation. Norepinephrine infusions performed by Frankenhauser and Jarpe (1962) and Vlachakis et al. (1974) were not panicogenic. Pyke and Greenberg (1986), however, in an open study of six patients, found norepinephrine infusion in higher doses to cause panic attacks.

Alkalosis

Grosz and Farmer (1972) were the first to argue that metabolic alkalosis is the mechanism of panic induction. They disproved the contention of Pitts and McClure (1967) that alkalosis occurs only after the onset of symptoms by showing that symptoms, lactate levels, and bicarbonate levels all rise simultaneously in normal subjects. Knowing that acute respiratory alkalosis is common in anxious patients who hyperventilate, they tested the effects of acute metabolic alkalosis by infusing their normal subjects with sodium bicarbonate. Lactate and bicarbonate caused equal numbers and intensity of symptoms in normals, including paresthesias, shakiness, tremors, dizziness, and palpitations. In contrast to exogenous sodium lactate administration, exercise-induced lactate production causes acidosis, not alkalosis. Stein et al. (unpublished data) recently demonstrated no difference in the anxiety between panic disorder patients and normal controls during a submaximal exercise test despite high lactate levels in both groups resulting from the exertion. Gorman et al. (1985a) showed that acute room air hyperventilation (respiratory alkalosis) is not panicogenic in patients with panic disorder, while inhalation of 5% CO_2, which induces hyperventilation without alkalsosi by stimulating respiratory chemoreceptors in the medulla, does induce panic. Bicarbonate infusions in patients with panic disorder as well as infusions of metabolically inactive 0.5 M D-lactate, which will produce the same osmolar load and calcium chelation without leading to alkalosis, will help to clarify these issues. Both studies are now underway in our center.

Central Noradrenergic Stimulation or Endogenous Opioid or 5-HT Dysregulation

The locus ceruleus is a noradrenergic center located in the pons. It contains approximately 70% of the brain's noradrenergic neurons and has inhibitory alpha-2-, 5-HT, and opiate innervations. Projections from the locus ceruleus innervate the cerebral and cerebellar cortices, limbic system, the brainstem, and the spinal cord (Judd et al., 1985). In animals this area is known to regulate level of arousal and to increase rate of discharge during stress (Cooper et al., 1982). Some evidence supports a physiologic defect in the locus ceruleus as being etiologic for panic attacks. Ko (1983), for example, found elevations in plasma 3-methoxy-4-hydroxyphenylglycol (MHPG) in agoraphobic patients during in vivo exposure.

Many pharmacologic agents alter locus ceruleus activity. Yohimbine is a presynaptic alpha-2-adrenergic antagonist that prevents inhibition of norepinephrine release. At high doses it provokes anxiety in most subjects, including normals (Holmberg and Gershon, 1961). Strangely, the effective antipanic medication imipramine appeared to augment rather than attenuate yohimbine-induced anxiety. However, at lower doses, yohimbine appears to produce anxiety symptoms in panic disorder patients and not in control subjects (Charney et al., 1984). The alpha-2, adrenergic agonist clonidine decreases firing of the locus ceruleus by increasing activity of inhibitory neurons. Clonidine has been shown to have some efficacy in the treatment of panic disorder (Liebowitz et al., 1981) and of opiate withdrawal (Gold et al., 1979). We know clonidine must have activity other than alpha-2-stimulation, as it also blocks the non-noradrenergic rhinorrhea and lacrimation associated with opiate withdrawal. There is also evidence that clonidine overdose can be treated successfully with naloxone (Qulig et al., 1982). Charney et al. (1986a) administered iv clonidine to 26 patients with agoraphobia and panic attacks and 21 normal controls. They found that clonidine produced significantly greater decreases in plasma MHPG levels and blood pressure in patients than in controls. Patients also had much smaller increases in growth hormone and drowsiness then did control subjects. Nutt (1986) also infused eight panic patients and eight normals with clonidine (1.5 µg/kg) and found that patients had a significantly greater fall in systolic and diastolic blood pressure and heart rate than did normals. If locus ceruleus discharge was solely responsible for panic, we would expect higher elevations in systolic blood pressure during attacks. Nevertheless, the increased sensitivity of noradrenergic centers to both yohimbine and clonidine in patients suggests some alteration in the alpha-adrenergic regulatory system (see Chapter 6, this volume, for extensive review).

Liebowitz et al. (unpublished data) took ten lactate panickers and reinfused them after pretreatment with intravenous clonidine. The lactate-induced panic was not prevented or attenuated by clonidine, but the time from the switch to lactate until the point of panic was prolonged. Therefore lactate probably does not work simply by alpha-2-receptor stimulation.

Antipanic drugs such as tricyclic antidepressants also change regulation of noradrenergic activity centrally, usually causing a decrease in locus ceruleus activity. Long-term administration of tricyclics does block lactate-induced panic effectively (Fyer et al., 1985; Rifkin et al., 1981).

Lingjaerde (1985) described lactate and pyruvate stimulation of serotonin reuptake and subsequent reduction of the inhibitory serotonergic influences on the locus ceruleus. The panic-blocking effects of tricyclics can be explained on the basis of inhibition of serotonin reuptake. On the other hand, Charney (1986c) infused patients and controls with tryptophan and found no panic and no difference in the degree of prolactin stimulation between patients and controls. This suggests that serotonin regulation is not abnormal in panic anxiety (see Chapter 8, this volume, for review).

Naloxone, an opiate antagonist known to precipitate withdrawal in opiate addicts, was administered by Liebowitz et al. (1984b) to 12 panic disorder patients both alone and in combination with sodium lactate. Naloxone is known to increase separation distress in animals. Morphine blocks the distress vocalization in animals separated from their mothers without sedating them. This suggests that endorphins may play some role in separation anxiety (Panksepp et al., 1978). Panic disorder is often accompanied by a history of childhood separation anxiety, another condition treatable with imipramine (Gittleman-Klein, 1975). Naloxone in iv doses of 22.5 mg did not produce panic attacks, and it did not alter the response to sodium lactate. It is possible that our dosage was too low to achieve blockade. Normal subjects given iv naloxone, 6 ml/kg of body weight, experience mild anxiety as well as panic-like physical symptoms (Cohen et al.,

1983). Charney et al. (1986b) found that combined infusions of naloxone and yohimbine in normals had a synergistic anxiogenic effect, suggesting some interaction between the two systems. Of course, many of the above provocations are acute stimulations or blockades and do not speak to effects of the long-term administration of beta-blockers, clonidine, or diazepam on lactate vulnerability.

Carbon Dioxide Sensitivity or Chemoreceptor Sensitivity

As discussed, patients panicking with sodium lactate show signs of acute hyperventilation with hypocapnea superimposed on their baseline chronic, compensated hyperventilation. Gorman et al. (1986) showed that low baseline phosphate, a marker of chronic alkalosis, predicts panic with lactate. There are two explanations for the chronic hypocapnea in panic patients: one, that hyperventilation leads to low CO_2, which leads to receptor hypersensitivity; and two, that receptor hypersensitivity leads to low CO_2. In normal women, central CO_2 sensitivity increases in the luteal phase under the influence of progesterone (Damas-Mora et al., 1980) and normal subjects tend to hyperventilate premenstrually. The clinical exacerbations of panic attacks in the late luteal phase in women with panic disorder and increases in anxiety and dysphoria premenstrually in women without panic disorder might be explained on this basis (Harrison et al., 1986; Sandberg et al., 1986). These observations lead one to consider the role of CO_2 sensitivity in panic (see Chapter 12, this volume).

Gorman et al. (1984a) challenged patients with room air hyperventilation and inhalation of 5% CO_2. Subjects remained supine throughout the procedure, with an indwelling radial arterial line. Their heads were sealed in a clear plastic canopy box to control the inspired gas mixture. The protocol was divided into five epochs: normal room air breathing for 15 min, 5% CO_2 inhalation for 20 min or until panic, normal room air breathing for 15 min, hyperventilation (30 deep breaths per minute) of room air for 15 min or until panic, and normal room air breathing for 15 min. Five percent CO_2 has been shown roughly to triple minute ventilation in normals, but does not result in hypocapnea or respiratory alkalosis.

The same subjects had a lactate infusion on another day. Eight of 12 patients had a panic attack with lactate, and 7 of 12 patients had a panic attack with CO_2 challenge. Six of 12 panicked with both CO_2 and lactate. Only three patients panicked with room air hyperventilation; these subjects panicked with lactate and CO_2 as well. They described the lactate and CO_2 panics as closely resembling their spontaneous attacks, but the room air attacks had mostly physical symptoms without anxiety.

Sodium lactate induces a peripheral alkalosis, but the effect on brain circulation is vasoconstriction with a resulting acidosis and relative CO_2 excess at the central chemoceptors (Carr and Sheehan, 1984). Lactate is metabolized to pyruvate, some of which enters the tricarboxylic acid cycle and is metabolized to HCO_3; however, HCO_3 ions cannot cross the blood–brain barrier. When bicarbonate joins with hydrogen ions, it forms carbonic acid, which dissociates to water and CO_2, and CO_2 readily crosses the blood–brain barrier. Therefore centrally perceived hypercarbia is a possible mechanism for hyperventilation and panic.

Another line of evidence supporting the CO_2 mechanism is the efficacy of breathing retraining in the treatment of panic disorder (Clark et al., 1985). Patients are taught to hyperventilate voluntarily and then to breath slowly and abdominally rather than thoracically. Patients practice the rhythmic abdominal breathing until they can voluntarily do it at the first sign of anxiety. The results in the open treatment of 19 patients showed substantial reductions in panic attack frequency and self-reported fear both within 2 weeks of treatment and at 6 month and 2 year follow-up (Clark et al., 1985). This study is uncontrolled, however, and some patients received concomitant therapies. Nevertheless, it supports a theory of feedback whereby increasing pCO_2 voluntarily will reset receptor sensitivity at a lower level over time.

Reiman et al. (1986) used the technique of positron emission tomography (PET scan) to assess regional blood flow in 16 patients with panic disorder and 25 normal controls. The eight patients who were vulnerable to lactate-induced panic showed several abnormalities in the resting, nonpanic state: abnormal hemispheric asymmetry of parahippocampal blood flow, high blood volume and oxygen metabolism, and abnormal susceptibility to episodic hyperventilation. It will be extremely informative to observe regional cerebral blood flow and metabolic activity during sodium lactate infusions and CO_2 inhalations in both patients and normal controls.

Alteration of NAD$^+$/NADH Ratio in Panic Patients

Carr and Sheehan (1984) wrote a comprehensive review of the "redox" hypothesis. According to this theory, the panic attack results from a shift in the redox state of the brainstem. The reduction of pyruvate to lactate involves the oxidation of the cofactor NADH to NAD$^+$ via the catalytic enzyme lactate dehydrogenase (LDH). The equation for the reaction is [lactate/pyruvate[$= K_{LDH} \times$ [NADH/NAD$^+$] $\times$ [H$^+$]. At physiologic pH, lactate is largely ionized and cannot cross the blood–brain barrier. However, there are breaks in the blood–brain barrier in the area of the medullary chemoceptors. The combination of passive rise in the lactate/pyruvate ratio plus vasoconstrictive cerebral ischemia and acidosis lowers pH in the medullary chemoceptors and thereby increases their firing rate. This hypothesis would explain both CO_2- and lactate-induced panic. The finding of Gorman et al. (1986) of low baseline phosphate in panic patients who are lactate-vulnerable also suggests some derangement in intracellular glycolysis in these individuals. However, as Rainey et al. (1985) point out in their review, there is some evidence against this hypothesis. Sacks (1965) found that less than 5% of iv-administered [^{14}C] sodium lactate was metabolized to [^{14}C]O$_2$ over 90 min. Furthermore, alterations in intracellular pH can change the lactate/pyruvate ratio 30-fold without changing the redox state of the cell. If either pyruvate infusion or 0.5 M D-sodium lactate infusion proves panicogenic, then the change in redox state will be excluded as a primary mechanism.

Nonspecific Stress That Frightens Patients

Behaviorists have long hypothesized a strong cognitive component to naturally occurring panic attacks, and their treatments have intervened in the cognitive area. It is possible that patients react with alarm to the physical symptoms induced by sodium lactate and that this explains the panicogenic effect. Views as to the relative importance of cognitive input vary: There are some who say patients with panic experience no different physical sensations than normals do and that they simply overreact; some say patients do have greater physical arousal than normals both spontaneously and during infusion, but that their cognitive interpretation is out of proportion; and some say that patients have a normal cognitive reaction to severe, pathological physical symptoms. Ehlers et al. (1986) performed lactate infusions in ten panic patients and ten normal controls and found no difference in anxiety reactions. Four patients and no controls, however, were distressed enough to request that the infusion be stopped. The setting was a sound attenuated room in which the subjects sat alone. Freedman et al. (1984) infused patients in a similar setting. Their panic rate of seven of eight patients and three of nine controls is much higher than the rates in our laboratory and that of Carr et al. (1985), in which staff sit with the subjects during the infusion. Such environmental changes could change the cognitive interpretation of symptoms and make subjects more fearful. Many times patients state "I would be panicky if this happened and you were not here." Although the study of Ehlers et al. has been criticized on methodologic grounds, such as low power, by Klein and Ross (1986), the possibility of a real finding from cognitive effects still remains.

Ackerman and Sachar (1974) were the first to propose a cognitive theory of panic, in which patients react phobicly to the physical symptoms induced by sodium lactate, while normals are not afraid. Margraf et al. (1986) wrote a review of all of the lactate studies to date with a cognitive theory in mind. They propose that the learning history of the subjects, along with their genetic endowment, baseline levels of arousal, and situational determinants form a dynamic positive feedback loop. Physical symptoms are interpreted as dangerous, and this anxiety reaction causes more physical symptoms, which increase anxiety further. In the words of Margraf et al.

(1986): "the appraisal of lactate anxiety as being genuine results in an ascending spiral of anxiety and arousal."

Empirical evidence for this theory is beginning to accumulate. In 1962, Schacter and Singer infused epinephrine into normal subjects and changed affective outcome according to the amount of instruction or explanation given, the demand of performing annoying tasks during the infusion, or the presence in the room of decoy subjects who freely discussed and demonstrated a supposed reaction. Their subjects responded with anger, euphoria, anxiety, or little response at all, depending on the manipulation of these variables. Bonn et al. (1971) administered lactate serially to patients concomitant with neutral stimuli and extinguished the panic response in a treatment-resistant group of patients. Improvement in spontaneous attacks extended into the period 6 weeks later.

van der Molen et al. (1986) studied the effect of lactate infusion in two differently instructed groups of normals in a double-blind, placebo-controlled cross-over design. Seven subjects told that infusions would produce anxiety had significant increases in anxiety during lactate, but not during glucose. Six subjects told that the infusion would produce a state of pleasurable excitement had no significant change in anxiety after either infusion. The individuals in the pleasure group, however, had variable reports. Two reported some mild anxiety and three reported pleasurable excitement. One mentioned pleasurable excitement initially but felt somewhat anxious by the end. Therefore, there is room for some biological effect and cognitive input to be working simultaneously in normal controls. This cannot automatically be extended to patients, however.

Rapee et al. (1987) administered one breath inhalations of a 50% CO_2/50% O_2 gas mixture to 16 subjects with panic disorder and 16 social phobics without spontaneous attacks. Half of each group was assigned to little or no explanation of what to expect versus a thorough explanation. A greater proportion of panic subjects receiving little explanation had catastrophic cognitions and panic than subjects who received a full explanation. The two groups of social phobics reported no difference in symptoms according to explanation. This suggests the specificity of cognitive mediation in spontaneous panic attacks. However, the investigators did not report analyses comparing panickers versus social phobics in the explanation group or panickers versus social phobics in the low explanation group. Therefore potentially important diagnostic differences have not been fully explored.

In pilot work, Shear and A. Fyer report blockade of lactate-induced panic using behavioral treatment without medication (Shear, 1986; see also Chapter 11, this volume).

There is also evidence against the influence of cognition in panic disorder. First of all, extreme relaxation induced by intravenous diazepam or clonidine pretreatment does not attenuate lactate panic. Also, reinfusion of lactate-vulnerable, remitted panic patients treated with tricyclic antidepressants and either maintained on medication or double blindly tapered to methscopalamine (Fyer et al., 1985) showed that patients remaining on tricyclics did not panic, but some patients tapered off tricyclic and reinfused on only the anticholinergic methscopalamine did panic. The panic rate in the tricyclic-free group appeared to be related to time off tricyclic. The longer someone was tricyclic free, the higher the likelihood of panicking with lactate. Preliminary unpublished data from Dillon also demonstrate that anxiety patients do not indiscriminately endorse symptom items during lactate infusion. Other nonspecific stressors such as EDTA, mental arithmetic (Kelly et al, 1971), or the cold pressor test (Grunhaus et al., 1983) induce marked physiologic change but do not cause anxiety attacks in patients with panic disorders.

CONCLUSIONS

The exact mechanism by which sodium lactate induces panic remains unclear. However, it appears that the peripheral effects are not the direct cause of panic. The central mechanisms of noradrenergic, opioid, and serotonergic regulation; acid–base and ventilatory regulation; and cognition seem to be major areas for further research. It may well be that sodium lactate's induction of panic attacks is a multidetermined phenomenon and reflects a multidetermined etiology for the illnesses themselves.

REFERENCES

Ackerman SH, Sachar EJ (1974): The lactate theory of anxiety: A review and reevaluation. Psychosom Med 36:69–81.

Arbab AJ, Bonn JA, Hicks DC (1971): Effects of propanolol in lactate induced phenomena in normal subjects. Br J Pharmacol 41:430.

Bonn JA, Harrison J, Rees WL (1971): Lactate induced anxiety: Therapeutic applications. Br J Psychiatry 119:468–471.

Carr D, Sheehan D (1984): Panic anxiety: A new biological model. J Clin Psychiatry 45:323–330.

Carr DB, Sheehan DV, Surman O, Coleman J, Greenblat D, Heninger G, Jones K, Levine P, Watkins W (1986): Neuroendocrine correlates of lactate induced anxiety and their response to chronic alprazolam therapy. Am J Psychiatry 143:283–494.

Charney DS, Heninger GR, Brier A (1984): Noradrenergic function in panic anxiety: Effects of yohimbine in healthy subjects and patients with agoraphobia and panic disorder. Arch Gen Psychiatry 41:751–763.

Charney D, Heninger G (1986a): Abnormal regulation of noradrenergic function in panic disorders. Arch Gen Psychiatry 43:1042–1054.

Charney DS, Heninger G (1986b): Alpha 2 adrenergic and opiate receptor blockade. Arch Gen Psychiatry 43:1037–1041.

Charney D, Heninger G (1986c): Serotonin function in panic disorders. Arch Gen Psychiatry 43:1059–1065.

Clark D, Salkovskis P, Chalkley A (1985): Respiratory control as a treatment for panic attacks. J Behav Ther Exp Psychiatry 16:23–30.

Cohen ME, White PD (1950): Life situations, emotions and neurocirculatory esthenia (anxiety neurosis, neuresthenia, effort syndrome). Proc Assoc Res Nervous Mental Dis 29:832–869.

Cohen MR, Cohen RM, Pichar D, Weingartner H, Murphy D (1983): High dose naloxone infusions in normals. Arch Gen Psychiatry 40:613–619.

Cooper JR, Bloom FE, Roth RH (1982): "The Biochemical Basis of Neuropharmacology." New York: Oxford University Press.

Curtis G, Buxton M, Lippman D, Nesse R, Wright J (1976): Flooding in vivo during the circadian phase of minimal cortisol secretion: Anxiety and therapeutic success without adrenal cortical activation. Biol Psychiatry 11:101–107.

Damas-Mora J, Davies L, Taylor W, Jenner FA (1980): Menstrual respiratory changes and symptoms. Br J Psychiatry 135:492–497.

Dillon D, Gorman JM, Liebowitz MR, Fyer AJ, Klein DF (1987): The measurement of lactate induced panic and anxiety. Psychiatry Res (in press).

Dimsdale JE, Moss J (1980): Plasma catecholamines in stress and exercise. JAMA 243:340–342.

Easton JD, Sherman DG (1976): Somatic anxiety attacks and propanolol. Arch Neurol 33:689–691.

Ehlers A, Margraf J, Roth W, Taylor C, Maddock R, Sheikh J, Kopell M, McClenahan K, Gossard D, Blowers G, Agras WS, Kopell B (1986): Lactate infusions and panic attacks: Do patients and controls respond differently? Psychiatry Res 17:295–308.

Fink M, Taylor MA, Volavka J (1969): Anxiety precipitated by lactate. N Engl J Med 281:1429.

Frankenhauser M, Jarpe G (1962): Psychophysiological reactions to infusions of a mixture of adrenaline and noradernaline. Scand J Psychol 3:21–29.

Freedman R, Ianni P, Ettedgui E, Pohl R, Rainey J (1984): Psychophysiological factors in panic disorder. Psychopathology 17[Suppl 1]:66–73.

Freedman R, Ianni P, Ettedgui E, Puthezhath N (1985): Ambulatory monitoring of panic disorder. Arch Gen Psychiatry 42:244–248.

Frohlich ED, Tarazi RC, Dustan HP (1969): Hyperdynamic beta adrenergic circulatory state. Arch Intern Med 123:1–7.

Fyer AJ, Gorman JM, Liebowitz MR, Levitt M, Danielson E, Martinez J, Klein DF (1984): Sodium lactate infusion, panic attacks, and ionized calcium. Biol Psychiatry 19:1437–1447.

Fyer AJ, Liebowitz MR, Gorman JM, Davies SO, Klein DF (1985): Lactate vulnerability of remitted panic patients. Psychiatry Res 14:143–148.

Gittelman-Klein R (1975): Pharmacotherapy and management of pathological separation anxiety. Int J Mental Health 4:255–271.

Gold MS, Redmond DE, Kleber HD (1979): Noradrenergic reversal of opiate withdrawal. Am J Psychiatry 136:100–102.

Gorman JM, Askanazi J, Liebowitz MR, Fyer AJ, Stein J, Kinney J, Klein DF (1984a): Response to hyperventilation in a group of patients with panic disorder. Am J Psychiatry 141:857–861.

Gorman JM, Cohen BS, Liebowitz MR, Fyer AJ, Ross D, Davies SO, Klein DF (1986): Blood gas changes and hypophosphatemia in lactate induced panic. Arch Gen Psychiatry 43:1067–1071.

Gorman JM, Davies M, Steinman R, Liebowitz MR, Fyer AJ, Coromilas J, Klein DF (1987): An objective marker of lactate induced panic. Psychiatry Res (in press).

Gorman JM, Dillon D, Fyer AJ, Liebowitz MR, Klein DF (1985a): The lactate infusion model. Psychopharmacol Bull 21:428–433.

Gorman JM, Fyer AJ, Gliklich J, King D, Klein DF (1981): Effect of sodium lactate on patients with panic disorder and mitral valve prolapse. Am J Psychiatry 138: 247–249.

Gorman JM, Levy GF, Liebowitz MR, McGrath P, Appleby I, Dillon D, Davies SO, Klein DF (1983): Effect of acute β-adrenergic blockade on lactate induced panic. Arch Gen Psychiatry 40:1079–1082.

Gorman JM, Liebowitz MR, Fyer AJ, Dillon DJ, Davies SO, Stein J, Klein DF (1985b): Lactate infusion in obsessive–compulsive disorder. Am J Psychiatry 142: 864–866.

Gorman JM, Liebowitz MR, Stein J, Fyer AJ, Klein DF (1984b): Insulin levels during lactate infusion. Am J Psychiatry 141:1621–1622.

Gorman JM, Martinez JM, Liebowitz MR, Fyer AJ, Klein DF (1984c): Hypoglycemia and panic attacks. Am J Psychiatry 141:101–102.

Grosz HJ, Farmer BB (1972): Pitts' and McClure's lactate anxiety study revisited. Br J Psychiatry 120:415–418.

Grunhaus L, Gloger B, Birmacher B, Palmer C, Menashe

BD (1983): Prolactin response to cold pressor test in patients with panic attacks. Psychiatry Res 8:171–177.

Harrison W, Gorman J, Sandberg D, Fyer M, Nee J, Endicott J (1986): Panic attacks after CO_2 inhalation in premenstrual dysphoric disorder. Presentation, American College of Neuropsychopharmacology.

Holmberg G, Gershon S (1961): Autonomic and psychic effects of yohimbine hydrochloride. Psychopharmacologia 2:92–106.

Holmgren A, Strom G (1959); Blood lactate concentration in relation to absolute and related work load in normal men, and in mitral storosis, atrial septal defect, and vasoregulatory asthenia. Acta Med Scand 163:186–193.

Jones M, Mellersh V, (1946): Comparison of exercise response in anxiety states and normal controls. Psychosom Med 8:180–187.

Judd F, Burrows G, Norman T (1985): The biological base of anxiety. J Affect Disorders 9:271–284.

Kelly D, Mitchell-Heggs N, Sherman D (1971): Anxiety and the effects of sodium lactate assessed clinically and physiologically. Br J Psychiatry 119:129–141.

Klein DF, Ross DC (1986): Response of panic patients and normal controls to lactate infusions. Psychiatry Res 19:163–164.

Knott V, Chaudhry R, LaPierre Y (1981): Panic induced by sodium lactate: Electrophysiological correlates. Prog Neuropsychopharmacol 5:511–514.

Ko GN, Elsworth JD, Roth RH, Rifkin B, Leigh H, Redmond E (1983): Panic induced elevation of plasma MHPG levels in phobic-anxious patients. Arch Gen Psychiatry 40:425–430.

Lapierre Y, Knott V, Gray R (1984): Psychophysiological correlates of sodium lactate. Psychopharmacol Bull 20:50–57.

Levin AP, Doran A, Liebowitz MR, Fyer AJ, Gorman J, Klein DF, Paul S (1987): Pituitary adrenocortical unresponsiveness in lactate induced panic. Psychiatry Res (in press).

Levin AP, Liebowitz MR, Fyer AJ, Gorman J, Klein DF (1984): Lactate induction of panic: Hypothesized mechanisms and recent findings. In "Biology of Agoraphobia." American Psychiatric Press, Washington APA Monogr, pp. 81–97.

Liebowitz MR, Fyer AJ, Gorman JM, Campeas R, Levin A, Davies S, Goetz D, Klein DF (1986a): Alprazolam in the treatment of panic disorders. J Clin Psychopharmacol 6:13–20.

Liebowitz MR, Fyer AJ, Gorman JM, Dillon D, Appleby I, Levy G, Anderson S, Levitt M, Palij M, Davies SO, Klein DF (1984a): Lactate provocation of panic attacks. I: Clinical and behavioral findings. Arch Gen Psychiatry 41:764–770.

Liebowitz MR, Fyer AJ, Gorman JM, Dillon D, Davies SO, Stein J, Cohen B, Klein DF (1985a): Specificity of lactate infusions in social phobia versus panic disorders. Am J Psychiatry 142:947–950.

Liebowitz MR, Fyer AJ, Gorman JM, Klein DF (1987): Comparability of clinical and lactate induced panic attacks. Ann Intern Med (in press).

Liebowitz MR, Fyer AJ, McGrath P (1981): Clonidine treatment of panic disorder. Psychopharmacol Bull 17:122–123.

Liebowitz MR, Gorman JM, Fyer AJ, Dillon D, Klein DF (1984b): Effects of naloxone in patients with panic attacks. Am J Psychiatry 141:995–997.

Liebowitz MR, Gorman JM, Fyer AJ, Levitt M, Dillon D, Levy G, Appleby I, Anderson S, Palij M, Davies SO, Klein DF (1985b): Lactate provocation of panic attacks. II: Biochemical and physiological findings. Arch Gen Psychiatry 42:709–719.

Lima D, Turner P (1983): Propanolol increases reduced beta receptor function in severely anxious patients. Lancet ii:1505.

Lindemann E, Finesinger JE (1938): The effects of adrenalin and mecholyl in states of anxiety in psychoneurotic patients. Am J Psychiatry 95:353–370.

Lingjaerde O (1985): Lactate induced panic attacks: Possible involvement of serotonin reuptake stimulation. Acta Psychiatr Scand 72:206–208.

Linko E (1950): Lactic acid response to muscular exercise in neurocirculatory asthenia. Ann Med Intern Fen 39:161–176.

Margraf J, Ehlers A, Roth W (1986): Sodium lactate infusions and panic attacks: A review and critique. Psychosom Med 48:23–51.

McGrath P, Stewart J, Harrison W, Quitkin F, Rabkin J (1985): Lactate infusions in patients with depression and anxiety. Psychopharmacol Bull 21:555–558.

Neftel KA, Adler RH, Kapelli L, Rossi M, Dolder M, Kaser H, Bruggesser H, Vorkauf H (1982): Stage fright in musicians: A model illustrating the effect of beta blockers. Psychosom Med 44:461–469.

Nesse RM, Cameron OG, Curtis GC, McCann D, Huber-Smith M (1984): Adrenergic function in patients with panic anxiety. Arch Gen Psychiatry 41:771–776.

Nutt D (1986): Increased central alpha 2 adrenoceptor sensitivity in panic disorder. Psychopharmacology 90:268–269.

Panksepp J, Herman B, Vilberg T (1978): Endogenous opioids and social behavior. Neurosci Behav Rev 4:473–487.

Pitts FN Jr, McClure JN (1967): Lactate metabolism in anxiety neurosis. N Engl J Med 277:1329–1336.

Pitts FN, Allen RE (1979): Biochemical induction of anxiety. In Fann WE, Karacan I, Pokorny AD, Williams RL (eds): Phenomenology and Treatment of Anxiety. New York: Spectrum Medical and Scientific Books.

Pyke RE, Greenberg HS (1986): Norepinephrine challenges in panic patients. J Clin Psychopharmacol 6:279–285.

Qulig K, Duffy J, Rumack DH (1982): Naloxone for treatment of clonidine overdose. Letter to the editor. JAMA 247:1697.

Rainey J, Frohman C, Freedman R, Pohl R, Ettedgui E, Williams M (1984a): Specificity of lactate infusion as a model of anxiety. Psychopharmacol Bull 20:45–49.

Rainey J, Pohl R, Williams M, Knitter E, Freedman R, Ettedgui E (1984b): A comparison of lactate and isoproterenol anxiety states. Psychopathology 17[suppl 1]:74–82.

Rainey JM, Frohman CE, Warner K, Bates S, Pohl R, Yeragani V (1985): Panic anxiety and lactate metabolism. Psychopharmacol Bull 21:434–437.

Rapee R, Mattick R, Murrell E (1987): Cognitive mediation in the affective component of spontaneous panic attacks. J Behav Ther Exp Psychiatry (in press).

Reiman E, Raichle M, Robins E, Butler K, Herscovitch P, Fox P, Perlmutter J (1986): The application of positron emission tomography to the study of panic disorder. Am J Psychiatry 143:469–477.

Rick S, Beckmann H, Muller W (1985): DL-sodium lactate reduces alpha-1 adrenergic receptor binding in rat and mouse brain. Psychiatry Res 16:241–247.

Rifkin A, Klein DF, Dillon D, Levitt M (1981): Blockade by imipramine or desipramine of panic induced by sodium lactate. Am J Psychiatry 138:676–677.

Sacks W (1965): The cerebral metabolism of L and D lactate ^{14}C in humans in vivo. Ann NY Acad Sci 119:1091–1108.

Sandberg D, Fyer A, Endicott J (1986): Premenstrual changes in anxiety patients. Presentation, American Psychiatric Association.

Schacter S, Singer J (1962): Cognitive social and physiologic determinants of emotional state. Psychol Rev 69:379–390.

Sheehan DV, Carr DB, Fishman S (1985): Lactate infusion in anxiety research: Its evolution and practice. J Clin Psychiatry 46:158–165.

Shear MK (1986): Pathophysiology of panic: A review of pharmacologic provocative tests and naturalistic monitoring data. J Clin Psychiatry 47:18–26.

Taylor CB, Sheikh J, Agras WS, Roth W, Margraf J, Ehlers A, Maddock R, Gossard D (1986): Ambulatory heart rate changes in patients with panic attacks. Am J Psychiatry 143:478–482.

Uhde TW, Vittone BJ, Post RM (1984): Glucose tolerance testing in panic disorder. Am J Psychiatry 141:1461–1463.

van der Molen GM, van den Hout MA, Vroemen J, Lousberg H, Griez E (1986): Cognitive determinants of lactate induced anxiety. Behav Res Ther 24:677–680.

Vlachakis ND, DeGuia D, Mendlowitz M, Antrom S, Wolf R (1974): Hypertension and anxiety: A trial with epinephrine and norepinephrine infusion. Mt. Sinai J Med 41:615–625.

11

Psychological Perspectives on Pharmacologic Challenge Testing

M. KATHERINE SHEAR, MD

Department of Clinical Psychiatry, The New York Hospital—Cornell Medical Center, New York, New York 10021

INTRODUCTION

The DSM III definition of panic is well known and consists of the sudden onset and rapid crescendo escalation of a feeling of fear or apprehension associated with endorsement of at least three from a list of somatic symptoms. This definition has been useful in identifying the clinical phenomenon of panic. Patients who meet diagnostic criteria for panic disorder represent a fairly uniform and clearly defined group. These patients have participated in research studies aimed at elucidating pathogenic mechanisms underlying panic and documenting treatment efficacy of specific pharmacologic (Ballenger, 1986; Zitrin et al., 1983; Charney and Heninger, 1985a; Ballenger et al., 1985; Johnston et al., 1988) and/or cognitive-behavioral (Waddell et al., 1984; Craske, 1988; Gitlin et al., 1986) treatments.

On the other hand, as has often been noted, the criteria-based definitions in DSM III fail to provide a conceptual framework needed for generation of hypotheses to elucidate pathogenesis. To this end, we prefer an ethologically based description of panic as a biobehavioral phenomenon characterized by a sudden sense of immediate (often catastrophic) danger. This subjective experience is accompanied by a stereotyped and automatic psychophysiologic defensive response. Flexibility of cognitive-behavioral defensive possibilities is compromised in the service of total commitment of available mental and physical resources to immediate escape from the danger. Seen from this vantage point, panic shares with other states of anxiety the sense of threat and associated mobilization of psychophysiologic defenses but differs in that panic occurs in response to threat perceived as immediate and catastrophic. Anxiety is elicited when the threat is more limited in scope and/or more distant in time. Anxiety stimulates a wider range of defensive possibilities. These include behavioral defenses such as passive avoidance, aggressive reactions, cognitive defense mechanisms, and interpersonal manipulations. Each of these may be associated with different physiologic responses, depending, in part, on the perceived degree of control.

Unlike the DSM III definition, the biobehavioral conception provides a model that can be used to generate and test hypotheses. Panic is seen as a potentially adaptive mechanism in some situations of real danger. Pathological panic can occur in response to activation of either biological or psychological systems. Similarly, compensatory psychological or biological processes can have a modifying effect on panic frequency, duration, or intensity. This model is consistent with the idea of an inborn neurobiologic panic mechanism, as postulated and studied by authors of other chapters in this book. We would add that pathological triggering of hypothetical brain panic mechanisms could occur as a result of psychological as well as physiological processes. Panic may occur with abnormal neurotransmitter activity or hormonal, metabolic, or impinging neurosecretory changes. Panic may also result from abnormal attentional, perceptual, appraisal, or behavioral mechanisms. The experience of "spontaneous" panic could oc-

Neurobiology of Panic Disorder, Pages 173–186

cur in connection with triggers that are either physiological or psychological events that are out of awareness.

A decade ago, reintroduction of the use of pharmacologic agents to probe biological aspects of panic disorder constituted a creative and promising research strategy, which seemed likely to elucidate the neurobiologic underpinnings of panic. Today, we are far less sanguine about our ability to build an explanatory neurophysiologic model of panic. Instead, we find ourselves faced with inconclusive and sometimes contradictory data. For example, studies by Liebowitz, Gorman, Fyer, Klein, and colleagues at Columbia (Liebowitz et al., 1985b) indicate that an abrupt heart rate elevation is the physiologic hallmark of a panic attack. On the other hand, these researchers and others (Taylor et al., 1986; Freedman et al., 1985; Shear et al., 1987) have demonstrated clearly that a substantial proportion of panic episodes occur in the absence of a tachycardic response. We now know that panic occurs when patients undergo room air hyperventilation (Hibbert, 1984a; Ley, 1988) or when they ventilate in a chamber containing 5% CO_2 (Gorman et al., 1984; Van den Hout and Griez 1985; Fyer et al., 1988). These two procedures have opposite physiologic effects. Intravenous infusion of the peripheral beta-adrenergic agonist isoproterenol has been reported to provoke panic (Rainey et al., 1984), but blockade of peripherral beta-receptors with propranolol does not block sodium lactate-provoked panic (Gorman et al., 1983). Furthermore, extensive studies of neuroendocrine and biochemical changes occurring during pharmacologically provoked panic have not revealed a consistent, pathognomonic pattern of neurophysiologic responses. Even attempts to characterize receptor function using specific central noradrenergic receptor agonists and antagonists yielded results that cannot be interpreted easily (Charney et al., 1984; Charney and Heninger, 1986).

One possible explanation for the confusion is that we have been measuring the wrong hormones and studying the wrong receptors. This would suggest that the basic approach is sound and will eventually produce the answers. Another possibility is that studies to date have been methodologically flawed by failure to control for important intervening variables. This hypothesis has been elaborated by Margraf, Ehlers, and Roth (1986a) in their excellent review of lactate infusion studies. They argue that cognitive parameters such as past experience, expectancy and anticipation, appraisal of external and internal cues, helplessness, uncertainty, and unpredictability and control, should be considered in studies of anxiety induction. In a second article, these authors point out that a psychophysiologic model of panic is better able to explain existing findings than a biological model (Margraf et al., 1986b). We support the view that the current difficulty in interpreting findings is based on lack of consideration of psychological factors operative in the testing procedures. In this chapter, we elaborate on this idea.

There are several specific issues of concern. First, to interpret the findings from a laboratory test, it must be clear that the experimental perturbation is the most salient manipulation of the subject. The possibility that stimuli associated with the experimental setting provide simultaneous, confounding psychological variables must be considered in conducting pharmacologic challenge experiments. Second, even if pharmacologic stimulation is primary, panic may be mediated by psychological factors rather than specific pharmacologic effects. Cognitive and conditioned responses to pharmacologically induced symptoms may play an important role in triggering or modifying panic reactivity. Finally, to explore the relationship between symptom production and physiologic changes, it is necessary to consider carefully and to delineate explicitly the criteria used to define panic. An attempt should be made to identify different types of panic and to discriminate clearly anxiety from panic reactions.

In 1974, Ackerman and Sachar published a paper in which they discussed the possible mechanisms of sodium lactate-induced panic. They included consideration of a psychological mechanism that they referred to as "nonspecific." The purpose of this chapter is to elaborate on the notion of psychological mechanisms that may be operative in pharmacologic challenge procedures. We further hope to influence readers to abandon the notion of nonspecific effects, since it is clear that psycholog-

TABLE 11–1.
Components of Panic

Cognitive	Behavioral	Perceptual	Physiologic
Fears: Losing control	Urge to flee	Somatic: heart palpitations	Tachycardia
Dying	Motor restlessness	Chest pain	Increased BP
Having a stroke	Changes in demeanor	Shortness of breath	Tachypnea
Having a heart attack	Help-seeking behavior	Tremulousness	Finger pulse changes
Fainting	Pill taking	Hot or cold sensation	Skin conductance
Going crazy	Social isolation	Numbness or tingling	Respiratory biochemical alterations (PCO_2, HCO_3, PH)
Mental confusion		Light-headedness or dizziness	Metabolic changes (lactate, HCO_3, CA^{++})
		Depersonalization or derealization	
		Perceptual distortions (visual, auditory)	

ical mechanisms should also be defined specifically and tested systematically. We address here the potential psychological issues in pharmacologic provocative testing in each of the following areas: 1) criteria for outcome assessment: the definition of panic, 2) specificity of the challenge procedure: psychological stimuli in the experimental situation, and 3) interpretation of response to pharmacologic challenge: contribution of psychological reactions. We end by presenting a psychosomatic model of panic that incorporates psychological and biological mechanisms in etiology and pathogenesis.

CRITERIA FOR OUTCOME ASSESSMENT: DEFINITION OF PANIC

The identification of panic as a discrete symptom and of panic disorder as a diagnostic category evolved from the work of Klein and colleagues (Klein 1964, 1981, 1982) in the early 1960s. Klein observed the specific pharmacologic effectiveness of imipramine in blocking panic, but not other anxiety symptoms, and proposed that panic represented a qualitatively discrete phenomenon. DSM III incorporated this view by developing a panic disorder category, different from generalized

anxiety or phobic disorders. Recurrent panic episodes are the central, pathognomonic feature. Anticipatory fear and phobic avoidance of panic-related situations occur as associated symptoms. Although there is continued debate about the panic–anxiety relationship (Turner et al., 1988; Tyrer, 1984), studies over the last 2 decades (Raskin et al., 1982; Crowe et al., 1980; Hoen Saric, 1982; Klein et al., 1985; Rapee, 1985) generally support the validity of the proposed distinction. Nevertheless, in actual clinical situations, it is sometimes difficult to tease apart symptoms that should be defined as panic and those that reflect high levels of anxiety. As noted, both are prominent in panic disorder patients. The blurring of this boundary represents a problem that must be addressed in pharmacologic challenge testing. Anticipatory fear of having a panic attack, or fears related to other aspects of the procedure, may be as intense as a panic episode, but the neurobiologic response may differ.

Panic is usually thought of as a unitary response. In other words, patients, clinicians, and researchers report the presence or absence of a panic attack. In fact, it is possible to identify separate cognitive, behavioral, perceptual, and physiologic components of a panic epi-

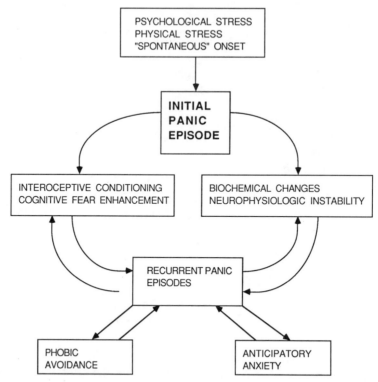

Figure 11–1. The figure illustrates a psychobiologic model of panic. According to this model, the first panic episode may occur in the context of disturbance of physiologic or psychologic equilibrium, or, with virtually no provocation, in a biologically vulnerable individual. The initial panic episode then induces a hypothesized state of neurophysiologic instability characterized by such changes as receptor modification, and hormonal and metabolic shifts. Psychological changes such as interoceptive conditioning and enhanced fearfulness also occur. These changes add to the effects of the initiating stressor(s) and increase the vulnerability to further panic episodes. More panic episodes then further increase psychological and physiologic vulnerability, creating a vicious cycle of more panic and more panic vulnerability. Secondly, cognitive and behavioral changes in the form of anticipatory anxiety and phobic avoidance then occur. These states also increase the vulnerability to panic.

sode (see Table 11–1). It is not yet clear if one of these components is central to the panic experience, or if panic occurs only if several or all of the components are present. Biological researchers have focused on the physiologic aspects of panic as central to pathogenesis. This has been disputed by psychological researchers, who see cognitive or conditioning processes as central. Our view is that the experience of panic is a manifestation of an integrated psychobiologic response that can be initiated by either psychological or physiologic stimuli (see Figure 11–1).

Another definitional issue relates to sub-types of panic. Researchers and clinicians identify several types of panic. First, panic may occur in a full-blown form (arbitrarily defined as attacks with three or more symptoms) or a limited-symptom form. The latter includes episodes of only one or two of the typical symptoms. Limited-symptom episodes are characterized by their abrupt onset and rapid crescendo peak as well as their similarity to full-blown panic. Although the importance of the distinction between full panic and limited-symptom episodes is not yet clear, the same criteria should be applied to laboratory-induced and clinical panic. A fuller view of panic vulnerability may emerge if limited-symptom episodes are scored in pharmacologic challenge testing. Both types of panic can begin in any of several ways. These include unexpected onset (also called "spontaneous"), situationally provoked panic, pharmacologically provoked panic, cognitively provoked panic, and voluntary hypertentilation. Situational provocation may occur in connection with stimuli associated with previous panic, in situations when the patient feels trapped and unable to escape or alone and unable to get help or in situations that provoke physiologic arousal (e.g., having an argument, watching a frightening movie or an exciting sports match, and physical exercise). Panic may also occur during relaxation (Heide and Forkovec, 1984; Cohen et al., 1985) or sleep (Barlow and Craske, 1988; Uhde et al., 1985; Hauri et al., 1985). Although descriptive analyses have failed to show differences in symptomatology based on type of onset, it is possible that there are differences in neurohormonal aspects of panic provoked in different ways. For example, it appears that anxiety related to social concerns is associated with epinephrine surges (Dimsdale and Moss, 1974; Liebowitz et al., 1985c), whereas fear of being trapped may be characterized by norepinephrine increases (Ballenger et al., 1988). Panic associated with sleep or relaxation may be associated with serotonergic or cholinergic instability. Thus panic occuring in different psychological contexts may differ in neurophysiologic and/or hormonal secretory patterns.

Psychological mechanisms involved in the onset of panic have not yet been thoroughly explored, but studies have identified specific thoughts and mechanisms of perception and attention to threat cues that characterize panic disorder patients. For example, work by Beck et al. (1974) and Hibbert (1984b) revealed that prominent anxiety-provoking ideation occurred in connection with panic episodes. Studies of attention processes reveal bias toward threat compared to neutral words (Matthews and McLeod, 1986; McLeod et al., 1986; Cambor et al., 1988; Ehlers et al., 1988; Matthews and McLeod, 1985). Another potentially important issue is the affective background from which panic emerges. Panic can begin in the context of mounting anxiety or of relaxation or in connection with frustration, anger, or depression. Subdiving panic episodes according to differences in onset and prepanic state may be important in identifying patterns of physiologic and/or neurohormonal reactivity.

SPECIFICITY OF THE CHALLENGE PROCEDURE: PSYCHOLOGICAL STIMULI IN THE EXPERIMENTAL SITUATION

There is an extensive literature documenting effects of experimental setting on physiologic reactivity in normal controls as well as patient populations. There is a need to differentiate panic provoked pharmacologically from anxiety related to the experimental setting. Patients' responses to the research setting depend on how the setting is constructed and how the patient is prepared for the testing as well as on the patient's personality and past experiences. For some subjects, an experimental laboratory is a more reassuring setting than the outside world, and this reassurance blocks panic. Some of our patients reported that they would have had a panic during sodium lactate infusion were it not for the presence of the supportive staff. This reaction is also documented in the literature (Kelly et al., 1971). On the other hand, some of our patients have reported that the presence of medical staff and elaborate monitoring equipment during lactate testing is frightening. They reported fears connected with the location of the procedure room (a hospital ward), the type and amount of monitoring equipment present, the presence or absence of multiple staff members, the presence of videotaping, and even the bodily position (lying down) the subject is asked to assume. Fear may be related to concerns about passivity, physical safety, dependency, loss of control, or a sense of embarrassment. The setting may be frightening because it serves as a reminder that the patient is ill. In addition, subjects may respond to unexpected or painful aspects of the procedures with feelings of anger.

There may also be differing reactions to the infusion itself. Unfamiliar physical sensations may be disturbing. There is evidence that unexplained physiologic arousal is aversive to normal subjects (Marshall and Zimbardo, 1979). Sodium lactate produces many noticeable physical sensations. Other issues include concerns about direct physical effects and/or long-term consequences or receiving the challenge agent. The method of administration of the pharmacologic agent may be disturbing. Intravenous needles provoked blood-injury phobia in patients we have seen. In others, indwelling catheters resulted in a feeling of being trapped. Inhalation procedures have provoke claustrophobic symptoms. Physiologic reactivity in a needle phobic is different from reactivity of subjects in other fearful situations. Comorbidity of blood-injury phobics in a subpopulation of subjects in a pharmacologic testing procedure may confuse results of physiologic monitoring. Subjects with claustrophobic concerns may have greater respiratory abnormalities. In our experience, a substantial number of panic disorder patients report a history of simple phobias.

The behavior of the research staff can also influence patient reactivity. Issues such as number of staff present; ability of the staff to provide a sense of safety; communication of interest, understanding, and competence all potentially play a role. In addition, studies have shown that the instructional set delivered to the patient influences response to pharmacologic testing. Van der Molen, Van den Hout, Vroeman, and colleagues (1986) and Clark and Salkovskis (Slakovskis, 1988) have demonstrated that normal subjects have widely variable reactions to CO_2 inhalation, hyperventilation, and sodium lactate infusion, depending on whether they are told that the symptoms are expected to be pleasurable or disturbing. Rapee, Mattick, and Murrell (1986) demonstrated that providing a detailed description of experimental procedures changed the rate of panic in panic disorder patients. Sanderson, Rapee, and Barlow (1988) documented a striking difference in panic rate with CO_2 based on whether the patient was told he had control over CO_2 flow rate.

There is a need to direct attention to each of these aspects of the experimental situation. The subject's level of anxiety in response to the experimental situation should be systematically measured and specific fears identified. Issues such as reassurance and instructional set should be considered potential experimental variables. Staff should be trained to provide a standardized degree of reassurance. Instruc-

tions should be standardized using scripts. Both should be varied systematically to test the reactivity of the patient population being studied.

INTERPRETATION OF RESPONSES TO PHARMACOLOGIC CHALLENGE: PSYCHOLOGICAL ASPECTS OF PANIC

Effects of Psychological Treatment on Sodium Lactate-Provoked Panic

Multiple studies have demonstrated that panic disorder patients are more likely to experience a panic attack during challenge testing than control groups of normal subjects (Pitts and McClure, 1967; Guttmacher et al., 1983; Liebowitz et al., 1984; Boulenger et al., 1984; Charney and Heninger, 1985b) and patients with other anxiety disorders (Gorman et al., 1985b); Liebowitz et al., 1985a). It is possible that heightened reactivity to the experimental setting plays a role in this vulnerability, as noted above. However, even if pharmacologic effects are primary, the possibility should be considered that psychological mechanisms mediate the observed panic response. There is evidence that psychological treatment can modify pharmacologic vulnerability. Bonn, Harrison, and Reese (1973) used repeated lactate infusions to carry out an effective behavioral desensitization treatment. Guttmacher (1984) reported reversal of lactate vulnerability in a patient undergoing behavioral treatment along with placebo medication.

We conducted an open prospective trial of cognitive behavioral treatment efficacy in 23 patients who met DSM III criteria for panic disorder. Patients were recruited, evaluated, and treated for a period of 8–24 weeks at Payne Whitney Anxiety Disorders Clinic. All subjects had had at least one full-blown panic episode in the month prior to beginning treatment. Nineteen of 23 subjects (83%) reported no full-blown panic attacks posttreatment. Two of the remaining four subjects showed a decrease in number of monthly panic episodes during the treatment, and two showed an increase. Ratings of anticipatory anxiety and phobic avoidance were also made, showing an associated decline during the treatment period.

Patients who participated in the cognitive behavioral treatment study were asked to participate in a collaborative study of sodium lactate vulnerability (Fyer, 1987; Shear, 1987). Sodium lactate infusions were conducted at the Biological Studies Unit and arranged through the Anxiety Disorders Clinic at New York State Psychiatric Institute. Twenty patients received pretreatment infusions, and six of them also underwent sodium lactate testing after treatment. The objective was to determine if patients undergoing cognitive behavioral treatment showed a decrement in vulnerability to pharmacologically provoked panic similar to that of those treated with medication (Liebowitz et al., 1985c).

Sodium lactate testing was carried out at the biological studies center of New York State Psychiatric Institute according to standard procedures that have been described previously (Liebowitz et al., 1984). According to this procedure, patients receive a 20 min infusion of normal saline followed by the sodium lactate. Patients are blind to infusion type. Lactate response is rated categorically by an observing physician as "panic" or "no panic." Five (25%) of the 20 subjects tested pretreatment had panic attacks during the saline infusion and did not receive sodium lactate pretreatment. Twelve of the remaining 15 (80%) had panic attacks during sodium lactate infusion.

Four of the six patients who returned for posttreatment sodium lactate infusion were rated by themselves and a blind rater as "no panic." One patient asked to terminate the infusion at 15 min (5 min before the infusion would be complete) and so was not formally rated. This patient had panicked in the first 5 min during her pretreatment infusion. One patient had a panic attack during the repeat lactate infusion. This patient had improved significantly on global measures and on phobic ratings during the cognitive behavioral treatment. However, she had reported only one panic episode in the month prior to beginning treatment and had experienced two panic episodes in the month prior to termination. Therefore, she was one of the two patients who showed an increase in panic episodes during the treatment period.

We obtained detailed reports of patients' experiences with the lactate infusions. Several types of reactions to pretreatment infusions were described. It is worth noting that, although there was a clear contribution of lac-

tate-induced somatic symptomatology in each of these types, the cognitive focus of concern differed in ways that may have implications for understanding the mechanism of lactate-induced panic. We will briefly describe four types of reactions we observed. One group of patients had reactions best described as typical of spontaneous panic episodes. These patients reported varying levels of anxiety during the preinfusion phase but did not remember any specific concern. They then experienced onset of a sudden, global panic episode during lactate infusion. Another group experienced panic qualitatively similar to anticipatory anxiety and probably closest to naturally occurring situational panic. This group reported preinfusion anticipatory anxiety specifically related to the possibility of having a panic episode. Fear increased quickly during the infusion to a level judged by patients and blind experimenter ratings as panic. The last two groups experienced panic that might best be conceptualized as related to claustrophobic and social anxiety, respectively. These patients reported preinfusion anxiety in response to the research situation. Testing is conducted using two indwelling iv lines; electrocardiogram (EKG) leads; finger pulse, skin conductance, and respiratory measuring devices; and electroencephalogram (EEG) recording electrodes. This setting led some patients to feel a sense of being trapped. The resulting claustrophobic-type anxiety esclated during the lactate infusion to levels described as panic. Other patients felt that the presence of the biochemical and physiologic recording machinery made them part of a "Frankenstein"-type situation in which some sort of bizarre experiment was being conducted. Their anxiety, related to concern about the trustworthiness of the experimenters, escalated to panic levels during the lactate phase of the procedure. These panic episodes seem closest to high levels of social anxiety.

The coping mechanisms used during the second infusion in the successfully treated patients are also of interest. Two patients, who had had global panic episodes pretreatment, reported that they were very aware of the specific somatic sensations during the posttreatment infusion. They knew the sensations were related to the lactate infusion and did not feel disturbed by them at all. One patient, who reported that she had had a "textbook panic" during pretreatment sodium lactate, stated that at posttreatment somatic sensations were much milder and different in quality from her previous experience. One patient who had felt frightened by the setting pretreatment reported using breathing techniques and a change in attitude to cope with sensations produced during posttreatment testing. This patient, a man, had decided that panic attacks should be viewed using an athletic analogy. This was a model he developed on his own after discussions with the therapist about the need for exposure to panic-provoking stimuli. He viewed the second lactate as a challenge to be anticipated with excitement and pleasure rather than a threat to be anticipated with fear. Following the infusion, he experienced a sense of triumph.

The proportion of patients in our study who panicked on inital infusion (80%) is similar to that reported by other investigators for panic disorder patients. The proportion who panicked on reinfusion (20%) is considerably lower. The posttreatment panic rate of one of five (20%) is similar to results reported for medication treated patients (four of 27; 15%) (Liebowitz et al., 1985c). These results support the hypothesis that psychological factors play a role modulating pharmacologic reponsiveness in panic patients.

A Review of Psychologically Based Theoretical Models

Biological researchers generally identify psychological reactivity as "nonspecific" effects (Levin et al., 1984). We believe that this term is unfortunate in that it discourages generation and testing of specific hypotheses related to psychological mechanisms for pharmacologic vulnerability. In fact, such hypotheses have been generated by cognitive behavioral researchers and include 1) conditioned reactivity to internal sensations, 2) cognitive misinterpretation of bodily sensations, 3) differences in perception of bodily sensations, 4) pathological accessibility of cognitive fear processing mechanisms, and 5) excessive behavioral tendency to hyperventilation. Other mechanisms that may play a role have not been as well studied or formulated. These include

the sense of predictability and controllability of situational threats (including panic episodes themselves), and an abnormality in attention processing in which attention is deployed selectively to threat-related perceptions. Here we briefly discuss each of these mechanisms.

The idea that panic occurs as a consequence of conditioned reactivity to internal sensations was suggested in the early 1970s by Ackerman and Sachar. This idea has been further elaborated by Barlow in a number of papers (1984, 1988) and by Seligman (1988) and by Van den Hout (1988). According to this model, an initial panic episode occurs as an unconditioned response in a patient with some underlying vulnerability. Further panic is then triggered by internal and external stimuli that are associated with the initial panic episode. The mechanism of pharmacologic provocation of panic predicted by this hypothesis would be through the generation of physical sensations similar to a naturally occurring panic episode. These sensations would act as stimuli for a conditioned panic reaction. The model predicts that a variety of pharmacologic agents would provoke panic. It is consistent with the observations that agents with opposite effects, e.g., CO_2 and hyperventilation (Van den Hout et al., 1987; Clark, 1986), or adrenalin and mecholyl (Lindemann and Finesinger, 1938), can both produce panic. The model also predicts that systematic, repeated exposure to panic-provoking stimuli would be effective in reducing panic vulnerability. There is some evidence to support this hypothesis. First, repeated exposure to sodium lactate (Bonn et al., 1973) or CO_2 (Wolpe, 1987) leads to decreased occurrence of panic. Second, cognitive behavioral therapy, which includes exposure to internal sensations as a central treatment strategy (see above), appears to be effective in treating panic.

A related model focuses on the importance of cognitive misinterpretation of bodily sensations as central to the development of a panic attack. Clark (1988) and Salkovskis (1988) are the main proponents of this theory. This model also emphasizes the importance of bodily sensations but focuses on cognitive mechanisms to explain the generation of panic. The bodily stimuli that are misinterpreted are related to autonomic activation. Anxiety generated by cognitive misinterpretation leads to further autonomic activation, creating a positive feedback situation. Studies using a contextual priming task (Fischler and Bloom, 1979) support the readiness of panic patients to interpret physical sensations catastrophically. In this paradigm, the subject is presented with an unfinished sentence followed by a letter string to finish the sentence. The subject is then asked to make a lexical decision (word or nonword) regarding the letter string as quickly as possible. Decision time is fastest, if the letter string constitutes a word that is expected to complete the sentence. The decrease in reaction time related to the match between the meaning of the sentence and the subsequent word is attributed to a cognitive process called contextual priming. In an innovative study, Clark et al. (1987) used this paradigm and found that panic patients react faster to the word "dying" than to the word "excited" in completing the phrase "John had palpitations because he was . . .". Other support for this model comes from studies of ideational components of panic (Beck, 1988; Hibbert, 1984b) showing higher frequency of catastrophic thoughts (e.g., loss of control, death or illness, anticipation of a heart attack, fainting, dying, or going mad) in panic disorder patients than in other patient groups. Hibbert (1984b) and Ley (1985) found that panic patients notice physical sensations and interpret them catastrophically. The cognitive misinterpretation hypothesis can be tested. Patients undergoing pharmacologic provocative testing could be questioned and rated for presence or absence of catastrophic cognitions. Detailed explanations could be used to prepare patients for physiologic reactions in order to decrease the likelihood of occurrence of catastrophic fears, and the effect of this manipulation on panic rate could be studied.

Margraf et al. (1986c) have suggested a psychophysiologic model based on altered perception and attention to bodily sensations. They cite studies showing differences between anxiety patients and controls in perception of bodily sensations (Tyrer et al., 1980; Katkin, 1985), but Margraf et al. have been unable to confirm this finding in panic disorder patients. This group also demonstrated that panic patients respond to false heart rate feedback with the generation of higher levels of anxiety than

a normal control group (Ehlers et al., 1988). Studies of attention bias have been carried out using a stroop-type paradigm. In this test, subjects are presented with a list of printed words. They are asked to react as quickly as possible to a task related to a characteristic of the words but unrelated to lexical content. The classic stroop entails reading a series of words written in different colors. The subject is asked to name the color of the word without paying attention to its meaning. However, in fact, the content of the word is impossible to ignore. Naming of words in which color is discrepant from content (e.g., the word "green" written in red ink) is delayed. Studies have shown that the words with more personally salient content will result in greater delay than neutral words in the color-naming task. This delay is thought to be related to automatic attention bias towards self-relevant words. Several studies of panic disorder patients demonstrate attention bias to threat compared to neutral words and delays in reaction times of patients compared to controls on threat words only (see above). The tendency of panic patients to attend preferentially to threat words has several potential consequences. First, the increased attention could lead to increased awareness of threat potential and greater anxiety. In addition, Beck (1988) notes that fixation of attention on the concept of impending disaster is associated with inability to apply reason or logic or to draw on past experience or knowledge. Thus a panic episode has the property of a closed or impermeable system, with a life of its own. Hypotheses about altered attention and perception could be tested during pharmacologic challenges. Stroop testing could be done during lactate infusion. Heart rate estimates could be compared in patients and controls. False heart rate feedback during lactate infusion could be provided.

A most interesting cognitive view of panic has been proposed by Lang (1988). This view involves a model of the mind best represented by a computer metaphor, with mentation as software and affective response (e.g., anxiety and panic) as system design outputs. Cognition is defined as a computation function in an organized, logical information processing system. Emotional responses are construed as efferent programs that mobilize the organism for fight or flight. An emotion program includes an information structure and an output production or efferent response. The information structure consists of a network of representations of stimuli, responses, and meanings. Output includes overt action, physiologic, and language components. Activation of the network occurs when there is a close enough match between input cues and network concepts. The model predicts that a network can be activated by a highly relevant stimulus representation or by a less relevant stimulus combined with activation of relevant response cues. For example, a sinuous stick would be more likely to provoke fear in a snake phobic during a period of sympathetic arousal from phsyical exertion than during relaxation. From this point of view, a panic response to a pharmacologic challenge procedure would be determined by a combination of 1) the degree and type of somatic symptoms produced by the pharmacologic agent itself, 2) the somatic symptoms associated affective states, and 3) the psychological stimuli that occur simultaneously. Considered independently, direct pharmacologic effects and associated psychological responses may each represent a subthreshold event. Lang postulates that cognitive processes in panic patients are characterized by a low degree of linkage of affective response dispositions to coherent affect networks (put the other way, a high degree of availability of affective response, prompted by many stimuli and linked to a variety of memory structures). If this is true, panic patients would be expected to have an overall lower threshold for activation of fear responses, which may account for the observed vulnerability to challenge procedures.

A fifth psychophysiologic model is based on the role of respiratory dysfunction and hyperventilation in producing panic symptoms. The fact that panic symptoms are similar to those produced by voluntary hyperventilation and that panic patients show a variety of respiratory abnormalities has attracted the interest of biological as well as psychological researchers. Panic patients have evidence for chronic hyperventilation (Salkovskis et al., 1986; Rapee, 1986), and hyperventilation is found during many panic episodes (Gorman et al., 1985a). Hyperventilation has a physiologic definition

of breathing in excess of metabolic requirements. Hyperventilation leads to a fall in arterial and alveolar pCO_2 below the normal range, with development of characteristic symptoms. A full discussion of respiratory physiology is beyond the scope of this chapter and is presented elsewhere in this volume. We wish to note here observations related to psychological effects on respiration. Bass and Gardiner (1985) reviewed the role of emotional influences on breathing and breathlessness. They note that, during quiet rest, a normal person breathes easily, without awareness. This automatic function is organized in the respiratory center in the pons and medulla and is controlled by a respiratory pacemaker. However, automatic or metabolic controls can be overridden by volitional or behavioral factors. The primary respiratory sensation is breathlessness, and this depends on psychological as well as physical factors. Patients with anxiety disorders have significantly higher respiratory rate, smaller tidal volume, and shorter breathholding times than controls. After exercise, there is a more marked increase in minute volume, which takes longer to return to resting values than in controls. Panic attacks can be provoked by hyperventilation in patients with panic disorder. However, normal individuals can hyperventilate with impunity and can maintain chronic hyperventilation with an occasional sigh and a paucity of symptoms. Psychological factors appear to account for the differences in tolerated hyperventilation and degree of development of symptoms. Evidence exists that voluntary control of respiration can modulate level of subjective anxiety experiences under a variety of circumstances. In particular, breathing retraining appears to be effective in managing panic attacks in some patients (Clark et al., 1985) and to enhance effects of behavioral treatment of agoraphobia (Bonn and Readhead, 1984). The role of respiratory dysfunction in panic is under active investigation. Studies in this area clearly should consider psychological parameters.

A final mechanism that might be considered in panic studies is the role of perceived self-efficacy in producing symptoms and physiologic reactivity. A series of studies by Bandura and colleagues have demonstrated strong effects of perception of predictability and controllability on physiologic responsiveness of phobic patients presented with phobic objects. The innovative study by Sanderson et al. (1988), discussed above, provides evidence that sense of control is an important mediating factor in panic provocation. Rachman and colleagues have studied effects of predictability and safety signals on stress-induced panic occurence in panic disorder and claustrophobic subjects. Bandura's studies (see Bandura et al., 1985) demonstrate that phobic patients with high or low degrees of perceived self-efficacy have little physiologic response to presentation of the phobic objects. The former group handles the exposure well; the latter avoids it completely. The situation in which control seems possible but uncertain provokes increases in plasma catecholamines and cardiovascular reactivity. This work suggests the hypothesis that the extent of phobic symptomatology and degree of perceived self-efficacy may differentiate physiologic subgroups of panic patients. It is possible to test effects of self-efficacy directly. Instructional sets in pharmacologic challenge tests could be varied to provide different degrees of control and predictability of the symptoms likely to be experienced.

A PSYCHOSOMATIC MODEL OF PANIC

The evidence from experimental studies of panic disorder patients strongly supports a role for both biological and psychological abnormalities in the pathogenesis of the syndrome. Thus it should be helpful to develop an integrated model to guide clinical and research efforts. The model we propose uses the paradigm developed by psychosomatic researchers. The psychobiologic model that has been used in studies of physical illness (Weiner 1977) predicts etiologic heterogeneity within an illness category and consequent difficulty in clearly identifying a single pathogenic mechanism. Psychological factors interact with physiologic disturbances to produce vulnerability to symptoms and illness onset. In general, a stressful situation will increase the likelihood of symptom formation. Stress may be nonspecific or specific, psychological or biological, or some combination of these.

Traditionally, psychobiologic studies of psychiatric disorders have focused primarily on discovering biological underpinnings of psychological syndromes. On the other hand, as was noted above, studies of physical illness have elucidated important psychological effects on biological processes. Clearly, a comprehensive psychobiologic approach must incorporate both these perspectives. In a systems approach to illness, biological and psychological forces are seen as interacting and influencing each other. This means that any particular biological finding represents the net outcome of a number of biological and psychological influences and vice versa. For example, a particular heart rate measurement reflects the anatomical and physiologic state of the heart itself, the neural tone of autonomic regulatory fibers, and the overall physiological, metabolic, behavioral, and emotional state of the organism. At any given time, an observed heart rate elevation may be due to emotional arousal, preparation for behavioral activation, actual physical activity, hyperventilation, autonomic nervous dysfunction, intrinsic cardiac pathology, or a toxic metabolic state (e.g., fever, lung disease, alcohol withdrawal, etc.). Heart rate always represents the net impact of a wide variety of factors. Neurobiological researchers have focused their efforts on identifying biological processes. This means that cognitive, behavioral, and affective changes are not always reported in study results or included in development of hypotheses to explain mechanisms of observed findings. In this chapter, we have outlined some psychological factors thought to be operant in panic patients and have suggested ways of including these factors in planning and understanding pharmacologic challenge studies.

CONCLUSIONS

Psychobiologic thinking focuses on the observation that brain and bodily physiologic systems can be perturbed by cognitive, affective, and behavioral interventions as well as by direct physiologic manipulations. Vicissitudes of social and environmental relationships may, in turn, have an impact on neurohormonal and autonomic nervous activity. Thus, for patients undergoing experimental physiologic tests, it may be as important to control for psychological variables as to be sure that subjects are free of interfering drugs or metabolic disturbance. Although ultimately psychological activities must themselves be determined by specific neural mechanisms, these mechanisms are not yet known. Studies are underway using brain imaging techniques (Reiman et al., 1984; Unde and Kellner, 1987; Reiman, 1987; Cameron, 1988), which show promise for elucidating neuroanatomical underpinnings of anxiety symptoms. In the meantime, incorporation of psychological measurements into biological testing procedures should enrich substantially our available database and allow us to test specific hypotheses related to psychogiologic functioning.

It seems clear that multiple features of panic and anxiety should be examined in each patient during pharmacologic testing procedures. Thus ratings might include 1) qualitative judgement by the clinician and patient of the presence or absence of panic; 2) number and type of symptoms in each area (listed in Table 11–1); 3) additional behavioral measures, such as changes in facial expression, motor restlessness, and verbalizations; and 4) reactions to the experimental setting and controllability of the situation. This approach would allow more meaningful exploration of the relationship between cognitive, behavioral, perceptual, and physiologic parameters and may facilitate elucidation of pathophysiologic mechanisms.

REFERENCES

Ackerman SH, Sachar EJ (1974): The lactate theory of anxiety: a review and reevaluation. Psychosom Med 36:39–79.

Ballenger J (1986): Pharmacotherapy of the panic disorders. J Clin Psychiatry 47 [suppl 6]:27–31.

Ballenger JC, Burrows GD, DuPont RL, Lesser IM, Noyes R, Pecknold JC, Rifkin A, Swinson RP (1985): Alprazolam in panic disorder and agoraphobia: results from a multicenter trial I. efficacy in short-term treatment. Arch Gen Psychiatry 45:413–422.

Ballenger JC, Laraia MT, Lydiard RB, Howell EF, Fossey MD (1988): Are plasma catecholamine increases in agoraphobia. Symposium Presentation 87E, Montreal, Canada, Proceedings of the American Psychiatric Association, p 251.

Bandura AC, Taylor B, Williams SL, Mefford IN, Barchas JD (1985): Catecholamine secretion as a function of perceived coping self-efficacy. J Clin Consult Psychol 53:406–414.

Barlow DH (1984): A psychological model of panic. In Shaw BF, Segal ZV, Valis TM and Cashman FE (eds): "Anxiety Disorders." New York: Plenum Press.

Barlow DH (1988): Current models of panic disorder and a view from emotion theory. In Frances AJ, Hales RE (eds): "Annual Review of Psychiatry." Washington, DC: American Psychiatric Press, pp 10–28.

Barlow DH, Craske MG (1988): The phenomenology of panic. In Rachman J, Mazer J (eds): "Panic: Psychological Perspectives." Hillsdale, NJ: Lawrence Erlbaum Associates, pp 11–35.

Bass C, Gardner W (1985): Emotional influences and breathing and breathlessness. J Psychosom Res 29:599–609.

Beck AT (1988): Cognitive approaches to panic disorder: theory and therapy." In Rachman J, Mazer J (eds): "Panic: Psychological Perspectives." Hillsdale, NJ: Lawrence Erlbaum Associates, pp 91–109.

Beck AT, Laude R, Bohnert N (1974): Ideational components of anxiety neurosis. Arch Gen Psychiatry 31:319–325.

Bonn JA, Harrison J, Rees L (1973): Lactate infusion in the treatment of "free-floating" anxiety. Can Psychiatr Assoc J 181:41–46.

Bonn JA, Readhead C (1984): Enhanced adaptive behavioral response in agoraphobic patients pretreated with breathing retraining. Lancet ii:665–669.

Boulenger JP, Uhde TW, Wolff EA III, et al. (1984): Increased sensitivity to caffeine in patients with anic disorder: Preliminary evidence. Arch Gen Psychiatry 41:1067–1071.

Cambor RL, Shear MK, Spielman LA, Bargh JA, Sweeney JA (1988): Attention bias in panic disorder. Abstract NR 309, New Research Proceedings of the American Psychiatric Association, p 146.

Cameron OG (1988): Caffeine, PET scanning and anxiety. Symposium Presentation 37D, Montreal, Canada, Proceedings of the American Psychiatric Association, p 173.

Charney DS, Heninger GR (1985a): II. Effect of long term imipramine treatment. Arch Gen Psychiatry 42:473–481.

Charney DS, Heninger GR (1985b): Noradrenergic function and the mechanism of action of antianxiety treatment. Arch Gen Psychiatry 42:458–485.

Charney D, Heninger G (1986): Abnormal regulation of noradrenergic function in panic disorders. Arch Gen Psychiatry 43:1042–1054.

Charney DS, Heninger GR, Breier A (1984): Noradrenergic function in panic anxiety. Arch Gen Psychiatry 41:751–763.

Clark DM (1986): A cognitive approach to panic. Behav Res Ther 24:461–470.

Clark DM (1988): A cognitive model of panic attacks. In Rachman J, Mazer J (eds): "Panic: Psychological Perspectives." Hillsdale, NJ: Lawrence Erlbaum Associates, pp 71–89.

Clark DS, Gelder M, Salkovskis P (1987): A cognitive approach to panic: theory and data. Symposium Presentation 68B, Chicago, Illinois, Proceedings of the American Psychiatric Association, p 130.

Clark DM, Salkovskis PM, Chalkey AJ (1985): Respiratory control as a treatment for panic attacks. J Behav Ther Exp Psychiatr 16:23–30.

Cohen AS, Barlow DH, Blanchard EB (1985): Psychophysiology of relaxation-associated panic attacks. J Abnormal Psychol 94:96–101.

Craske MS (1988): Cognitive behavioral treatment of panic. In Frances AJ, Hales RE (eds): "Annual Review of Psychiatry. Washington, DC: American Psychiatric Press, pp 121–137.

Crowe RR, Pauls DC, Slymen DJ, Noyes R (1980): Family study of anxiety neurosis. Arch Gen Psychiatry 37: 77–79.

Dimsdale J, Moss (1974): Short term catecholamine response to psychological stress. Psychosom Med 42: 493–497.

Ehlers A, Margraf J, Roth WT, Taylor CB, Birbaumer N (1988): Anxiety induced by false HR feedback in patients with panic disorder. Behav Res Ther 26:1–11.

Fischler I, Bloom PA (1979): Automatic and attentional processes in the effects of sentence contexts on word recognition. J Verbal Learning Verbal Behav 18:1–20.

Freedman RR, Ianni P, Ettedgui E, Puthezhath N (1985): Ambulatory monitoring of panic disorder. Arch Gen Psychiatry 42:244–248.

Fyer A (1987): Effects of cognitive behavior therapy on sodium lactate vulnerability in panic patients. Paper presented at the second conference on panic and phobic disorders, Ringberg, Federal Republic of Germany.

Fyer MR, Uy J, Martinez J, Goetz R, Klein DF, Liebowitz MR, Fyer AJ, Gorman JM (1988): Carbon dioxide challenge in patients with panic disorder. Am J Psychiatry 144:1080–1082.

Gitlin B, Martin J, Shear MK, Frances AJ, Ball G, Josephson S (1986): Behavior therapy for panic disorder. J Nervous Mental Dis 173:742–743.

Gorman JM, Askanzai J, Liebowitz MR, Fyer AJ, Stein J, Kinney J, Klein DF (1984): Response to hyperventilation in a group of patients with panic disorder. Am J Psychiatry 41:857–861.

Gorman JM, Fyer AJ, Ross DC, Cohen BS, Martinez JM, Liebowitz MR, Klein DR (1985a): Normalization of venous pH, pCO_2, and bicarbonate levels after blockade of panic attacks. Psychiatr Res 14:57–65.

Gorman JM, Levy GF, Liebowitz MR, et al. (1983): Effect of acute β-adrenergic blockade on lactate-induced panic. Arch Gen Psychiatry 40:1079–1082.

Gorman JM, Liebowitz MR, Fyer AJ (1985b): Lactate infusions in obsessive–compulsive disorder. Am J Psychiatry 142:864–866.

Guttmacher LB (1984): In Vivo desensitization alteration of lactate-induced panic: A case study. Behav Ther 15:369–372.

Guttmacher LB, Murphy DL, Insel TR (1983): Pharmacologic models of anxiety. Comp Psychiatry 24:312–326.

Hauri P, Friedman M, Ravaris R, Fisher J (1985): In Chafe MH, McGinty DJ, Wilder-Jones R (eds): "Sleep Research. Vol 14." p. 128.

Heide FJ, Borkovec TD (1984): Relaxation induced anxiety: Mechanisms and theoretical implications. Behav Res Ther 22:1–12.

Hibbert GA (1984a): Hyperventilation as a cause of panic attacks. Br Med J 288:263–264.

Hibbert GA (1984b): Ideational components of anxiety: Their origin and content. Br J Psychiatry 144:618–624.

Hoen Saric R (1982): Comparison of generalized anxiety disorder with panic disorder patients. Psychopharmacol Bull 18:104–108.

Johnston DG, Troyer IE, Whitsett SF (1988): Chlomipramine treatment of agoraphobic women. Arch Gen Psychiatry 45:453–459.

Katkin ES (1985): Blood sweat and tears: Individual differences in autonomic self perception. Psychophysiology 22:125–137.

Kelly D, Mitchell-Heggs M, Sherman D (1971): Anxiety and the effects of sodium lactate assessed clinically and physiologically. Br J Psychiatry 119:129–141.

Klein DF (1964): Delineation of two drug-responsive anxiety syndromes. Psychopharmacology 5:397–408.

Klein DF (1981): Anxiety reconceptualized. In Klein DF, Rabkin JG (eds): "Anxiety New Research and Changing Concepts." New York: Raven Press.

Klein DF (1982): Medication in the treatment of panic attacks and phobic states. Psychopharmacol Bull 18: 85–90.

Klein DF, Rabkin JG, Gorman JM (1985): Etiologic and pathophysiologic inferences from the pharmacologic treatment of anxiety. In Tuma AH, Maser J (eds): "Anxiety and the Anxiety Disorders." Hillsdale, NJ: Lawrence Erlbaum Associates.

Lang RJ (1988): Fear, anxiety and panic: Context, cognition, and visceral arousal. In Rachman J, Maser J (eds): "Panic: Psychological Perspectives." Hillsdale, NJ: Lawrence Erlbaum Associates, pp 219–236.

Levin AP, Liebowitz MR, Fyer AJ, Gorman JM, Klein DF (1984): Lactate induction of panic: hypothesized mechanisms and recent findings. In Ballenger JC (eds): "Biology of Agoraphobia." Washington DC: American Psychiatric Association Press, pp 81–99.

Ley R (1985): Agoraphobia, eht panic attack, and the hyperventilation syndrome. Behav Res Ther 23:79–81.

Ley R (1988): HYperventilation and lactate infusion in the production of panic attacks. Clin Psychol Rev 8: 1–18.

Liebowitz MR, Fyer AJ, Gorman JM (1985a): Specificity of lactate infusions in social phobia versus panic disorder. Am J Psychiatry 142:947–950.

Liebowitz MR, Fyer AJ, Gorman JM, et al. (1984): Lactate provocation of panic attacks. I. Clinical and behavioral findings. Arch Gen Psychiatry 41:764–770.

Liebowitz MR, Gorman JM, Fyer AJ, Klein DF (1985b): Social phobia: A review of a neglected anxiety disorder. Arch Gen Psychiatry 42:729–736.

Liebowitz MR, Gorman JM, Fyer AJ, Levitt M, Dillon D, Levy G, Appleby IL, Anderson S, Paley M, Davies SO, Klein DF (1985c): Lactate provocation of panic attacks. II. Biochemical and physiological findings. Arch Gen Psychiatry 42:709–718.

Lindemann E, Finesinger JE (1938): The effect of adrenalin and mecholyl in states of anxiety in psychoneurotic patients. Am J Psychiatry 95:353–370.

Margraf J, Ehlers A, Roth WT (1986a): Biological models of panic disorder and agoraphobia, a review. Behav Res Ther 24:553–567.

Margraf J, Ehlers A, Roth WT (1986b): Sodium lactate infusions and panic attacks: A review and critique. Psychosom Med 48:23–51.

Margraf J, Ehlers A, Roth WT (1986c): Panic attacks: Theoretical models and empirical evidence. In Hand I, Wittchen HU (eds): "Panic and Phobias." New York: Springer Verlag, p 31–43.

Marshall GD, Zimbardo PG (1979): Affective consequences of inadequately explained physiologic arousal. J Person Soc Psychol 37:970–988.

Matthews A, McLeod C (1985): Selective processing of threat cues in anxiety states. Behav Res Ther 23:563–569.

Matthews A, McLeod C (1986): Discrimination of threat cues without awareness in anxiety states. J Abnormal Psychol 95:131–138.

McLeod C, Matthews A, Tata P (1986): Attentional bias in emotional disorders. J Abnormal Psychol 95:15–20.

Pitts RN, McClure JN (1967): Lactate metabolism in anxiety neurosis. N Engl J Med 25:1329–1336.

Rachman SJ, Levitt K (1985): Panics and their consequences. Behav Res Ther 23:585–600.

Rainey JM, Pohl RB, Williams M, Knitter E, Freedman RR, Ettedgui E (1984): A comparison of lactate and isoproterenol anxiety states. Psychopathology 17 [Suppl 1]:74–82.

Rapee RM (1985): Distinction between panic disorder and generalized anxiety disorder. Aust NZ J Psychiatry 19:227–232.

Rapee R (1986): Differential response to hyperventilation in panic and generalized anxiety disorder. J Abnormal Psychol 95:24–28.

Rapee RM, Mattick R, Murrell E (1986): Cognitive mediation in the affective component of spontaneous panic attacks. J Behav Res Exp Psychiatry 17:245–253.

Raskin M, Peeke HVS, Dickman W, Pinsker H (1982): Panic and generalized anxiety disorders: Developmental antecedants and precipitants. Arch Gen Psychiatry 39:687–689.

Reiman EM (1987): The study of panic disorder using positron emission tomography. Psychiatr Dev 1:63–78.

Reiman EM, Raichle ME, Butler KF, Herskovita P, Robbins E (1984): A focal brain abnormality in panic disorder, a severe form of anxiety. Nature 310:683–685.

Salkovskis PM (1988): Phenomenology, assessment and the cognitive model of panic. In Rachman J, Maser J (eds): "Panic: Psychological Perspectives." Hillsdale, NJ: Lawrence Erlbaum Associates.

Salkovskis PM, Jones DR, Clark DM (1986): Respiratory control in the treatment of panic attacks: Replication and extension with concurrent measures of behavior and pCO_2. Br J Psychiatry 148:526–532.

Sanderson WS, Rappee RM, Barlow DH (1988): Influence of perceived control on carbon dioxide panic. Abstract NR 297, Montreal, Canada, New Research Proceedings of the American Psychiatric Association, p 142.

Seligman MEP (1988): Competing theories of panic. In Rachman J, Maser J (eds): "Panic: Psychological Perspectives." Hillsdale, NJ: Lawrence Erlbaum Associates, pp 321–329.

Shear MK (1987): Cognitive behavior therapy efficacy for panic disorder. Paper presented at American Association for Behavioral Therapy, Boston.

Shear MK, Kligfield P, Harshfield G, Devereux RB, Polan JJ, Mann JJ, Pickering T, Frances AJ (1987): Cardiac rate and rhythm in panic disorder patients. Am J Psychiatry 144:633–637.

Taylor CB, Sheikh J, Agras WS, Roth WT, Margraf J, Ehlers A, Maddock RJ, Gossard D (1986): Ambulatory heart rate changes in patients with panic attacks. Am J Psychiatry 143:478–480.

Turner SM, Beidel DC, Jacob RG (1988): Assessment of panic. In Rachman J, Maser J (eds): "Panic: Psychological Perspectives." Hillsdale, NJ: Lawrence Erlbaum Associates, pp 37–50.

Tyrer P (1984): Classification of anxiety. Br J Psychiatry 144:78–83.

Tyrer P, Lee I, Alexander J (1980): Awareness of cardiac function in anxious, phobic and hypochondrical patients. Psychol Med 10:171–174.

Uhde TW, Kellner CH (1987): Cerebral ventricular size in panic disorder. J Affect Disorders 12:175–178.

Uhde TW, Roy-Byrne PP, Vittone BJ, Boulenger JP, Post RM (1985): Phenomenology and Neurobiology of Panic. In Tuma AH, Maser J (eds): "Anxiety and the Anxiety Disorders." Hillsdale, NJ: Lawrence Erlbaum Associates, pp 557–576.

Van den Hout MA (1988): The explanation of experimental panic. In Rachman J, Maser J (eds): "Panic: Psychological Perspectives," pp 237–257.

Van den Hout MA, Griez E (1985): Peripheral Panic symptoms occur during changes in alveolar CO_2. Comp Psychiatry 26:381–387.

Van den Hout MA, Griez E, Van der Molen GM (1987): pCO_2 and panic sensations after inhalation of 35% CO_2. J Behav Ther Exp Psychiatry 18:19–23.

Van der Molen GM, Van den Hout MA, Vroeman J, Lousberg J, Griez E (1986): Cognitive determinants of lactate induced anxiety. Behav Res Ther 24:677–680.

Waddell MT, Barlow DH, O'Brien GT (1984): A preliminary investigation of cognitive and relaxation treatment of panic disorder: Effects on intense anxiety vs. 'background' anxiety. Behav Res Ther 22:393–402.

Weiner H (1977): Psychobiologic contributions to human disease. In Weiner H (ed): "Psychobiology and Human Disease." New York: Elsevier.

Wolpe J (1987): Carbon dioxide inhalation treatments of neurotic anxiety: an overview. J Nervous Mental Dis 175:129–133.

Zitrin CM, Klein DF, Woerner MG, Ross DC (1983): Treatment of phobias: I. Comparison of imipramine hydrochloride and placebo. Arch Gen Psychiatry 40:125–138.

12

Respiratory Physiology of Panic

JACK M. GORMAN, MD, AND **LASZLO A. PAPP**, MD

Department of Psychiatry, Columbia University College of Physicians and Surgeons, New York, New York 10032

INTRODUCTION

Compared to the extensive literature on cardiovascular function in anxiety disorders, relatively little research or theory has been produced on respiratory physiology. This is surprising in that anxious patients almost invariably complain of a choking sensation or rapid and uncontrolled breathing rate. A familiar sight in the emergency room is a patient furiously breathing into a brown paper bag in the belief that rebreathing CO_2 will abort the episode of "psychogenic" hyperventilation.

To the surprise of many, however, it is increasingly apparent that inhalation of CO_2 induces anxiety in patients with a history of panic disorder much more reliably than does hyperventilation. Inhalation of CO_2 in fact is becoming a safe and reliable model of laboratory-induced panic.

Specifically, it now appears that hyperventilation is an important component of acute panic attacks but is not the primary cause. Stimulation of areas of the nervous system that secondarily provoke hyperventilation appears to cause panic attacks in patients suffering from panic disorder. Patients with panic disorder may have hypersensitive respiratory control mechanisms that, when triggered by CO_2, among other possible stimuli, fire at abnormally low threshold and initiate a cascade of events ultimately resulting in a panic attack.

In addition to an increased understanding of the pathophysiology of panic, respiratory physiology studies can potentially yield objective clinical parameters of anxiety. Grossman (1983) has suggested that indices of respiratory function may correlate with the subjective sense of anxiety better than any other physiological function, including heart rate. Indeed, in a recent study in which patients with social phobia underwent intravenous (iv) epinephrine infusion, increased minute ventilation, but not plasma epinephrine level or heart rate, was highly correlated with subjective ratings of anxiety (Papp et al., 1988).

This chapter, after giving a brief historical background, reviews the basic physiology of respiration. It details the evidence that hyperventilation is associated with pathological anxiety and also work using the sodium lactate method of panic induction indicating that hyperventilation occurs during acute panic attacks. Next, this chapter summarizes the findings from studies using the CO_2 challenge test and theories of the pathophysiology of panic generated by these studies. Finally, it discusses some of the clinical implications and treatment considerations based on new knowledge of respiratory physiology of anxiety.

HISTORY

Since it was first isolated in pure form by Priestly about 1770, CO_2 has been forgotten and rediscovered several times in medicine. After it was first promoted as an analgesic by Hickman in the early 19th century, the inhalation of CO_2 resurfaced in 1929 (Loevenhart et al., 1929) as a "treatment" for "dementia precox," "manic depressive insanity," and "involutional melancholia."

The dominance of psychoanalysis in psychiatry temporarily halted further CO_2 research until the early 1950s, when Cohen and White (1951) and Meduna (1950) independently published their observations on CO_2 and anxiety. Cohen and White found that rebreathing up to 4% CO_2 caused anxiety attacks in patients with

Neurobiology of Panic Disorder, Pages 187–203

"neurocirculatory asthenia," and Meduna reported significant clinical improvements in stutter and "anxiety neurosis" in response to CO_2 inhalation.

The results prompted the American Psychiatric Association to elect a special committee on CO_2 research, which, in 1953, became the "Carbon Dioxide Research Association," with an active membership of close to 200. After a few years and some controversial studies, enthusiasm for work with CO_2 abated, and, with the exception of some behavioral therapists, CO_2 treatment was again abandoned by psychiatrists. A few behavioral therapists continued to use repeated inhalation of CO_2 as a method of desentitization of phobias (Wolpe, 1973).

Not until a few years ago did the investigation of the role of CO_2 in anxiety become legitimate again in mainstream psychiatry. The pharmacological dissection of the formerly homogeneous diagnostic category of "anxiety neurosis" (Klein, 1964) gave new momentum and meaning to thorough description of physiological and biochemical changes during panic anxiety.

Anecdotal, traditional, and casual clinical claims regarding various respiratory derangements in panic have now become the subject of rigorous scientific investigations. The first significant observation was that the symptoms of acute hyperventilation have a great deal of overlap with the symptoms commonly found in patients with panic disorder, generalized anxiety disorder, and phobias. Subsequently, a number of studies found respiratory and acid–base parameters in panic patients that were characteristic of both chronic and acute hyperventilation. Thus the seemingly simple physiological derangement of hyperventilation and its complex relationship with CO_2 concentration changes has become the focus of intensive biomedical investigation.

PHYSIOLOGY OF RESPIRATION

Respiratory Control

The partial pressure of CO_2 in arterial blood is maintained between 35 and 45 torr. Three factors influence this function, called the $PaCO_2$, the amount of CO_2 produced by cellular metabolism, the amount of CO_2 exhaled, and the concentration of CO_2 in the inhaled air. Normally, room air contains almost no CO_2.

Increases in CO_2 (hypercapnia) are detected in the body by at least three highly developed and sensitive receptors: the intrapulmonary receptors, the peripheral chemoreceptors of the aortic arch and carotid bodies, and the chemosensitive area of the medullary reticular activating system in the brain stem.

Relatively little is known about the intrapulmonary receptors, and it is doubtful that their contribution to the overall control of respiration is as significant as that of the peripheral or medullary chemoreceptors. Increases in CO_2 level in arterial blood are detected by the peripheral chemoreceptors, which send efferent fibers via the vagus nerve to the nucleus solitarius in the medulla (Errington and Dashwood, 1979). Similarly, increases in central carbon dioxide concentration are detected by rostral and caudal medullary chemoreceptors (Fig. 12–1).

Projections from these medullary centers reach higher portions of the brainstem, including the pontine noradrenergic nucleus, the locus ceruleus. Hypercapnia also causes trachael constriction mediated by vagal cholinergic efferent mechanisms. This response is under the influence of the ventral surface of the medulla (Deal et al., 1986). Once the medullary chemoreceptors are stimulated by increased CO_2 concentration, they initiate a rapid, reflexive increase in ventilation.

Physiology of Hyperventilation

An increase in the rate of breathing (frequency), the amount of air inhaled and exhaled at each breath (tidal volume), or both (minute ventilation) is properly called "hyperventilation" only if overall ventilation exceeds the demand of cellular metabolism. In this case, more CO_2 is exhaled than is produced. The resulting drop in $PaCO_2$ below 35 torr is called hypocapnia.

During exercise, the increased alveolar ventilation leading to increased exhalation of CO_2 is in synchrony with increased cellular metabolism. Hyperventilation does not occur, therefore, because the partial pressure of CO_2 in blood remains constant.

CO_2 exists in dynamic equilibrium with hy-

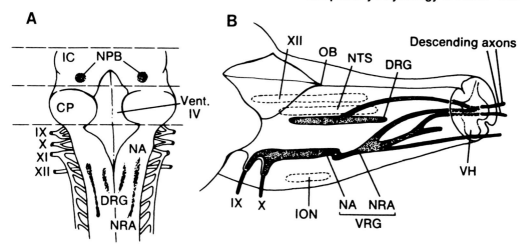

Fig. 12–1. Respiratory centers in the medulla. Dorsal **(A)** and dorsolateral **(B)** views of cat brainstem to show the dorsal (DRG) and ventral (VRG) respiratory groups and their projections. NPB, nucleus parabrachialis; IC, inferior collicu-lus; CP, cerebellar peduncle; NA, nucleus am-biguus; NRA, nucleus retroambigulis, OB, OBEX; NTS, nucleus tractus solitarius; ION, in-ferior olivary nucleus; VH, ventral horn.

drogen ion according to the following equa-tion.

$$H^+ + HCO_3^- = H_2CO_3 = CO_2 + H_2O$$

The conversion of carbonic acid (H_2CO_3) to CO_2 and back is catalyzed by the enzyme car-bonic anhydrase. As CO_2 is lost through alve-olar hyperventilation, the entire equation is shifted to the right, resulting in a reduction of free hydrogen ion. Thus alkalosis is induced as pH rises above 7.45. Because the increase in pH in this case is caused by increase in venti-lation, the situation is known as respiratory al-kalosis (Fig. 12–2).

The hypocapnic, alkalotic state induces a number of important secondary physiological changes that are crucial in understanding the pathophysiology of hyperventilation (Missri and Alexander, 1978). First, hemoglobin binds O_2 more tightly, a phenomenon known as the Bohr effect. In essence, this means that, al-though the subject is breathing very deeply and very fast, and usually generates a higher than normal PaO_2, there is less efficient deliv-ery of O_2 to the tissues. Second, hypocapnia is a potent stimulus to vascular constriction. Dur-ing hyperventilation, there is marked decrease in cerebral blood flow (Plum et al., 1968),

which may account for many of the symptoms reported by the hyperventilating subject, in-cluding lightheadedness, dizziness, derealiza-tion, and anxiety. Finally, the kidney attempts to compensate for the alkalotic state by in-creasing the excretion of bicarbonate and de-creasing the excretion of titratable acid (Stan-burg and Thomson, 1952). This tends to bring pH back toward the normal range of 7.35–7.45.

For complex reasons, plasma inorganic phosphate levels are also routinely lowered by hyperventilation. Two possible mechanisms for this have been proposed (Knochel, 1977; Okel and Hurst, 1961). Phosphate may enter cells in exchange for acids that leave cells to enter the extracellular compartment. This ef-fectively buffers the loss of hydrogen ion from plasma. Second, alkalosis may stimulate gly-colysis. This would result in the catalysis of several glycolytic enzymes, such as hexoki-nase and glyceraldehyde-3-phosphate dehy-drogenase, facilitating phosphate movement into the cells. In both cases, the result is loss of inorganic phosphate from plasma and there-fore hypophosphatemia.

As hyperventilation increases, the reduction in cerebral blood flow creates a situation of relative cerebral hypoxia (Hange et al., 1980; Kennealy et al., 1980). This stimulates dilata-

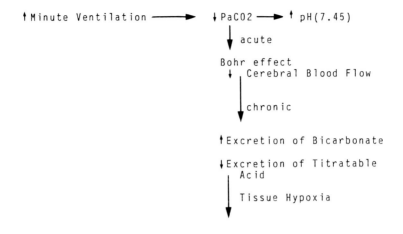

```
↑Minute Ventilation ─────────►  ↓PaCO2 ───►  ↑pH(7.45)

                                   │ acute
                                   ▼
                                Bohr effect
                                 ↓ Cerebral Blood Flow


                                   │ chronic
                                   ▼

                                ↑Excretion of Bicarbonate

                                ↓Excretion of Titratable
                                   Acid
                                   │
                                   │  Tissue Hypoxia
                                   ▼


  ↓PaCO2; ↓HCO3; Normal pH; Normal Cerebral Blood Flow
```

Fig. 12–2.   Physiological changes caused by hyperventilation.

tion of the cerebral vasculature and restores blood flow to nearly normal levels. Once chronic hyperventilation is in place, relatively few deep breaths per hour have been shown sufficient to maintain the state (Salzman et al., 1963).

The acute hyperventilator, then, will manifest decreased $PaCO_2$, increased pH, decreased plasma phosphate, and decreased cerebral blood flow. The chronic hyperventilator will also have low $PaCO_2$ and low phosphate, but bicarbonate will be low, pH nearly normal, and cerebral blood flow nearly normal (Berger et al., 1977). If the chronic hyperventilator increases ventilation even slightly, the acute hyperventilatory state is rapidly reestablished (Kerr et al., 1937; Lum, 1976).

"HYPERVENTILATION SYNDROME"

The list of subjective symptoms of acute hyperventilation is so long it probably includes symptom clusters from a number of different medical conditions. It includes dizziness, breathlessness, tingling in hands and feet, dry mouth, unsteadiness, nausea, disorientation, depersonalization, feeling faint, palpitations, panic, flushing, etc. (Rapee, 1986) (Table 12–1). The overlap between these symptoms and those commonly encountered in patients with panic disorder generated a number of studies documenting that patients with "anxiety dis-

TABLE 12–1.
Symptoms of Hyperventilation

Shortness of breath	Depersonalization
Dizziness, faintness	Tremor
Paresthesias	Dry mouth
Carpal spasm	Apprehension
Palpitation	Tightness in chest
Disorientation	Nausea
Derealization	Flushing

order" have faster resting respiratory rates, higher minute ventilation, and greater tidal volume than normal controls (Garssen, 1980; Goldstein, 1964). End tidal CO_2, an indirect but accurate measure of $PaCO_2$, has also been found to be low in these patients, indicating hyperventilation (Suess et al., 1980). Anxious patients have also been found to make more frequent sighs than normal controls at rest (Lum, 1976; Rice, 1950).

These studies suffer from two main drawbacks. First, most were conducted before operationalized criteria were developed for psychiatric diagnosis. Hence it is unclear exactly what kind of anxiety disorder the subjects had. Second, it could not be ascertained whether the patients were chronic hyperventilators or simply hyperventilating acutely to the stress of being in a laboratory.

An additional type of study attempted to learn whether enforced hyperventilation under laboratory circumstances can cause an anxious patient to become symptomatic (Compernolle et al., 1979). The patient is asked to "hyperventilate" and subsequent complaints are recorded. The so-called "hyperventilation test" was used clinically to determine which patients might respond to breathing retraining techniques.

A problem with this approach is that it does not distinguish symptoms that are produced by the mechanical discomfort and fatigue of breathing fast from those actually produced by hypocapnic alkalosis. It is likely that many patients stopped hyperventilating and complained of a variety of symptoms during these tests simply because they were tired. Despite these criticisms, the studies outlined suggested that patients with anxiety disorders are prone to hyperventilate and to complain of physical symptoms that may well be the result of hyperventilation.

Lum and others formulated various theories based on this work to explain the relationship of hyperventilation to anxiety and, most particularly, to panic attacks (Hill, 1979; Lum, 1976). According to Lum, for example, patients with panic disorder are chronic hyperventilators who have developed the "bad habit" of thoracic breathing. Normally, adults breathe predominantly abdominally, using the diaphragm, but Lum observed that his patients with panic disorder used intercostal muscles excessively to expand the chest cavity during inspiration. This produces a greater force of expiration than diaphragmatic breathing and thus leads to greater amounts of exhaled CO_2 at each breath. When stressed, according to this hypothesis, the chronic hyperventilator quickly becomes an acute hyperventilator, thus decreasing cerebral blood flow and delivery of O_2 to tissues as described above. The hypothesized result is symptoms of panic.

RESPIRATORY CHANGES DURING ACUTE PANIC

Most recent work on these ideas has focused specifically on patients with panic disorder or agoraphobia with panic attacks (Rapee, 1986). These patients very often complain of dyspnea and hyperventilation during acute panic attacks and can be differentiated from patients with generalized anxiety disorder by the de-

gree to which their complaints are of a physical and somatic nature.

Biophysiology of Lactate-Induced Panic

Infusion of half molar sodium lactate over 20 min has been shown reliably to induce panic in patients with panic disorder but to have little effect on patients with other psychiatric disorders or on normal controls (Liebowitz et al., 1985; see also Chapter 10, this volume). Investigation of the physiological and biochemical components of lactate-induced panic has shed some light on the respiratory physiology of panic disorder patients. At baseline, just before the lactate infusion is begun, patients with panic disorder have lower pCO_2 and lower bicarbonate levels than normal controls but normal pH. This is evidence specifically of chronic hyperventilation in these patients.

One study showed that patients with panic disorder who went on to panic with lactate infusion had lower plasma inorganic phosphate levels than nonpanicking patients or normal controls (Gorman et al., 1986a) (Fig. 12–3). In fact, a phosphate level of less than 2.25 mg/dl virtually ensured that the subject would go on to panic. The most likely explanation for this finding is, again, that the patients were hyperventilating.

Infused lactate is first metabolized to pyruvate in the liver. Much of this pyruvate then enters the tricarboxylic acid cycle, ultimately generating bicarbonate. Thus the infusion of sodium lactate produces an increase in bicarbonate level, which raises pH. This situation is known as metabolic alkalosis. Substantial metabolic alkalosis causes pulmonary compensation in which ventilation is decreased to conserve CO_2 and hydrogen ion, thus restoring pH to normal (Javaheri et al., 1982). Hence, lactate infusion should lead to a decrease in overall ventilation. A number of research findings suggest, however, that exactly the opposite is the case, especially for lactate panickers.

In most laboratories, the lactate infusion is stopped as soon as the panic attack occurs. Because lactate is usually given in a dose of 10 cc/kg over 20 min during this procedure, the patient who panics actually gets a smaller dose of lactate than the nonpanicking patient or normal control who receives the full 20 min dose.

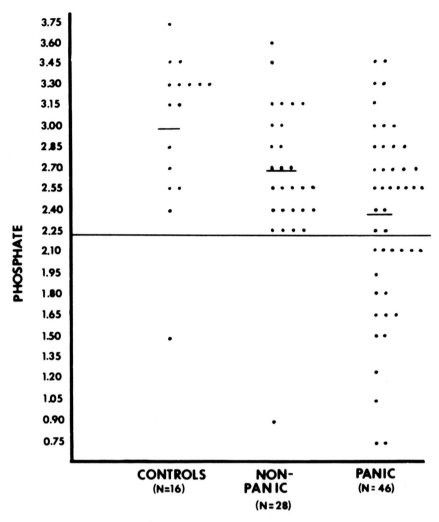

Fig. 12–3. Distribution of phosphate values at time 0 (beginning of lactate infusion) for three groups, with posthoc cut-off of 2.25 mg/dl (0.73 mmol/liter).

This makes statistical analysis of many dependent variables difficult.

One solution is to compare only the nonpanicking patients to the normal controls. In this way, patient–control differences may emerge without the necessity of adjusting for different amounts of received lactate. In making this comparison, it was observed that the nonpanicking patients developed a higher level of lactate and also of pyruvate than the normal controls, even though both groups received the same amount of infused lactate (Liebowitz et al., 1985). This could be because patients do not metabolize lactate as readily as normal individuals, although the metabolic defect would have to be beyond the level of lactate conversion to pyruvate, because patients also developed a higher pyruvate level than normals.

Hyperventilation During Lactate-Induced Panic

Another method of increasing lactate levels is by hyperventilation. Indeed the difference in

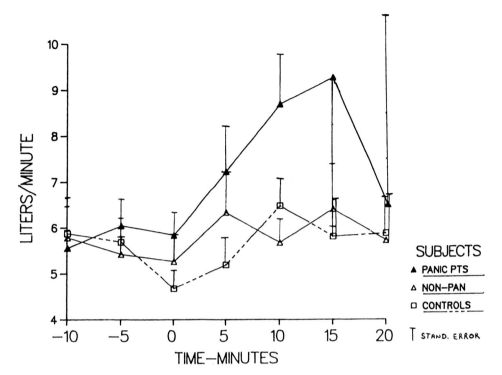

Fig. 12–4. Minute ventilation (±SEM) (liter/min) for the period 10 min prior to starting lactate (−10 to 0) and the period of lactate infusion (0–20) in three groups; panic disorder patients who had panic attacks during the infusion (solid triangles), panic disorder patients who did not panic (open triangles), and controls (open squares).

lactate level between the nonpanicking patients and the normal controls was exactly the amount of lactate increase observed during room air hyperventilation in another experiment. Hence higher lactate levels in nonpanicking patients may be secondary to greater hyperventilation during the infusion. Furthermore, even though no actual panic attack occurs, nonpanicking patients develop significantly more somatic complaints during lactate infusion than normal controls. These have been shown to be attributable to hyperventilation (Gorman et al., 1987).

The panicking patients develop lower pCO_2 and lower bicarbonate than nonpanicking patients or controls (Gorman et al., 1986a), indicating that the lactate-induced panic is accompanied by acute hyperventilation. This finding was later confirmed from arterial blood assays (Papp et al., 1989). Most recently, using a non-invasive method of respiratory monitoring, it was shown that the panicking patients develop a greater increase over baseline in minute ventilation rates than nonpanicking patients or controls, even though there is no difference in minute ventilation rate among the three groups at baseline (Gorman et al., unpublished data) (Fig. 12–4). The panicking patients thus clearly appear to be hyperventilating acutely at the point of lactate-induced panic.

There are two important considerations in understanding the finding that lactate-induced panic involves acute hyperventilation. First, the increase in minute ventilation observed is due almost entirely to an increase in the average tidal volume per breath, not in the respiratory rate. Thus simply counting the number of breaths per minute during a lactate infusion—or probably during any form of anxiety provocation—will yield misleading information. The change is in the amount of air inhaled and exhaled during each breath, not in the number of breaths. Second, as was explained above, hyperventilation during a procedure that causes metabolic alkalosis is obviously paradoxical. Bicarbonate levels probably rise more slowly during the infusion in the panicking patient than in the nonpanicking subject, probably because renal compensation for respiratory alkalosis causes an enhanced excretion of bicarbonate (Gorman et al., 1986a). Thus, in the panicking patients, the effect of respiratory alkalosis overrides the effect of metabolic alkalosis.

An explanation for the observation of hyperventilation during lactate-induced panic may lie in further knowledge about the metabolism of lactate. The bicarbonate that lactate generates does not readily cross the blood–brain barrier (Rapoport, 1976). Peripherally, this bicarbonate is further metabolized by carbonic anhydrase to CO_2. CO_2, of course, rapidly traverses the blood–brain barrier and enters the central nervous system. It is possible, then, that the CO_2 generated by lactate has the effect of stimulating respiration and causing an increase in minute ventilation. Thus lactate infusion studies suggest that increasing CO_2 level may cause both panic and hyperventilation.

Two other studies using lactate infusion also highlighted the importance of hyperventilation in panic attacks. Among a group of 20 patients with panic disorder, it was found that successful treatment with antipanic medication—including imipramine, desipramine, and clonidine—lead to a normalization of venous pH, pCO_2, and bicarbonate at baseline before a second lactate infusion (Gorman et al., 1985). The variance of these measures was greater in the patients than in controls before treatment, but after treatment the patients' variance equalled that of normal controls. Thus the evidence of respiratory abnormality seen prior to a first infusion when the subjects were drug-free and still clinically symptomatic disappeared prior to a second infusion when the patients were on effective medication and in clinical remission. Interestingly, Clark et al. (1985) observed the same normalization of respiratory indices at baseline following successful behavioral treatment of panic disorder.

As was mentioned above, nonpanicking patients develop more somatic symptoms and anxiety during lactate infusion than normal controls, even though they do not panic (Gorman et al., 1987). After successful pharmacologic treatment of panic disorder, a group of these patients who did not actually panic during the first infusion were reinfused. A complex statistical analysis of their reported complaints during the infusions indicated that antipanic medication specifically ameliorated symptoms referable to hyperventilation. The most powerful drug effect was on the complaint of difficulty breathing experienced by the patients during the first infusion (Gorman et al., 1987).

The CO_2 Challenge Test

The evidence described thus far indicates that hyperventilation is an important component of panic disorder and panic attacks. Furthermore, it suggests that both behavioral and pharmacological treatments of panic disorder also act to eliminate both chronic hyperventilation and the tendency to hyperventilate during acute panic.

Much of this evidence, however, was collected under the special circumstance of lactate-induced, rather than spontaneously occurring, panic attacks. Also, the question of whether hyperventilation is actually the cause of panic, as Lum (1976) contends, or is simply an important concomitant of panic remains unanswered. Here the literature is misleading. As was mentioned above, there are no systematic attempts to clarify whether the anxiety attacks induced by so-called "hyperventilation tests" are due to actual induction of respiratory alkalosis or merely to the fatigue and discomfort of breathing fast. A control for hyperventilation is needed in which the subject must breathe fast without becoming hypocapnic or alkalotic. This can be accomplished by the inhalation of 5% CO_2.

THE 5% CO_2 INHALATION CHALLENGE

Increasing CO_2 concentration to approximately 10% in room air results in linear increases in minute ventilation. With each increase in level of inhaled CO_2, steady-state minute ventilation is usually achieved within 10 min. Administering 5% CO_2 roughly triples the minute ventilation of a normal subject.

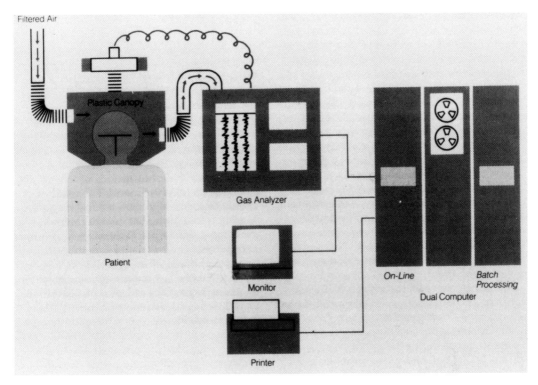

Fig. 12–5.   Canopy-spirometer system to measure gas exchange.

However, because CO_2 is continuously added to the inspired air, there is no net loss of CO_2, so hypocapnic alkalosis does not develop. Thus CO_2 administration increases ventilation similarly to room air hyperventilation and causes the same degree of mechanical effort but is a control for the hyperventilatory induction of alkalosis.

Patients with panic disorder and other anxiety disorders and normal controls were placed in a clear, rigid, plastic head canopy, which was sealed from outside air. Unlike various mouthpiece and noseclip arrangements, the canopy induces neither anxiety nor hyperventilation in normal subjects (Kinney et al., 1964) (Fig. 12–5). The canopy is connected to a spirometer and a gas analyzer, both of which transmit data to the laboratory computer on line on a breath-by-breath basis.

The system provides the following respiratory parameters for every breath: frequency, tidal volume, minute ventilation, O_2 consumption, CO_2 production, respiratory quotient, and inspiratory drive. The subject undergoes several respiratory challenges during the study, including 5% CO_2 in room air for 20 min and breathing room air at a rate of 30 breaths per minute. The latter is sufficient to induce significant hypocapnia and alkalosis. Finally, depending on whether the subject panicked on 5% CO_2, 3% or 7% CO_2 is administered in room air for 20 min.

In 1984, the somewhat surprising findings of this experiment were reported. Contrary to the original hypothesis (Lum, 1976), inhalation of CO_2 and not room air hyperventilation induced panic attacks in patients with panic disorder (Gorman et al., 1984). Normal controls did not panic with either intervention. For patients with panic disorder, CO_2 inhalation proved almost as reliable a panicogenic agent as sodium lactate infusion.

In retrospect, this finding should not have been surprising. Cohen and White (1951) had shown that rebreathing up to 4% CO_2 caused anxiety attacks in patients with "neurocirculatory asthenia." These patients did not have panic attacks during room air hyperventilation. CO_2 has also been found to induce anxiety in patients with "irritable heart" (Drury, 1919) and "neurotic anxiety" (Singh, 1984). These conditions overlap to a considerable extent with DSM III-R panic disorder.

Also, CO_2 inhalation has been used by behavioral therapists to treat anxiety disorders (Wolpe, 1973). In this case, the CO_2 caused anxiety that habituated with repeated administration. Hence, CO_2 inhalation has been used to desensitize patients to anxiety reactions much as exposing phobics to phobic stimuli serves to desensitize them.

In an extension of the first study of CO_2 inhalation, which included determination of a number of respiratory and biochemical variables, the finding that CO_2 inhalation causes panic in patients with panic disorder was further substantiated (Gorman et al., 1988). Twelve of 31 patients with panic disorder had panic attacks during 5% CO_2 inhalation, compared to one of 13 normal controls and none of 12 patients with other anxiety disorders (i.e., social phobia, obsessive–compulsive disorder, and generalized anxiety disorder).

Only seven of 30 patients with panic disorder had attacks with room air hyperventilation. Interestingly, two of these patients reported having panic attacks even though arterial pH did not exceed 7.45. Furthermore, panic disorder patients who did not report panic attacks during room air hyperventilation stopped hyperventilating because of fatigue significantly more quickly than normal volunteers. None of the 13 normal volunteers had panic attacks during room air hyperventilation, whereas one of the 12 patients with other anxiety disorders had panic attacks during room air hyperventilation.

Taking the patients with panic disorder and other anxiety disorders together, women were marginally more likely to panic during room air hyperventilation than men. Almost all (9 of 12) patients with panic disorder who panicked during 5% CO_2 inhalation also had attacks during sodium lactate infusion. However, room air hyperventilation panic did not correlate with lactate panic. Furthermore, patients who gave histories of respiratory complaints during naturally occurring panic attacks were especially

likely to panic with room air hyperventilation but not to 5% CO_2. Thus the study potentially identified a subgroup of panic disorder patients who panic with both lactate and 5% CO_2 and are distinct from a second subgroup who panic during room air hyperventilation.

In a small pilot study, increasing the CO_2 level to 7% increased the proportion of panic patients who had panic attacks during the procedure. At the 7% level, patients with social phobia also appeared susceptible to having anxiety attacks, but normal controls remained unaffected.

Panic with 5% CO_2 was associated with a more rapid rise in minute ventilation (see Fig. 12–6) compared to nonpanicking patients and normal controls and with an increase in the plasma norepinephrine level. Interestingly, as is the case with sodium lactate-induced panic, there was no increase in either plasma cortisol or plasma epinephrine level during CO_2-induced panic. The fact that patients who had panic attacks during 5% CO_2 had a more rapid rise in minute ventilation than nonpanicking patients or normal controls may indicate that these patients have a basic hypersensitivity to CO_2.

Another function of respiratory physiology, called inspiratory drive, was also measured. This function is expressed as

$$\frac{\text{tidal volume}}{\text{time in inspiration}}$$

and is believed by respiratory physiologists to represent the portion of respiratory response that is under the control of brainstem chemoreceptors (Milic-Emili and Grunstein, 1976). Inspiratory drive also increased significantly more rapidly in panicking patients than nonpanicking patients or normal controls during CO_2 inhalation. This was interpreted as suggesting that a subgroup of patients with panic disorder has hypersensitive medullary chemoreceptors for CO_2 (Gorman et al., 1986b).

In addition to delineating some aspects of respiratory physiology in patients with panic disorder, these experiments may point in the direction of a typology of panic disorder. Thus the group of patients with supersensitive CO_2

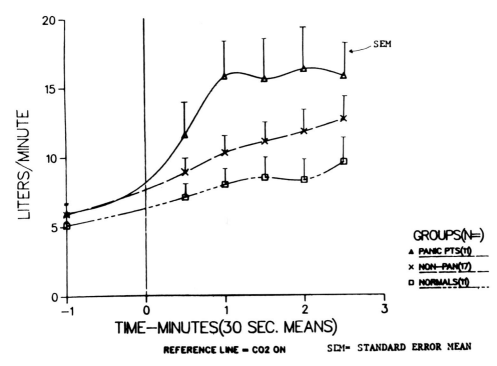

Fig. 12–6.   Minute ventilation (liters/min) at baseline and during the first 2.5 minutes of 5% CO_2 inhalation for panicking patients, nonpanicking patients, and controls.

detectors who panic during CO_2 inhalation are distinct from a group of patients who actually complain of respiratory-related symptoms during panic attacks and panic in the laboratory during room air hyperventilation. It is possible that both sodium lactate infusion and CO_2 inhalation cause panic attacks by triggering brainstem receptors sensitive to CO_2.

Antipanic drugs may decrease the sensitivity of these receptors so that panic is less likely during attempts at laboratory provocation. Indeed, Woods et al. (1986) found that alprazolam treatment markedly reduced CO_2-induced anxiety in panic disorder patients.

CO_2 INHALATION BY REBREATHING

The finding that CO_2 inhalation can cause panic attacks was replicated by Woods et al. (1986), who used the modified Read method (Read, 1967) of rebreathing (Fig. 12–7). In this experiment, the subject, while his nose is occluded with a clip, breathes in and out of a spirometer filled with a mixture of 5% CO_2 and

95% O_2. This results in a continuous rise in CO_2 concentration. The rebreathing essentially continues until the subject becomes anxious. At the end of an average of 5 min rebreathing, the inhaled CO_2 level is approximately 9%. The ventilatory response is determined as the slope of the regression line representing the correlation between the increase of end tidal pCO_2 and the increase of minute ventilation. Woods et al. did not find evidence of CO_2 hypersensitivity in panic disorder patients. However, they measured minute ventilatory response to CO_2 inhalation between CO_2 concentrations of 5% and 9%, rather than between 0% and 5% as in the study previously described. Since the earlier study found that CO_2 hypersensitivity was evident in the first 3 min of exposure to CO_2 (Gorman et al., 1988), it may be that levels of CO_2 greater than 5% produce such extreme minute ventilation increases that group differences were obscured in the Woods et al. study. Furthermore, Woods et al. did not discriminate between panicking and nonpanicking patients

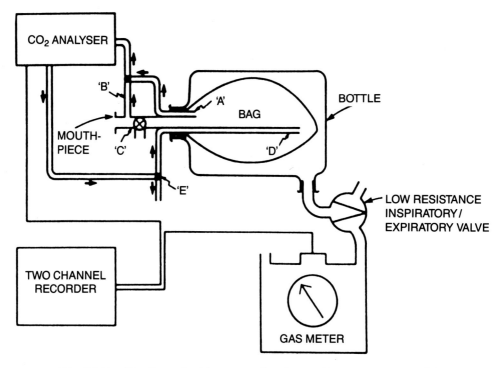

Fig. 12–7. Circuit required for measuring the ventilatory response to CO_2 by rebreathing. The short, thick arrows indicate the direction of gas flow to and from the CO_2 analyzer.

in assessing CO_2 sensitivity, although Gorman et al. (1988) found that only the panicking patients manifested increased CO_2 sensitivity compared to normal controls. Hence, methodologic differences may explain the discrepancy between the Gorman et al. and the Woods et al. studies. Indeed a recent rebreathing experiment, using a starting CO_2 concentration of 0%, found significant sensitivity difference between panicking patients and normal controls (Carr et al., 1987).

THE 35% CO_2 INHALATION CHALLENGE

The Dutch scientists Griez and van den Hout (1985; van den Hout and Griez, 1984) have worked for several years with CO_2 induction of panic attacks, using a method different from those described above. In the Dutch experiments, patients are fitted with a face mask rather than being placed in a canopy. Instead of continuous inhalation of CO_2 at relatively low concentrations for 20 min, the subjects in the Griez and van den Hout studies receive one or two vital capacity inhalations of a mixture of 35% CO_2 and 65% O_2 (van den Hout and Griez, 1984). This is counterbalanced by one or two vital capacity breaths of room air to act as placebo.

Griez and van den Hout have shown, using their relatively simple and inexpensive method, that patients with panic disorder have attacks during CO_2 inhalation but not during room air inhalation (Griez et al., 1987a). In these experiments, normal volunteers did not panic to either air or CO_2. Griez and van den Hout originally reported that panic attacks occur immediately after the cessation of CO_2 inhalation, during the period when pCO_2 is rapidly declining but before any hyperventilatory overshoot into hypocapnia has occured (Griez and van den Hout, 1985). They believed that the change in CO_2 level causes panic. More recently however, Griez and van den Hout,

(1987) supported the finding of Gorman et al. (1984), Woods et al. (1986), and Carr et al. (1987) that panic occurs while the patients are still inhaling CO_2.

Rapee et al. (1986) have also used the Griez and van den Hout method, but with higher concentration of CO_2 (i.e., 50% CO_2/50% O_2). In their work, ten of 16 panic disorder patients, but only three of 16 social phobics, had attacks during single-breath inhalation of CO_2. Rapee further showed that altering the cognitive set of the patients with panic disorder influenced the intensity of panic during CO_2 inhalation. Thus patients given no explanation about what to expect had more intense panic attacks than those given explanations. Cognitive factors may then modulate either the experienced or reported intensity of panic to higher concentration of CO_2. The Dutch method of panic induction was also used by Fyer et al. (1987). As with Rapee et al. and Griez and van den Hout, it was found that double breath inhalation of 35% CO_2 causes panic in a majority of patients with panic disorder but not in normal controls.

In addition to studying patients with anxiety disorders, the ease of this procedure allowed the investigation of the CO_2 response in women with late luteal phase dysphoric disorder. Premenstrual anxiety symptoms may be related to hyperventilation, because CO_2 sensitivity increases in the luteal phase under the influence of progesterone (Damas-Mora et al., 1980). Carr et al. (1987) reported that normal women had significantly greater ventilatory and anxiogenic response to CO_2 inhalation premenstrually than postmenstrually.

Of 13 women meeting stringent criteria for late luteal phase dysphoric disorder studied by Harrison et al. (1986), ten experienced acute panic attacks during 35% CO_2 inhalation compared to none of ten controls. The attacks occurred in both luteal and follicular phases of the cycle in nine patients and only in the luteal phase in the tenth. None of the subjects ever met criteria for panic disorder, but six of the ten panickers had experienced panic attacks in the past compared to only two of the ten non-panickers. This work suggests that premenstrual dysphoria and panic disorder may have a common biological diathesis.

As a laboratory challenge test of panic, CO_2 inhalation offers a number of advantages. Unlike lactate or isoproteronol, CO_2 crosses the blood–brain barrier readily. It is relatively simple, safe, noninvasive, and well tolerated by patients. As opposed to iv infusion methods, there is no volume overload to obscure subtle biochemical changes, such as increase of plasma catecholamine levels.

The 35% CO_2/65% O_2 method is specifically far simpler than the canopy method, although it does not offer the opportunity for sophisticated spirometric assessment. Only patients with serious pulmonary disease need routinely be excluded. The specificity and sensitivity of this test, as well as the biological concomitants of panic induced with this method, require further investigation. Conceivably, if the 35% CO_2/65% O_2 method proves reliable and specific, it could someday become a clinically useful diagnostic test for panic disorder.

THEORETICAL CONSIDERATIONS

The mechanism of action by which CO_2 induces panic is unknown, but a number of theories have been proposed.

Biological Theories

Elam et al. (1981) have shown that CO_2 inhalation produces a dose-dependent increase in firing rate of the pontine nucleus locus ceruleus in rat. This nucleus, which contains at least 50% of all central nervous system neurons that use norepinephrine as the neurotransmitter, has been cited as a possible locus for the generation of panic attacks (Charney and Redmond, 1984). The involvement of neurotransmitter systems other than noradrenergic mechanisms cannot be ruled out. One preclinical study (Prous et al., 1977) found increased serotonin and decreased dopamine turnover in response to CO_2.

In their original report on CO_2 induction of panic, Gorman et al. (1984) suggested that the mechanism of action of CO_2-induced panic may be through CO_2-provoked increase in locus ceruleus firing and central nervous system noradrenergic activity. This was also the explanation invoked by Woods et al. (1986).

Two factors mitigate against this idea, however. First, CO_2-induced panic was not associated with increases in plasma 3-methoxy-4-hydroxyphenylglycol (MHPG), a metabolite of norepinephrine believed to reflect central noradrenergic activity (Woods et al., 1985). MHPG does increase during induction of panic with yohimbine, the alpha-2-antagonist that is known to stimulate the locus ceruleus. Second, cells in the locus ceruleus have not been shown to be specifically sensitive to changes in CO_2 or hydrogen ion concentration.

It is plausible, therefore, that CO_2 stimulates receptors in the medulla, which then secondarily stimulate the locus ceruleus. This in turn would increase autonomic nervous system activity throughout the body, creating symptoms typical of a spontaneous panic attack. Panic disorder patients may have congenitally hypersensitive CO_2 chemoreceptors; therefore, according to this theory, these patients hyperventilate chronically to keep CO_2 levels as low as possible. Increasing the inhaled CO_2 concentration triggers these hypersensitive receptors, causing an inappropriately prolonged phase of hyperventilation even after the stimulus is stopped. An additional potential mechanism is that the low CO_2 level maintained by chronic hyperventilation further sensitizes these CO_2 receptors according to a deafferentation hypersensitivity model. Blunting the exaggerated ventilatory response, either by antipanic drugs, which may reregulate the CO_2 receptors, or behavioral intervention, which teaches the patient not to overbreathe, could have the effect of blocking the full-blown attack.

Looking for commonalities among various panicogenic maneuvers, Carr and Sheehan (1984) proposed a "neuroendocrine or redox model" for panic anxiety. They speculate that panic is the result of a shift in the intraneural redox state determined by the ratio of reduced to oxidized NAD. This ratio is proportional to the ratio of pyruvate reduced to lactate according to the following equation.

$$[\text{lactate/pyruvate}] = {}^K\text{LDH} \times [\text{NADH/NAD}^+] \times [\text{H}^+]$$

^{K}LDH refers to a group of isoenzymes (lactate dehydrogenase) catalyzing this reaction.

Rise in the lactate/pyruvate ratio will lower intraneural pH in medullary chemoreceptors, increasing their firing rate. Since lactate, as opposed to CO_2, does not cross the blood–brain barrier, Carr and Sheehan hypothesize that the endothelium of certain areas of the medulla is fenestrated. These "leaky" areas would directly respond to elevation of the lactate/pyruvate ratio and the subsequent acidosis during lactate infusion. Carr and Sheehan suggest that the systemic alkalosis caused by acute hyperventilation would decrease cerebral blood flow, produce cerebral ischemia, and therefore also lower brain pH and raise lactate/pyruvate ratio. This model would explain the effect of the three most frequently used laboratory maneuvers of panic induction; however, no experimental test exists to substantiate its validity.

Cognitive Theories

Cognitive therapists suggest that the inhalation of CO_2 provokes a set of somatic sensations that by prior association is connected by the patient with the conditioned response of panic anxiety. The cognitive model would not fit if it is shown that some panic disorder patients actually have a physiologic hypersensitivity to CO_2.

CLINICAL CONSIDERATIONS

For the practicing clinician, these studies in respiratory physiology of anxiety have a number of implications. Most important, they give renewed scientific basis to the long held belief that hyperventilation is a major component of anxiety reactions. Although room air hyperventilation is not a robust method for inducing panic, the data indicate that a small subgroup of patients will have acute anxiety attacks if asked to hyperventilate.

Patients who appear to overbreathe or who experience typical anxiety symptoms during a hyperventilation provocation can then be instructed in breathing retraining techniques (Lum, 1981, 1983). Some authorities advise the patient to use relaxation techniques before practicing breathing retraining. Patients may benefit from such treatment in less than 2 weeks. There are claims that breathing retraining is sufficient to block panic attacks (Clark et al., 1985; Bonn et al., 1984). This remains open to study; at present, it appears that breathing retraining is useful in reducing a number of distressing symptoms that occur during anxiety attacks but does not actually block the attack. The use of antipanic medications, such as imipramine, phenelzine, and alprazolam, is still recommended for treating panic disorder.

The question is often asked whether in fact the tactic of having the patient in the midst of an acute attack breathe into a paper bag is effective. It is possible, of course, that this is merely a form of "distraction therapy" that occupies the patient's attention while the panic attack runs its usual 10–30 min course. On the other hand, it may be that, once the attack has begun and the hypocapnic, alkalotic state is secondarily induced, rebreathing CO_2 is indeed ameliorative up to the point that $PaCO_2$ returns to normal range. Theoretically, continued rebreathing of CO_2 after normal $PaCO_2$ and pH have been restored would lead to more anxiety and even panic. This has never been studied empirically.

It now seems clear that, although there is great symptomatic overlap between what has been called "hyperventilation syndrome" and panic disorder, the two are not the same condition. There probably is a small group of anxious patients for whom simple hyperventilation is the pathogenesis of their symptoms. For patients with panic disorder, however, it is more likely that hyperventilation is an important concomitant of the acute panic attack that reflects, rather than represents, the underlying primary etiology. One important research strategy is to investigate whether panic attacks provoked by stimuli other than CO_2 or lactate infusion—such as yohimbine, isoproterenol, and phobic exposure—also produce changes in ventilation.

The possibility that ventilatory studies will shed light on the neural mechanisms underlying acute panic has attracted great attention. It is now possible that a laboratory diagnostic test for panic disorder employing both hyperventilation and CO_2 challenges will emerge from this work and that new adjunctive methods of treating anxiety disorder will be defined. The results further indicate that the inhalation of CO_2 should be considered among the most valuable and convenient anxiogenic challenge tests.

ACKNOWLEDGMENTS

This work was supported in part by Research Scientist Development Awards MH 00416 (J.M.G.) MH 903-1301A and MH 903-C003I from the National Institute of Mental Health. The authors thank Barbara Barnett for editorial assistance.

REFERENCES

Berger AJ, Mitchell RA, Severinghause JW (1977): Regulation of respiration. N Engl J Med 297:92–97.

Bonn JA, Redhead CPA, Timmons BH (1984): Enhanced behavioural response in agoraphobic patients pretreated with breathing retraining. Lancet ii:665–669.

Carr DB, Fishman SM, Systrom D, Beckett A, Sheehan DV, Rosenbaum JF (1987): Carbon dioxide in panic disorder and premenstrually normals. Paper presented at the 140th annual meeting of the American Psychiatric Association, Chicago.

Carr DB, Sheehan DV (1984): Panic anxiety: A new biological model. J Clin Psychiatry 45:323–330.

Charney DS, Redmond DE (1984): Neurobiologic mechanisms in human anxiety: Evidence supporting central noradrenegic hyperactivity. Neuropharmacology 22:1531–1536.

Clark DM, Salkovski PM, Chalkly AJ (1985): Respiratory control as a treatment for panic attacks. J Behav Ther Exp Psychiatry 16:23–30.

Cohen ME, White PD (1951): Life situations, emotions and neurocirculatory asthenia. Psychsom Med 13:335–357.

Compernolle T, Hoogduin K, Joele L (1979): Diagnosis and treatment of the hyperventilation syndrome. Psychosomatics 20:612–625.

Damas-Mora J, Davies L, Taylor W, Jenner FA (1980): Menstrual respiratory changes and symptoms. Br J Psychiatry 135:492–497.

Deal CE, Haxkin MA, Norcia MP, Mitra J, Cherniack N (1986): Influence of the ventral surface of the medulla on tracheal responses to CO_2. J Appl Physiol 61:1091–1097.

Drury AN (1919): The percentage of carbon dioxide in the alveolar air and the tolerance to accumulating carbon dioxide in cases of so-called "irritable heart" of soldiers. Heart 7:165–173.

Elam M, Yao T, Thoren P, Svensson TH (1981): Hypercapnia and hypoxia chemoreceptor-mediated control of locus ceruleus neurons and splanchnic sympathetic nerves. Brain Res 222:373–381.

Errington ML, Dashwood MR (1979): Projections to the ventral surface of the cat brainstem demonstrated by horseradish peroxidase. Neurosci Lett 12:153–158.

Fyer MR, Uy J, Martinez J, Goetz R, Klein DF, Liebowitz MR, Fyer AJ, Gorman JM (1987): Carbon dioxide challenge of patients with panic disorder. Am J Psychiatry 144:1080–1082.

Garssen B (1980): Role of stress in the development of the hyperventilation syndrome. Psychother Psychosom 33:214–225.

Goldstein IB (1964): Physiological responses in anxious women patients. Arch Gen Psychiatry 10:382–388.

Gorman JM, Askanazi J, Liebowitz MR, Fyer AJ, Stein J, Kinney J, Klein DF (1984): Response to hyperventilation in a group of patients with panic disorder. Am J Psychiatry 41:857–861.

Gorman JM, Cohen BS, Liebowitz MR, Fyer AJ, Ross D, Davies SO, Klein DF (1986a): Blood gas changes and hypophosphatemia in lactate-induced panic. Arch Gen Psychiatry 43:1067–1071.

Gorman JM, Fyer MR, Goetz R, Askanazi J, Liebowitz MR, Fyer AJ, Kinney J, Klein DF (1988): Ventilatory physiology of patients with panic disorder. Arch Gen Psychiatry 45:31–39.

Gorman JM, Fyer AJ, Ross DC, Cohen BS, Martinez J, Liebowitz MR, Klein DF (1985): Normalization of venous pH, pCO_2 and HCO_3 levels after blockade of panic attacks. Psychiatry Res 14:57–65.

Gorman JM, Liebowitz MR, Dillon D, Fyer AJ, Cohen BS, Klein DF (1987): Anti-panic drug effects during lactate infusion in lactate refractory panic patients. Psychiatry Res 21(3):205–212.

Gorman JM, Liebowitz MR, Fyer AJ, Fyer MR, Klein DF (1986b): Possible respiratory abnormalities in panic disorder. Psychopharmacol Bull 22:797–801.

Griez E, Lousberg H, van den Hout MA, van der Molen GM (1987): CO_2 vulnerability in panic disorder. Psychiatry Res 20:87–95.

Griez E, van den Hout MA (1985): Peripheral panic symptoms occur during changes in alveolar carbon dioxide. Comp Psychiatry 26:381–387.

Griez E, van den Hout MA (1987): Blood gases and panic. Paper presented at the 140th annual meeting of the American Psychiatric Association, Chicago.

Grossman P (1983): Respiration, stress and cardiovascular function. Psychophysiology 20:284–300.

Hange A, Thoresen M, Walloe L (1980): Changes in cerebral blood flow during hyperventilation and CO_2 rebreathing in humans by a bidirectional, pulsed ultrasound doppler blood velocity meter. Acta Physiol Scand 110:167–173.

Harrison W, Gorman J, Sandberg DP, Endicott J (1986): Provocation of panic attacks with CO_2 in premenstrual dysphoric disorder. ACNP poster, Washington DC.

Hill O (1979): The hyperventilation syndrome. Br J Psychiatry 135:367–368.

Javaheris S, Shore NJ, Rose B, Kazemi H (1982): Compensatory hypoventilation in metabolic alkalosis. Chest 81:296–301.

Kennealy JA, McLennan JE, London RG, McLaurin RL (1980): Hyperventilation-induced cerebral hypoxia. Am Rev Respir Dis 122:407–411.

Kerr WJ, Dalton JW, Gliebe PA (1937): Some physical phenomena associated with the anxiety states and their relation to hyperventilation. Ann Intern Med 11: 961–992.

Kinney JM, Morgan AP, Domingues FJ (1964): A method for continuous measurement of gas exchange and expired radioactivity in acutely ill patients. Metabolism 13:205–211.

Klein DF (1964): Delineation of two drug responsive anxiety syndromes. Psychopharmacologia 5:396–408.

Knochel JP (1977): Pathophysiology and clinical characteristics of severe hypophosphatemia. Arch Intern Med 137:203–209.

Liebowitz MR, Gorman JM, Fyer AJ, Levitt M, Dillon D,

Levy G, Appleby I, Anderson S, Palij M, Davies SO, Klein DF (1985): Lactate provocation of panic attacks. II. Biochemical and physiologic findings. Arch Gen Psychiatry 42:709–719.

Loevenhart AS, Lorenz WF, Waters R: (1929): Cerebral stimulations. J Am Med Assoc 11:880–883.

Lum LC (1976): The syndrome of habitual chronic hyperventilation. In Hill OW (ed): "Modern Trends In Psychosomatic Medicine, Vol 3." London; Butterworths.

Lum LC (1981): Hyperventilation and anxiety states. J R Soc Med 74:1–4.

Lum LC (1983): Physiological considerations in the treatment of hyperventilation syndromes. J Drug Res 8:1867–1872.

Meduna LJ (1950): "Carbon Dioxide Therapy: A Neurophysiological Treatment of Nervous Disorders." Springfield, IL: Charles C. Thomas.

Milic-Emili J, Grunstein MM (1976): Drive and timing components of ventilation. Chest 70 [Suppl 1]:131–133.

Missri JC, Alexander S (1978): Hyperventilation syndrome. J Am Med Assoc 240:2093–2096.

Okel BB, Hurst JW (1961): Prolonged hyperventilation in man: Associated electrolyte changes and subjective symptoms. Arch Intern Med 108:757–762.

Papp LA, Liebowitz MR, Klein DF, Fyer AJ, Cohen B, Gorman JM (1988): Epinephrine infusion in patients with social phobia. Am J Psychiatry 145:733–736.

Papp LA, Martinez JM, Klein DF, Liebowitz MR, Fyer AJ, Hollander E, Gorman JM (1989): Arterial blood gas changes during lactate-induced panic. Psychiatry Res 28:171–180.

Plum F, Posner JB, Smith WW (1968): Effect of hyperbaric-hypoxic hyperventilation on blood, brain and CSF lactate. Am J Physiol 215:1240–1244.

Prous GYJ, Carlsson A, Gomez MMA (1977): The effect of CO_2 on monoamine metabolism in rat brain. Naunyn-Schmiedebergs Arch Pharmacol 301:11–15.

Rapee R (1986): Differential response to hyperventilation in panic disorder and generalized anxiety disorder. J Abnormal Psych 95:24–28.

Rapee R, Mattick R, Murrell E (1986): Cognitive mediation in the affective component of spontaneous panic attack. J Behav Ther Exp Psychiatry 17:245–253.

Rapoport SI (1976): "Blood–Brain Barrier in Physiology and Medicine." New York: Raven Press.

Read DJC (1967): A clinical method for assessing the ventilatory response to CO_2. Aust Ann Med 16:20–32.

Rice RL (1950): Symptom patterns of hyperventilation syndrome. Am J Med 8:691–700.

Salzman HA, Heyman A, Sicker HJ (1963): Correlation of clinical and physiological manifestations of sustained hyperventilation. N Engl J Med 268:1431–1436.

Singh BS (1984): Ventilatory response to CO_2: II. Studies in neurotic psychiatric patients and practitioners of transcendental meditation. Psychosom Med 46:347–362.

Stanburg SW, Thomson AE (1952): The renal response to respiratory alkalosis. Clin Sci 11:357–374.

Suess WM, Alexander AB, Smith DD, Sweeney HW, Marion RJ (1980): The effects of psychological stress on respiration: A preliminary study of anxiety and hyperventilation. Psychophysiology 17:535–540.

Wolpe J (1973): "The Practice of Behavior Therapy, 2nd ed. "New York: Pergamon Press.

Woods SW, Charney DS, Heninger GR (1985): Comparison of drug induced and phobic exposure-induced anxiety states. Paper presented at Annual Meeting of the American Congress of Neuropsychopharmaology, December, Honolulu.

Woods SW, Charney DS, Lake J, Goodman WK, Redmond DE, Heninger DR (1986): Carbon dioxide sensitivity in panic anxiety: Ventilatory and anxiogenic response to carbon dioxide in healthy subjects and panic anxiety patients before and after alprazolam treatment. Arch Gen Psychiatry 43:900–909.

van den Hout MA, Griez E (1984): Panic symptoms after inhalation of CO_2. Br J Psychiatry 144:503–507.

13

Biologic Responses to Panic Anxiety Elicited by Nonpharmacologic Means

SCOTT W. WOODS, MD, AND DENNIS S. CHARNEY, MD

Clinical Neuroscience Research Unit, Connecticut Mental Health Center, and Department of Psychiatry, Yale University School of Medicine, New Haven, Connecticut 06508

INTRODUCTION

Although an increasing number of studies have examined biologic responses to panic anxiety induced by pharmacologic challenges, relatively few attempts have been made to make biological measurement during non-pharmacologically induced panic attacks. The studies that have been performed fall into three general groups: those that experimentally induce situational panic attacks by exposing patients to phobic situations, those that utilize ambulatory monitoring techniques to record naturally occurring situational and spontaneous attacks, and those that wait in the laboratory for spontaneous attacks to occur or observe them serendipitously.

The aim of this chapter is to review the biologic findings from studies of panic attacks in panic disorder patients in which the panic was not elicited by a pharmacologic challenge. This chapter also reviews biologic findings from phobic exposure studies of simple phobia and social phobia patients, although the degree of similarity between panic attacks in panic disorder patients and the severe anxiety experienced by these patients has not been established. These findings are here integrated with those from studies of pharmacologically induced panic attacks and of experimentally induced or naturally occurring stress in laboratory animals and humans in an attempt to increase understanding of the pathophysiology of the panic state. Finally, directions for further research in this area are proposed.

Neurobiology of Panic Disorder, Pages 205–217
© 1990 Alan R. Liss, Inc.

RESEARCH FINDINGS

Studies meeting review criteria are described in detail below. Their findings are also summarized in Tables 13–1 and 13–2.

Panic Disorder and Agoraphobia

PHOBIC EXPOSURE STUDIES

Only two phobic exposure studies in panic disorder/agoraphobia patients have been published. Ko et al. (1983) measured plasma free 3-methoxy-4-hydroxyphenylglycol (MHPG), an index of peripheral and central norepinephrine turnover (Crawley et al., 1978; Kopin et al., 1984) 30 min after six patients placed themselves in typical phobic situations. All six patients apparently had panic attacks induced by this procedure. These single panic-day determinations were compared to single determinations made in the same patients on two separate days when they did not have panic attacks. All six patients underwent repeat exposure after 3 weeks' treatment with clonidine and also after 3 weeks' treatment with imipramine. The phobic stimuli during repeat exposure were of greater intensity than the patients had tolerated initially during placebo treatment. Ko et al. reported that plasma free MHPG concentrations on panic days were a mean 56% higher than on nonpanic days during placebo treatment. MHPG was also significantly higher on exposure days than on nonexposure days during imipramine treatment but not during clonidine treatment.

Woods et al. (1987) reported biological findings in 18 panic disorder patients and 13 normal controls undergoing structured exposure to agoraphobic situations. The research psychiatrist conducting the phobic exposure test determined that 15 patients and no healthy subjects had a panic attack during the test. Table 13–1 shows that this study reported the largest number of nonpharmacologically induced attacks of any to date, with the exception of one ambulatory monitoring study that recorded only heart rate. Each patient was accompanied to and from the exposure site by the research psychiatrist. Most patients were also accompanied during exposure; however, if the patient believed that the physician's presence during exposure would prevent an attack from occurring, the patient then entered the phobic situation alone. When accompanying the patients during exposure, the psychiatrist kept a careful log documenting the time of onset and end of panic attacks, the severity of panic rated subjectively by the patients on a scale from 1 to 10, and what physical activity the patients were performing. During exposure periods in which the patient was not accompanied, the patient was asked to note the exact times at which a panic attack began and ended. The patient was then interviewed in detail immediately after exposure. Each control subject was matched to a panicking patient for age within 2 years; sex; and exact procedure before, during, and after the exposure period. Eleven patients who had panic attacks and nine healthy subjects wore ambulatory electrocardiogram (EKG) (Holter monitor) recorders throughout the test day. The recordings were reviewed by a cardiologist who was blind to subject diagnosis. All patients and healthy subjects wore ambulatory blood pressure recorders. Blood pressure was recorded automatically at 6 min intervals throughout the test session. Blood samples were obtained at 30 and 5 min before the phobic exposure; at midexposure; at the end of exposure; and 15, 30, 45, 60, 90, 120, and 150 min after the end of the exposure period.

The panic attacks averaged 6.3 on a 0 to 10 scale (moderately severe) and lasted a mean of 20.5 min. Heart rate responses during phobic exposure were significantly higher in patients having panic attacks than in the healthy subjects. The mean heart rate during panic attacks was 32% greater than during the baseline period. Only part of this increase can be attributed to the attack itself, however, because heart rate increased 17% during exposure in the healthy subjects. Blood pressure responses during phobic exposure were modest and were similar in patients and healthy subjects. The plasma MHPG findings of Ko et al. (1983) were not replicated. Plasma MHPG increased by a peak of only 13% in the panicking patients. Moreover, the healthy subjects showed a similar maximal plasma free MHPG increase of 17%. Cortisol increased significantly in the panicking patients at midexposure by 38% over baseline. However, because of a 22% increase in the healthy subjects, the patient-healthy subject comparison was not statistically significant. The exposure period had significant effects on plasma human growth hormone that tended to be smaller in patients experiencing situational panic attacks than in healthy subjects and a slightly greater effect on plasma prolactin level in healthy subjects than in panicking patients.

Methodologic differences exist between these two studies, but it is difficult to account for the conflicting MHPG results on the basis of methodology. Woods et al. (1987) compared MHPG to a same-day baseline when the patients were experiencing anticipatory anxiety, whereas Ko et al. (1983) used a nonexposure day baseline when the patients were presumably not unusually anxious, raising the question of whether patients in the more recent study might have been so anxious at baseline that MHPG levels could not rise further as a result of a panic attack. The similar baseline MHPG values in the two studies, however, suggest that this methodologic difference does not explain the disparate results. It is possible that the patients in the Ko et al. study experienced attacks that were more severe or more prolonged than those in the second study. The behavioral measures in the two studies were sufficiently different that they cannot be compared directly; however, the attacks elicited by Woods et al. were similar in severity to typical situational panic attacks. The weight of the evidence would tend to point away from major effects of situational panic attacks on plasma MHPG, because of the larger number of subjects, the use of controls, and the use of a same-day baseline design in the more recent study.

One additional study, a pilot study, of biologic responses to phobic exposure in panic patients has recently been reported. Sellew et al. (1987a,b) exposed four patients to phobic situations in imagination; two of these patients experienced panic attacks. Two additional patients reported apparent spontaneous panic attacks during recovery from an exercise test. Samples for plasma norepinephrine and epinephrine were obtained in the seated position immediately upon report of a panic attack and at rapid intervals thereafter. The peak of these levels was compared to a supine baseline measurement. Sellew et al. report that peak norepinephrine and epinephrine increases over baseline were 254% and 77%, respectively, during these four panic attacks.

AMBULATORY MONITORING

Four published studies have reported on physiologic changes during panic attacks in panic disorder patients as determined by ambulatory monitoring. Freedman et al. (1985) studied 12 panic disorder patients and 11 healthy subjects who underwent 12 hr of monitoring on each of two consecutive days. Heart rate and finger temperature were recorded continuously. Data were presented by a visual comparison of values for each minute during a period from 5 min before to 5 min after patients pressed an event marker indicating the onset of a panic attack. Eight attacks occurred in five patients. In all cases the heart rate increases during the panic attack exceeded those during a control period when the patient was quite anxious but no panic attack occurred. From the range of heart rate increases and the baselines reported, it is possible to calculate that heart rate increased by a maximum of approximately 35% during these attacks. The authors report that patients attributed five of the eight attacks to emotional upset but do not classify the attacks as either spontaneous or situational. Finger temperature also increased during panic attacks.

Taylor et al. (1983, 1986) reported two studies in which heart rate was recorded by ambulatory monitor in panic patients. In the first study, eight panic attacks were recorded in seven of ten patients who underwent monitoring for 24 hr. Peak heart rates (a mean of 110 beats per minute during attacks) but not baselines were reported. Peak heart rates in the first study were very similar to those in the second study, in which 17 spontaneous and eight sit-

uational attacks were recorded in 12 panic patients who underwent monitoring for 120–144 hr. The mean maximum heart rate was 37% greater than a baseline measurement taken 10 min before the onset of the attacks. Heart rate increases were similar in spontaneous and situational attacks.

Shear et al. (1987) found similar but smaller heart rate increases (peak heart rate 19% higher than the peak of the 15 min interval preceding the attack) in five of 23 panic patients who experienced a panic attack during 21–27 hr of recording.

LABORATORY OBSERVATION OF SPONTANEOUS PANIC

Spontaneous panic attacks have been observed serendipitously during laboratory experiments equipped to make biological measurements as described in three reports. Lader and Mathews (1970) reported on three spontaneous attacks occurring during psychophysiological monitoring in the laboratory. The panic attacks were accompanied by heart rate increases of roughly 52%, 59%, and 67%. Skin conductance also increased during attacks. Electromyographic (EMG) changes were inconsistent. Cohen et al. (1985) reported two patients who experienced panic attacks during muscle relaxation exercises. Because the patients were not described as having previously been fearful of relaxation, these attacks do not appear to have been precipitated by phobic exposure. Whether they are best classified as spontaneous or as induced by relaxation is unclear. Heart rate increased by approximately 42% and 68%. Frontalis EMG tracings and hand-surface temperature also increased during the attacks. Sellew et al. (1987a,b) observed panic attacks in two patients recovering from an exercise tolerance test. Again, the attacks are probably best not considered situational attacks, in that the patients had not been previously phobic of exercise. Increases in plasma norepinephrine and epinephrine were observed.

Cameron and colleagues (1987) demonstrated that it is feasible to study spontaneous attacks prospectively if patients with a relatively high spontaneous panic rate are selected. These investigators recorded heart rate, blood pressure, oral temperature, and plasma

MHPG, norepinephrine, epinephrine, cortisol, growth hormone, and prolactin before, at the peak of, immediately following, and at multiple time points after nine spontaneous panic attacks occurring during 36 hr of bedrest in four of eight patients whose baseline panic frequency was at least one episode daily. The changes observed were relatively modest and inconsistent. Peak mean effects of the nine attacks are shown in Table 13–1. None of these changes were statistically significant in comparison to preattack baselines. The apparently robust growth hormone effects were not significant, probably because increases occurred during only two attacks.

Social Phobia

No biological studies of anxiety in social phobia patients have yet been published to our knowledge. Levin, Liebowitz, and colleagues (Levin et al., 1986; Levin and Liebowitz, 1987) studied 23 social phobia patients and 14 healthy subjects in a phobic exposure paradigm involving 10 min videotaped simulated public speaking sessions. Heart rate was measured throughout using a continuous EKG R-wave detector. Plasma norepinephrine, epinephrine, and cortisol were measured at baseline and at several time points during and after exposure. Although patients experienced significantly greater increases in anxiety during exposure, when the full sample of control subjects was studied, it was apparent that responses on biological measures were similar in the two groups. Heart rate increased by approximately 12 beats per minute, and plasma norepinephrine and epinephrine increased roughly 30% and 70%, respectively, both in patients and in healthy subjects. No ambulatory monitoring studies of social phobia patients have been conducted.

Simple Phobia

A number of phobic exposure studies have been performed in simple phobia patients. Edmondson et al. (1972) measured heart rate and plasma catecholamines in 11 dental phobia patients and 11 nonphobic dental patients before, during, and after dental surgery. The dental phobia subjects but not controls received intravenous diazepam 0.2 mg/kg before their procedures. Heart rate and epinephrine levels were higher in the phobic patients at baseline and throughout the experimental session. Changes from baseline during dental surgery appear to have been approximately equal in the two groups. Norepinephrine levels were described as similar in the two groups. The interpretation of the results of the phobic exposure is impaired by the use of diazepam in the phobic patients and a difficulty with the baseline measurements. Since no behavioral ratings were obtained, it is not clear whether the phobic patients were anxious at the time of the baseline measurements and consequently whether the increases during dental surgery represent changes from a true baseline.

Curtis, Nesse, and colleagues in a series of papers reported on the plasma catecholamine, neuroendocrine, and cardiovascular responses to phobic exposure of patients with animal phobias. Measurements obtained during exposure to the feared animal were compared to measurements obtained in the same laboratory when patients were not thus exposed. No subjects without phobias were studied. These studies found modest increases in heart rate and systolic and diastolic blood pressure (Nesse et al., 1985); increases in plasma norepinephrine and epinephrine of 46% and 87%, respectively (Nesse et al., 1985); modest (Nesse et al., 1985) or no (Curtis et al., 1976, 1978) increases in plasma cortisol; increases of plasma growth hormone of 72–157% (Curtis et al., 1979; Nesse et al., 1985); modest increases in insulin levels (Nesse et al., 1985); and no increase in prolactin (Nesse et al., 1980), thyrotropin (Nesse et al., 1982), or glucagon or pancreatic polypeptide levels (Nesse et al., 1985).

The same group is currently conducting a study of the effects of phobic exposure on regional cerebral blood flow (CBF) in simple phobia patients (Curtis et al., 1987). Regional CBF is being determined by positron emission tomography (PET) using the $H_2^{15}O$ technique during phobic exposure and compared to scans obtained during nonexposure times on the same day in the same patients. Additional studies of this type would be very useful.

Comparisons Across Studies

Examination of Table 13–1 shows that relatively little is known about the biological events underlying panic attacks not produced by pharmacologic challenges. The total number of attacks described in these studies is fairly small, and the only variables measured in more than two studies of panic patients are heart rate and plasma MHPG.

Additional information is gained by including studies of social phobia and (see Table 13–2) simple phobia patients, but these comparisons must be made with caution because the degree of similarity between the anxiety experienced by these patients and panic attacks in panic patients is not well established. Aimes et al. (1983) showed that the proportion of social phobic and agoraphobic patients experiencing specific somatic symptoms was similar for 17 of 23 symptoms. The social phobics experienced more blushing and the agoraphobics more limb weakness, dyspnea, dizziness, fainting, and tinnitus. Munjack et al. (1987) reported that social phobia patients scored lower on the somatization and higher on the interpersonal sensitivity subscales of the SCL 90-R than did patients with panic disorder.

Only a few studies have included normal control subjects who were placed in situations identical to those in which the patients experienced panic attacks or severe anxiety. These studies have shown that increases in a number of variables of interest can occur in healthy subjects in these experimental situations in the absence of reported anxiety (Levin et al., 1986; Levin and Liebowitz, 1987; Woods et al., 1987) and raise questions about the accuracy of concluding, if no such control group is studied, that a biological finding observed during anxiety-provoking situations in anxious patients is due to the anxiety. Studies of spontaneous attacks in patients at bedrest may not require this sort of control group.

PANIC DISORDER STUDIES

With these caveats in mind, what do the data suggest about the biological accompaniments of nondrug-induced panic? The strongest findings suggest that such panic attacks appear in general to be characterized by increases in heart rate. Changes in other biological measures to date have been relatively modest or nonexistent (see Table 13–1).

Heart rate changes during nondrug-induced panic attacks average roughly a 30–60% maximal increase above baseline. The precise fraction of this increase that is due to the attack or that is due to physical activity during but incidental to the attack is difficult to establish from the ambulatory monitoring studies. The studies of spontaneous attacks that occurred when patients were at rest do suggest that some part of the observed heart rate increases are due to the attacks. These heart rate increases, however, can be quite variable. For example, Cameron et al. (1987) observed a heart rate increase in only one of their four patients during attacks. Since the eight attacks occurring in their remaining three patients did not affect heart rate, the mean increase across attacks was quite small in this study. This variability in the heart rate response to panic attacks suggests some heterogencity in the pathophysiology of panic disorder. The anxiety experienced by simple phobic patients may not affect heart rate as strongly as do panic attacks in panic patients.

The weight of the data does not support a large increase in plasma MHPG during situational or spontaneous panic attacks. Preliminary work with plasma catecholamines in one study (Sellew et al., 1987a,b) but not in another (Cameron et al., 1987) suggests that these hormones may increase during nondrug-induced attacks. Blood pressure may be only modestly affected or not affected during most panic attacks.

The neuroendocrine effects of panic attacks appear fairly modest. Cortisol increased slightly in two studies, but the increase was not statistically significant in comparison to controls (Woods et al., 1987) or to the patients' own baselines (Cameron et al., 1987) with the relatively small sample sizes studied. Growth hormone increases in the same studies, though larger in mean magnitude than the cortisol increases, were more variable and thus also are not statistically significant. Prolactin increases also were not significant in either study.

COMPARISON WITH SOCIAL AND SIMPLE PHOBIA STUDIES

The anxiety experienced by social phobia patients (Levin et al., 1986; Levin and Liebowitz, 1987) and by simple phobia patients (see Table 13–2) seems to affect heart rate less than do panic attacks in panic disorder patients. There is too little information to permit a comparison

TABLE 13–1.
Biological Findings From Studies in Panic Disorder Patients of Panic Attacks not Induced by Pharmacologic Challenge†

Study	N	Method	HR	SBP	DBP	MHPG	NE	E	CORT	GH	PRL	Comments
Lader and Mathews, 1970	3	S	59									1,2a
Ko et al., 1983	6	PE				56						2b,3
Taylor et al., 1983	8	AM	T									—
Cohen et al., 1985	2	S	55									1,2a
Freedman et al., 1985	8	AM	35									2a,3
Taylor et al., 1986	25	AM	37									2a,3
Shear et al., 1987	5	AM	19									2a,3
Woods et al., 1987	15	PE	32*	14	6	13			38	260	0	2c
Sellew et al., 1987a,b	4	PE/S					254	77				2a,3
Cameron et al., 1987	9	S	4	1	0	−5	11	0	37	415	37	2d

†Abbreviations: N, number of panic attacks measured in panic patients; HR, heart rate; SBP, systolic blood pressure; DBP, diastolic blood pressure; MHPG, plasma 3-methoxy-4-hydroxyphenylglycol; NE, plasma norepinephrine; E, plasma epinephrine; CORT, plasma cortisol; GH, plasma human growth hormone; PRL, serum prolactin; S, probable spontaneous attacks occurring in the laboratory; PE, phobic exposure; AM, ambulatory monitoring.

Numbers under findings indicate mean maximal percent increase above baseline. Comments: 1, Statistical analysis was not performed. 2, "Mean maximal percent increases" are not necessarily comparable across studies because of differing methods of presentation of the data and varying numbers of time points at which to identify the peaks; the specific methods used to calculate the mean maximal percent increases were: a, mean of individual peak increases; b, only one measurement made; compared to nonexposure days; c, group mean of average values obtained during individual panic attacks for HR, SBP, and DBP; largest mean increase of time points reported for other variables; d, largest mean increase of time points reported. 3, Study used no nonanxious control group exposed to the same situations as the anxious patients.

*The finding was significantly greater than any changes occurring in controls or significantly higher than baseline in studies of spontaneous attacks occurring in patients during bedrest when no controls appear to be necessary.

of noradrenergic function in these patients with that during panic attacks. The substantial increases in norepinephrine and epinephrine seen during phobic exposure in simple phobics (Nesse et al., 1985) must be viewed with caution because of the lack of a control group. Similar changes in these hormones were observed by Levin and Liebowitz (1987) in both their social phobic and healthy subject groups during simulated public speaking. The neuroendocrine effects of phobic exposure in simple phobics appear relatively modest.

COMPARISON WITH PHARMACOLOGICALLY INDUCED PANIC

The conclusions reached earlier about the cardiovascular, noradrenergic, and neuroendo-crine effects of nonpharmacologically elicited panic attacks in general correspond to those from recent reviews of studies of panic attacks induced by pharmacologic challenges (for review, see Woods and Charney, 1988). Heart rate was increased to a greater degree in panickers than in nonpanickers in five of ten studies of drug-induced panic. The five studies showing greater increases in heart rate involved administration of sodium lactate (Lapierre et al., 1984; Liebowitz et al., 1985), carbon dioxide (Woods et al., 1988), yohimbine (Charney et al., 1987a), and caffeine (Charney et al., in press). Studies showing similar heart rate effects involved administration of sodium lactate (Freedman et al., 1984; Kelly et al., 1971), isoproterenol (Freedman et al., 1984), norepinephrine (Pyke and Greenberg, 1986),

TABLE 13–2.
Biological Findings From Studies of Induced Anxiety in Simple Phobia Patients*

Study	N	Method	HR	SBP	DBP	NE	E	CORT	GH	PRL	TSH	Com-ments
Edmondson et al., 1972	11	PE	10				10					1a,2
Curtis et al., 1976	7	PE						~0				1a,3
Curtis et al., 1978	6	PE						~0				1a,3
Curtis et al., 1979	11	PE							157			1a,3
Nesse et al., 1980	8	PE								0		1a,3
Nesse et al., 1982	9	PE									~0	1a,3
Nesse et al., 1985	10	PE	15	10	8	46	87	24	72			1b,3

*Abbreviations: N, number of simple phobia patients participating; TSH, thyroid stimulating hormone. Other abbreviations as for Table 13–1. Numbers under findings indicate mean maximal percent increase above baseline. Comments: 1, "Mean maximal percent increases" are not necessarily comparable across studies because of differing methods of presentation of the data and varying numbers of time points from which to identify the peaks; the specific method used to calculate the mean maximal percent increases were: a, largest mean increase of time points reported; b, group mean of average values obtained during individual anxiety episodes; 2, Value suspect because true baseline was uncertain (see text); 3, Study used no group of nonanxious controls exposed to the same situations as the anxious patients.

and the serotonin agonist m-chlorophenylpi-perazine (MCPP) (Charney et al., 1987b).

Systolic blood pressure increased to a greater degree in panickers in only one of seven studies of drug-induced panic. The greater increase was observed in a study of yohimbine-induced panic (Charney et al., 1987a), whereas the negative studies involved panic attacks induced by caffeine (Charney et al., in press), MCPP (Charney et al., 1987b), CO_2 (Gorman et al., 1988; Woods et al., 1988), sodium lactate (Liebowitz et al., 1985), and norepinephrine (Pyke and Greenberg, 1986). Diastolic blood pressure also increased to a greater degree in panickers in only one of the same seven studies, a study of sodium lactate (Liebowitz et al., 1985).

Plasma MHPG increased to a greater degree in panicking patients only in the study of yohimbine-induced panic attacks (Charney et al., 1987a) and not in studies of attacks induced by sodium lactate (Pohl et al., 1987), CO_2 (Woods et al., 1988), isoproterenol (Pohl et al., 1987), caffeine (Charney et al., in press), or MCPP (Charney et al., 1987b). Plasma norepinephrine rose significantly higher in panickers in one (Liebowitz et al., 1985) of two (Appleby et al., 1981) sodium lactate studies and tended to rise higher in a CO_2 study (Gorman et al., 1988), whereas plasma epinephrine increases were greater in the panickers in the Appleby et al. (1981) study but not in the Liebowitz et al. (1985) or Gorman et al. (1988) studies.

Plasma cortisol was more strongly affected in the panicking group in one (Liebowitz et al., 1985) of two lactate studies (Appleby et al., 1981) and in yohimbine (Charney et al., 1987a) and caffeine (Charney et al., in press) but not CO_2 (Gorman et al., 1988; Woods et al., 1988) or MCPP studies (Charney et al., 1987b). Prolactin changes were similar in panicking and nonpanicking groups in six studies of lactate-induced (Appleby et al., 1981; Liebowitz et al., 1985), yohimbine-induced (Charney et al., 1987a), MCPP-induced (Charney et al., 1987b), caffeine-induced (Charney et al., in press), and CO_2-induced (Woods et al., 1988) panic. Growth hormone changes were similar in panickers and nonpanickers in four drug-induced panic studies involving administration of yohimbine, MCPP, caffeine, and CO_2, respectively (Charney et al., 1987a,b, in press; Woods et al., 1988).

DISCUSSION

The major goal of the search for abnormal biological findings during panic attacks is to disclose abnormalities of neuronal function during panic attacks. The remainder of this review focuses on the neurobiologic implications of the findings described above and on directions for future research.

Panic Attacks and Noradrenergic Function

The generally negative plasma MHPG results from studies of situational, spontaneous, and drug-induced panic attacks could suggest that large increases in central and peripheral noradrenergic function do not generally accompany panic attacks. It is conceivable that dysfunction of endogenous benzodiazepine (Ferrero et al., 1984) or other neurotransmitter or neuromodulator systems is more critically involved than noradrenergic dysfunction. The neurobiologic mechanisms underlying panic attacks may differ from those underlying other types of acute anxiety for which there is abundant evidence that noradrenergic hyperactivity plays a role, such as anxiety in research volunteers (Uhde et al., 1982; Ward et al., 1983), public speaking anxiety (Bolm-Audorff et al., 1986; Dimsdale and Moss, 1980), opiate withdrawal (Charney et al., 1984), and stressful circumstances such as aircraft carrier landings (Rubin et al., 1970) and parachute jumping (Bloom et al., 1963; Hansen et al., 1978). Evidence suggests that it is unlikely that acute effects of panic attacks on plasma MHPG would diminish as attacks recur because under normal conditions noradrenergic systems appear to adapt to chronic stress by mechanisms other than a decrease in norepinephrine turnover (Dunn and Kramarcy, 1984; Mason, 1968), such as increased norepinephrine synthesis (Dunn and Kramarcy, 1984; Kvetansky and Mikulaj, 1970; Weiss et al., 1975) and postsynaptic receptor down-regulation (Dunn and Kramarcy, 1984; Stone, 1983).

The MHPG results, however, do not prove an absence of association between central noradrenergic function and panic attacks. A compelling clinical and preclinical literature suggests that this association may exist (Dunn and Kramarcy, 1984; Glavin, 1985; Mason, 1968; Redmond, 1979). More recently, work involving the effects of stress on single neuron firing in the noradrenergic nucleus locus ceruleus in freely moving animals has corroborated an association between brain noradrenergic function and stress and fear. A variety of anxious or physiologically stressful situations reliably increase locus ceruleus single unit activity in freely moving animals (Jacobs, 1986). Psychologically stressful or fear-inducing situations also increase locus ceruleus firing. In the freely moving cat, exposure to a dog or loud noise increases locus ceruleus cell firing by 100–200% (Abercrombie et al., 1986; Jacobs et al., in press). Firing of cells in the serotonergic dorsal raphe nucleus is unaffected by these situations (Jacobs et al., in press; Wilkinson et al., 1986). Arousing but nonstressful stimuli, such as presentation of nonavailable food or a rat, do not increase locus ceruleus cell firing (Abercrombie et al., 1986; Jacobs et al., in press).

An increase in central noradrenergic function could occur during typical panic attacks in the absence of MHPG changes if the increase were either too brief or too restricted in regional localization to affect MHPG in plasma. These possibilities receive some support from rat studies indicating that stress can increase norepinephrine turnover differentially in different brain regions. After 15–30 min of restraint stress, brain tissue MHPG was elevated only in the hypothalamus, and not until after 60 min did increases in other regions such as the amygdala and cerebral cortex occur (Nakagawa et al., 1981; Tanaka et al., 1982). Most panic attacks may be too brief for MHPG to accumulate in a sufficient mass of neuronal tissue to permit plasma MHPG levels to rise. The increases in plasma MHPG produced in patients experiencing oral yohimbine-induced panic attacks were first observed 2 hr after yohimbine administration (Charney et al., 1987a). Phobic stimuli, spontaneous attacks, or panicogenic drugs other than yohimbine might activate only a limited subset of noradrenergic neurons insufficient to raise MHPG in plasma, whereas yohimbine might activate a larger proportion of noradrenergic neurons.

Measurement of plasma catecholamines in a larger number of nondrug-induced panic attacks may help to clarify these issues. Catecholamine levels increase more quickly in plasma than do MHPG levels (Kopin, 1984). Plasma catecholamines may provide an index of central noradrenergic function, despite the inability of these molecules to cross the blood–brain barrier (Minneman, 1983), since central and peripheral noradrenergic function may change in parallel under many circumstances (Crawley et al., 1980; Maas, 1984; Peyrin et al., 1985).

Research results reviewed above support the possibility that plasma norepinephrine increases during some situational (Sellew et al., 1987a,b), spontaneous (Cameron et al., 1987; Sellew et al., 1987a,b), and drug-induced panic attacks (Gorman et al., 1988; Liebowitz et al., 1985) and support the view of panic attack as a state mediated at least in part by noradrenergic hyperactivity. Care must be taken, however, in attributing such elevations to the panic attack, at least in comparisons of panicking patients with nonpanicking healthy subjects. Sothmann et al. (1987) recently observed greater norepinephrine responses to psychologic stressors in a low cardiovascular fitness group of healthy subjects than in a high fitness group. The reported exercise intolerance of panic patients is well known (Cohen and White, 1950).

Neuroendocrine Effects of Panic Attacks

Panic attacks appear to have no major effect on the hormones measured in studies to date. Modest cortisol increases may result from some situational (Woods et al., 1987), spontaneous (Cameron et al., 1987), or drug-induced (Charney et al., 1987a,b; Liebowitz et al., 1985) attacks. The results suggesst that the large cortisol increase previously reported in a single case during an apparent spontaneous panic attack (Bliss et al., 1956) may not be a consistent feature of all or even most panic attacks. Growth hormone and prolactin appear to be unaffected by panic attacks.

The generally negative neuroendocrine effects of panic attacks are somewhat surprising in view of the large bodies of clinical and preclinical evidence that indicate that hypothalamic-pituitary-adrenal cortical function (Brown and Heninger, 1976; Dunn and Kramarcy, 1984; Greene et al., 1970; Levine, 1978; Mason, 1968; Mills, 1985; Miyabo et al., 1979; Newsome and Rose, 1971; Rose, 1984; Yokota et al., 1977), growth hormone levels (Brown and Heninger, 1975, 1976; Brown et al., 1978; Greene et al., 1970; Johnston et al., 1985; Kosten et al., 1984; Mills, 1985; Miyabo et al., 1977, 1979; Newsome and Rose, 1971; Noel et al., 1972; Pinter et al., 1979; Quabbe, 1985; Salter et al., 1972; Weitzman and Ursin, 1978),

and prolactin levels (Armario et al., 1986; Frantz et al., 1972; Miyabo et al., 1977; Noel et al., 1972; Pinter et al., 1979; Siegel et al., 1982; Wolinska-Witort et al., 1986; Yokota et al., 1977) are all increased by a variety of acute anxiety-producing or stressful situations and experimental manipulations. Although, there is a paucity of studies on the neuroendocrine effects of isolated episodes of acute fear in healthy subjects, panic attacks appear to have less marked endocrine effects than were observed in these few studies. For example, increases in mean plasma cortisol (150% to 15 μg/dl) were observed after the first jump in parachute trainees (Levine, 1978; Weitzman and Ursin, 1978), and increases in mean plasma growth hormone (to approximately 7.5 ng/ml) and prolactin levels (by about 53%) were observed in inexperienced passengers during aerobatic airplane flight (Pinter et al., 1979).

Studies of repeated exposure to stressors in laboratory animals and human studies of chronic stress suggest that chronic stress causes an adaptation of the neuroendocrine effects of acute stress. Preclinical studies generally show that the hormonal effects of acute stressors diminish and disappear with repeated applications of the same stressor (Brown et al., 1978; Johnston et al., 1985; Mason et al., 1968; Pollard et al., 1976; Sakellaris and Vernikos-Danellis, 1975; Weiss et al., 1975; Wolinska-Witort et al., 1986). In addition, individuals employed in chronically stressful occupations, such as wartime medical evacuation helicopter flying or firefighting, typically show no elevations of urinary cortisol (Bourne et al., 1967; Dutton et al., 1978) or plasma cortisol (Cullen et al., 1979), growth hormone (Pinter et al., 1979), or prolactin (Cullen et al., 1979; Pinter et al., 1979) as a result of work stress.

Considered together, studies of acute and chronic stress and the panic attack studies reviewed earlier suggest the hypothesis that stress-responsive neuroendocrine mechanisms may be activated acutely by panic attacks but then undergo adaptation as a result of repetition of the attacks (Woods et al., 1987). Consistent with this hypothesis are studies showing decreased cortisol responses to corticotropin-releasing hormone (Roy-Byrne et al., 1986a),

decreased growth hormone responses to clonidine (Charney and Heninger, 1986), and decreased prolactin responses to thyrotropin-re-
leasing hormone (Roy-Byrne et al., 1986b) in
panic disorder patients. The relatively modest
neuroendocrine effects of phobic exposure in
simple phobia patients may also be consistent
with this hypothesis if the patients studied
were confronted by their phobic stimuli relatively frequently in their lives. This hypothesis
could be tested in emergency wards by studying patients experiencing their first attacks.

Implications

The relatively unimpressive evidence supporting the existence of abnormal neurobiologic function during panic attacks in studies
to date should engender a search for methodologies capable of providing more sensitive assessment of neuronal function during panic attacks. Unless one rejects philosophical notions
of materialism, the abnormal cognitions and
somatic experiences well documented during
panic attacks must be mediated by abnormal
neuronal function. New methods should be developed that are able to assess serotonergic,
endogenous opioid, benzodiazepine–gamma
aminobutyric acid, and respiratory system
neuronal function during panic attacks, and
noradrenergic function should be assessed
more sensitively during panic attacks. Variables other than heart rate should be measured
in future ambulatory monitoring studies. Brain
imaging methods currently being developed
offer the hope of an eventual ability to conduct
studies indicating the anatomical localization
of abnormal neuronal function during panic attacks. Already such methods have been applied to the anxiety experienced by simple
phobia patients (Curtis et al., 1987) and, very
recently, to panic attacks induced by sodium
lactate (Reiman et al., 1988; Stewart et al.,
1988) and yohimbine (Koster et al., 1988;
Woods et al., 1988). It may soon be possible to
adapt these methods to the study of nonpharmacologically induced panic attacks in panic
disorder patients.

REFERENCES

Abercrombie ED, Wilkinson LO, Jacobs BL (1986): Environmental stress and activity of dorsal raphe serotonergic neurons in the freely moving cat. Soc Neurosci Abstr 12:1134.

Aimes PL, Gelder MG, Shaw PM (1983): A comparative
clinical study. Br J Psychiatry 142:174–179.

Appleby I, Klein DF, Sachar E, Levitt M (1981): Biochemical indices of lactate-induced panic: A preliminary report. In Klein DF, Rabkin J (eds): "Anxiety:
New Research and Changing Concepts." New York:
Raven Press.

Armario A, Lopez-Calderon A, Jolin T, Castellanos JM
(1986): Sensitivity of anterior pituitary hormones to
graded levels of psychological stress. Life Sci 39:471–
475.

Bliss EL, Migeon CJ, Branch CH, Samuels LT (1956):
Reaction of the adrenal cortex to emotional stress.
Psychosom Med 18:56–76.

Bloom G, VonEhler NS, Frankenhaeuser M (1963): Catecholamine excretion and personality traits in para-
troop trainees. Acta Physiol Scand 58:77–89.

Bolm-Audorff U, Schwammle J, Ehlenz K, Koop H, Kaf-
farnik H (1986): Hormonal and cardiovascular variations during a public lecture. Eur J Appl Physiol 54:
669–674.

Bourne PG, Rose RM, Mason JW (1967): Urinary 17-
OHCS levels: Data on seven helicopter ambulance
medics in combat. Arch Gen Psychiatry 17:104–110.

Brown GM, Seggie JA, Chambers JW, Ettigi PG (1978):
Psychoendocrinology and growth hormone: A review.
Psychoneuroendocrinology 3:131–153.

Brown WA, Heninger G (1975): Cortisol, growth hormone, free fatty acids and experimentally evoked affective arousal. Am J Psychiatry 132:1174–1176.

Brown WA, Heninger G (1976): Stress-induced growth
hormone release: Psychologic and physiologic correlates. Psychosom Med 38:145–147.

Cameron OG, Lee MA, Curtis GC, McCann DS (1987):
Endocrine and physiologic changes during "spontaneous" panic attacks. Psychoneuroendocrinology 12:
321–331.

Charney DS, Heninger GR (1986): Abnormal regulation
of noradrenergic function in panic disorders: Effects
of clonidine in healthy subjects and patients with agoraphobia and panic disorder. Arch Gen Psychiatry
43:1042–1058.

Charney DS, Redmond DE Jr, Galloway MP, Kleber HD,
Heninger GR, Murberg M, Roth RH (1984): Naltrexone
precipitated opiate withdrawal in methadone addicted human subjects: Evidence for noradrenergic
hyperactivity. Life Sci 35:1263–1272.

Charney DS, Woods SW, Goodman WK, Heninger GR
(1987a): Neurobiological mechanism of panic anxiety:
Biochemical and behavioral correlates of yohimbine-
induced panic attacks. Am J Psychiatry 144:1030–
1036.

Charney DS, Woods SW, Goodman WK, Heninger GR
(1987b): Serotonin function in anxiety: II. Effects of
the serotonin agonist, MCPP, in panic disorder patients and healthy subject. Psychopharmacology 92:
14–24.

Charney DS, Woods SW, Heninger GR (in press): Neurobiologic mechanisms of panic anxiety: A review of
the behavioral, biochemical, and cardiovascular effects of three different panicogenic stimuli. In Lerer B,
Gershon S (eds): "New Directions in Affective Disorders." New York, Alan R. Liss, Inc.

Cohen AS, Barlow DH, Blanchard EB (1985): Psychophysiology of relaxation-associated panic attacks. J Abnormal Psychol 94:96–101.

Cohen ME, White PD (1950): Life situations, emotions, and neurocirculatory aesthenia (anxiety neurosis, neuraesthenia, effort syndrome). Assoc Res Nervous Mental Dis Proc 29:832–869.

Crawley JN, Hattox SE, Maas JW, Roth RH (1978): 3-Methoxy-4-hydroxyphenethylene glycol increase in plasma after stimulation of the nucleus locus coeruleus. Brain Res 141:380–384.

Crawley JN, Maas JW, Roth RH (1980): Evidence against specificity of electrical stimulation of the nucleus locus coeruleus in activating the sympathetic nervous system in the rat. Brain Res 183:301–311.

Cullen J, Fuller R, Dolphin C (1979): Endocrine stress responses of drivers in "real life" heavy-goods vehicle driving task. Psychoneuroendocrinology 4:107–115.

Curtis GC, Buxton M, Lippman D, Nesse RM, Wright J (1976): 'Flooding in vivo' during the circadian phase of minimal cortisol secretion: Anxiety and therapeutic success without adrenal cortical activation. Biol Psychiatry 11:101–107.

Curtis GC, Mountz J, Modell J, Wilson M, Koeppe R (1987): Personal communication.

Curtis GC, Nesse RM, Buxton M, Lippman D (1978): Anxiety and plasma cortisol at the crest of the circadian cycle: Reappraisal of a classical hypothesis. Psychosom Med 40:368–378.

Curtis GC, Nesse R, Buxton M, Lippman D (1979): Plasma growth hormone: Effect of anxiety during flooding in vivo. Am J Psychiatry 136:410–414.

Dimsdale JE, Moss J (1980): Plasma catecholamines in stress and exercise. J Am Med Assoc 243:340–342.

Dunn AJ, Kramarcy NR (1984): Neurochemical responses to stress: Relationships between the hypothalamic-pituitary-adrenal and catecholamine systems. In Iversen L, Iversen S, Snyder S (eds): "Handbook of Psychopharmacology." New York: Plenum Publishing Corp, pp 455–515.

Dutton LM, Smolensky MH, Leach CS, Lorimor R, Hsi BP (1978): Stress levels of ambulance paramedics and fire fighters. J Occup Med 20:111–115.

Edmondson HD, Roscoe B, Vickers MD (1972): Biochemical evidence of anxiety in dental patients. Br Med J 4:7–9.

Ferrero P, Guidotti A, Conti-Tronconi B, Costa E (1984): A brain octadecaneuropeptide generated by tryptic digestion of DBI (diazepam binding inhibitor) functions as a proconflict ligand of benzodiazepine recognition sites. Neuropharmacology 23:1359–1362.

Frantz AG, Kleinberg DL, Noel GL (1972): Studies on prolactin in man. Rec Prog Horm Res 28:527–590.

Freedman RR, Ianni P, Ettedgui E, Pohl R, Rainey JM (1984): Psychophysiological factors in panic disorder. Psychopathology 17:66–73.

Freedman RR, Janis P, Ettedgui E, Puthezhath N (1985): Ambulatory monitoring of panic disorder. Arch Gen Psychiatry 42:244–248.

Glavin GB (1985): Stress and brain noradrenaline: A review. Neurosci Biobehav Rev 9:233–243.

Gorman JM, Fyer MR, Goetz R, Askanazi J, Liebowitz MR, Fyer AJ, Kinney J, Klein DF (1988): Ventilatory physiology of patients with panic disorder. Arch Gen Psychiatry 45:31–39.

Greene WA, Conron G, Schalch DS, Schreiner BF (1970): Psychologic correlates of growth hormone and adrenal secretory responses of patients undergoing cardiac catheterization. Psychosom Med 32:599–614.

Hansen JR, Stoa KF, Blix AS, Ursin H (1978): Urinary levels of epinephrine and norepinephrine in parachutist trainees. In Ursin H, Band E, Levine S (eds): "Psychobiology of Stress." Orlando: Academic Press Inc, pp 63–74.

Jacobs BL (1986): Single unit activity of locus coeruleus neurons in behaving animals. Prog Neurobiol 27:183–194.

Jacobs BL, Abercrombie ED, Morilak DA, Fornal CA (in press): Brain norepinephrine and stress: Single unit studies of locus coeruleus neurons in behaving animals. Paper presented at the Fourth Symposium on Catecholamines and Other Neurotransmitters in Stress, Smolenice Castle, Czechoslovakia, 1987.

Johnston DG, Davies RR, Prescott RWG (1985): Regulation of growth hormone secretion in man: A review. J R Soc Med 75:319–327.

Kelly D, Mitchell-Heggs N, Sherman D (1971): Anxiety and the effects of sodium lactate assessed clinically and physiologically. Br J Psychiatry 119:129–141.

Ko GN, Elsworth JD, Roth RH, Rifkin BG, Leigh H, Redmond DE Jr (1983): Panic-induced elevation of plasma MHPG levels in phobic-anxious patients. Arch Gen Psychiatry 40:425–430.

Kopin IJ (1984): Avenues of investigation for the role of catecholamines in anxiety. Psychopathology 17 [Suppl 1]:83–97.

Kopin IJ, Jimerson DC, Markey SP, Ebert MH, Polinsky RJ (1984): Disposition and metabolism of MHPG in humans: Application to studies in depression. Pharmacopsychiatry 17:3–8.

Kosten TR, Jacobs S, Mason J, Wahby V, Atkins S (1984): Psychological correlates of growth hormone response to stress. Psychosom Med 46:49–58.

Koster V, Woods SW, Smith EO, Zubal IG, Krystal JH, Charney DS, Hoffer PB (1988): Regional cerebral blood flow changes in patients with panic disorder. J Nuclear Med 29:1317.

Kvetnansky R, Mikulaj L (1970): Adrenal and urinary catecholamines in rats during adaptation to repeated immobilization stress. Endocrinology 87:738–743.

Lader M, Mathews A (1970): Physiologic changes during spontaneous panic attacks. J Psychiatry Res 17:261–266.

Lapierre YD, Knott VJ, Gray R (1984): Psychophysiological correlates of sodium lactate. Psychopharmacol Bull 20:50–57.

Levin A, Liebowitz MR (1987): Personal communication.

Levin A, Liebowitz MR, Gorman JM, Fyer AJ, Klein DF, Crawford R (1986): Pathophysiology of social phobia. In: "Proceedings of The Annual Meeting of the American Psychiatric Association." Washington, DC: APA, 158.

Levine S (1978): Cortisol changes following repeated experiences with parachute training. In Ursin H, Bande E, Levine S (eds): "Psychobiology of Stress." Orlando: Academic Press, Inc., pp 51–56.

Liebowitz M, Gorman J, Fyer A, Levitt M, Dillon D, Levy G, Appleby I, Anderson S, Palij M, Davies S, Klein DF (1985): Lactate provocation of panic attacks: II. Biochemical and physiological findings. Arch Gen Psychiatry 42:709–719.

Maas JW (1984): Relationships between central nervous system noradrenergic function and plasma and urinary concentrations of norepinephrine metabolites. In Usdin E, Asberg M, Bertilsson L, Sjoqvist F (eds): Frontiers in Biochemical and Pharmacological Research in Depression, New York: Raven Press, pp 45–55.

Mason JW (1968): A review of psychoendocrine research on the sympathetic adrenal medullary system. Psychosom Med 30:631–653.

Mason JW, Brady JV, Tolliver GA (1968): Plasma and urinary 17-hydroxycorticosteroid responses to 72-hr avoidance sessions in the monkey. Psychosom Med 30:608–630.

Mills FJ (1985): The endocrinology of stress. Aviat Space Environ Med 56:642–650.

Minneman KP (1983): Peripheral catecholamine administration does not alter cerebral β-adrenergic receptor density. Brain Res 264:328–331.

Miyabo S, Asato T, Mizushima N (1977): Prolactin and growth hormone responses to psychological stress in normal and neurotic subjects. J Clin Endocrinol Metab 44:947–951.

Miyabo S, Asato T, Mizushima N (1979): Psychological correlates of stress-induced cortisol and growth hormone releases in neurotic patients. Psychosom Med 41:515–522.

Munjack DJ, Brown RA, McDowell DE (1987): Brief communication: Comparison of social anxiety in patients with social phobia and panic disorder. J Nervous Mental Dis 175:49–51.

Nakagawa R, Tanaka M, Kohno Y, Noda Y, Nagasaki N (1981): Regional responses of rat brain noradrenergic neurones to acute intense stress. Pharmacol Biochem Behav 14:729–732.

Nesse RM, Curtis GC, Brown GM (1982): Phobic anxiety does not affect plasma levels of thyroid stimulating hormone in man. Psychoneuroendocrinology 7:69–74.

Nesse RM, Curtis GC, Brown GM, Rubin RT (1980): Anxiety induced by flooding therapy of phobias does not elicit prolactin secretory response. Psychosom Med 41:25–31.

Nesse RM, Curtis GC, Thyer BA, McCann DS, Huber-Smith MJ, Knopf RF (1985): Endocrine and cardiovascular responses during phobic anxiety. Psychosom Med 47:320–332.

Newsome HH, Rose JC (1971): Response of human adrenocorticotrophic hormone and growth hormone to surgical stress. J Clin Endocrinol Metab 33:481–487.

Noel GL, Suh HK, Stone JG, Frantz AG (1972): Human prolactin and growth hormone release during surgery and other conditions of stress. J Clin Endocrinol Metab 35:840–851.

Peyrin L, Pequignot JM, Chauplannaz G, Laurent B, Aimard G (1985): Sulfate and glucuronide conjugates of 3-methoxy-4-hydroxyphenylglycol (MHPG) in urine of depressed patients: Central and peripheral influences. J Neural Transmiss 63:255–269.

Pinter EJ, Tolis G, Guyda H, Katsarkas A (1979): Hormonal and free fatty acid changes during strenuous flight in novices and trained personnel. Psychoneuroendocrinology 4:79–82.

Pohl R, Ettedgui E, Bridges M, Lycaki H, Jimerson D, Kopin I, Rainey JM (1987): Plasma MHPG levels in lactate and isoproterenol anxiety states. Biol Psychiatry 22:1127–1136.

Pollard I, Bassett JR, Cairnscross KD (1976): Plasma glucocorticoid elevation and ultrastructural changes in the adenohypophysis of the male rat following prolonged exposure to stress. Neuroendocrinology 21:312–330.

Pyke RE, Greenberg HS (1986): Norepinephrine challenges in panic patients. J Clin Psychopharmacol 6:279–285.

Quabbe H-J (1985): Hypothalamic control of GH secretion: Pathophysiology and clinical implications. Acta Neurochir 75:60–71.

Redmond DE Jr (1979): New and old evidence for the involvement of a brain norepinephrine system in anxiety. In Fann WE, Karacan I (eds): "Phenomenology and Treatment of Anxiety." Jamaica, NY: Spectrum Publishers Inc., pp 153–203.

Reiman EM, Mintun MA, Raichle ME, Robins E, Price JL, Fusselman F, Hackman KA (1988): Neuroanatomical correlates of lactate-induced panic. Washington, DC: American Psychiatric Association, New Research Abstracts, NR9, 1988.

Rose RM (1984): Overview of endocrinology of stress. In Brown GM, Koslow SH, Reichlin S (eds): "Neuroendocrinology and Psychiatric Disorder." New York: Raven Press, pp 95–131.

Roy-Byrne P, Uhde TW, Post RM, Gallucci W, Chrousos GP, Gold PW (1986a): The corticotropin-releasing hormone stimulation test in patients with panic disorder. Am J Psychiatry 143:896–899.

Roy-Byrne P, Uhde TW, Rubinow DR, Post RM (1986b): Reduced TSH and prolactin responses to TRH in patients with panic disorder. Am J Psychiatry 143:503–507.

Rubin RT, Miller RG, Clark BR, Poland RE, Arthur RJ (1970): The stress of aircraft carrier landings: II. 3-Methoxy-4-hydroxyphenylglycol excretion in naval aviators. Psychosom Med 32:589–597.

Sakellaris P, Vernikos-Danellis J (1975): Increased rate of response of the pituitary-adrenal system in rats adapted to chronic stress. Endocrinology 97:597–602.

Salter C, Fluck DC, Stimmler L (1972): Effect of open-heart surgery on growth-hormone levels in man. Lancet ii:853–854.

Sellew AP, Low JA, Shear MK, Mann JJ, James G (1987a): Norepinephrine increase during panic attacks. In: "Proceedings of The Annual Meeting of the American Psychiatric Association." Washington, DC: APA, 232.

Sellew AP, Low JA, Shear MK, Mann JJ, James G (1987b): Personal communication.

Shear MK, Kligfield P, Harshfield G, Devereux RB, Polan

JJ, Mann JJ, Pickering T, Frances AJ (1987): Cardiac rate and rhythm in panic patients. Am J Psychiatry 144:633–637.

Siegel RA, Chowers I, Conforti N, Weidenfeld J (1982): Effects of naloxone on basal and stress-induced prolactin secretion, in intact, hypothalamic deafferentated, adrenalectomized, and dexamethasone-pretreated male rats. Life Sci 30:1691–1699.

Sothmann MS, Horn TS, Hart BA (1987): Comparison of discrete cardiovascular fitness groups on plasma catecholamine and selected behavioral responses to psychological stress. Psychophysiology 24:47–54.

Stewart RS, Devous MD Sr, Rush AJ, Lane L, Bonte FJ (1988): Cerebral blood flow changes during sodium-lactate-induced panic attacks. Am J Psychiatry 145:442–449.

Stone EA (1983): Adaptation to stress and brain noradrenergic receptors. Neurosci Biobehav Rev 7:503–509.

Tanako M, Kohno Y, Nakagawa R, Yoshishige I, Takeda S, Nagasaki N (1982): Time-related differences in noradrenaline turnover in rat brain regions by stress. Pharmacol Biochem Behav 16:315–319.

Taylor CB, Sheikh J, Agras WS, Roth WT, Margrat J, Ehlers A, Maddock RJ, Gossard D (1986): Ambulatory heart rate changes in patients with panic attacks. Am J Psychiatry 143:478–482.

Taylor CB, Telch MJ, Haavik D (1983): Ambulatory heart rate changes during panic attacks. J Psychiatry Res 17:261–266.

Uhde TW, Boulenger J, Post RM, Siever LJ, Vittone BJ, Jimerson DJ, Roy-Byrne PP (1984): Fear and anxiety: Relationship to noradrenergic function. Psychopathology 17 [suppl 3]:8–23.

Uhde TW, Siever LJ, Post RM, Jimerson DC, Boulenger JP, Buchsbaum MS (1982): Relationship of plasma-free MHPG to anxiety and psychophysical pain in normal volunteers. Psychopharmacol Bull 18:129–132.

Ward MM, Mefford IN, Parker SD, Chesney MA, Taylor B, Keegan DL, Barchas JD (1983): Epinephrine and norepinephrine responses in continuously collected human plasma to a series of stressors. Psychosom Med 45:471–486.

Weiss JM, Glazer HI, Pohovecky LA, Brick J, Miller NE (1975): Effects of chronic exposure to stressors on avoidance-escape behavior and on brain norepinephrine. Psychosom Med 37:522–534.

Weitzman ED, Ursin H (1978): Growth hormone. In Ursin H, Bande E, Levine S (eds): Psychobiology of Stress, Orlando, Fla: Academic Press, Inc, pp 91–97.

Wilkinson LO, Abercrombie ED, Jacobs BL (1986): Environmental stress and activity of dorsal raphe serotonergic neurons in the freely moving cat. Soc Neurosci Abstr 12:1134.

Wolinska-Witort E, Przekop F, Mateusiak K, Domanski E (1986): Effect of repeated and prolonged stress stimuli on the plasma prolactin concentration in sheep. Exp Clin Endocrinol 87:265–276.

Woods SW, Charney DS (1988): Applications of the pharmacologic challenge strategy in panic disorders research. J Anxiety Disorders 2:31–49.

Woods SW, Charney DS, Goodman WK, Heninger GR (1988): Carbon Dioxide-Induced Anxiety. Behavioral, physiologic, and biochemical effects of carbon dioxide in patients with panic disorders and healthy subjects. Arch Gen Psychiatry 45:43–52.

Woods SW, Charney DS, McPherson CA, Gradman AH, Heninger GR (1987): Situational panic attacks: Behavioral, physiologic, and biochemical characterization. Arch Gen Psychiatry 44:365–375.

Woods SW, Koster K, Krystal JH, Smith EO, Zubal IG, Hoffer PB, Charney DS (1988): Yohimbine alters regional cerebral blood flow in panic disorder (Letter). Lancet ii:678.

Yokota H, Kawashima Y, Hashimoto S, Manabe H, Onishi T, Aono T, Matsumoto K (1977): Plasma cortisol, luteinizing hormone (LH), and prolactin secretory responses to cardiopulmonary bypass. J Clin Endocrinol Metab 44:947–951.

14

Caffeine Provocation of Panic: A Focus on Biological Mechanisms

THOMAS W. UHDE, MD

Section on Anxiety and Affective Disorders, Biological Psychiatry Branch, National Institute of Mental Health, Bethesda, Maryland 20892

INTRODUCTION

Panic disorder is a neuropsychiatric syndrome characterized by episodes of profound anxiety. These episodes of anxiety, particularly early in the course of illness, are often perceived by the patient as being "unexpected," "unprovoked," "spontaneous," or coming "out-of-the-blue." These unexpected attacks are associated with myriad somatic symptoms (e.g., shortness of breath, lightheadedness or vertigo, diaphoresis, choking, atypical angina, tachycardia, palpitations, marked psychosensory perceptual alterations (Boulenger et al., 1986; Uhde et al., 1985), and typically frightening cognitions (e.g., "I'm going to die"). No specific set of symptoms or physiologic or biochemical measures have been discovered that can accurately and consistently document the validity of panic attacks as a distinct entity from a wide spectrum of other subjective experiences of anxious dysphoria. Although several lines of epidemiologic, pharmacologic, and biochemical data suggest that panic disorder and simple phobias are qualitatively distinct disorders, considerable controversy remains regarding the phenomenological and neurobiological overlap among panic disorder, generalized anxiety disorder, social phobia (Stein et al., 1987), major depressive disorder (Leckman et al., 1983; Stein and Uhde, 1988a; Uhde et al., 1985, 1986), and, to a lesser extent, obsessive–compulsive disorder (Cloninger et al., 1981; Mellman and Uhde,

1987; Rasmussen and Tsuang, 1986) and post-traumatic stress disorder (Rainey et al., 1987). Although most investigators concur that agoraphobia develops as a secondary complication of panic attacks (Freud, 1959; Klein and Rabkin, 1981; Uhde et al., 1985), there remains a small cohort of experts that argue that context-specific fears, rather than panic attacks, represent the fundamental pathogenesis in most agoraphobic syndromes.

An even larger number of investigators still view panic attacks as simply an extreme form of generalized anxiety. In fact, recent findings from independent drug trials raise important questions regarding the validity of Klein's hypothesis (Klein, 1964) that panic and generalized anxiety disorders preferentially respond to tricyclic antidepressants (e.g., imipramine) and benzodiazepines (e.g., diazepam), respectively. It was this differential responsivity to pharmacologic agents that provided the greatest impetus to the theory that panic disorder could be separated not only from affective disorders but also from other anxiety syndromes. Whereas the validity of the pharmacological basis of Klein's original theory is currently being challenged, emerging genetic and family pedigree data seem to support the diagnostic specificity of panic disorder from generalized anxiety disorder. For example, in an important study by Crowe et al. (1983), the risk of panic disorder was found to be 24.7% in the first-degree relatives of probands with panic disorder compared to 2.3% for the relatives of a control group. There was no difference in the rate of generalized anxiety disorder in the relatives

Neurobiology of Panic Disorder, Pages 219–242
Published 1990 by Alan R. Liss, Inc.

of panic disorder patients (4.8%) vs. the control group (3.6%). These findings suggested that panic disorder and generalized anxiety disorder could be distinguished in terms of differential rates of familial transmission. Several subsequent studies have largely supported these findings, suggesting a qualitative difference between panic and generalized anxiety disorders (Cloninger et al., 1981; Harris et al., 1983; Noyes et al., 1986). Moreover, preliminary findings from a twin study (Torgersen, 1983) indicate a significantly greater coincidence of panic disorder in adult, same-sexed twins. In all these studies, a clear, but as yet not totally proved pattern begins to emerge. First, agoraphobia indeed appears to aggregate with panic disorder. Second, panic disorder appears to be qualitatively distinct from generalized anxiety disorder. Thus, although Klein's original notion that the two disorders can be differentiated on the basis of pharmacologic response has been increasingly challenged, the aforementioned family and genetic studies actually support his conceptualization. It should also be noted, however, that all these lines of evidence can be interpreted from the perspective of a "continuum model" of anxiety, with generalized anxiety disorder simply representing a milder or earlier stage in the development of panic disorder or agoraphobia with panic attacks. Although neurobiological studies are in an early phase of investigation, no single biological test or group of tests has been able to discriminate among the anxiety disorders (for reviews, see Barlow, 1988; Uhde and Nemiah, 1988; Uhde et al., 1986).

At present, these viewpoints can best be understood within the context of the neverending battle between "lumpers" vs. "splitters," although, of course, the future may elucidate a continuum of phenotypic expression (e.g., severity) within several dichotomous anxiety disorders. Although molecular genetics and brain imaging technologies may ultimately provide answers regarding the precise nature of the neurobiological abnormalities within and across anxiety syndromes, one of the most productive research strategies during the past several years arguably has been the use of chemical agents to induce panic attacks in panic disorder patients.

The basic hypothesis with the chemical models paradigm is that, if panic disorder is an illness distinct from other anxiety syndromes, then panic disorder patients should demonstrate a qualitatively or quantitatively different behavioral and biochemical response to the probe under study compared to normal controls and nonpanic psychiatric patients. However, even with the demonstration of a differential sensitivity to a particular anxiogenic drug, a secondary and, scientifically, logically more problematic assumption becomes manifest. That is, one operates on the assumption that the mechanisms that mediate chemically induced anxiety states have some relevance to the neurobiological substrates that underlie natural panic attacks. Of course, this simply may not be true, and this represents one of the more problematic, yet often overlooked, aspects of this research strategy. Despite this and other potential flaws with chemical models (Uhde and Tancer, 1988), the induction of panic with chemical agents has proved a popular and useful tool in the study of panic and related anxiety disorders. Moreover, data from several chemical models, including caffeine-induced panic, have led to the development of practical guidelines for the assessment and management of panic disorder patients (Uhde, in press).

This chapter presents the rationale, historical development, and current status of the caffeine model of panic. When relevant, the caffeine model is discussed within the context of other chemical models and neurotransmitter-neuromodulatory (i.e., noradrenergic, dopaminergic, benzodiazepine–gamma-aminobutyric acid (GABA)-ergic, and adenosinergic) systems implicated in the neurobiology of panic disorder.

CAFFEINE: AN ANCIENT DRUG

As reviewed elsewhere (Uhde and Tancer, 1988), several agents, including epinephrine-norepinephrine (Breggin, 1964; Garfield et al., 1967; Pyke and Greenberg, 1982), yohimbine (Charney et al., 1982, 1983, 1985; Garfield et al., 1967; Uhde et al., 1984a), isoproterenol (Frohlich et al., 1969; Nesse et al., 1984; Rainey et al., 1984a,b), lactate (Carr et al., 1986; Dillon et al., 1987; Kelly et al., 1971; Liebowitz et al., 1984; Pitts and McClure, 1967; Rainey et al.,

1984b, 1987), carbon dioxide (Cohen and White, 1949; Gorman et al., 1984a; Griez et al., 1987; Latimer, 1977; Woods et al., 1986; van den Hout and Griez, 1984), metaclorophenylpiperazine (Charney et al., 1987; Mueller et al., 1985; Zohar et al., 1987), and FG 7142 (Dorow et al., 1983) have been used to induce pathological degrees of anxiety, including panic attacks. However, probably the oldest psychotropic agent consistently used by humans throughout history, which is currently being employed as a chemical model of panic, is caffeine or 1,3,7-trimethylxanthine.

It is believed that humans have consumed caffeinated beverages for centuries (Barone and Roberts, 1984). Although the first reliable written reference to tea, probably the oldest caffeine-containing beverage, was in a Chinese dictionary of Kuo P'o from around 350 AD (Barone and Roberts, 1984), humans have probably ingested caffeine since the late stone age (Rall, 1985). In South America, ancient caffeine-containing beverages, such as guarana, yoco, and mate, were made from the seeds of *Paullinia sorbilis*, *P. yoco*, and from *Ilex paraguariensis*, respectively (Rall, 1985). The Aztec Indians drank a caffeinated chocolate drink, and Indians in North America enjoyed a "black" caffeinated beverage made from yaupon. Many of these ancient drinks have persisted until modern times. Even today, inhabitants of the Amazon region in South America take seeds of the *Paullinia cupana* to make *Guarana* paste, which is hardened by baking and consumed later after mixing with hot or cold water. As was noted by Emboden (1979), this practice is as "indispensable to these people as is our morning cup of coffee." The central role that caffeinated beverages have played in human history is also illustrated by the practice of measuring distance in terms of consumption, e.g., the distance between two villages being the quantity of tea or cocoa required to provide sufficient sustenance for the trip. Also noted by Emboden (1979) is that the practical or recreational uses of the methylxanthines have not been limited to humans; fatigued mules in Tibet are given large amounts of tea to increase their capacity to work.

So far, this review of caffeine has emphasized its positive psychotropic attributes. In fact, it can be documented that, during some historical periods, the positive attributes of caffeine were considered to be so unique and beneficial that its consumption was exclusively limited to religious events or was made accessible to only the most privileged individuals within society. Eventually, however, issues regarding possible negative effects of caffeinated beverages were raised within western cultures. For example, in the sixth century, it was thought that caffeine induced a syndrome probably similar to what modern psychiatric nomenclature would refer to as hypomania. In several European countries, this was apparently thought to be of such a potentially serious problem that, according to Emboden (1979), the Prince of Waldeck offered rewards to anyone who could identify a coffee consumer. During the eighth century, both public beatings and taxation were supposedly levied against nonaristocratic consumers who illegally consumed caffeinated beverages. Of interest, most of the early literature fails to mention consistently any significant anxiogenic effects related to caffeine. In fact, it is unclear when the first mention of caffeine as a possible anxiogenic substance was recorded.

CAFFEINE AND ANXIETY

In the past 20 years, there has been increasing concern regarding the effects of both illicit (e.g., heroin, marijuana, lysergic acid diethylamide, cocaine) and licit (e.g., nicotine, caffeine) drug abuse. In relation to caffeine, most scientific research has focused on the possible relationship between caffeine and cardiovascular and gastrointestinal disease, infertility, cancer, and teratogenesis (for reviews, see Gilbert, 1976). Given the large number of new scientific studies on caffeine (approximately 650 citations in *Index Medicus* during the past 2 years), relatively little attention has been paid to the behavioral and anxiogenic effects of caffeine except, perhaps, as related to the anxiogenic consequences of the abrupt discontinuation of caffeine in the chronic consumer (for review, see Uhde, 1988).

Nonetheless, both anecdotal reports and emerging systematic studies of caffeine strongly suggest that caffeine intoxication states can mimic both panic and generalized anxiety disorders and that adult panic disorder patients have an increased sensitivity to caffeine's panicogenic effects compared to normal controls. The following sections review the indirect and direct evidence that supports these conclusions.

Indirect Evidence

Greden (1974) reported three cases of caffeine intoxication in patients whose caffeine consumption was between 1,200 and 1,500 mg daily. Greden (1974) noted that these patients' symptoms of caffeinism were "indistinguishable" from anxiety neurosis. In Greden's report, all three patients improved after a reduction in caffeine consumption. Although Greden did not explicitly address the relationship of caffeinism to panic attacks, it is interesting that the one individual who had only recently consumed excessive amounts of caffeine reported palpitations, lightheadedness, tremulousness, breathlessness, chest discomfort, and irregular heartbeat on a sporadic basis approximately two or three times per day. In contrast, the two individuals who had consumed large amounts of caffeine for years reported symptoms more reminiscent of generalized anxiety disorder. These data suggest that *acute* caffeine intoxication may mimic panic disorder whereas *chronic* toxicity may mimic generalized anxiety. Our unit had previously reported two cases (Uhde, 1988) in support of this conclusion. These two original reports (cases 1 and 3) plus two additional cases (cases 2 and 4) that have recently come to our attention are reported in this chapter to substantiate further the similarity between caffeine intoxication states and anxiety disorders. Cases 1 and 3 have been reported in greater detail elsewhere (Uhde, 1988) and are presented here only in synopsis to provide a broad overview.

CASE 1

An 18-year-old college student consumed up to 1,800 mg of caffeine while preparing for final examinations. This student, who had no previous psychiatric history, developed an acute panic attack associated with pounding chest, tachycardia, sweating in his hands and feet, and paresthesia. Because of his fear of having a heart attack, he went to a local emergency room, where he was misdiagnosed as having examination anxiety. Except for minimal insomnia on the following three nights,

his symptoms totally remitted after discontinuation of his caffeine intake. He has not subsequently developed pathological degrees of anxiety or other psychiatric syndromes.

CASE 2

A 32-year-old professional woman was self-referred for evaluation and treatment of panic attacks that had been occurring for 4 weeks. The patient had recently moved to the Washington, DC, metropolitan area and, although she experienced the geographical relocation as moderately stressful, had never previously experienced panic attacks or prolonged periods of free-floating or situational anxiety. A paternal uncle had a probable diagnosis of recurrent major depressive episodes, melancholic subtype, but otherwise her family history was negative. She had been a low caffeine consumer for years (<100 mg daily) until her recent move to the area. Because of the considerable amount of unpacking and making arrangements for decorating her home, she began to drink several caffeinated cola drinks and coffee to give her energy. Her first panic attack awakened her from sleep following an evening when she had consumed eight cups of coffee. The patient was told that she probably suffered from caffeinism and to discontinue her newly acquired coffee habit. She did and has remained free of panic attacks for 6 months.

CASE 3

Mr. B. is a 43-year-old married male who was referred to a psychopharmacologist by his family physician for evaluation and treatment of his anxiety symptoms. Mr. B. complained of insomnia, "hot flashes," abdominal "uneasiness," anxiety, marked psychomotor agitation, and restless legs. These symptoms had increased in severity during the past 2 months, but he had had frequent intermittent problems with tension, nervousness, and tachycardia for the past 2 years. He denied any history of panic attacks, agoraphobia, obsessions, or compulsions.

A review of his dietary habits revealed that he consumed an average of 20 cups of coffee per day. Although he had consistently consumed two to five cups of coffee per day since adolescence, he had gradually increased his coffee consumption up to 25 cups daily over the past 3 years. A taper schedule was recommended and the number of daily cups of coffee was gradually decreased from 20 to three per day. This decrease was accomplished over 2 months and was well tolerated except for intermittent early morning headache and insomnia.

CASE 4

Mr. R is a 16-year-old high school student who was referred for evaluation of poor school performance. He also had complaints of nervousness, jitteriness, sweating, insomnia, and periodic hand tremor. The patient denied panic attacks but did report dysphoria of several months' duration. According to the mother, patient, and school principal, he had previously been a "straight A" student. During this school year, however, he had received Fs in several subject areas in three consecutive grading periods. Although the subject matter of his current courses was considered difficult, his poor performance was judged to represent a dramatic change uncharacteristic of students with his advanced potential.

There had been longstanding marital discord within the family, but neither the mother nor the patient attributed his current school problems to this situation. In fact, the patient stated, "My parents have always fought, and I have never had trouble with school before." The patient, obviously bright and articulate, was at a loss to explain his school problems and anxious symptomatology.

Upon further questioning, Mr. R. related that he had typically consumed two cola drinks daily (lunch and dinner) until several months ago when he began to consume seven or eight 12-ounce cola drinks in order to stay up to study. He occasionally also had taken No Doz on nights before examinations. Thus his caffeine consumption had gradually increased from approximately 45–90 mg daily to as much as 500 mg daily over several months during the current school year. He was instructed to taper and discontinue his caffeine consumption over a 4 week period. He complied with these recommendations and had no untoward side effects except for the development of a transient headache. Within several weeks after discontinuation of caffeine, there was a noticeable improvement in his school performance and a total resolution of his anxious symptomatology.

In the differential diagnosis of panic and generalized anxiety disorders, the presence of symptoms such as marked diarrhea, restless legs, widely distributed motor tics, and acute psychomotor agitation should increase the clinician's index of suspicion of possible caffeine intoxication. Obviously, a history of excessive caffeine consumption is a key requirement for making the diagnosis. The recognition of an association between high caffeine consumption and anxiety states is hardly a new observation (Charney et al., 1985; Fontaine et al., 1978; Gilliland and Andress, 1981; Greden et al., 1974; Rapoport et al., 1981a,b; Victor et al., 1981; Uhde et al., 1984b). An association between high caffeine consumption and state anxiety (Winstead, 1976) or both state and trait anxiety (Greden et al., 1978) has been reported in groups of psychiatric inpatients with unspecified disorders. However, our suggestion that *acute* and *chronic* caffeine consumption can specifically mimic panic and generalized anxiety disorders, respectively, is a novel hypothesis. Whether additional research will confirm this specific hypothesis is unknown, but, at the very least, our observations extend previous findings indicating that caffeine can induce pathological states of anxiety when consumed in excessive quantities. Moreover, although most individuals probably self-select their caffeine consumption to control for its psychoactive properties (Rapoport et al., 1981a), accumulating evidence suggests that some patients can unwittingly develop clinically significant symptoms of caffeine-induced anxiety.

Even more controversial than the hypothesis that acute and chronic caffeinism can mimic specific anxiety disorders is the question of whether there are truly different degrees of individual sensitivity to caffeine's behavioral and biochemical effects. The ability to address such a question is complicated by the fact that many parameters, such as patterns of usage (acute vs. intermittent vs. chronic), time-of-day, dosage, physical health, drug interactions, and weight of the consumer can influence the behavioral effects of caffeine. No study investigating the behavioral effects of caffeine has adequately controlled for all these variables. Nonetheless, converging lines of evidence suggest that panic disorder patients are more sensitive to the anxiogenic effects of caffeine than normal controls.

In the early 1980s, our group began examining patterns of daily caffeine consumption and the relation between these patterns and degree and type of anxiety in patients with well defined DSM III diagnoses of agoraphobia with panic attacks or major depressive disorder (Boulenger and Uhde, 1982). Results in each patient group were compared to normal controls matched for age, gender, and socioeconomic status.

Although neither panic nor depressed patients consumed significantly lower amounts of caffeine than their respective normal controls in this initial survey, a subsequent, ongoing assessment in a larger sample of patients has revealed that panic disorder ($P < 0.05$) patients but not depressed patients consume significantly smaller amount of caffeine. Moreover, even in our initial study, a significantly lower percentage of patients with panic disorder (67%) had given up coffee compared to the patients with major depressive disorders (22%) or normal controls (13–20%) (Boulenger et al., 1984). In most cases, the panic disorder patients reported that they had given up coffee consumption because of its psychostimulant or related properties. Unlike the depressed patients, the panic disorder patients also reported that the consumption of one cup of coffee produces significantly greater increases in measures of anxiety ($P < 0.001$), alertness ($P < 0.01$), and insomnia ($P < 0.01$) but not well-being compared to the normal control group (see Fig. 14–1A,B). There was also a significant

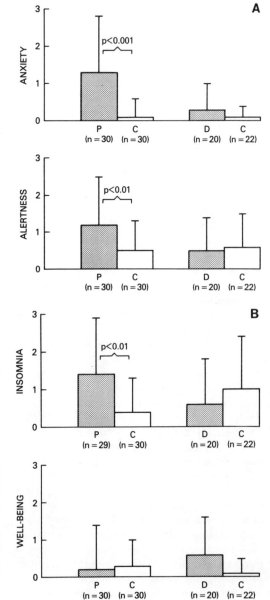

Fig. 14–1. A,B: Patients with panic disorder (P) or major affective disorder (D) and their respective age- and sex-matched normal controls (C) rated the degree to which one cup of coffee induced symptoms of anxiety, alertness, insomnia, and a sense of well-being. Ratings were made on a five-point scale. Means, standard deviations, and P values (reflecting significance of two tailed t tests between patients and their respective controls) are presented; these indicate that the consumption of one cup of coffee was associated with significantly greater ratings of anxiety, alertness, and insomnia, but not well-being, in panic disorder patients compared to their normal controls. This increased sensitivity does not appear to be a consequence of psychiatric illness per se; the patients with affective disorders did not respond to one cup of coffee in a manner significantly different from the normal controls. (Reproduced from Boulenger et al., 1984.)

correlation between daily caffeine consumption and measures of trait anxiety (r = 0.50, P = 0.006), depression (r = 0.56, P = 0.02) and the SCL-90 subscales for general symptomatic index (r = 0.44, P = 0.02), positive symptom distress (r = 0.44, P = 0.02), retarded depression (r = 0.45, P = 0.01), and agitated depression (r = 0.37, P = 0.04). There were no significant correlations between daily caffeine consumption and any of these measures in either the depressed patients or normal control groups. Using a questionnaire format, Lee et al. (1985) essentially confirmed our observations. In their study, daily caffeine consumption and subscale scores on the SCL 90-R (Derogatis, 1977) were evaluated in 124 medical inpatients without a psychiatric illness and 43 outpatients with a primary anxiety disorder (79% of whom had panic disorder or agoraphobia with panic attacks by DSM III diagnostic criteria). The panic disorder patients were found to have a different distribution of daily caffeine consumption compared to the medical comparison group (P < 0.001). Eighty-four percent of the panic disorder patients compared to 41% of the medical inpatients were low consumers of caffeine, defined in this study as ≤249 mg/day according to the criteria of Victor et al. (1981). In contrast, only 2% of the anxiety disorder patients were high consumers (≥750 mg/day), whereas 16% of the medical comparison group were found to be high consumers. Although this study failed to find a significant correlation between subscale scores of the SCL 90-R and daily caffeine consumption, the anxiety disorder patients reported a significantly higher rate of anxiety in response to drinking one cup of coffee compared to the group of medical inpatients. The authors controlled for the amount of daily caffeine consumption by comparing only those patients within each group who were low caffeine consumers. Thus the study by Lee et al. (1985) confirmed our earlier observations suggesting that anxiety disorder patients, perhaps particularly panic disorder patients, were more sensitive to the anxiogenic effects of caffeine and, as a result, self-impose a diet low in caffeine content. Both our study (Boulenger and Uhde, 1982; Boulenger et al., 1984) and the study of Lee et al. (1985) provided strong but indirect evidence that panic disorder patients were more sensitive to the anxiogenic effects of caffeine.

Direct Evidence

As a result of these retrospective studies, we examined our hypothesis by directly testing the effects of caffeine under double-blind, placebo-controlled conditions in panic disorder patients compared to normal controls. Results of this direct challenge study, presented below, indicate that panic disorder patients, indeed, are more sensitive than controls to the anxiogenic effects of caffeine. In the initial study (Uhde et al., 1984b), three doses of caffeine 240, 480, and 720 mg of caffeine base and placebo were administered orally to eight normal controls. Even in this small sample (n = 8), there was a significant dose-related increase in Zung anxiety (F = 8.84, df = 1.36/9.49, P < 0.01), with a nonsignificant increase in Spielberger state anxiety values (F = 1.84, df = 1.49/10.44, P < 0.19). Two of the eight normal volunteers had unequivocal panic attacks after receiving the 720 mg dose. This suggested that caffeine, in sufficient doses, could be anxiogenic and even panicogenic in normal controls. To study possible differential effects of caffeine in panic disorder patients and in normal controls, we chose a dose of caffeine (480 mg) that produced moderate anxiogenic effects but failed to induce panic attacks in normal controls. Thus the 480 mg dose was used in a subsequent study involving 24 panic disorder patients and 14 normal controls. In this second study, only single-dose caffeine (480 mg) or placebo was administered to subjects. Nine of the 24 patients (37.5%) and none of the 14 (0%) controls had panic attacks following caffeine administration (X^2, P < 0.05). Subjects had to be fearful and experience symptoms very similar to natural panic symptoms to be counted as panicking. None of the patients or normal controls reported panic attacks after placebo, although not all subjects received placebo in this latter study.

These preliminary findings suggested that panic disorder patients were more sensitive to the panicogenic effects of caffeine than normal controls. In a similar study, Charney et al. (1985) used a caffeine paradigm in which 10 mg/kg of caffeine citrate was also administered orally to panic disorder patients and normal controls. Twenty-one patients meeting DSM III criteria for panic disorder or agoraphobia with panic attacks and 17 normal controls participated in the study. Fifteen of the 21 patients (71%) and none of the controls had panic attacks in response to the caffeine. Charney (personal communication) has indicated that none of the patients had panic attacks during the placebo administration. These findings provided further evidence that caffeine produces severe anxiety, including panic attacks, in panic-prone individuals.

In both our study and that of Charney et al. (1985), the caffeine-induced panic attacks were very similar to spontaneous panic attacks, although some of our patients experienced waves of panic attacks after caffeine. Of interest, the caffeine doses used in our laboratory (Uhde et al., 1984b) are not comparable to those used by Charney et al. (1985). For example, Charney et al. (1985) used caffeine citrate, which is 50% caffeine by weight, whereas Uhde et al. (1984b) used 480 mg of caffeine base. Although the explanation for the differences in panic rates is unclear, both studies provided direct evidence that panic disorder patients are significantly more sensitive to the anxiogenic effects of caffeine than normal controls. Despite these findings of a greater sensitivity in panic disorder patients, some critics of chemical models of anxiety have suggested that the increased rate of panic in panic disorder patients is simply due to the overreporting of normal changes in interoceptive cues and biochemical function (Margraf et al., 1986).

Furthermore, Margraf et al. (1986) have pointed out that, despite the dramatic differences in subjective measures of lactate-induced anxiety, only subtle or unimpressive changes in physiological or biochemical variables are noted between panic disorder patients and normal controls. It has been argued that, if there are significantly different biological (as well as behavioral) responses to a specific chemical agent, then this would provide a substantive basis for an underlying biological disturbance in panic disorder. As reviewed elsewhere (Uhde and Tancer, 1988), this interpretation itself is not without problems. Nonetheless, given the lack of biochemical correlates associated with some models of panic (Margraf et al., 1986), our group was particularly interested in whether there were different physiological (blood pressure) or biochemical (cortisol, glucose, lactate) responses to caffeine in panic disorder patients vs. normal controls.

Compared to baseline values, our group found that 480 mg of caffeine induced significant increases in mean arterial pressure, cortisol, glucose, and lactate in both panic disorder patients and normal controls. Although the caffeine-induced increases in mean arterial pressure were similar, there was a significantly greater main effect increase in cortisol in the panic disorder group compared to controls ($P < 0.02$). There was also a significant (group $\times$ time) interaction between the panic patients and normal controls with significantly greater glucose ($P < 0.05$) and lactate ($P < 0.04$) levels at 90 min following caffeine administration. Moreover, the "panicking" vs. "nonpanicking" panic disorder patients had significantly greater increases in lactate ($P < 0.03$).

Considered together, these data suggest that the quality, duration, and type of panic attacks induced by caffeine are similar to naturally occurring panic attacks. Moreover, caffeine induces a greater increase in lactate, glucose, and cortisol in panic disorder patients than in normal controls, perhaps providing added validity to the concept that the primary disturbance in panic disorder is not simply a perceptual-cognitive abnormality that culminates in the biased reporting or overreaction to the same biochemical and physiological alterations experienced by normal controls.

A word of caution, however, is indicated regarding the interpretation of our data. Despite the significantly different behavioral and biochemical responses to caffeine in panic disorder patients and normal controls, it remains conceivable that the experience of panic itself might induce secondary feedback changes in cortisol, lactate, and glucose. Even if this is a viable explanation, our findings do suggest that this type of anxiety (i.e., panic) is associated with alterations in several different indices of neurobiological function. That is, there are definitive changes in the biological environment associated with caffeine-induced panic. Several other lines of investigation also suggest that panic disorder patients can be differentiated from normal healthy controls on a number of other biological measures (for re-

TABLE 14–1.
Ideal Chemical Model of Panic

Symptom convergence: The quality, duration, and severity of symptoms of an induced panic attack must closely mimic those of the patient's spontaneous panic attacks; the extreme fear and the physiologic symptoms must be present

Specificity: The challenge stimulus should exhibit either "complete" or "threshold" specificity for panic disorder patients; complete specificity implies that only panic disorder patients and no other psychiatric or normal control subjects experience panic attacks in response to the challenge stimulus; threshold specificity, a less stringent criteria, implies that healthy and psychiatric controls as well as panic disorder patients can have panic attacks in response to the challenge, but the controls require a larger stimulus

Clinical validation: Clinically effective panic-reducing agents, such as imipramine, phenelzine, and alprazolam, should either reduce the frequency or raise the threshold of chemically induced panic attacks; conversely, the frequency or threshold should not be altered by treatments known to be relatively ineffective in panic disorder, such as propranolol

Replicability: A susceptible patient should predictably respond to repeated challenges in the absence of changing clinical status

views, see Stein and Uhde, 1988a; Uhde et al., 1986). The fact that caffeine induces panic attacks similar in quality and duration to "spontaneous" panic attacks and produces a differentially greater increase in lactate, cortisol, and glucose does not itself prove that the mechanisms that mediate caffeine-induced anxiety are identical or inclusive in terms of those processes that precipitate natural panic attacks. For example, it appears that natural panic attacks are not associated with marked changes in blood glucose. Moreover, lactate-induced panic attacks are not associated with significant changes in glucose (Gorman et al., 1984b), and neither glucose-induced (Uhde et al., 1984d) nor insulin-induced (Schweizer et al., 1986) hypoglycemia produces symptoms of anxiety typical of spontaneous panic attacks. That panic disorder patients have greater caffeine-induced lactate is intriguing and consistent with other lines of evidence (Cohen and White, 1949; Liebowitz et al., 1984; Rainey et al., 1984b), suggesting that abnormalities in lactate metabolism may be indirectly connected to the neuropathology of panic disorder. The relation of natural panic attacks to changes in hypothalamic-pituitary-adrenal function remains controversial (for review, see Uhde et al., 1988; Stein and Uhde, 1988a); therefore, the significance of the modest but significant increase in cortisol following caffeine-induced panic requires further investigation.

As was suggested by Gorman et al. (1987) and Guttmacher et al. (1983), an ideal chemical model of anxiety or panic should have clinical validity (see Table 14–1). That is, drugs that are effective in reducing "spontaneous" panic attacks should also either reduce the frequency or raise the threshold of chemically induced panic attacks. Our group has begun to address this question. In a preliminary study (Uhde et al., 1986), we administered an acute challenge of caffeine to 16 panic disorder patients participating in a double-blind, placebo-controlled, alprazolam treatment study. Each patient received an acute challenge of caffeine (480 mg) while receiving, in random order, either placebo or alprazolam as a part of a crossover treatment study of alprazolam. Seven of the 16 (43.7%) patients had panic attacks during the placebo phase whereas none of the panic disorder patients had panic attacks during the alprazolam phase of the study. Compared to placebo, alprazolam also significantly reduced measures of anxiety on the Zung Anxiety Scale and significantly reduced at 90 min postcaffeine administration the rise in both lactate and cortisol. Thus this preliminary study demonstrated clinical validity as reflected by a known antipanic agent's (i.e., alprazolam) ability to block the behavioral (i.e., panicogenic) and biochemical (i.e., lactate, cortisol) effects of the chemical probe (e.g., caffeine). Of course, future studies with other clinically effective agents are indicated to address the extent to which caffeine's mechanism of action simulates the final common pathway of panicogenesis. Our preliminary findings with imipramine, conducted by Dr. Murray Stein in our Unit on Anxiety and Affective Disorders, are mixed. That is, although some previously caffeine-sensitive patients have demonstrated blockade of both natural and caffeine-induced panic attacks after being treated with imipramine, other imipramine responders have continued to experience panic attacks after a second challenge of caffeine while on therapeutic doses of imipramine. These preliminary findings are complex, and a number of mechanisms can be hypothesized to explain the results. For example, it is unclear to what extent the failure of some patients to panic following the second caffeine challenge can be explained on the basis of tolerance to caffeine's panicogenic effects. In fact, the issues of tolerance to both panicogenic stimuli and therapeutic drugs have been inadequately addressed within the chemical-model literature. It is also a problem that will require additional research before a consensus about its implications can be achieved.

As is noted in Table 14–1, Gorman et al. (1987) suggested that an ideal chemical model of panic should be characterized by the ability of the panicogenic substance (e.g., caffeine) to produce panic attacks predictably with repeated exposure to the chemical probe. Were this concept to be widely accepted, it is of interest that two well known panicogenic agents would fail to meet this criteria of an ideal chemical model; both lactate (Bonn et al., 1973) and carbon dioxide (Griez and van den Hout, 1983) given over time have actually been associated with desensitization. For this and other reasons discussed in greater detail elsewhere (Uhde and Tancer, 1988), we believe that the "replicability" of a chemical agent to produce panic is not a particularly useful condition for a satisfactory chemical model. In fact, several lines of evidence suggest that the investigation of responses to repeated exposure to both autonomic and chemical stimuli may provide clues to the pathogenesis of panic disorder or mechanism that mediate the therapeutic response to a wide spectrum of different pharmacologic agents. As was mentioned previously, it is intriguing that agents that are initially panicogenic, such as lactate (Carr et al., 1986; Dillon et al., 1987; Kelly et al., 1971; Liebowitz et al., 1984; Pitts and McClure, 1967; Rainey et al., 1984b, 1987), carbon dioxide (Gorman et al., 1984a; Griez et al., 1987; Latimer, 1977; Woods et al., 1986), and even imipramine (Aronson and Logue, 1988; Uhde, 1986a), can later reduce anxiety after repeated administration. Moreover, Lader and Matthews (1970) have shown that anxious patients demonstrate a delayed habituation to autonomic stimuli.

For these reasons, our group has conducted, in collaboration with Dr. Thomas Mellman, a preliminary study investigating the effects of repeated exposure to caffeine. In this study, ten panic disorder patients and eight normal controls gave informed consent to receive oral caffeine 7 mg/kg on 8 consecutive days. All of the normal controls but only six of ten (60%) patients completed the study. The four patients who dropped out of the study clearly had more severe anxiogenic responses to their initial exposure to caffeine. That is, these patients became too frightened to complete the study despite the presence of a safe environment and empathic professional staff. Despite the exclusion of these patients from the analysis, the six panic disorder patients who completed the study still demonstrated a delayed and, perhaps, diminished pattern of habituation to caffeine compared to the normal controls. At the present time, we have not determined whether the patients who completed the study involving repeated exposure to caffeine had a significant change in the frequency of their panic attacks after the repeated caffeine challenge compared to their baseline frequency before participation in the study. Nonetheless, these preliminary findings suggest that mechanisms that underlie the processes of both sensitization (Post and Uhde, 1984) and habituation may be important in elucidating the neurobiology of panic and related anxiety conditions.

THEORETICAL IMPLICATIONS

As discussed in this chapter and elsewhere (Uhde and Tancer, 1988), chemical models of panic provide conceptual frameworks for investigating the biochemical, physiological, and neuroendocrine correlates of both normal and pathological degrees of anxiety. By extrapolation from the mechanisms that mediate chemically induced anxiety states one hopes to derive new information regarding the pathogenesis of "spontaneous" or "unprovoked" panic attacks. This section discusses the possible role of various neurotransmitter-neuromodulatory and physiological systems that regulate the behavioral effects of caffeine. It must be emphasized, however, that caffeine-induced panic, like all chemical models of heuristic value, may not necessarily replicate the precise underlying processes involved in "spontaneous" panic attacks.

Neurotransmitter-Neuromodulatory Systems

NORADRENERGIC FUNCTION

Several neurobiological systems may be relevant in caffeine's anxiogenic effects. Given our long-standing interest in the possible role of adrenergic systems in the mood and anxiety disorders (Siever and Uhde, 1984; Uhde et al., 1984a), our group first studied the possible role of noradrenergic hyperactivity in caffeine-induced anxiety states. Several lines of basic science evidence had suggested that noradrenergic mechanisms might be relevant to caffeine's psychostimulant properties. For example, stimulation of the nucleus locus ceruleus and noradrenergic overactivity have been linked to fear behaviors in animals (Redman and Huang, 1979) and anxiety in humans (Charney et al., 1983; Uhde et al., 1984a), respectively, and caffeine has been reported to increase the firing of the locus ceruleus in animals (Olpe et al., 1983) at doses (10 mg/kg) that induce anxiety in normal human subjects (for review, see Uhde, 1988). Methylxanthines, including caffeine, had been reported to increase norepinephrine release and turnover in animal brains and, at high doses, to increase 3-methoxy-4-hydroxyphenylglycol (MHPG) levels in rat brains (Berkowitz et al., 1970; Galloway and Roth, 1983; Gagnon and Boucher, 1972; Waldeck, 1971). Whereas caffeine appears reliably to increase noradrenergic activity in animals, the literature on humans regarding the effects of methylxanthines on norepinephrine and other catecholamines and their metabolites has been suggestive, but

less convincing, of a noradrenergic overactivity model of anxiety (Atuk et al., 1967; Bellet et al., 1969; Elkins et al., 1981; Levi, 1967; Robertson et al., 1978).

For the reasons mentioned above, we predicted that caffeine's anxiogenic effects would be associated with activation of central noradrenergic systems in humans (Uhde et al., 1984). Moreover, we hypothesized that caffeine would produce an increase in plasma levels of norepinephrine and its metabolites and that ratings of anxiety would correlate with plasma levels of caffeine.

In our first study of normal controls (Boulenger et al., 1987; Uhde et al., 1982), we investigated the effects of caffeine on several indices of catecholaminergic function. Subjects received placebo and three oral doses of caffeine (240, 480, and 720 mg). Drugs were given in the morning after 30 min of bed rest. Blood samples were obtained at baseline and at $+30$, $+60$, $+90$, $+120$, and $+150$ min, and a urine sample was obtained for the 3 hr period immediately after drug administration. As expected, there were dose-related increases in plasma caffeine levels from $16.8 \pm 5.0 \mu M$ (range $6.5-23.0 \mu M$) with 240 mg to $56.8 \pm 10.3 \mu M$ (range $43.8-73.3 \mu M$) with 720 mg. To assess the relation between caffeine plasma levels and caffeine-induced anxiety, the slopes of the best fitting lines to the bivariate plot of Spielberger and Zung anxiety scores and caffeine levels were determined for each subject. As is illustrated in Figures 14–2 and 14–3, a significantly greater number of subjects showed a positive linear relationship between their caffeine levels and changes in Zung (sign test, $P < 0.0064$) and Spielberger state (sign test, $P < 0.035$) anxiety than would be predicted by the binomial equation.

Despite the increase in ratings of anxiety and a positive association between plasma levels of caffeine and ratings of anxiety, a one-way ANOVA indicated that there was no significant change in urinary measures (n = 6) of MHPG, normetanephrine, and metanephrine or plasma levels (n = 14) of MHPG or norepinephrine. In a similar study, Charney et al. (1985) also found that caffeine citrate at 10 mg/kg did not produce significant increases in plasma MHPG. At first glance, these findings suggest that caffeine probably does not mediate its

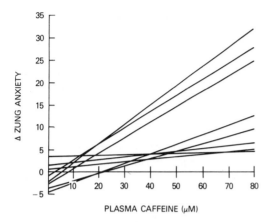

Fig. 14–2. Positive correlations of plasma caffeine levels and Zung anxiety ratings in all subjects. (Reproduced from Boulenger et al., 1987).

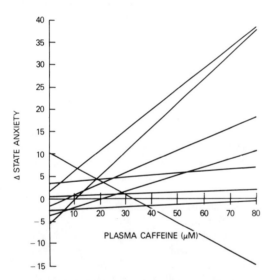

Fig. 14–3. Positive correlations of plasma caffeine levels and state anxiety in seven of eight normal controls. (Reproduced from Boulenger et al., 1987).

anxiogenic effects via activation of the noradrenergic system. However, such a mechanism cannot be totally excluded for two reasons: First, it is quite possible that caffeine might selectively activate central noradrenergic pathways in a localized fashion. In this situation, a small increase in localized brain MHPG may not be reflected in the total plasma pool. Second, although we failed to find a significant

increase in plasma norepinephrine, this negative finding was due to an atypical (i.e., not generally observed in our other challenge studies) increase in plasma norepinephrine following placebo and a large variance in the norepinephrine values at the +30, +60, and +90 min time points. In fact, if the values at these time points are dropped, a reanalysis of the data comparing precaffeine baseline measures of norepinephrine with the latest time point, our data demonstrate a clear dose-response increase of norepinephrine at +150 min. Of interest, the degree of increase of norepinephrine at this time point is almost identical to the increase demonstrated by Robertson and colleagues (1978) at 3 hr after 250 mg of caffeine given to nine normal controls. Thus our negative findings with norepinephrine might represent a statistical artifact obscuring significant increases in norepinephrine, as demonstrated by Robertson and coworkers, at later time points. It is noteworthy, however, that we also failed to find an increase in plasma MHPG up to +150 min postcaffeine. Because one can anticipate a delay of approximately 60–120 min in the increase in MHPG after peak changes in the norepinephrine, it is possible that our methodology also failed to uncover a later rise in both plasma and urinary MHPG. This, however, seems unlikely; Charney et al. (1985) also failed to find significant increases in plasma MHPG after placebo or caffeine in either normal controls or panic disorder patients up to 4 hr after drug administration.

Taken together, it is difficult to invoke noradrenergic hyperactivity as the principal mechanism that mediates caffeine's anxiogenic or panicogenic effects in humans. Given the complexity of our data and the noradrenergic system, as well as the inconsistent findings with norepinephrine, MHPG, normetanephrine, and metanephrine reported in the literature, it is also premature to exclude totally noradrenergic overactivity as a relevant mechanism in caffeine-induced anxiety states.

DOPAMINERGIC FUNCTION

Dopaminergic function has received very little attention in the investigation of panic disorder. In part, this lack of interest is founded on the knowledge that tricyclic antidepressants and some high-potency benzodiazepines are very effective in the treatment of panic disorder (for reviews, see Ballenger, 1986; Katon et al., 1988; Uhde, 1987a) and the unsubstantiated suspicion that neuroleptic agents might actually exacerbate anxiety symptomatology (Klein, 1964; Klein and Rabkin, 1981). However, emerging lines of evidence suggest that alterations in dopaminergic function may be relevant to the study of panic disorder (Gurguis and Uhde, in press; Roy-Byrne et al., 1986b). Both basic science and clinical data suggest that methylxanthines may have important effects on dopaminergic function. For example, methylxanthines increase dopamine-induced motor activity (Anden and Jackson, 1975) and rotational behavior induced by apomorphine in animals with lesions of the nigrostriatal systems (Fredholm et al., 1983). Stoner et al. (1988) also demonstrated that caffeine significantly depresses the firing rate of dopamine neurons in the ventral tegmental area of rats. These authors also found that caffeine had no effect on the nigrostriatal dopaminergic systems. In short, caffeine appears selectively to affect those mesolimbic dopaminergic systems that have been implicated in the pathophysiology of panic disorder (for review, see Post and Uhde, 1984; Uhde et al., 1984c). Caffeine (McManamy and Schube, 1936; Mikkelsen, 1978) and many other psychostimulants that exacerbate psychosis in schizophrenic patients also tend to precipitate nonpsychotic panic attacks in panic disorder patients. Of interest, cholecystokinin (CCK), a peptide that is often colocalized and cosecreted with dopamine in the brain, recently has been found in its tetrapeptide form to induce panic attacks in panic disorder patients (Bradwejn et al., 1988). Thus the effects of caffeine on dopaminergic systems would appear to be at least indirectly relevant in the study of panic disorder and will probably play an increasingly important role in future research.

ADENOSINERGIC FUNCTION

Initially, caffeine's behavioral and biochemical effects were thought to be directly linked to an increase in brain cyclic adenosine monophosphate (cAMP) via inhibition of phosphodiesterase activity (Butcher and Sutherland, 1962; Sutherland and Rall, 1958). The antagonism of adenosine analogs by methylxanthines at adenosine receptors, however, occurs at concentrations that have little or no effect on phosphodiesterase activity (Fredholm, 1980). This and other lines of evidence suggest that caffeine's antagonism of adenosinergic receptors may be the principal mechanism by which methylxanthines mediate their physiological, biochemical, and behavioral effects in animals and humans (Daly et al., 1981; Phillis and Kostopoulos, 1975; Phillis and Wu, 1981; Sattin and Rall, 1970; Snyder et al., 1981; Stone, 1981). If so, then caffeine might be expected to have neurobiological and behavioral effects opposite those of adenosine. Of interest, adenosine and/or its analogs, N_6 cyclohexyladenosine (CHA), N_6 (R-phenylisopropyl) adenosine (PIA), and 2-chloradenosine (2-Clad), produce sedation (Crawley et al., 1981, 1983), hypotension without rebound hypertension (Hoffman et al., 1982; Newberg et al., 1985), and bradycardia (Berne et al., 1984; Di Marco et al., 1984). Adenosine is one of several endogenous agents with natural anticonvulsant properties (for review, see Dragunow et al., 1985).

In contrast, the adenosine antagonist caffeine has been reported to increase verbal and motor output and decrease fatigue and induce insomnia in humans (Battig and Buzzi, 1986; Brezinova, 1974; File et al., 1982; Rapoport et al., 1981b; Saletu et al., 1974). Methylxanthines, including caffeine, have also been reported to increase blood pressure and pulse and both to induce and to augment seizures (Coffey et al., 1987; Shapira et al., 1987; Vestal et al., 1983; Yarnell and Chu, 1975). Caffeine, therefore, does appear to have behavioral and physiological effects opposite those of adenosine.

Stress-mediated responses, which are probably similar but not identical to anxiety states (Uhde et al., 1988), and chronic exposure to methylxanthines also up-regulate central adenosinergic receptors (Boulenger et al., 1983). That both caffeine and stress up-regulate adenosine receptors is interesting in relation to several reports in animals and humans (Henry and Stephens, 1980) that caffeine augments the neurobiological effects of stress. For example, caffeine has been reported to increase the rate of death in mice exposed to head and cold stressors (Muller and Vernikos-Danellis, 1970) and caffeine potentiates nephropathy in mice subjected to chronic "psychosocial" stress (Bennett et al., 1983; Henry and Stephens, 1980). Caffeine also augments the development of gastric lesions in rats exposed to restraint plus cold (Doreen, 1977) or restraint plus water immersion (Yano et al., 1982) stressors. The data in humans (Cobb, 1974; Stillner et al., 1978) are less compelling but nonetheless are suggestive that caffeine might potentiate the effects of stress. In a study by Cobb (1974), caffeine-drinking males exposed to the natural stress of losing their jobs appeared to have increased urinary excretion of norepinephrine compared to either noncaffeine consumers experiencing the same stress or caffeine consumers or abstainers in a nonstressed control group of male workers. In a controlled laboratory study of ten healthy college students, Lane (1983) found that caffeine, in clinically relevant doses of 250 mg, produced an increase in blood pressure over the increase already associated with the psychological stress of a mental arithmetic test.

Given these converging lines of evidence suggesting that caffeine might induce anxiety or mediate stress responses via adenosine receptor blockade, our group recently explored the effects of caffeine on plasma adenosine levels. The recent development of a reliable method for measuring physiological levels of adenosine (Boulenger et al., 1987; Klabunde and Althouse, 1981; Klabunde, 1983; Sollevi et al., 1984; Von Borstel et al., 1983) made it possible to investigate the relation between caffeine-induced anxiety and changes in plasma adenosine. As discussed elsewhere (Boulenger et al., 1987; Uhde et al., 1984b), and in this chapter (see above under "Direct Evidence"), eight normal controls (five females, three males; mean age 35 years) participated in a double-blind, placebo-controlled study involving the random administration of three oral doses of base caffeine (240, 480, and 720 mg) or placebo. All subjects had been instructed to maintain a caffeine-free diet for a minimum of 1 week before and during the duration of the study. As was previously indicated, there was a dose-related increase in ratings of Zung anxiety. However, caffeine had no effect on plasma samples of adenosine obtained 1 hr after drug administration. Adenosine levels after placebo (1.22 ± 1.19 μM) were similar to val-

ues obtained at 240 mg (0.96 ± 0.66 μM), 480 mg (1.26 ± 0.81 μM) and 720 mg (2.18 ± 2.88 μM) of caffeine. Although we had hoped to demonstrate that caffeine increased endogenous levels of adenosine, our negative findings were not totally unexpected; the reuptake of adenosine displaced from brain adenosinergeic receptors is probably too rapid to reflect changes in the plasma. There was also no association between levels of adenosine after placebo, presumably reflecting typical baseline levels under relatively nonstressful conditions, and vulnerability to caffeine-induced anxiety. Despite these negative findings, our results were not inconsistent with the concept of adenosine receptor blockade as a mechanism of caffeine-induced anxiety, since the caffeine levels (44–73 μM) achieved after the 720 mg dose [the only dose that produced panic attacks in the normal controls (see Boulenger et al., 1987; Uhde et al., 1984b; see also above under "Direct Evidence")] are in the range known to compete with the binding of ligands to adenosine receptors in human brain (Ki = 35–115 μM) (Boulenger et al., 1982).

Considered together, these data from both animal and human investigations suggest that caffeine induces anxiety, in part, via blockade of adenosinergic receptors. At the present time, two types of adenosinergic receptors, referred to as A_1 and A_2 according to their ability to mediate a decrease or increase in cAMP at low and high concentrations of adenosine analogs, respectively, (Londos et al., 1988), have been identified. Both A_1 and A_2 receptors are blocked by caffeine; however, the A_2 receptor is currently thought to mediate most of caffeine's behavioral effects. Thus it appears that the adenosinergic neuromodulatory system, perhaps particularly the A_2 receptor, plays an important role in the neurobiology not only of panic disorder but, perhaps, of other stress-related medical conditions as well (Kaminkawa et al., 1983; Watt, 1984, 1985).

BENZODIAZEPINE-GABA-ERGIC FUNCTION

The identification of the benzodiazepine-GABA recepter complex and the linkage of this system to animal and human fear have firmly established benzodiazepine-GABA-ergic function as playing a central role in the neurobiology of anxiety, fear, and arousal (for reviews, see Haefley, 1983; Skolnick et al., 1984). Particularly provocative in terms of panic disorder has been the work of Insel et al. (1984) and Dorow et al. (1983). Insel et al. (1984) used B-CCE, a benzodiazepine inverse agonist to produce dose-dependent activation of fear-related behaviors and increases in blood pressure, pulse, and cortisol in rhesus monkeys. Diazepam, a benzodiazepine agonist, blocked these behavioral and biochemical effects. These findings indicated that fear-related behaviors could be precipitated and reversed by agents that bind in a stereospecific, saturable, and reversible manner to benzodiazepine receptors. Insel and coworkers (1984) also provided evidence that beta-carbolines do not directly mediate these effects via secondary changes in other neurotransmitter systems. For example, whereas diazepam blocked both the behavioral and biochemical effects of B-CCE, clonidine (an alpha-2-adrenergic agonist that decreases locus ceruleus firing) blunted only the biochemical and physiological effects but did not prevent B-CCE-induced behavioral activation. In addition, propranolol, a beta-adrenergic antagonist, diminished the heart rate increase associated with B-CCE but had little effect on B-CCE-mediated fear behaviors or cortisol secretion. Since inverse agonists, such as B-CCE, can induce seizures, few studies have investigated the effects of beta-carbolines in humans. The one exception to this rule has been investigations using FG 7142, a potent benzodiazepine inverse agonist. FG 7142 has been shown to produce fear-related behaviors in both animals (Ninan et al., 1982) and humans (Dorow et al., 1983). In the study by Dorow and coworkers (1983), two of five normal volunteers had panic-like symptoms after administration of FG 7142. Because of the severity of these symptoms, the authors decided to discontinue the study on ethical grounds. Collectively, these and other studies (for reviews, see Gurguis and Uhde, in press; Skolnick et al., 1984; Uhde and Tancer, 1988) provide firm but indirect evidence for benzodiazepine-GABA-ergic abnormalities in the human emotions of anxiety and fear. This theoretical orientation and the fact that caffeine-induced panic is nearly identical to spontaneous panic attacks raise issues regarding caffeine's effects on the benzodiazepine-GABA complex.

At present, most investigators have concluded, perhaps prematurely, that caffeine's anxiogenic effects are not mediated via the benzodiazepine-GABA system. The rationale for this belief is based on the observation that caffeine binds to benzodiazepine receptors in vitro (Marangos et al., 1981) only at concentrations comparable to those reached in humans after near-fatal or fatal suicide attempts (see Uhde, 1988). Moreover, caffeine binds to and up-regulates adenosine receptors at much lower concentrations (Boulenger et al., 1983; Fredholm, 1982) but has weak and inconsistent effects on benzodiazepine receptors (Boulenger et al., 1982; Daval et al., 1984; Marangos et al., 1984). Despite these observations, several lines of evidence suggest that caffeine's effects on benzodiazepine receptor function should not be totally dismissed. First, it remains unclear what degree of occupancy at the benzodiazepine receptor site is required to induce physiological changes. That is, whereas caffeine may bind to adenosine receptors at lower concentrations, it is possible that a partial binding at benzodiazepine receptors might mediate a clinically relevant response. Although this is highly speculative, other lines of animal and human evidence also suggest at least a nonspecific interaction between the benzodiazepine-GABA-ergic and adenosinergic systems. In animals, methylxanthines blunt the effects of benzodiazepines on neuronal firing and neurotransmitter release (Phillis and Wu, 1981), and the pure benzodiazepine antagonist Ro 15-1788 has been found to antagonize caffeine-induced seizures (Seale et al., 1987; Velluci and Webster, 1984).

In humans, several studies have suggested that caffeine or theophylline can block the behavioral and physiological effects of benzodiazepines. For example, caffeine or theophylline blocks many of the behavioral and physiological effects of lorazepam (File et al., 1982), temazepam (Okuma et al., 1982), and diazepam (Mattila et al., 1982; Niemand et al., 1984; Stirt, 1981). The blockade of caffeine-induced panic by alprazolam is consistent with a putative benzodiazepine mechanism, but only the demonstration of a similar blockade by the pure (inactive) antagonists such as Ro 15-1788 would confirm a role for an inverse agonist-like effect of caffeine in its panicogenic activity.

It remains unclear, therefore, to what extent, if any, caffeine mediates its panicogenic, neuroendocrine, biochemical, and physiological effects via the benzodiazepine-GABA system. It appears that the benzodiazepine-GABA neurotransmitter-neuromodulatory system influences human behavior and emotions, perhaps especially vigilance and arousal. Of interest, this receptor system is widely distributed in the brain and in peripheral systems. Such a widespread distribution would not be surprising in a system that mediates a human emotion (i.e., anxiety) whose basic nature involves changes in the function of multiple organ systems. To the extent that any chemical model replicates the pathophysiology of spontaneous panic attacks, it also would not be unexpected if caffeine directly or indirectly influenced several neurotransmitter systems, including, but not limited to, the benzodiazepine-GABA-ergic, adenosinergic, noradrenergic, and dopaminergic neurotransmitter systems.

Limbic System Function

One of the most provocative and controversial subjects in the area of anxiety research is the putative relation between panic disorder and complex partial seizures. Several observations have suggested a possible connection between the two disorders. For example, it has been long recognized that panic disorder patients, especially during panic attacks, experience many of the symptoms found in complex partial seizures (Roth, 1959; Uhde et al., 1984c, 1985). In our study of 64 patients with DSM III-R-defined panic disorder, with or without agoraphobia, (Boulenger et al., 1986; Uhde et al., 1985), the most common psychosensory symptoms reported by patients during panic attacks were distortions in light (56%) or sound (44%) intensity, derealization (41%), strange visceral feelings (41%), vestibular sensations (31%), speeding up of thoughts (31%), distortion of distance (20%), J'amais vu experiences (19%), and the sense that time had suddenly slowed (19%). Of interest, many of these symptoms (e.g., distortions of light and sound intensity) are actually more common than

many symptoms, including psychosensory disturbances (e.g., depersonalization), incorporated in the DSM III-R criteria for panic attacks. Except for a small number of symptoms that are clearly more prevalent in complex partial seizures (i.e., motor automatisms, aphasia, and tactile or gustatory hallucinations) (Roth, 1959; Stein, 1986; Uhde et al., 1985), there is, therefore, considerable overlap between the two syndromes. The similarity of symptoms, including the secondary development of agoraphobic symptoms in patients with complex partial seizures, is intriguing given the fact that electrical stimulation of temporal lobe-limbic and amygdaloid regions in humans induces symptoms of fear, apprehension, anxiety, depersonalization, and derealization (Gloor, 1972; Jasper and Rasmussen, 1958; Mullan and Penfield, 1959). Intravenous procaine hydrochloride, an agent that has been reported to activate limbic substrates (Adamec et al., 1985), produces fear and anxiety in many patients with epilepsy (Adamec et al., 1980). In addition to ictal fear, anxiety is a common interictal experience in patients with temporal lobe epilepsy (Currie et al., 1971; Hermann, 1979; Roth and Harper, 1962). These data have led some investigators to suggest that both panic disorder and complex partial seizures may share in common a dysfunction within the temporal lobe substrate (Post and Uhde, 1984; Uhde et al., 1984c). It should be emphasized, however, that it has yet to be proved or disproved that the natural panic attacks of panic disorder are linked to electrical discharges in deep limbic substrates. In two separate studies (Roy-Byrne et al., 1986a; Stein and Uhde, 1989), our group found panic disorder patients to have normal electroencephalographic (EEG) activity after sleep deprivation with both standard and nasopharyngeal leads. We also failed to find any association between EEG activity and the experience of psychosensory symptoms (Stein and Uhde, 1989). Consistent with these observations, our group recently found carbamazepine, an anticonvulsant with particular efficacy in inhibiting limbic discharges, to be ineffective in the treatment of panic disorder patients with normal EEGs (Uhde et al., 1988). However, several case reports have been published of patients with atypical panic disorder plus abnormal

EEGs who have responded to anticonvulsants (Brodsky et al., 1985; Edlund et al., 1987; Weilburg et al., 1987). Thus it remains possible that a subgroup of panic disorder patients have a disturbance in limbic system function, including the possibility of abnormal discharges or excessive activation of neuronal firing within the temporal lobe and limbic substrates during panic attacks. Based on this conceptualization, one would predict that caffeine stimulates firing of limbic neurons and/or lowers seizure thresholds. This section therefore reviews both animal and human evidence in support of this prediction.

Extensive studies with a number of different animal models have consistently found caffeine and other methylxanthines, usually at high doses, to have proconvulsant properties (Ault and Wong, 1986; Greene et al., 1985; Ault et al., 1987; Seale et al., 1987; Velluci and Webster, 1984). Xanthine derivatives, including caffeine, also enhance amygdala kindling (Cain, 1981) and prolong amygdala-kindled seizures (Cain, 1981; Dragunow and Goddard, 1984). In humans, both caffeine and theophylline (Yarnell and Chu, 1975; for review, see Uhde, 1988) have been associated with seizures. In fact, caffeine's proconvulsant properties in humans have led some investigators to test its utility in the clinical setting. Two recent studies have found that caffeine increases seizure duration and may reduce the electrical current required to induce seizures in patients undergoing electroconvulsive therapy (Shapira et al., 1987; Coffey et al., 1987). As with the behavioral (i.e., panicogenic) effects of caffeine, both adenosinergic (Popoli et al., 1987) and benzodiazepine-GABA-ergic (Seale et al., 1987; Velluci and Webster, 1984) receptor systems have been implicated in the proconvulsant action of caffeine. Of interest, it has recently been shown that caffeine induces epileptiform activity in mouse hippocampal preparations (Ault et al., 1987), particularly the CA_3 area, which has a high density of both adenosine and benzodiazepine receptors. These latter findings are particularly provocative in that the CA_3 area has been described as the "primary generator" of epileptiform activity (Ault et al., 1987; Schneiderman, 1986; Wong and Traub, 1983) within the hippocampus. Thus it is possible that caffeine-induced panic attacks are associated with hippocampal discharges induced by caffeine's binding to adenosine receptors or benzodiazepine receptors or both.

CONCLUSIONS

This chapter presents an overview of the historical development and current use of the caffeine model of anxiety as a research tool in the investigation of panic disorder. Four criteria of an ideal chemical model of anxiety or panic have been proposed by two separate research teams (Gorman et al., 1987; Guttmacher et al., 1983).

As reviewed in Table 14–1, the criteria include "symptom convergence," "specificity," "clinical validation," and "replicability." Although these criteria have been partially criticized (Uhde and Tancer, 1988), they provide a pragmatic framework for evaluating chemical models of panic. In terms of symptom convergence, caffeine-induced panic attacks appear to resemble closely, if not mimic exactly, the quality of spontaneous panic attacks. Of course, few studies have systematically evaluated with objective measures the symptomatic overlap between chemically induced panic attacks and natural panic attacks. Even fewer studies have compared the quality and duration of panic attacks across a number of different chemical models. In a recent study conducted in our Section (Klein et al., unpublished manuscript), we compared the behavioral effects of metachlorophenylproperazine (mCPP), a serotonergic agonist, to the effects of caffeine. A self-rating scale was used to assess the similarity of both mCPP- and caffeine-induced anxiety states to each patient's own spontaneous panic attacks. Preliminary findings suggest that, whereas the caffeine-induced panic attacks were generally more severe than mCPP-induced panic attacks, the quality of both drug-induced anxiety states was similar to each patient's spontaneous-natural panic attacks. These data suggest that *different* chemical models can induce qualitatively *similar* panic attacks, presumably via different mechanisms of action.

In sufficient doses, caffeine and other methylxanthines can induce panic attacks in normal controls. However, panic disorder patients are more sensitive to the anxiogenic effects of caffeine. In another study conducted in our Section (Zohar et al., unpublished), we were unable to produce either panic attacks or an increase in obsessions or compulsions in obsessive–compulsive patients after the administration of caffeine. These findings support the concept of threshold specificity for caffeine-induced panic attacks in panic disorder, although additional studies will be required to confirm these preliminary findings.

In terms of clinical validation, both alprazolam and, perhaps, imipramine block caffeine-induced panic attacks. Obviously, additional studies with clinically effective and ineffective antipanic drugs will be necessary to evaluate extensively the caffeine model according to this criterion. Of interest, carbamazepine, a tricyclic anticonvulsant with a chemical structure similar to that of imipramine, was recently found by our group (Uhde et al., 1988) to be ineffective in the treatment of EEG-normal panic disorder patients. Carbamazepine, like caffeine, has a biochemical profile consistent with an adenosine antagonist and up-regulates adenosinergic receptors. Considered together, these observations provide both indirect evidence for the importance of adenosinergic systems in the anxiety disorders and further validation of the caffeine model of panic.

The criterion that chemical models should consistently induce panic attacks with repeated administration is particularly vulnerable to criticism (Uhde and Tancer, 1988). Nonetheless, our data indicate that panic disorder patients probably habituate more slowly than normal controls to the repeated administration of caffeine. Thus, to the extent that this represents a legitimate criterion of an ideal chemical model of panic disorder, our preliminary findings indicate that panic disorder patients have a response over time different from that of normal controls to the repeated administration of caffeine.

More important, perhaps, is the fact that acute and chronic caffeinism can mimic anxiety disorders. It is therefore important to evaluate all patients with anxiety symptomatology for the presence of excessive caffeine use, keeping in mind that both caffeine-intoxication and caffeine-withdrawal states (Uhde, 1988) are associated with many of the symptoms characteristic of panic and generalized anxiety disorders. Although current evidence suggests that panic disorder patients are more sensitive than normal controls to the panicogenic effects of caffeine, the mechanisms underlying this increased vulnerability have yet to be determined. Of interest, a recent study found that nonpanic patients with mitral valve prolapse syndrome are at greater risk than normal controls for developing caffeine-induced arrhythmias (Dobmeyer et al., 1983). Thus, just as the controversy regarding the relationship between mitral valve prolapse and panic disorder began to subside (Boudoulas et al., 1980; Dager et al., 1986; Gorman et al., 1981), a new twist to an old theme emerged: Are panic disorder patients with mitral valve prolapse at greater risk for developing caffeine-induced panic attacks and arrhythmias than panic disorder patients without mitral valve prolapse? The scientific process that stimulates such a hypothesis underscores a certain reality about this neuropsychiatric syndrome. That is, the psychological, behavioral, and neurobiological aspects of this illness are intertwined in an intimate and delicate matrix. Future research involving a multidisciplinary approach certainly will be required to unlock the pathogenetic secret of panic disorder.

In terms of the neurobiology of panic disorder, the data reviewed in this chapter suggest that caffeine-induced anxiety and panic represent an excellent chemical model of anxiety and panic disorder. As such, the model provides a valuable clinical investigative tool with great clinical and research potential. New techniques should soon be available to make it possible to dissect which of caffeine's effects (i.e., noradrenergic, dopaminergic, adenosinergic, or benzodiazepine) are responsible for its panicogenic effects. The comparison of caffeine-induced panic with other chemical models of panic should greatly enhance our understanding of the anatomical and neurotransmitter pathways mediating pathological anxiety.

REFERENCES

Adamec RE, Stark-Adamec C, Perrin R, Livingston KE (1980). In Girgis M, Kiloh LG (eds): "Limbic Epilepsy and the Dyscontrol Syndrome." Amsterdam: Elsevier North Holand, p 117.

Adamec R, Stark-Adamec C, Saint-Hilaire J, Livingston K (1985): Basic science and clinical aspects of procaine HCl as a limbic system excitant. Prog. Neuropsychopharmacol. Biol. Psychiatry 9:109–119.

Anden N-E, Jackson DM (1975): Locomotor activity stimulation in rats produced by dopamine in the nucleus accumbens: Potentiation by caffeine. J Pharm Pharmacol 27:666–670.

Aronson TA, Logue CM (1988): Phenomenology of panic attacks: A descriptive study of panic disorder patients' self-reports. J Clin Psychiatry 49:8–13.

Atuk NO, Blaydes MC, Westervelt FB Jr, Wood JE Jr (1967): Effect of aminophylline on urinary excretion of epinephrine and norepinephrine in man. Circulation 35:745–753.

Ault B, Olney MA, Joyner JL, Boyer CE, Notrica MA, Soroko FE, Wong CM (1987): Proconvulsant actions of theophylline and caffeine in the hippocampus: Implications in the management of temporal lobe epilepsy. Brain Res 426:92–102.

Ault B, Wong CM (1986): Adenosine inhibits epileptiform activity arising in hippocampal area CA3. Br J Pharmacol 87:695–703.

Ballenger JC (1986): Pharmacotherapy of the panic disorders. J Clin Psychiatry 47:27–32.

Barone JJ, Roberts H (1984): Human consumption of caffeine. In Dews PB (ed): "Caffeine: Perspectives From Recent Research." New York: Springer-Verlag, pp 59–73.

Barlow DH (1988): "Anxiety and Its Disorders: The Nature and Treatment of Anxiety and Panic." New York: The Guilford Press.

Battig K, Buzzi R (1986): Effect of coffee on the speed of subject-paced information processing. Neuropsychobiology 16:126–130.

Bellet S, Roman L, DeCastro O, Kim KE, Kershbaum A (1969): Effect of coffee ingestion on catecholamine release. Metabolism 18:288–291.

Bennett WM, Walker RG, Henry JP, Kincaid-Smith P (1983): Chronic interstitial nephropathy in mice induced by psychosocial stress potentiation by caffeine. Nephron 34:110–113.

Berkowitz BA, Tarver JH, Spector S (1970): Release of norepinephrine in the central nervous system by theophylline and caffeine. Eur J Pharmacol 10:64–71.

Berne RM, Di Marco JP, Belardinelli L (1984): Dromotropic effects of adenosine and adenosine antagonists in the treatment of cardiac arrhythmias involving the atrioventricular node. Circulation 69:1195–1197.

Bonn JA, Harrison J, Rees L (1973): Lactate infusion in the treatment of 'free-floating' anxiety. J Can Psychiatr Assoc 18:41–46.

Boudoulas H, Reynolds JC, Mazzaferri E, Wooley CF (1980): Metabolic studies in mitral valve prolapse syndrome: A neuroendocrine-cardiovascular process. Circulation 61:1200–1205.

Boulenger J-P, Bierer LM, Uhde TW, Silberman EK, Post RM (1986): Psychosensory phenomena in panic and affective disorders. In Shagass C, Josiassen RC, Bridger WH, Weiss KJ, Stoff D, Simpson GM (ed): "Biological Psychiatry 1985." New York: Elsevier Science Publishing Co., pp 463–465.

Boulenger J-P, Patel J, Marangos PJ (1982): Effects of caffeine and theophylline on adenosine and benzodiazepine receptors in human brain. Neurosci Lett 30: 161.

Boulenger J-P, Patel J, Post RM, Parma AM, Marangos PJ (1983): Chronic caffeine consumption increases the number of brain adenosine receptors. Life Sci 32: 1135–1142.

Boulenger J-P, Salem N Jr, Marangos PJ, Uhde TW (1987): Plasma adenosine levels: Measurement in humans and relationship to the anxiogenic effects of caffeine. Psychiatry Res 21:247–255.

Boulenger J-P, Uhde TW (1982): Caffeine consumption and anxiety: Preliminary results of a survey comparing patients with anxiety disorders and normal controls. Psychopharmacol Bull 18:53–57.

Boulenger J-P, Uhde TW, Wolff EA III, Post RM (1984): Increased sensitivity to caffeine in patients with panic disorder. Arch Gen Psychiatry 41:1067–1071.

Bradwejn J, Meterissian GB, Koszycki D (1988): Cholecystokinin tetrapeptide induces panic attacks in patients suffering from panic disorder. Paper presented at the 141st Annual Meeting of the American Psychiatric Association, May 10, 1988.

Breggin PR (1964): The psychophysiology of anxiety: With a review of the literature concerning adrenaline. J Nervous Mental Dis 139:558–568.

Brezinova V (1974): Effects of caffeine on sleep: EEG study in late middle age people. Br J Pharmacol 1: 203–208.

Brodsky L, Zuniga JS, Casenos ER, et al. (1985): Refractory anxiety: a masked epileptiform disorder? Psychiatr J Univ Ottawa 8:42–45.

Butcher RW, Sutherland EW (1962): Adenosine 3',5'-phosphate in biological materials. J Biol Chem 237: 1244–1250.

Cain DP (1981): Kindling: Recent studies and new directions. In Wada JA (ed): "Kindling 2." New York: Raven Press, pp 55–66.

Carr DB, et al. (1986): Neuroendocrine correlates of lactate-induced anxiety and their response to chronic alprazolam therapy. Am J Psychiatry 143:483–494.

Charney DS, Heninger GR, Jatlow PI (1985): Increased anxiogenic effects of caffeine in panic disorder. Arch Gen Psychiatry 42:233–243.

Charney DS, Heninger GR, Redmond DE Jr (1983): Yohimbine induced anxiety and increased noradrenergic function in humans: effects of diazepam and clonidine. Life Sci 33:19–29.

Charney DS, Heninger GR, Sternberg DE (1982): Assessment of alpha-2 adrenergic autoreceptor function in humans: Effects of oral yohimbine. Life Sci 30:2033–2041.

Charney DS, Woods SW, Goodman WK, Heninger GR (1987): Serotonin function in anxiety. II. Effects of the serotonin agonist mCPP in panic disorder patients and healthy subjects. Psychopharmacology 92:14–24.

Cloninger CR, Martin RL, Clayton P, et al. (1981): A blind follow-up and family study of anxiety neurosis: Preliminary analysis of the St Louis 500. In Klein DF, Rabkin J (eds): "Anxiety: New Research and Changing Concepts." New York, Raven Press.

Cobb S (1974): Physiologic changes in men whose jobs were abolished. J Psychosom Res 18:245–258.

Coffey CE, Weiner RD, Hinkle PE, Cress M, Daughtry G, Wilson WH (1987): Augmentation of ECT seizures with caffeine. Biol Psychiatry 22:637–649.

Cohen ME, White PD (1949): Life situations, emotions and neurocirculatory asthenia (anxiety neurosis, neurasthenia, effort syndrome). Res Nervous Mental Dis 29:832–869.

Crawley JN, Patel J, Marangos PJ (1981): Behavioral characterization of two long lasting adenosine analogs: Sedative properties and interaction with diazepam. Life Sci 29:2623–2630.

Crawley JN, Patel J, Marangos PJ (1983): Adenosine uptake inhibitors potentiate the sedative effects of adenosine. Neurosci Lett 36:169–174.

Crowe RR, Noyes R, Pauls DL, Slymen DJ (1983): A family study of panic disorder. Arch Gen Psychiatry 40:1065–1069.

Currie S, Heathfield KWG, Henson RA, Scott DR (1971): Clinical course and prognosis of temporal lobe epilepsy: A survey of 666 patients. Brain 94:173.

Dager SR, Comess KA, Saal AK, Dunner DL (1986): Mitral valve prolapse in a psychiatric setting: Diagnostic assessment research and clinical implications. Integr Psychiatry 4:211–223.

Daly JW, Bruns RF, Snyder SN (1981): Adenosine receptors in the central nervous system: Relationship to the central actions of methylxanthines. Life Sci 28:2083–2097.

Daval JL, Barberis C, Verp P (1984): In vitro and in vivo displacement of [^{3}H]diazepam binding by purine derivatives in developing rat brain. Dev Pharmacol Ther 7:169–176.

Derogatis LR (1977): "SCL-90-R Manual: I. Scoring and Procedure Manual for the SCL-90-R." Baltimore: Clinical Psychometrics Research Unit.

Dillon DJ, Gorman JM, Liebowitz MR, Fyer AJ, Klein DF (1987): Measurement of lactate-induced panic and anxiety. Psychiatry Res 20:97–105.

Di Marco JP, Sellers TD, Berne RM, West GA, Belardinelli L (1983): Adenosine: Electrophysiologic effects and therapeutic use for terminating paroxysmal supraventricular tachycardia. Circulation 68:1254–1263.

Dobmeyer DJ, Stine RA, Leier CV, Greenberg R, Schaal SF (1983): The arrhythmogenic effects of caffeine in human beings. N Engl J Med 308:814–816.

Doreen B (1977): Effects of drugs on rats exposed to cold-restraint stress. J Pharm Pharmacol 29:748–751.

Dorow R, Horowski R, Paschelke G, Amin M, Braestrup C (1983): Severe anxiety induced by FG 7142, a beta-carboline ligand for benzodiazepine receptors. Lancet ii:98–99.

Dragunow M, Goddard GV (1984): Adenosine modulation of amygdala kindling. Exp Neurol 84:654–656.

Dragunow M, Goddard GV, Laverty R (1985): Is adenosine an endogenous anticonvulsant? Epilepsia 26:480–487.

Edlund MJ, Swann AC, Clothier J (1987): Patients with panic attacks and abnormal EEG results. Am J Psychiatry 144:508–509.

Elkins RN, Rapoport JL, Zahn TP, Buchsbaum MS, Weingartner H, Kopin IJ, Langer D, Johnson C (1981): Acute effects of caffeine in normal prepubertal boys. Am J Psychiatry 138:178–183.

Emboden (1979): "Narcotic Plants." New York: Macmillan Publishing Company.

File SE, Bond AJ, Lister RG (1982): Interaction between effects of caffeine and lorazepam in performance tests and self-ratings. J Clin Psychopharmacol 2:102–106.

Fontaine P, Lubetsky M, Chamberlin K (1978): Anxiety and depression associated with caffeinism among psychiatric inpatients. Am J Psychiatry 963–966.

Fredholm BB (1980): Are methylxanthine effects due to antagonism of endogenous adenosine. Trends Pharmacol Sci 1:129–132.

Fredholm BB (1982): Adenosine actions and adenosine receptors after one week treatment with caffeine. Acta Physiol Scand 115:283–286.

Fredholm BB, Herrera-Marschitz M, Jonzon B, Lindstrom K, Ungerstedt U (1983): On the mechanism by which methylxanthines enhance apomorphine induced rotation in the rat. Pharmacol Biochem Behav 19:535–541.

Freud S (1959): On the grounds for detaching a particular syndrome from neurasthenia under the description "anxiety neurosis." In: "The Standard Edition of the Complete Psychological Works of Sigmund Freud, Vol 3," London: Hogarth Press, p 90.

Frohlich ED, Tarazi RC, Duston HP (1969): Hyperdynamic beta-adrenergic circulatory state: Increased beta-receptor responsiveness. Arch Intern Med 123:1–7.

Gagnon DJ, Boucher P (1972): Effects of caffeine on central monoamine neurons. J Pharm Pharmacol 24:155–158.

Galloway MP, Roth RH (1983): The neuropharmacology of 3-isobutylmethylxanthine: Effects on central noradrenergic systems in vivo. J Pharmacol Exp Ther 227:1–8.

Garfield SI, Gershon S, Sletten I, Sundland DM, Ballou S (1967): Chemically induced anxiety. Int J Neuropsychiatry 3:426–33.

Gilbert RM (1976): Caffeine as a drug of abuse. In Gibbons RJ, Israel Y, Kalant H, Popham R, Schmidt W, Smart R (eds): "Research Advances in Alcohol and Drug Problems." Wiley: New York. Vol III, pp 49–176.

Gilliland K, Andress D (1981): Ad lib caffeine consumption symptoms of caffeinism and academic performance. Am J Psychiatry 131:512–514.

Gloor P (1972): In Eleftheriou BE (ed): "The Neurobiology of the Amygdala, Advances in Behavioral Biology, Vol 2." New York: Plenum, p 423.

Gorman JM, et al. (1984a): Response to hyperventilation in a group of patients with panic disorder. Am J Psychiatry 141:857–861.

Gorman JM, Fyer AF, Glocklich J, King D, Klein DF (1981): Effects of sodium lactate on patients with panic disorder and mitral valve prolapse. Am J Psychiatry 138:247–249.

Gorman JM, Fyer MR, Liebowitz MR, Klein DF (1987): Pharmacologic provocation of panic attacks. In Meltzer HY (ed): "Psychopharmacoloty: A Third Generation of Progress." New York: Raven Press, pp 985–998.

Gorman JM, Martinez JM, Liebowitz MR, et al. (1984b): Hypoglycemia and panic attacks. Am J Psychiatry 141:101–102.

Greden JF (1974): Anxiety or caffeinism: A diagnostic dilemma. Am J Psychiatry 131:1089–1092.

Greden JF, Fontaine P, Lubetsky M, Chamberlin K (1978): Anxiety and depression associated with caffeinism among psychiatric inpatients. Am J Psychiatry 135:963–966.

Green RW, Haas HL, Herman A (1985): Effects of caffeine on hippocampal pyramidal cells in vitro. Br J Pharmacol 85:163–169.

Griez EJL, Lousberg H, van den Hout MA, van der Molen GM (1987): CO$_2$ vulnerability in panic disorder. Psychiatry Res 20:87–95.

Griez E, van den Hout MA (1983): Treatment of phobophobia by exposure to CO^2-induced anxiety symptoms. J Nervous Mental Dis 171:506–508.

Gurguis G, Uhde TW (in press): Panic disorder: New research directions In Norton GR, Walker JR, Ross C (ed): "Panic Disorder and Agoraphobia: A Guide for the Practitioner." New York: MacMillan.

Guttmacher LB, Murphy DL, Insel TR (1983): Pharmacologic models of anxiety. Comp Psychiatry 24:312–326.

Haefley W (1983): The biological basis of benzodiazepine actions. J Psychoactive Drugs 15:19–39.

Harris EL, Noyes R, Crowe RR, Chaudhry DR (1983): Family study of agoraphobia. Arch Gen Psychiatry 40:1061–1064.

Henry JP, Stephens PM (1980): Caffeine as an intensifier of stress-induced hormonal and pathophysiological changes in mice. Pharmacol Biochem Behav 13:719–727.

Hermann BP (1979): Psychopathology in epilepsy and learned helplessness. Med Hypoth 5:723–729.

Hoffman WE, Satinover I, Miletich DJ, Albrecht RF, Gans BJ (1982): Cardiovascular changes during sodium nitroprusside or adenoside triphosphate infusion in the rat. Anesth Analg (Cleveland) 61:99–103.

Insel TR, Ninan PT, Aloi J, Jimerson DC, Skolnick P, Paul SM (1984): A benzodiazepine receptor-mediated model of anxiety: Studies in nonhuman primates and clinical implications. Arch Gen Psychiatry 41:741–750.

Jasper HH, Rasmussen T (1958): Res Publ Assoc Nervous Mental Dis 36:316.

Kaminkawa Y, Cline WH Jr, Su C (1983): Possible roles of purinergic modulation in pathogenesis of some diseases: Hypertension and asthma. In Daly JW, Kuroda Y, Phillis JW, Shimizu H, Ui M (eds): "Physiology and Pharmacology of Adenosine Derivatives." New York: Raven Press, pp 189–196.

Katon W, Sheehan DV, Uhde TW (1988): Panic disorder: A treatable problem. Patient Care 22:148–173.

Kelly D, Mitchell-Heggs N, Sherman D (1971): Anxiety and the effects of sodium lactate assessed clinically and physiologically. Br J Psychiatry 119:129–141.

Klabunde RE (1983): Dipyramidole inhibition of adenosine metabolism in human blood. Eur J Pharmacol 93:21–26.

Klabunde RE, Althouse DG (1981): Adenosine metabolism in dog whole blood: Effects of dipyridamole. Life Sci 28:2631–2641.

Klein DF (1964): Delineation of two drug-responsive anxiety syndromes. Psychopharmacologia 5:397–408.

Klein DF, Rabkin J (1981): "Anxiety: New Research and Changing Concepts." New York: Raven Press.

Klein E, Zohar J, Geraci MF, Murphy DC, Uhde TW (in press): Anxiogenic effects of mCPP in patients with panic disorder: Comparison to caffeine's anxiogenic effects.

Lader M, Matthews A (1970): Physiological changes during spontaneous panic attacks. J Psychosom Res 14:377–382.

Lane JD (1983): Caffeine and cardiovascular responses to stress. Psychosom Med 45:447–451.

Latimer P (1977): Carbon dioxide as a reciprocal inhibitor in the treatment of neurosis. J Behav Ther Exp Psychiatry 8:83–85.

Leckman JF, Weissman MM, Merikangas KR, Pauls DL, Prusoff BA (1983): Panic disorder and major depression: increased risk of depression, alcoholism, panic and phobic disorders in families of depressed probands with panic disorder. Arch Gen Psychiatry 40:1055–1060.

Lee MA, Cameron OG, Greden JF (1985): Anxiety and caffeine consumption in people with anxiety disorders. Psychiatry Res 15:211–217.

Levi L (1967): The effect of coffee on the function of the sympathoadrenomedullary system in man. Acta Med Scand 181:431–438.

Liebowitz MR, et al. (1984): Lactate provocation of panic attacks: I. Clinical and behavioral finding. Arch Gen Psychiatry 41:764–770.

Londos CD, Cooper MF, Wolff J (1980): Subclasses of external adenosine receptors. Proc Natl Acad Sci USA 77:2551–2554.

Marangos PJ, Boulenger J-P, Patel J (1984): Effects of chronic caffeine on brain adenosine receptors: Anatomical and ontogenetic studies. Life Sci 34:899–907.

Marangos PJ, Martino AM, Paul SM, Skolnick P (1981): The benzodiazepines and inosine antagonize caffeine-induced seizures. Psychopharmacology 72:269–273.

Margraf J, Ehlers A, Roth WT (1986): Sodium lactate infusions and panic attacks: a review and critique. Psychosom Med 48:23–51.

Mattila MJ, Palva E, Savolamen K (1982): Caffeine antagonizes diazepam effect in man. Med Biol 60:121–123.

McManamy MC, Schube PG (1936): Caffeine intoxication: Report of a case the symptoms of which amounted to a psychosis. N Engl J Med 215:616–620.

Mellman TA, Uhde TW (1987): Obsessive-compulsive symptoms in panic disorder. Am J Psychiatry 144:1573–1576.

Mikkelsen EJ (1978): Caffeine and schizophrenia. J Clin Psychiatry 39:732–735.

Mueller EA, Murphy DL, Sunderland T (1985): Neuroendocrine effects of M-Chlorophenylpiperazine, a serotonin agonist in humans. J Clin Endocrinol Metab 61:1179–84.

Mullan S, Penfield W (1959): Illusions of comparative

interpretation and emotion. Arch Neurol Psychiatry 81:269.

Muller PJ, Vernikos-Danellis J (1970): Effect of environmental temperature on the toxicity of caffeine and dextroamphetamine in mice. Pharmacol Exp Ther 171:153–158.

Nesse RM, Cameron OG, Curtis GC, McCann DS, Huber-Smith MJ (1984): Adrenergic function in patients with panic anxiety. Arch Gen Psychiatry 41:771–776.

Newberg LA, Milde JW, Michenfeldar JD (1985): Cerebral and systemic effects of hypotension induced by adenosine or ATP in dogs. Anesthesiology 62:429–436.

Niemand DS, Martinell S, Arvidsson S, Svedmyr N, Ekstrom-Jodal B (1984): Aminophylline inhibition of diazepam sedation: Is adenosine blockade of GABA-receptors the mechanism? Lancet i:463–464.

Ninan PT, Insel TM, Cohen RM, Cook JM, Skolnick P, Paul SM (1982): Benzodiazepine receptor-mediated experimental "anxiety" in primates. Science 218: 1332–1334.

Noyes R Jr, Crowe RR, Harris EL, Hamra BJ, McChesney CM, Chaudhry DR (1986): Relationship between panic disorder and agoraphobia: A family study. Arch Gen Psychiatry 43:227–232.

Okuma T, Matsuoka H, Matsue Y, Toyomura K (1982): Model insomnia by methylphenidate and caffeine and use in the evaluation of temazepam. Psychopharmacology 76:201–208.

Olpe HR, Jones RSG, Steinmann MW (1983): The locus coeruleus: Actions of psychoactive drugs. Experientia 39:242–249.

Phillis JW, Kostopoulos GK (1975): Adenosine as a putative transmitter in the cerebral cortex. Studies with potentiators and antagonists. Life Sci 17:1085–1094.

Phillis JW, Wu PH (1981): The role of adenosine and its nucleotides in central synaptic transmission. Prog Neurobiol 16:187–239.

Pitts FN Jr, McClure JN (1967): Lactate metabolism in anxiety neurosis. N Engl J Med 277:1329–1336.

Popoli PS, Sagratella, Scotti de Carolis A (1987): An EEG and behavioural study on the excitatory properties of caffeine in rabbits. Arch Int Pharmacodyn 290:5–15.

Post RM, Uhde TW (1984): Carbamazepine in the treatment of mood and anxiety disorders: implications for limbic system mechanisms. In Trimble M, Zarifian E (eds): "Psychopharmacology of the Limbic System." New York: Oxford University Press, pp 134–147.

Rainey JM, Aleem A, Ortiz A, Yergamio V, Pohl R, Berchou R (1987): A laboratory procedure for the induction of flashbacks. Am J Psychiatry 144:1317–1319.

Rainey JM, Ettedgui E, Pohl B, Balon R, Weinberg P, Yelonek S, Berchou R (1984a): The beta-receptor. Isoproteranol anxiety states. Psychopathology 17[Suppl 3]:40–51.

Rainey JM, Pohl RB, Williams M, Knitter E, Freedman RR, Ettedqui E (1984b): A comparison of lactate and isoproteranol anxiety states. Psychopathology 17 [Suppl 3]:74–82.

Rall TW (1985): Central nervous system stimulants: The methylxanthines. In Gilman AG, Goodman LS, Rall TW, Murad FS (eds): "Goodman and Gilman's The Pharmacological Basis of Therapeutics." New York: MacMillan Publishing Co., pp 589–603.

Rapoport JL, Elkins R, Neims A, Zahn T, Berg C (1981a): Behavioral and autonomic effects of caffeine in normal boys. Dev Pharmacol 3:74–82.

Rapoport JL, Jensvold M, Elkins R, Buchsbaum MS, Weingartner H, Ludlow C, Zahn TP, Berg CJ, Neims AH (1981b): Behavioral and cognitive effects of caffeine in boys and adult males. J Nervous Mental Dis 169:726–732.

Rasmussen SA, Tsuang MT (1986): Clinical characteristics and family history in DSM-III obsessive-compulsive disorder. Am J Psychiatry 143:317–322.

Redmond DE Jr, Huang YH (1979): New Evidence for a locus coeruleus connection with anxiety. Life Sci 25: 2149–2162.

Robertson D, Frolick JC, Carr RK, Watson JT, Hollifield JW, Shand DG, Oates JA (1978): Effects of caffeine on plasma renin activity, catecholamines, and blood pressure. N Engl J Med 298:181–185.

Roth M (1959): The phobic-anxiety-depersonalization syndrome. Proc R Soc Med 52:587–596.

Roth M, Harper M (1962): Compr Psychiatry 3:215.

Roy-Byrne PP, Uhde TW, Post RM (1986a): Effects of one night's sleep deprivation on mood and behavior in patients with panic disorder: Comparison with depressed patients and normal controls. Arch Gen Psychiatry 43:899.

Roy-Byrne PP, Uhde TW, Sock DA, Linnoila M, Post RM (1986b): Plasma HVA and anxiety in patients with panic disorder. Biol Psychiatry 21:849–853.

Saletu B, Allen M, Itil TM (1974): The effect of Coca-Cola, caffeine antidepressants, and chlorpromazine on objective and subjective sleep parameters. Pharmakopsychiatr Neuropsychopharmakol 254:307–321.

Sattin A, Rall TW (1970): The effect of adenosine and adenine nucleotides on the cyclic AMP content of guinea-pig cerebral cortex slices. Mol Pharmacol 6: 13–23.

Schneiderman JH (1986): Differences in penicillin-induced synchronous bursts in the CA1 and CA3 regions of the hippocampus. Epilepsia Vol. 27:3–9.

Schweizer E, Winokur A, Rickels K (1986): Insulin-induced hypoglycemia and panic attacks. Am J Psychiatry 143:654–655.

Seale TW, Carney JM, Rennert OM, Flux M, Skolnick P (1987): Coincidence of seizure susceptibility to caffeine and to the benzodiazepine inverse agonist, DMCM, in SWR and CBA inbred mice. Pharmacol Biochem Behav 16:381–387.

Shapira B, Lerer B, Gilboa D, Drexler H, Kugelmass S, Calev A (1987): Facilitation of ECT by caffeine pretreatment. Am J Psychiatry 144:1199–1202.

Siever LJ, Uhde TW (1984): New studies and perspectives on the noradrenergic receptor system in depression: Effects of the alpha-2-adrenergic agonist clonidine. Biol Psychiatry 19:131–156.

Skolnick P, Crawley JN, Glowa JR, Paul SM (1984): Beta-carboline-induced anxiety states. Psychopathology 17 [Suppl 3]:52–60.

Snyder SH, Katims JJ, Annau Z, Bruns RF, Daly JW (1981): Adenosine receptors and the behavioral actions of methylxanthines. Proc Natl Acad Sci USA 78:3260–3264.

Sollevi A, Ostergren J, Hjemdahl P, Fredholm BB, Fagrell B (1984): The effect of dipyridamole on plasma adenosine levels and skin micro-circulation in man. Adv Exp Med Biol 165:363.

Stein MB (1986): Panic disorder and medical illness. Psychomatics 27:833–838.

Stein MB, Shea CA, Uhde TW (1989): Social phobic symptoms in patients with panic disorder: Clinical and theoretical implications. Am J Psychiatry 146: 235–238.

Stein MB, Uhde TW (1988a): Panic disorder and major depression: A tale of two syndromes. In Coryell W, Winokur G (eds): "Psychiatric Clinics of North America." Philadelphia: W.B. Saunders Co., Vol 11, pp 441–461.

Stein MB, Uhde TW (1988b): Cortisol response to clonidine in panic disorders: Comparison with depressed patients and normal controls. Biol Psychiatry 24:322–330.

Stein MB, Uhde TW (1989): Infrequent occurrence of EEG abnormalities in panic disorder. Am J Psychiatry 146:517–520.

Stillner VM, Popkin MK, Pierce CM (1978): Caffeine-induced delirium during prolonged competitive stress. Am J Psychiatry 135:855–856.

Stirt JA (1981): Aminophylline is a diazepam antagonist. Anesth Analg (Paris) 60:767–768.

Stone TW (1981): Physiological roles for adenosine and adenosine-5′-triphosphate in the nervous system. Neuroscience 6:523–555.

Stoner GR, Skirboll LR, Werkman J, Hommer DW (1988): Preferential effects of caffeine on limbic and cortical dopamine systems. Biol Psychiatry 23:761–768.

Sutherland EW, Rall TW (1958): Fractionation and characterization of cyclic adenine rebonueotide formed by tissue particles. J Biol Chem 232:1077–1091.

Torgersen S (1983): Genetic factors in anxiety disorders. Arch Gen Psychiatry 40:1085–1089.

Uhde TW (1986a): Treating panic and anxiety. Psychiatr Ann 16:536–541.

Uhde TW (1986b): Caffeine and yohimbine challenges in patients with panic disorder. Paper presented at the Panic Disorder Biological Research Workshop, Washington, DC, April 14–16, 1986 (Abstract 4418).

Uhde TW (1987a): Panic disorder and agoraphobia. In Rakel RE (ed): "Conn's Current Therapy." Philadelphia: W.B. Saunders, pp 949–953.

Uhde TW (1987b): Noradrenergic studies in anxiety. In Sen AK, Lee T (eds): "Receptors and Ligands in Psychiatry and Neurology." London: Cambridge University Press, Vol III, pp 375–387.

Uhde TW (1988): Caffeine: Practical facts for the psychiatrist. In Roy-Byrne PP (ed): "Anxiety: New Research Findings for the Clinician." Washington, DC: American Psychiatric Press.

Uhde TW, Boulenger J-P, Post RM, Siever LJ, Vittone BJ, Jimerson DC, Post RM (1984a): Fear and anxiety: Relationship to noradrenergic function. Psychopathology 17(3):8–23.

Uhde TW, Boulenger J-P, Roy-Byrne PP, Vittone BJ, Post RM (1985): Longitudinal course of panic disorder: Clinical and biological considerations. Prog Neuropsychopharmacol Biol Psychiatry 9:39–51.

Uhde TW, Boulenger J-P, Vittone B, Jimerson DC, Post RM (1984b): Caffeine: Relationship to human anxiety, plasma MHPG and cortisol. Psychopharmacol Bull 20: 426–430.

Uhde TW, Joffe RT, Jimerson DC, Post RM (1988): Normal urinary free cortisol and plasma MHPG in panic disorder: Clinical and theoretical implications. Biol Psychiatry 23:575–585.

Uhde TW, Nemiah J (1988): Panic and generalized anxiety disorders. In Kaplan HI, Sadock BJ (eds): "Comprehensive Textbook of Psychiatry, 5th ed." Baltimore: Williams and Wilkins.

Uhde TW, Post RM, Ballenger JC, Boulenger J-P (1984c): Carbamazepine (Tegretol®) in the treatment of neuropsychiatric disorders. In Emrich HM, Okuma T, Miller A (eds): "Anticonvulsants in Affective Disorders." Amsterdam: Excerpta Medica International Congress Series 626, pp 116–113.

Uhde TW, Stein MB, Post RM (1988): Lack of efficacy of carbamazepine in panic disorder. Am J Psychiatry 145:1104–1109.

Uhde TW, Tancer ME (1988): Chemical models of panic: A review and critique. Tyrer P (ed): "Psychopharmacology of Anxiety." Oxford, England: Oxford University Press, pp 110–131.

Uhde TW, Vittone BJ, Post RM (1984d): Glucose tolerance testing in panic disorder. Am J Psychiatry 141: 1461–1463.

Uhde TW, Roy-Byrne PP, Post RM (1986): Panic disorder and major depressive disorder: Biological relationship. In Shagass C, Josiassen RC, Bridger WH, Weiss KJ, Staff D, Simpson GM (eds): "Biol Psychiatry 1985." New York: Elsevier Science Publishing Co., pp 472–474.

van den Hout MA, Griez E (1984): Cardiovascular and subjective responses to inhalation of carbon dioxide: A controlled test with anxious patients. Psychotherapy and Psychosomatics 37:75–82.

Vellucci SV, Webster RA (1984): Antagonism of caffeine-induced seizures in mice by RO 15-1788. Eur J Pharmacol 97:289–293.

Vestal RE, Eriksson CE, Musser B, Ozaki L, Halter JB (1983): Effect of intravenous aminophylline on plasma levels of catecholamines and related cardiovascular and metabolic responses in man. Circulation 67:162–171.

Victor B, Lubetsky M, Greden J (1981): Somatic manifestation of caffeinism. J Clin Psychiatry 42:185–188.

Von Bortsel RW, Wurtman RJ, Conlay LA (1983): Chronic caffeine consumption potentiates the hypotensive action of circulating adenosine. Life Sci 32: 1151–1158.

Waldeck B (1971): Some effects of caffeine and aminophylline on the turnover of catecholamines in the brain. J Pharm Pharmacol 23:824–830.

Watt AH (1984): Hypertrophic cardiomyopathy: A disease of impaired adenosine-mediated autoregulation of the heart. Lancet i:1271–1273.

Watt AH (1985): Hypothesis. Sick sinus syndrome: An adenosine-mediated disease. Lancet i:786–788.

Weilburg JB, Bear DM, Sachs G (1987): Three patients with concomitant panic attacks and seizure disorder: possible clues to the neurology of anxiety. Am J Psychiatry 144:1053–1056.

Winstead DK (1976): Coffee consumption among psychiatric inpatients. Am J Psychiatry 133:1447–1450.

Wong RKS, Traub RI (1983): Synchronized burst discharge in disinhibited hippocampal slice. I. Initiation in the CA2-CA3 region. J Neurophysiol 49:442–458.

Woods SW, Charney DS, Loke J, Goodman WK, Redmond DE, Heninger GR (1986): Carbon dioxide sensitivity in panic anxiety: Ventilatory and anxiogenic responses to carbon dioxide in healthy subjects and patients with panic anxiety before and after alprazolam treatment. Arch Gen Psychiatry 43:900–909.

Yano S, Isobe Y, Harada M (1982): The etiology of caffeine-induced aggravation of gastric lesions in rats exposed to restraint plus water-immersion stress. J Pharmacobiodyn 5:485–494.

Yarnell PR, Chu NJ (1975): Focal seizures and aminophylline. Neurology 25:819–822.

Zohar J, Mueller EA, Insel TR, Zohar-Kadouch RC, Murphy DL (1987): Serotonergic responsivity in obsessive-compulsive disorder. Arch Gen Psychiatry 44:946–951.

Brain Imaging Studies

15

PET, Panic Disorder, and Normal Anticipatory Anxiety

ERIC M. REIMAN, MD

Department of Psychiatry, Washington University School of Medicine, St. Louis, Missouri 63110

INTRODUCTION

To establish the pathophysiology of psychiatric disorders, researchers must be able to investigate the local functions of the living human brain. Positron emission tomography (PET) is a brain imaging technique that safely provides quantitative, regional measurements of biochemical and physiological processes. Because of its capabilities, PET is well suited to the study of psychiatric disorders.

PET may have particular promise in the study of panic disorder. It has been demonstrated that sodium lactate and several other agents can precipitate an anxiety attack in patients with panic disorder (Pitts and McClure, 1967; Fink et al., 1971; Kelly et al., 1971; Liebowitz et al., 1984, 1985; Reiman et al., 1984; Gorman et al., 1984; Rainey et al., 1984; Charney et al., 1984, 1985). It has also been shown that, when antipanic medications block naturally occurring anxiety attacks, they also block the attacks induced by lactate (Liebowitz et al., 1984, 1986). Lactate and other panicogenic agents thus provide an experimental framework for investigating the elements necessary for the generation and treatment of anxiety attacks. This chapter reviews PET—its components, capabilities, and limitations—and its application to the study of panic disorder and normal anticipatory anxiety. (Thus, it extends an earlier review of these topics [Reiman, 1987].)

This chapter is decidedly parochial: It emphasizes the research now being conducted in our PET laboratory at Washington University. For a more complete review of the field, the reader is encouraged to examine the perspectives of other PET researchers (see, for instance, Reivich and Alavi, 1985) and to review other functional brain imaging studies of anxiety and anxiety disorders [for instance, PET studies of anticipatory anxiety (Reivich et al., 1983), phobic anxiety (Mountz et al., 1988), obsessive–compulsive disorder (Baxter et al., 1987, 1988), and generalized anxiety disorder (Buchsbaum et al., 1987) as well as single photon emission computed tomography (SPECT) studies of lactate-induced panic (Stewart et al., 1988) and yohimbine-induced anxiety (Woods et al., 1988)].

PET

To understand the prospects for studying panic disorder and other psychiatric conditions with PET, it is helpful to understand the major components of PET studies (Table 15–1). In reviewing these components, this chapter emphasizes those issues that have been particularly important to the functional brain mapping studies performed in our laboratory.

Positron-Emitting Radiotracers

PET requires the use of positron-emitting radiotracers. These are pharmacological and physiological compounds that are labeled with positron-emitting radionuclides, such as ^{15}O, ^{13}N, ^{11}C, and ^{18}F. Although a large number of radiotracers have been synthesized, some are more suitable than others for the computation of valid biochemical and physiological processes in the brain. Some well known examples include ^{15}O-water, which is used in our laboratory to measure cerebral blood flow (Raichle, 1983a; Herscovitch et al., 1983);

Neurobiology of Panic Disorder, Pages 245–270

TABLE 15–1.
Important Components of PET Studies

Positron-emitting radiotracer
PET imaging system
Tracer-kinetic model
Anatomical localization
Data analysis
Experimental design

[18]F-fluorodeoxyglucose, which is used by many laboratories to measure the cerebral metabolic rate for glucose (Sokoloff et al., 1977; Huang et al., 1981; Reivich et al., 1983); and ^{11}C-raclopride, which is used to measure dopamine D_2 receptor binding characteristics (Farde et al., 1985; Sedvall et al., 1986). Measurements that carry promise in the study of panic disorder and other forms of anxiety are summarized in Table 15–2 and are discussed below.

The synthesis of each positron-emitting radiotracer requires the use of a cyclotron and often complicated radiochemistry techniques. Since most of the radionuclides decay with short half-lives (2 min for ^{15}O, 10 min for ^{13}N, 20 min for ^{11}C, and 110 min for ^{18}F), the cyclotron and radiochemistry facilities must be in close proximity to the PET imaging system.

Our laboratory makes extensive use of radiotracers labeled with [15]O. The rapid decay of these radiotracers permits the performance of multiple, sequential studies in the same subject during a single scanning session. Thus, an individual can be studied before and during the performance of increasingly complex behavioral tasks, before and during a pharmacological challenge, or before and during the production of anxiety. In each case, the subject can serve as his or her own control. A number of radiotracers have been synthesized for the purpose of measuring the characteristics of neurotransmitters and neuroreceptors. Characteristics of the ideal radioligand for the measurement of neuroreceptor characteristics are described below.

Once the tracer is synthesized, it is rapidly transported to the PET laboratory and administered to the subject intravenously or by inhalation. The administered radiotracer decays by the emission of a positron from the unstable nucleus of the radioisotope (Fig. 15–1). A positron is a subatomic particle with the mass of an electron and a positive charge. Each positron travels about 1–6 mm before it comes to rest and interacts with an electron in the surrounding tissue (Phelps et al., 1975). The positron-electron pair undergoes annihilation, converting its combined mass into two high-energy photons (i.e., gamma-rays), which travel in virtually opposite directions. These photons are detected by the PET imaging system, described below.

The PET Imaging System

After the radiotracer is administered, an imaging system is employed to make regional measurements of PET counts in the brain (Fig. 15–2). Available PET systems consist of one or more concentric rings of detectors into which the head can be placed (Ter-Pogossian, 1985a) (Fig. 15–3). Each detector is connected to multiple opposing detectors by coincidence circuits. Coincidence circuits record those events in which the opposing detectors sense two annihilation photons simultaneously. Coincidence circuits thus record the number of annihilation events that have occurred anywhere along a straight line joining the two detectors. (These circuits also record a relatively small number of random events in which unrelated photons strike opposing detectors simultaneously.) Typically, PET systems record at least 1,000,000 coincidence events per PET slice during a single scan. Measurements of regional PET counts in the head are reconstructed from the record of coincidence events by means of a computer-applied mathematical reconstruction algorithm, similar to that employed for computed tomography (CT) (Ter-Pogossian, 1985a; Herman, 1985). The principle of coincidence detection is diagrammed in Figure 15–3.

Most available PET systems can simultaneously record regional PET counts in multiple, horizontal sections of the brain. The acquired data can also be reconstructed into sagittal and coronal sections.

PET systems differ in their spatial resolution (a term related to the ability to image small objects), their temporal resolution (a term related to the ability to acquire data quickly), and their sensitivity (a term related to the ability to acquire data from small amounts of

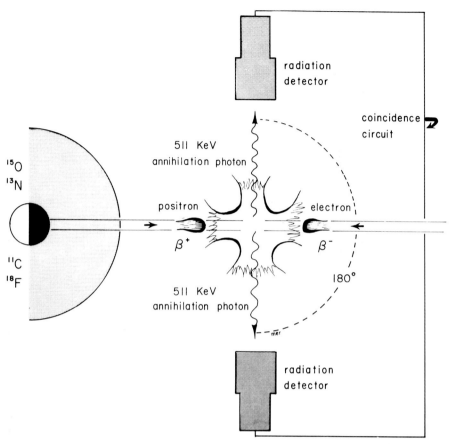

Fig. 15–1. Radioisotopes employed in PET studies decay by the emission of positrons (β+) or positive electrons from a nucleus unstable because of a deficiency of neutrons. Positrons lose their kinetic energy in matter after traveling about 1–6 mm and, when they are brought to rest, interact with electrons (β−). The two particles undergo annihilation, and their mass is converted to two annihilation photons traveling at approximately 180° from each other, each with an energy of 511 keV. The paired annihilation photons are detected by the imaging device, using opposing radiation detectors connected by electronic circuits (coincidence circuits) that record an event only when these two photons arrive simultaneously. (Reproduced, with permission, from the Annual Review of Neuroscience, Volume 6, © 1983 by Annual Reviews, Inc.)

radioactivity) (Ter-Pogossian, 1985a). PET systems differ in other specifications, including the size of the aperture into which the head or body is placed, the number of horizontal PET slices for which data are simultaneously acquired, the distance between contiguous slices, and the "thickness" of each slice.

The spatial resolution of an imaging system can be defined as the smallest distance between two point sources that permits a distinction to be made between their respective images. The latest generation of PET systems has a spatial resolution of about 3–8 mm in the plane of each slice, although the mathematical reconstruction process typically limits the resolution further (Ter-Pogossian, 1985a). This resolution is close to the best that can be expected from PET studies, since the positron must travel a short distance from the radionuclide before it interacts with an electron (Phelps et al., 1975). PET's spatial resolution imposes a limitation on the ability to detect and represent accurately data from very small structures, such as brainstem nuclei. The ex-

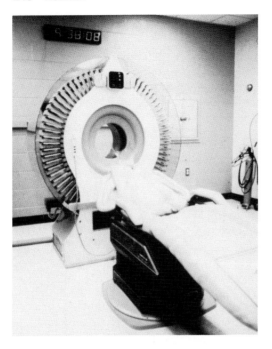

Fig. 15–2. The PETT VI system currently employed in our laboratory. This system simultaneously records regional measurements of radioactivity in seven horizontal slices with an in-plane resolution of 12–14 mm and an interslice distance of 14.4 mm. This system permits scanning times as brief as 40 sec, making it feasible to study patients during a brief and uncomfortable episode of anxiety. New generation systems can simultaneously record regional measurements of radioactivity in many more slices and with an in-plane resolution of 3–8 mm.

tent of this limitation depends on the resolution of the system; the size, shape, and orientation of the structure of interest; and the contrast in radioactivity between the structure of interest and its neighbors (Mazziotta et al., 1981).

Despite the PET system's spatial resolution, experimental studies can be designed to discriminate regional *changes* in PET measurements that are as close as 1–2 mm apart (Fox et al., 1986; Mintun et al., 1989). (This capability depends upon the acquisition of sequential images in the same subject and upon the use of "image subtraction," a data analysis technique described below.) Thus, it has been possible to map the somatotopic organization of supple-

mentary motor cortex and the retinotopic organization of visual cortex (Fox et al., 1987a, b).

A PET system's temporal resolution is partly related to its ability to tolerate high radioactivity counting rates. The PET systems employed in our laboratory tolerate unusually high counting rates and, consequently, permit scanning times as brief as 40 sec (Ter-Pogossian et al., 1982; Yamamoto et al., 1982; Ter-Pogossian, 1985a); these systems permit us to study an individual during a brief and uncomfortable episode of anxiety. (For comparison, the measurement of the metabolic rate for glucose typically involves data acquisition and scanning times of more than 45 min.)

The sensitivity of the typical PET system is quite high compared to other brain imaging techniques such as magnetic resonance imaging (MRI) and SPECT. This characteristic gives PET special promise in the study of neurotransmitters and neuroreceptors, compounds that exist in such minute tissue concentrations (Brownell et al., 1982; McGeer, 1984; Ter-Pogossian, 1985b).

Tracer-Kinetic Models

The imaging system provides an image of regional PET counts, corresponding to the local concentration of radionuclides in the brain. To convert PET counts into biochemical and physiological processes, a tracer-kinetic model must be employed. Tracer-kinetic models consist of mathematical equations that account for the behaviors of the radiotracer in the body, including its radioactive half-life, its rate of transport to the brain, its distribution into various tissue compartments, its active and labeled metabolites, and in the case of neurotransmitter and neuroreceptor measurements its specific and nonspecific binding.

Tracer-kinetic models often require the acquisition of peripheral measurements during the performance of PET scans. For instance, the tracer-kinetic models employed in our laboratory typically rely on multiple, sequential measurements of radioactivity through a radial artery catheter to estimate the rate of radiotracer delivery to the brain. (There is at least one notable exception: We recently began to analyze of images of regional PET counts following the intravenous bolus injection of ^{15}O-water to map the local functions of the hu-

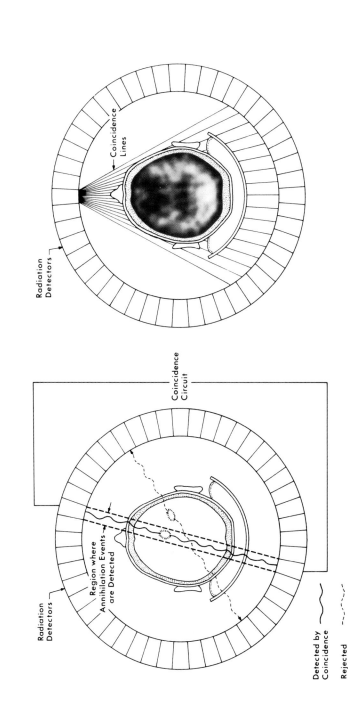

Fig. 15–3. Schematic representation of the arrangement of radiation detectors in a PET imaging system. Because the radioactive decay of a positron-emitting radionuclide results in two annihilations photons traveling at approximately 180° from each other (Fig. 15–1), coincidence detection is employed to localize the event in the tissue. A coincidence circuit between pairs of de-tectors arrayed about the imaged object records an event only if both detectors in the circuit record an event simultaneously. To increase the number of such coincidence lines through the imaged object, each radiation detector is in coincidence with many opposing radiation detectors. (Reproduced, with permission, from the Annual Review of Neuroscience, Volume 6, © 1983 by Annual Reviews, Inc.)

TABLE 15–2.
Promising PET Measurements in the Study of Anxiety

PET Measurement[a]	Radiotracer(s) employed[b]
Cerebral blood flow	^{15}O-water
Cerebral blood volume	^{15}O-carbon monoxide
Cerebral metabolic rate for oxygen	^{15}O-oxygen, ^{15}O-water, and ^{15}O-carbon monoxide
Cerebral metabolic rate for glucose	^{18}F-fluorodeoxyglucose
Permeability-surface area product for water	^{15}O-water and ^{11}C-butanol
Acid-base chemistry in brain tissue	^{11}C-carbon dioxide and ^{15}O-carbon monoxide
Benzodiazepine receptor characteristics[c]	^{11}C-RO 15-1788

[a]Each PET measurement relies on the radiotracer(s) indicated and a tracer-kinetic model. The accuracy of PET measurements depends on the validity of the tracer-kinetic model and its underlying assumptions. (Some of these measurements have also been made with radiotracers other than those shown).

[b]Some PET measurements rely on sequential measurements, using different radiotracers in the same subject. For instance, the measurement of the cerebral metabolic rate for oxygen is derived from measurements of blood flow using ^{15}O-water, blood volume using ^{15}O-carbon monoxide, and ^{15}O-uptake using ^{15}O-oxygen. The tracer-kinetic model employed in this measurement assumes that the physiological state remains unchanged throughout the entire period of data acquisition.

[c]Characteristics assayed in this procedure include the maximum density of benzodiazepine-binding receptors (Bmax) and the ligand-receptor equilibrium dissociation constant (Kd).

man brain. In comparison to blood flow images (in ml/min per 100 g), these images do not require an arterial catheter or tracer-kinetic model and produce virtually identical results in the detection of state-dependent regional changes Fox and Minutn, 1989.) Ultimately, the accuracy of biochemical and physiological measurements with PET depends on the validity of the tracer-kinetic model and its underlying assumptions. Efforts to develop and validate tracer-kinetic models remain vitally important to PET research.

Promising PET Measurements in the Study of Panic Disorder

Several radiotracer techniques have particular promise in the study of panic disorder and other forms of anxiety. These techniques provide regional measurements of cerebral blood flow (CBF) (Raichle et al., 1983; Herscovitch et al., 1983), the cerebral blood volume (CBV) (Grubb et al., 1978), the cerebral metabolic rate for oxygen (CMRO$_2$) (Mintun et al., 1984b), the cerebral metabolic rate for glucose (CMRgl) (Sokoloff et al., 1977; Huang et al., 1981; Reivich et al., 1983), the permeability-surface area product for water (PS$_w$) (Herscovitch et al., 1984, 1987), acid-base chemistry in the brain, and characteristics of benzodiazepine receptor binding (Pappata et al., 1987).

Regional CBF, CBV, and CMRgl have been shown to reflect local neuronal activity (Raichle et al., 1976; Yarowski and Ingvar, 1981; see Raichle, 1987). [The relationship between regional CMRO$_2$ and local neuronal activity is less clear (Fox and Raichle, 1986).] These measurements can be used to map those regions of the brain involved in the production of cognitions, emotions, and behaviors; those regions involved in the pathophysiology of psychiatric disorders; and those regions that are selectively affected by pharmacological and psychological therapies.

As was mentioned above, our laboratory uses ^{15}O-water to map the local functions of the human brain. This radiotracer permits us to make images of regional blood flow in a single subject during both a baseline state and an experimental state in a single scanning session. Thus each subject can be utilized as his or her own control in the attempt to identify state-dependent changes in regional blood flow.

Investigators in our laboratory are now using this radiotracer technique to establish the relation between specific behaviors, cognitions, and emotions and specific regions of the brain. So far, it has been used to identify primary somatosensory cortex (Fox et al., 1987a), primary visual cortex (Fox et al., 1987b), primary motor cortex (Fox et al., 1985a), supplementary motor area (Fox et al., 1985b), frontal eye fields (Fox et al., 1985b), and cortical regions involved in several components of language (Petersen et al., 1988). As is described below, it has also been used to identify regions of the brain involved in the production of lactate-induced anxiety attacks (Reiman et al., 1989b) and normal anticipatory anxiety (Reiman et al., 1989a).

Investigators have employed PET and other functional brain imaging techniques in an effort to identify abnormalities in regional blood flow and metabolism in patients with psychiatric disorders. Regional abnormalities have been reported in patients with panic disorder (Reiman et al., 1984, 1986b), obsessive–compulsive disorder (Baxter et al., 1987, 1988), generalized anxiety disorder (Buchsbaum et al., 1987), and schizophrenia (Ingvar and Franzen, 1974a,b; Franzen and Ingvar, 1975; Mathew et al., 1982; Buchsbaum et al., 1982, 1984; Ariel et al., 1983; Gur et al., 1983, 1985; Sheppard et al., 1983; Widen et al., 1983; Farkas et al., 1984; DeLisi et al., 1985; Wolkin et al., 1985; Garnett et al., 1985; Berman et al., 1986; Weinberger et al., 1986; Volkow et al., 1986; Early et al., 1987). Our studies of panic disorder and normal anticipatory anxiety are described below.

Finally, investigators can begin to map the neuroanatomical regions that are related to the therapeutic or adverse effects of psychotropic medications (see, for instance, Mathew et al., 1985; Buchsbaum et al., 1987). Perhaps these studies will serve as a bridge between information derived from basic and clinical studies.

PS_w, a measure of blood–brain barrier permeability to small molecules like water (Eichling et al., 1974), also has promise in the study of panic disorder. Animal studies indicate that PS_w is actively regulated by the central adrenergic system arising in the locus ceruleus (Raichle, 1983b) and that PS_w is consistently increased by antidepressant medications (Preskorn et al., 1980). Other studies suggest that the central adrenergic system may be involved in the generation of anxiety attacks and other forms of anxiety (Redmond and Huang, 1979; Charney et al., 1984). Still, other studies indicate that antidepressants effectively block anxiety attacks (Klein, 1967; McNair and Kahn, 1981; Sheehan et al., 1980). An interesting exception to these observations is the investigational antidepressant bupropion. This medica-

tion does not increase PS_w in animals (Winsky et al., 1982) and does not appear to block anxiety attacks in patients with panic disorder (Sheehan et al., 1983). Thus, PS_w may have an important role in the generation and treatment of anxiety attacks.

Although our technique for measuring PS_w with PET has promise in the study of panic disorder, it does have one important limitation: It requires two separate measurements of CBF (with a minimum interval of 10 min between scans), the first with the diffusion-limited tracer ^{15}O-water and the second with the freely diffusible tracer ^{11}C-butanol (Herscovitch et al., 1987). The accurate measurement of PS_w depends on the assumption that the subject is in the same physiological state during the two scans. It may be difficult to comply with this assumption during the production of an anxious response.

The measurement of acid-base chemistry in the brain also has promise in the study of panic disorder. Acid-base chemistry in the brain appears to be regulated in part by the beta-adrenergic system (through its effect on carbonic anhydrase activity in glial cells) (Church et al., 1980; Winsky et al., 1982). Theories implicate the beta-adrenergic system in the generation and treatment of anxiety attacks (Pitts et al., 1984), although the evidence is not particularly strong (Gorman et al., 1983; Reiman, 1987). In addition, it has been postulated that lactate-induced anxiety attacks lead to the development of a cerebral acidosis to which patients with panic disorder are hypersensitive (Gorman et al., 1984; Carr and Sheehan, 1984).

If one considers that lactate causes a metabolic alkalosis peripherally, then the suggestion that it causes an acidosis centrally might seem paradoxical. Carr and Sheehan (1984) speculate that the metabolic alkalosis induced by lactate leads to the development of a central acidosis. However, PET research conducted in our laboratory (Reiman et al., 1986a) and SPECT studies conducted elsewhere (Stewart et al., 1988) indicate that lactate does not cause a cerebral ischemia; instead, it causes a cerebral hyperemia, at least in nonpanicking subjects. Alternatively, Klein and his colleagues note that lactate is rapidly metabolized to bicarbonate which, in turn, is in equilibrium with carbon dioxide and water (Gorman et al., 1984). Since carbon dioxide penetrates the blood–brain barrier much more rapidly than bicarbonate, these investigators have suggested that a central acidosis could be established in conjunction with a peripheral alkalosis. Nonetheless, it remains difficult to reconcile this theory with the observation that carbon dioxide is quickly removed by the lungs due to hyperventilation.

Despite the problems with these acid-base theories, several observations are consistent with the possibility that alkaline infusions such as lactate might induce a central acidosis. Previous studies have shown that bicarbonate infusions lead to the development of an acidosis in cerebral spinal fluid (Leusen, 1972). Furthermore, the reports of a lactate-induced hyperemia in nonpanicking patients and control subjects are consistent with the possibility that lactate causes a central acidosis. Finally, analyses of arterial blood samples in our laboratory and elsewhere (Gorman et al., 1986) indicate that lactate leads to a respiratory alkalosis in addition to a metabolic alkalosis, even in normal volunteers. This finding is consistent with the possibility that lactate causes a central acidosis.

PET studies can determine whether lactate induces a central acidosis. These studies can also investigate the role of acid-base chemistry in the pathophysiology and treatment of panic disorder.

In addition to these and other physiological measurements, PET has the potential to provide quantitative, regional measurements of neurotransmitter and neuroreceptor characteristics in the living human brain. The prospects for measuring these characteristics depend on the development and testing of valid radiotracer techniques.

Already a number of radioligands have been synthesized, administered, and imaged in human subjects. However, the resulting images (in units of PET counts) do not provide quantitative measurements of receptor characteristics. These images can even be misleading; the distribution of PET counts may be sensitive to other variables, such as regional differences in blood–brain barrier permeability to the ligand and its labeled metabolites, regional differences in radioligand metabolism, and regional differences in nonspecific receptor binding.

The accurate measurement of neuroreceptor characteristics ultimately depends on the suitability of the radioligand and the validity of the tracer-kinetic model employed. The ideal radioligand has several characteristics (Sedvall et al., 1986). It should be synthesized rapidly and with high specific activity. It should be highly selective for the receptor or receptor subtype of interest. It should bind with high affinity to these specific receptors and with minimal affinity to nonspecific binding sites. It should readily cross the blood–brain barrier. It should have minimal side effects. Other features of the ligand, including its radioactive half-life, its saturability of binding, and its rate of receptor association and disassociation should satisfy the requirements of the tracer-kinetic model. Thus far, radioligands have been developed for the visualization of dopamine D_1 and D_2, serotonin S_2, opiate, cholinergic, estrogen, and benzodiazepine receptors (Sedvall et al., 1986). However, many of these ligands are not suitable for quantitative measurements of receptor binding properties in the living human brain.

The development of tracer-kinetic models and their validation under normal and pathological circumstances constitute great challenges to PET researchers interested in neurotransmitter and neuroreceptor characteristics. At present, the greatest advances have been related to the measurement of dopamine D_2 receptor characteristics (Mintun et al., 1984a; Sedvall et al., 1986; Wong et al., 1986; Perlmutter et al., 1986; Huang et al., 1986, 1987; Farde et al., 1987). Currently, three different strategies have been developed for the measurement of dopamine D_2 characteristics (Perlmutter et al., 1986; Sedvall et al., 1986; Wong et al., 1986). These strategies employ different radioligands and different tracer-kinetic models; they also measure different characteristics of D_2 receptors. The validity of these approaches remains open to controversy (Perlmutter et al., 1986; Huang et al., 1986, 1987; Farde et al., 1987).

More recently, a strategy was developed by investigators at the Karolinska Institute for measuring the regional concentrations of specifically bound RO 15-1788, a benzodiazepine antagonist with very favorable characteristics as a radioligand (Pappata et al., 1987). Although the assumptions of the tracer-kinetic model merit additional testing, their strategy offers promise in efforts to study the therapeutic actions of sedative-hypnotic medications. Although the efficacy of most benzodiazepines in the treatment of panic disorder remains open to question, at least when these medications are employed at lower doses (McNair and Kahn, 1981; Noyes et al., 1984), the measurement of benzodiazepine receptor binding characteristics may be helpful in understanding the pathophysiology and treatment of panic disorder.

Data Analysis

To this point, this chapter has discussed the steps involved in making accurate regional measurements with PET. PET studies also require an appropriate method of data analysis. Four major challenges to the analysis of PET data are localizing anatomical regions of interest within the PET image, minimizing the contribution of variable whole brain measurements in the assessment of regional brain function, utilizing as much of the acquired data as possible while addressing the statistical problem of multiple comparisons, and detecting potentially subtle differences in regional PET measurements. Each of these issues is discussed here.

ANATOMICAL LOCALIZATION

To relate functional brain measurements to neuroanatomy, PET studies require an accurate method of anatomical localization. Since PET images consist of low- resolution physiological data that lack precise anatomical landmarks, it is difficult to identify neuroanatomical regions of interest (ROIs) within the PET image. PET laboratories have employed several strategies to localize anatomical ROIs within the PET image; each approach has certain limitations.

Some laboratories attempt to identify ROIs based on visual inspection of the PET image. Unfortunately, this approach is likely to be inaccurate and unreliable. Furthermore, the choice of brain regions relies on visual inspection of the data, increasing the chance of observer bias.

Some laboratories attempt to obtain PET images in horizontal planes that are parallel to a standard craniofacial reference such as the or-

bitomeatal line; subsequently, the PET images are compared to a tomographic atlas of the brain. Unfortunately, this approach fails to account for the variable relationship between standard craniofacial landmarks and the brain (Mazzochi and Vignolo, 1978; Fox et al., 1985a).

Some laboratories localize ROIs by comparing the PET image to a CT or MR image obtained in the same horizontal planes (Evans et al., 1988). This approach has great advantages over earlier efforts, particularly in its ability to localize regions of interest in an individual subject. However, it is expensive, limited in its ability to distinguish between regions not separated by clear anatomical boundaries, and uncertain in its ability to provide reliable comparisons among different subjects.

Our laboratory employs a stereotactic method of anatomical localization (Fox et al., 1985b). This method is based on the finding that a line between the glabella and inion of the skull is parallel to and a predictable distance below a line between the anterior and posterior commissures of the brain. The glabella and inion are cranial landmarks that can be identified on a lateral skull radiograph; the anterior and posterior commissures are reference landmarks for some stereotactic atlases of the brain. This method employs a lateral skull radiograph on which the levels of each PET slice are recorded, a brain atlas, and a computer program to identify ROIs within the PET image. It records data from these regions without visual inspection of the image and thus is free from observer bias. This method permits regional comparisons among different subjects and different laboratories. It has served as the basis for a new data analysis strategy for functional brain mapping, which is discussed below.

Our stereotactic method of anatomical localization has been an indispensable part of our studies. However, its use is limited to the study of brains that are free from gross antomical distortion or significant atrophy. In addition, the small variations between morphologically normal brains impose a limitation on the precision of this method: Currently, our anatomical localization procedure has a standard deviation of about 5 mm in each axis (Fox et al., 1985b).

In the opinion of this author, the decision to

localize anatomical regions of interest with an MR reference or stereotactic method depends in part on the nature of the study. I look forward to the development and evaluation of a localization technique that combines the use of an MR image with our stereotactic method.

IMAGE NORMALIZATION

Efforts to study regional brain processes such as CBF and CMRgl have been confounded by variability in whole brain measurements. Investigators have attempted to minimize the contribution of whole brain measurements by analyzing regions as ratios of regional-to-whole brain, left-to-right, or anterior-to-posterior measurements. Regional-to-whole brain ratios have demonstrated utility in mapping the cognitive-behavioral functions of the brain (Fox et al., 1985a–c, 1986, 1987a,b; Fox and Raichle, 1986). Left-to-right regional ratios enabled us to identify a local brain abnormality in certain patients with panic disorder (Reiman et al., 1984, 1986b). Anterior-to-posterior ratios have been employed in the study of schizophrenia and other psychiatric conditions.

Physiologically, it appears to make sense to investigate state-dependent changes in regional CBF and CMRgl independent of whole brain variations. Functional brain mapping studies in our laboratory indicate that the distribution of regional measurements within an image varies independently of whole brain measurements. For instance, there is a predictable relationship between the frequency of a visual stimulus and the increase in visual cortex-to-whole brain blood flow (Fox and Raichle, 1984). Our laboratory routinely investigates state-dependent changes in blood flow by comparing a baseline control image to an experimental image, both of which have been "normalized" to the same whole brain CBF.

THE PROBLEM OF MULTIPLE COMPARISONS

PET investigators would like to analyze as much of their data as possible. After all, potentially significant group differences in regional PET measurements could be centered around nearly 50,000 voxels of information within our seven-slice PET images. At the same time, they want their findings to be statistically meaningful. Unfortunately, analysis of numerous regions leads to the statistical problem of multiple comparisons: As the number of comparisons increase, it becomes more likely that a regional difference will achieve "significance" by chance alone. In other words, the likelihood of type I errors (i.e., "false positives") increases with the number of comparisons made.

Perhaps the most scrupulous approach to the multiple comparison problem is application of a statistical correction such as the Bonferroni procedure to account for the number of comparisons made (Hays, 1980). The Bonferroni correction dictates that one should divide alpha, ordinarily set at 0.05, by the number of comparisons made in order to avoid a larger proportion of type I errors. Unfortunately, implementation of the Bonferroni procedure produces an unreasonably high probability of type II errors (i.e., false negatives) when a large number of comparisons are made.

A second approach to the problem is to restrict the data analysis to a small number of preselected regions. Unfortunately, this approach fails to utilize a wealth of potentially meaningful data. It may be unwise to restrict the investigation to a few preselected regions, especially in the study of psychiatric disorders so poorly understood. Despite this limitation, we employed this strategy in our initial studies of panic disorder (Reiman et al., 1984, 1986b).

A third approach is to conduct a two-part study: first, an exploratory study that analyzes numerous regions to generate a few specific hypotheses; second, a replication study that tests the newly generated hypotheses. This approach was utilized in our study of never-medicated patients with schizophrenia (Early et al., 1987).

Recently, we developed and tested a method for investigating the entire population of regional differences in blood flow between two sets of images. This method, summarized below, partially addresses the problem of multiple comparisons. (Even so, a separate replication study could address this problem more fully.)

A New Strategy for the Analysis of PET Data

We recently developed and tested an automated data analysis technique to maximize our ability to detect and localize state-dependent changes in regional blood flow (Fox et al.,

1988). This technique has great utility in functional brain mapping. Indeed, it enabled us to identify neuroanatomical correlates of lactate-induced panic and normal anticipatory anxiety.

This data analysis technique is currently restricted to paired images of regional blood flow obtained in the same subject without head movements between scans. One image corresponds to a baseline state; the other image corresponds to an experimental state. (We currently use the PETT VI system to make seven-slice images of regional blood flow.)

First, each image is normalized to the same mean blood flow by multiplying every pixel in the image by the same linear correction factor. As was noted above, this technique enables us to investigate state-dependent changes in regional blood flow independent of the variation in whole brain measurements.

Second, an image of regional blood flow changes is computed in each subject as the pixel-by-pixel subtraction of the baseline image from the experimental image (Fig. 15–4). The resulting "subtraction image" consists of a large number of changes in regional blood flow, some of which may be state-dependent, but most of which are random (i.e., "noise"). An individual subtraction image permits us to localize a large state-dependent change in regional blood flow within 1–2 mm despite the limited resolution of PET (Mintun et al., 1986; Fox et al., 1986). It also improves our ability to detect these changes. However, it is still difficult to distinguish subtle state-dependent changes from noise in a single subtraction image. The next few steps are used to reduce the noise.

A linear interpolation is performed on each seven-slice image of blood flow changes to generate data for voxels existing between the imaged planes (Mintun et al., 1989). Next, our computer algorithm for anatomical localization is employed to transform each interpolated image of blood flow changes into standard spatial coordinates (Fig. 15–5). Once the data from each subject have been transformed into the same spatial coordinates, the data are averaged on a voxel-by-voxel basis. This procedure produces an image of mean state-dependent changes in regional blood flow. In the averaged image, random changes in regional

blood flow tend to cancel out, whereas the magnitude of state-dependent changes in regional blood flow is preserved (Fox et al., 1988). Thus image averaging improves our ability to distinguish state-dependent changes in regional blood flow from noise.

Next, an automated program computes the magnitude and stereotactic location of all the mean changes in regional blood flow. State-dependent regional changes, defined as significant "outliers" in the distribution of mostly random blood flow changes, are established by computation of the gamma-2 statistic from the population of mean regional blood flow changes. This statistic characterizes the shape of the population of blood flow changes. It is performed independent of the issue of multiple comparisons. A significantly positive gamma-2 statistic is specific for populations that contain nonrandom changes in regional blood flow. For populations characterized by a significantly positive gamma-2, Z scores (response magnitude/standard deviation) are employed to characterize the nonrandom changes in regional blood flow (Fox et al., 1988). Finally, paired t tests are used to assess the consistency of the state dependent changes in regional blood flow related to the production of anxiety (Reiman et al., 1989a, b).

Although this technique has great utility in the detection of state-dependent changes in regional blood flow, its use is currently limited to cases when there is no head movement between scans. We recently developed a screening procedure to identify and exclude from subsequent data analysis paired images with significant interscan movements (Reiman et al., 1989b). We are now refining our technique to analyze the difference in regional blood flow between scans performed on separate days (i.e., to evaluate the differences in regional blood flow between patients and control and the changes in regional blood flow due to various treatments).

One last note to readers regarding the interpretation of PET data: Carefully inspect the quantitative measurements and statistical analyses employed in the derivation of findings. Individual PET images—such as our image of the parahippocampal asymmetry in a patient who was vulnerable to lactate-induced panic (Fig. 15–6)—are interesting and attrac-

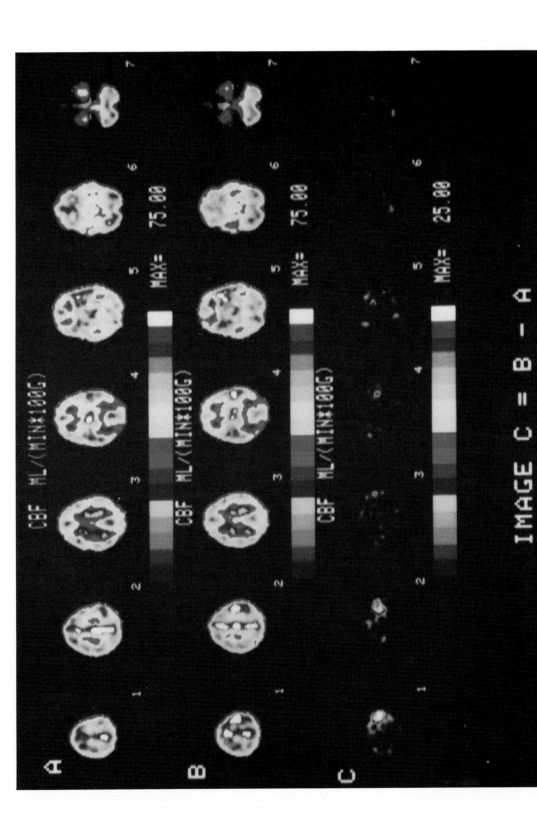

IMAGE C = B - A

tive illustrations, but they should not distract the reader from critical assessment of the data.

Experimental Design

In addition to the technical details discussed above, PET studies demand careful consideration of experimental design. Well designed psychiatric studies are characterized by the selection of homogeneous patient populations and appropriate control groups; by successful efforts to control or account for potentially confounding variables such as medication history, presence of coexisting psychiatric or neurological disorders, and the subject's cognitive-emotional-behavioral state at the time of the study; by success in tailoring the study to the PET laboratory's particular strengths; and by the ability to address specific, testable hypotheses. Our laboratory has capitalized on the use of experimental procedures to induce anxiety in the PET laboratory; on the use of ^{15}O-labeled tracers to permit studies before and during the production of anxiety; and on the use of a fast imaging system to study patients during a brief and uncomfortable episode of anxiety.

Fig. 15–4.   Application of image subtraction to functional brain mapping. Row A is a seven-slice image of cerebral blood flow (CBF), which was obtained in a normal volunteer who was resting quietly with eyes closed and with minimal sensory stimulation. Row B is a CBF image from the same volunteer, which was obtained in the identical head position during left hand vibration. Row C is a "subtraction image," derived from the pixel-by-pixel subtraction of image A from image B. The subtraction image indicates the regional increases in CBF due to left hand vibration. The white area in slice 1 of this row indicates a large CBF increase in a region of right somatosensorycortex (as determined by our stereotactic method of anatomical localization). Each row of color-coded slices corresponds to the scale below it. In each row, the horizontal slices proceed from higher to lower sections of the brain. In each slice, the subject's left is to the reader's left, and anterior is at 12 o'clock. Image subtraction improves our ability to detect and localize functionally activated brain regions. Unfortunately, more subtle state-dependent changes in CBF may be difficult to distinguish from noise in an individual subtraction image. (Reproduced courtesy of Peter Fox; reproduced in color in Color Figure Section.)

Risks to Human Subjects

An important consideration in the performance of PET studies is the risk to human subjects. The usual risks to subjects who participate in PET studies can be attributed to radiation exposure and vascular catheterization.

Positron-emitting radiotracers produce low level, low linear-energy transfer (LET) radiation, that consists of positrons and gammarays. In our laboratory, the total radiation dose to any research subject must be lower than the limits established by the Food and Drug Administration (United States Code of Federal Regulations).

The main risk of low level, low LET radiation is the development of cancer much later in life. This risk is too small to measure directly, but a conservative estimate of 10^{-4} lethal cancers per whole body rem has been derived from a linear-quadratic extrapolation of the high-dose radiation effects in atomic bomb survivors (BEIR, 1980). The radiation risk from participation in a PET study is based on a calculation of the radiation exposure to individual organs and the whole body. Based on several estimates a typical multiscan PET study in our laboratory produces a risk of developing a lethal cancer that is roughly equivalent to the estimated risk of developing a lethal cancer due to smoking about a half carton of cigarettes or the risk due to exposure to air pollution while living in a city such as Boston or New York for 2 months (Wilson, 1979; BEIR, 1980; Brill et al., 1982; Hall, 1984; Harber and Pollimia, 1984).

Experts have studied additional risks of low level LET radiation. The risk to the developing embryo (Beir, 1980) makes it necessary to exclude pregnant women from participating in PET studies. The risk of genetic abnormalities in subsequent generations (due to irradiation of germ cells) is immeasurably small (Beir, 1980). Finally, the risks of infertility, aging, cataract formation, skin or blood changes, and radiation sickness require much higher levels of radiation exposure than is received in PET studies (BEIR, 1980).

Most PET studies require venous catheterization for the purpose of radiotracer administration or blood sampling. This procedure is associated with only transient discomfort.

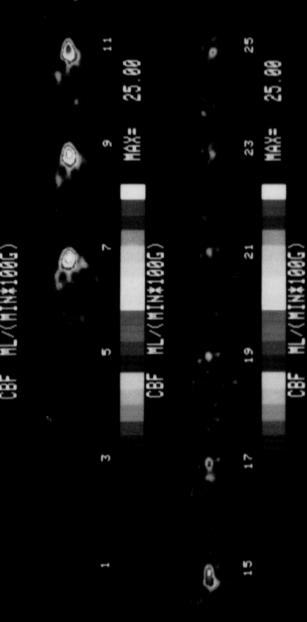

Many PET studies also require arterial catheterization, usually in an effort to estimate the rate of radiotracer transport to the brain. Our laboratory has inserted radial artery catheters in over 1,200 medically stable subjects, producing only transient discomfort and occasional bruises—far less discomfort than volunteers from the health professions typically expect.

Although the risks of PET are limited, they must always be weighed against the potential benefits of the particular study.

Expense and Availability

Another consideration in the performance of PET studies is the cost. PET studies are expensive. The cost of installing a cyclotron and imaging system has been estimated to be about $3,000,000 (Evens et al., 1983), but can be considerably greater. In addition, the major PET centers rely on numerous personnel. Important members of the PET team can include physicists, engineers, mathematicians, radiation scientists, nuclear medicine technologists, computer scientists, physiologists, physicians, and researchers from related fields. The break-even cost of each PET procedure has been estimated to be between $615 and $2780, depending on procedure volume (Evens et al., 1983). Because of its expense, limited availability (about 60 centers worldwide), and lack of clear therapeu-

tic or prognostic implications, PET's utility in clinical psychiatry remains to be demonstrated. (However, some investigators have touted the clinical utility of PET in other areas, such as cardiology and neurology.) In my opinion, it is more reasonable for psychiatrists to think of PET as a research tool with enormous promise.

Capabilities and Limitation of PET

As a technique that can be employed to investigate a variety of regional brain processes, PET has a great promise in the study of psychiatric disorders. The extent to which PET fulfills its promise will depend on the ability of investigators to address several methodological challenges. To reiterate, these challenges include the development of suitable radiotracers, the development and application of PET imaging systems with ever more desirable performance characteristics, the development and validation of useful tracer-kinetic models, the use of an accurate technique for anatomical localization, the development and application of powerful data analysis techniques, and the implementation of careful experimental design.

STUDIES OF PANIC DISORDER AND NORMAL ANTICIPATORY ANXIETY

Our laboratory is now using PET to investigate the neurobiology of panic disorder (Reiman et al., 1984, 1986b, 1989). Patients with panic disorder and normal volunteers are studied before and during the infusion of sodium (DL) lactate. (Lactate is infused at an undisclosed time and the subjects are told that it may or may not precipitate an anxiety attack.) After this scanning session, the patients are treated with an antipanic medication for several weeks and are then restudied before and during lactate. These studies are designed to investigate the elements involved in the production and treatment of anxiety attacks.

In these studies, our criteria for a lactate-induced anxiety attack were the report of an unequivocal anxiety attack during the infusion or the presence of at least 15 symptoms from an inventory of 21 anxiety symptoms originally utilized by Pitts and McClure (1967). These criteria were chosen to minimize heterogeneity in the group of panicking patients.

Fig. 15–5. Transformation of a subtraction image into standard spatial coordinates. Figure shows every other slice of a 49-slice subtraction image, corresponding to coordinates from an atlas of the brain (Talairach and Szilka, 1967), and representing the regional increase in CBF induced by left hand vibration. This image was derived from the subtraction image in Figure 15–4, row C, but depicts only CBF increases. The maximal change in CBF was localized to right somatosensory cortex utilizing an automated search routine; this maximal change is located in slice 10. Once transformed into the standard spatial coordinates, the data from each subject can be averaged. Image averaging reduces noise and improves our ability to detect small changes in regional blood flow. This strategy was employed to identify neuroanatomical correlates of lactate-induced panic and normal anticipatory anxiety. (Reproduced in color in Color Figure Section.)

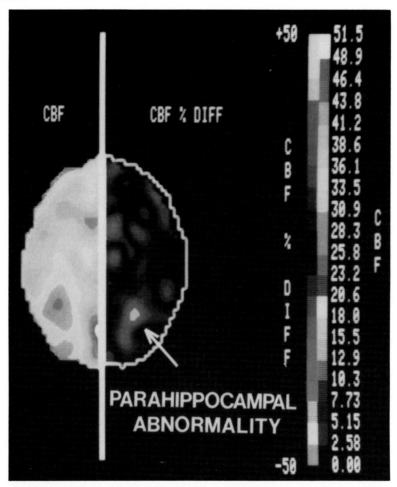

Fig. 15–6. Illustration of the abnormal parahippocampal asymmetry in a patient with panic disorder who was vulnerable to a lactate-induced anxiety attack. This is a horizontal PET slice obtained in the nonpanic state prior to lactate infusion. The patient's left is to the reader's left and anterior is at 12 o'clock. The left side of the image is a color-coded map of cerebral blood flow (ml/min per 100g). The right side of the image is a color-coded map of the percent difference in blood flow between homologous regions on the left and right sides. Areas with no difference appear black. Areas of increase on the right appear red to white. Areas of decrease on the right appear green and blue. The arrow points to a bright yellow area, which corresponds to the abnormal parahippocampal region. The abnormal asymmetry was identified in the resting, nonpanic state and was demonstrated independent of the visual inspection of the image. Other asymmetries analyzed in the image varied randomly from subject to subject. The abnormality was identified independent of the visual inspection of the image. (Reprinted by permission from *Nature*, Volume 310:683–685, © 1984, Macmillan Magazines Limited. Reproduced in color in Color Figure Section.)

Analysis of the Nonpanic State Prior to Lactate Infusion

In a preliminary study, we analyzed measurements of regional CBF obtained during the resting, nonpanic state prior to lactate infusion (Reiman et al., 1984). For the purpose of data analysis, the subjects were divided into three groups: seven patients with panic disorder who were vulnerable to lactate-induced panic, three patients with panic disorder who were not vulnerable to lactate-induced panic, and six control subjects. To address the statistical problem of multiple comparisons, the analysis was restricted to seven regions of the brain that had been alleged to mediate symptoms of panic, anxiety and vigilance. These regions were identified using our stereotactic method of anatomical localization and investigated independent of the visual inspection of the PET images. To explore the possibility of regional abnormalities independent of variations in whole brain measurements, these regions were analyzed in terms of left-to-right ratios.

The patients who were vulnerable to lactate-induced panic had an abnormal asymmetry of CBF (left less than right) in Economo's TH region (1929) of the parahippocampal gyrus (Reiman et al., 1984). An image depicting the parahippocampal abnormality is shown in Figure 15–6.

Quite frankly, we were a little surprised to find a regional brain abnormality during the nonpanic state. We performed this initial analysis as a "dress rehearsal" for the investigation that really interested us: analysis of the blood flow changes corresponding to a lactate-induced anxiety attack. (Indeed, that is the reason that we divided the patients into those who were vulnerable to a lactate-induced anxiety attack from those who were not.) We were even more surprised to find no overlap between the left-to-right CBF ratios of the patients who were vulnerable to lactate induced panic and the ratios of the other subjects, especially given the limitation in the resolution of our images, some imprecision in our localization method, and some variability in the relation between the region of interest and the plane of the relevant PET slice. In contrast to our initial report, we later found some overlap between groups.

In an extension of this work, we analyzed measurements of CBF, CBV, and CMRO$_2$ from the nonpanic state prior to lactate infusion in a larger number of subjects: eight patients with panic disorder who were vulnerable to lactate-induced panic, eight patients with panic disorder who were not vulnerable to lactate-induced panic, and 25 normal control subjects (Reiman et al., 1986b). The subjects included the participants from our original analysis. Based on our earlier study, the data analysis was restricted to parahippocampal and whole brain measurements.

The patients who were vulnerable to lactate-induced panic had an abnormal asymmetry of parahippocampal CBF, CBV, and CMRO$_2$ (Table 15–3) (Reiman et al., 1986b). Analysis of absolute regional measurements suggested that the abnormal asymmetry reflects increased blood flow and metabolism in the right parahippocampal region rather than decreased measurements in the left. In addition to the parahippocampal abnormality, these patients had abnormally high whole brain CMRO$_2$ (Table 15–3). Finally, these patients exhibited abnormal episodic hyperventilation, as indicated by a mild respiratory alkalosis during the resting scans (Table 15–3). The parahippocampal and whole brain abnormalities were not attributable to group differences in age, sex, handedness, medications, history of phobic avoidance, arterial pH or PCO$_2$, number of anxiety symptoms, or number of severe anxiety symptoms during the resting scans.

From a biological standpoint, the parahippocampal abnormality could reflect an asymmetry in neuronal activity, neuroanatomy, or PS$_w$ (Reiman et al., 1986): If the abnormality reflects increased neuronal activity in the right parahippocampal region, it is likely to reflect increased activity of terminal neuronal fields that innervate the parahippocampal region rather than increased activity in the cell bodies that arise there (Schwartz et al., 1979). Thus the abnormality could reflect increased activity in one of the projections to the parahippocampal region. Projections to the parahippocampal region arise in local interneurons, hippocampus, subiculum, entorhinal cortex, multimodal sensory association areas, amygdala, raphe nuclei, and locus ceruleus (Nieuwenhuys et al., 1981; Price and Marall, 1981; Van Hoesen, 1982). Two of these regions, the hippocampus and locus ceruleus, have been implicated in the neurobiology of anxiety (Charney et al., 1984; Redmond and Huang, 1979).

Recent studies in our laboratory indicate that regional CMRO$_2$ is not coupled to state-dependent increases in neuronal activity, at least not those increases that last on the order of a few minutes (Fox et al., 1986). Thus, if the abnormality is related to an alteration in local neuronal activity, we suspect that the alteration is long-lasting.

It is also possible that the regional abnormal-

TABLE 15–3.
Abnormalities in Patients Who Were Vulnerable to Lactate-Induced Panic*

	Left-to-right parahippocampal ratios			Whole brain $CMRO_2$	Arterial pH	Arterial PCO_2
	CBF	CBV	$CMRO_2$			
Patients vulnerable to lactate-induced panic (N = 8)	0.88 ± 0.04[a]	0.82 ± 0.08[a]	0.93 ± 0.06[a]	3.28 ± 0.55[a]	7.44 ± 0.04[a]	33.3 ± 5.1[a]
Patients not vulnerable to lactate-induced panic (N = 8)	0.97 ± 0.05	0.98 ± 0.10[b]	1.00 ± 0.04[b]	2.57 ± 0.36[b]	7.41 ± 0.03	35.0 ± 2.8
Normal control subjects (N = 25)	0.98 ± 0.07	0.98 ± 0.12	1.01 ± 0.07[c]	2.74 ± 0.41[c]	7.42 ± 0.03	36.8 ± 2.8
F (df)	7.20 (2,38)	4.62 (2,26)	3.42 (2,26)	4.47 (2,26)	5.30 (2,38)	3.37 (2,38)
P	.0022	.019	.048	.021	.0093	.045

*Identified in the resting stage, prior to lactate infusion (Mean ± SD). (Adapted from Reiman et al.; 1986, with permission of the publisher.)

[a]Abnormal measurement on the basis of pairwise comparisons.

[b]N = 6.

[c]N = 15.

ity reflects an asymmetry in microscopic or macroscopic neuroanatomy. The possibility that the abnormality reflects a hemispheric asymmetry in the size, shape, or orientation of structures in the vicinity of the parahippocampal region can now be investigated using MRI. Although MR images need to be interpreted cautiously in light of well recognized problems with spatial distortion (Zhu et al., 1986; Schad et al., 1987), MRI offers promise as a complement to PET studies. In a preliminary MRI study, investigators recently reported right temporal lobe abnormalities and temporal atrophy in an unusually large proportion of patients with panic disorder (Fontaine, 1987).

Finally, we suspected that the abnormality might reflect an asymmetry in parahippocampal PS_w (see Reiman et al., 1986b, for an explanation). However, a preliminary analysis of parahippocampal PS_w does not support this possibility.

From a functional standpoint, the parahippocampal abnormality could be related to a genetic predisposition to panic, a conditioned predisposition to panic, or a state of anticipatory anxiety in the patients who are vulnerable to lactate-induced panic. If the abnormality is related to a genetic predisposition to panic—and there does appear to be a genetic contribution to panic disorder (see Crowe, 1985)—we might expect to find this abnormality in an unusually large percentage of a patient's first-degree relatives. If the abnormality is related to a conditioned predisposition to panic, we might expect to find this abnormality in patients with a simple phobia. Finally, if the abnormality is related to a state of anticipatory anxiety, we might expect to reproduce the parahippocampal asymmetry in healthy volunteers during the production of anticipatory anxiety.

We do not believe that the parahippocampal abnormality is related to a state of anticipatory anxiety in the patients who were vulnerable to lactate-induced panic. First, it would be difficult to reconcile our finding of an abnormal asymmetry in $CMRO_2$ with a brief state of anticipatory anxiety. Second, we failed to induce the parahippocampal asymmetry in healthy volunteers during the production of anticipatory anxiety (Reiman et al., 1989a).

The analysis of data from the nonpanic state led us to develop a provisional model for the initiation of an anxiety attack (Reiman et al., 1986). We proposed that the parahippocampal abnormality was involved in a predisposition to panic. We suggested that a triggering event— say, for heuristic purposes, activation of the noradrenergic projections to the abnormal region—leads the parahippocampal abnormality to initiate an anxiety attack through sequential efferent projections (Reiman, 1987).

This model predicted that the production of a lactate-induced anxiety attack would be associated with increased CBF in one of the regions that receives a projection from the parahippocampal region (Reiman, 1987). (Remember that an increase in regional CBF seems to reflect increased activity in terminal neuronal fields.) At the time, we expected to see increased blood flow in the septoamygdalar region (Gray, 1982; Swanson, 1983; Reiman, 1987). Instead, we identified a robust CBF increase in another region that receives a projection from the TH region of the parahippocampal gyrus, temporopolar cortex (Reiman et al., 1988).

One last point about our analysis of the nonpanic state: it was limited to seven preselected regions. We do not yet know if other regional abnormalities exist in patients with panic disorder. We do not even know if the abnormality identified in the preselected parahippocampal region is centered in this location or, instead, in a neighboring structure. In the latter case, we might have identified an abnormality in the parahippocampal region due to the limited resolution of the image. (In other words, the parahippocampal region might reside at the periphery of a blurred focus). We are currently working on a data analysis technique that will enable us to address these issues better.

The Effects of Lactate Infusion on Whole Brain Blood Flow

We are now evaluating the effects of lactate infusion on whole brain CBF. We find that lactate infusion causes a significant increase in CBF in nonpanicking patients and normal control subjects but does not cause a significant change in the panicking patients (Reiman et al., 1986a). These findings are consistent with those of Stewart and her colleagues (1988), who measured the hemodynamic effects of lactate infusion using SPECT.

In preliminary studies we compared the effects of lactate to those of an equiosmolar infusion of glucose-in-saline on CBF; the hyperemic effect of lactate seems to be partly but perhaps not completely attributable to hemodilution. Studies have demonstrated that hemodilution increases CBF because of decreased blood viscosity or decreased availability of oxygen to the brain (Thomas et al., 1977; Humphrey et al., 1979). As was noted above, the hyperemic effect of lactate is consistent with the possibility that it induces a cerebral acidosis.

Based on our measurements of arterial pH and blood gases, we believe that the absence of a hyperemic effect of lactate in panicking patients is at least partly attributable to their greater degree of hyperventilation. Studies have demonstrated a direct relationship between arterial PCO_2 and cerebral flow (Grubb et al., 1974).

It is possible that the lack of a hyperemic effect in the panicking patients is also partly attributable to a reduction in PS_w, since such a reduction would lead to an underestimation of CBF using our technique (Herscovitch et al., 1984, 1987). Indeed, preliminary studies in our laboratory suggest that PS_w may be reduced during a lactate-induced anxiety attack. However, this observation is based on the assumption that CBF remains constant during lactate-induced panic; this assumption requires further study.

Neuroanatomical Correlates of Lactate-Induced Panic

More recently, we investigated the regions of the brain involved in the production of a lactate-induced anxiety attack (Reiman et al., 1989b). PET was employed to measure regional blood flow in 24 patients with panic disorder and 18 normal control subjects before and during lactate infusion. (Many of these subjects were included in our analysis of the nonpanic state prior to lactate infusion.) Initially, the subjects were divided into three groups: the 14 patients who had a lactate-induced anxiety attack; the ten patients who did not have a lactate-induced anxiety attack; and the 18 control subjects, none of whom had a lactate-induced anxiety attack.

An automated procedure for the detection of interscan head movements was used to exclude from subsequent data analysis all subjects who moved more than 1 pixel (2 mm) or 1° in any direction. Based on this screen, eight patients who had a lactate-induced anxiety attack, nine patients who did not have a lactate-induced anxiety attack, and 15 normal control subjects were included in the final data analysis.

Our new technique for the analysis of PET data was employed to compute an image of mean changes in regional blood flow related to lactate infusion in each subject group. The statistical procedures described earlier were employed to establish populations with significant increases or decreases in regional blood flow.

During the production of a lactate-induced anxiety attack, there were significant increases in regional blood flow; there were no significant decreases. There were large and significant blood flow increases in bilateral temporal poles and smaller but significant blood flow increases bilaterally in insular cortex, claustrum, or lateral putamen, bilaterally in the vicinity of the superior colliculi and in the vicinity of the left anterior cerebellar vermis. (Our data analysis strategy has a standard deviation of about 5 mm in each axis.)

The increases in regional blood flow seem to be related to the production of an anxiety attack rather than the other effects of lactate infusion. There were no significant changes in regional blood flow related to lactate infusion in the nonpanicking patients or nonpanicking control subjects.

The findings are consistent with the possibility that the parahippocampal abnormality is involved in a predisposition to panic and that it interacts with some triggering event in the initiation of an anxiety attack. The elaboration of an anxiety attack could be mediated through projections to other regions, including the temporal poles.

Neuroanatomical Correlates of Normal Anticipatory Anxiety

Most recently, we investigated the regions of the brain involved in a normal form of anxiety (Reiman et al., 1989a). Eight normal volunteers were studied before, during, and after the anticipation of a painful electric shock, a well established method for inducing anxiety (see

Lader, 1981). The subjects were informed that no shock would be delivered during the first and third scans, but that a painful electric shock would be delivered to their hands some time within a 2 min period following the start of the second scan. To produce a sustained episode of anxiety, the subjects were told that the severity of the stimulus was likely to increase with the passage of time before its arrival. A brief electric shock was delivered immediately after the second 40-sec scan to maintain our credibility for the remainder of the study. The severity of the stimulus was predetermined on the basis of its ability to produce a tingling sensation or mild discomfort in the researchers themselves. The subjects typically stated that the shock was much less uncomfortable than they imagined; their anxiety quickly abated.

Four of the subjects had three additional scans to investigate the possibility that the blood flow increases related to the production of anxiety might be related to voluntary movements or increases in motor tone independent of anxiety. They were studied during repetitive opening and closing of the right hand, during a motionless control state, and during tonic contraction of the right fist.

During anticipation of the shock, there were large and significant increases in subjective and physiological measurements of anxiety (a 0–10 analog scale, the S-Anxiety scale of the Spielberger State-Trait Anxiety Inventory, mean heart rate, and number of nonspecific fluctuations in skin conductance). The same data analysis technique used in our study of lactate-induced panic was employed to investigate the regions of the brain involved in the production of anticipatory anxiety. During the production of anticipatory anxiety, there were large and significant blood flow increases in bilateral temporal poles, the same regions previously implicated in the production of lactate-induced panic. The increases were unrelated to scan order, anticipation, voluntary movements, or increased motor tone independent of the anxious state.

Temporal Poles in the Production of Anxiety

We have now demonstrated involvement of the temporal poles in pathological and normal forms of human anxiety, at least those forms that we have studied so far. These data are compatible with a number of previous studies. Penfield and Jasper (1954) reported that temporopolar stimulation was associated with the experience of anxiety in epileptic patients. Temporopolar stimulation also affects the cardiovascular, respiratory, and gastrointestinal responses that we often associate with the anxious state (Kaada, 1960). Finally, bilateral lesions of the temporal poles attenuate expressions of fear in nonhuman primates in response to normally threatening stimuli (Kluver and Bucy, 1929; Kling and Steklis, 1976). Fear is commonly experienced in association with temporal lobe seizures (Halgren and Walter, 1978; Gloor et al., 1982; Strauss et al., 1982). In addition, anxiety attacks sometimes develop in association with anterior temporal lobe pathology (Wall et al., 1985, 1986; Ghadirian et al., 1986).

Based on the connections with sensory association areas and the amygdala, Mesulam and his colleagues suggest that the temporal poles are involved in interpreting the relevance of environmental information (Mesulam and Mufson, 1982; Moran et al., 1987). In regard to the production of anxiety, the temporal poles could be involved in the evaluation process that characterizes a situation with a sense of uncertainty, helplessness, or danger.

Pathological Versus Normal Forms of Anxiety

What is the relationship between these pathological and normal forms of anxiety? Panic disorder seems to be distinguished by the presence an abnormality in the vicinity of the parahippocampal region. This abnormality could interact with some triggering event in the initiation of an anxiety attack. In contrast to this distinguishing feature of panic disorder, lactate-induced panic and normal anticipatory anxiety appear to share a common pathway involving the temporal poles.

Future Directions

Our studies of panic disorder and normal anticipatory anxiety raise important challenges for the future. One set of challenges pertains to PET methodology. We need to enhance our ability to detect and localize state-dependent changes in regional blood flow. We need to develop and test radiotracer techniques for the measurement of other biochemical processes that are relevant to the pathophysiology and treatment of anxiety disorders.

Another set of challenges pertains to the mechanisms by which various treatments exert their therapeutic effects. If a particular medication or psychotherapy is effective in the treatment of panic disorder, does it work by correcting the parahippocampal abnormality? Does it work, instead, by interfering with some triggering event that interacts with the parahippocampal region in the initiation of an anxiety attack? Or does it work by interfering with the progression of an anxiety attack, perhaps through some action on the temporal poles?

Finally, we need to recognize that anxiety is a multifaceted condition (Reiman, 1988). Eventually, we will need to dissect the various forms of anxiety into their elementary operations: the evaluation procedure that leads to that sense of uncertainty, helplessness, or danger; those processes involved in the conscious experience of anxiety; and those processes involved in the cognitive, behavioral, and autonomic expressions of anxiety. Ultimately, we need to relate these elementary aspects of anxiety to specific pathways in the brain (LeDoux, 1987).

ACKNOWLEDGMENTS

This work was supported by Health and Human Services Physician Scientist Award MH-00615 from NIMH and the McDonnell Center for Studies of Higher Brain Function. The author thanks Sylvia Sirkin for her secretarial services.

REFERENCES

Ariel RN, Golden CJ, Berg RA, Quaife MA, Dirksen JW, Forsell T, Wilson J, Graber B (1983): Regional cerebral blood flow in schizophrenics. Arch Gen Psychiatry 40:258–263.

Baxter LR, Phelps ME, Mazziotta JC, Guze BH, Schwartz JM, Selin CE (1987): Local cerebral glucose metabolic rates in obsessive-compulsive disorder. Arch Gen Psychiatry 44:211–218.

Baxter LR, Schwartz JM, Mazziotta JC, Phelps ME, Pahl JJ, Guze BH, Fairbanks L (1988): Cerebral glucose metabolic rates in nondepressed patients with obsessive–compulsive disorder. Am J Psychiatry 145:1560–1563.

Beir (1980): The effects of populations of exposure to low levels of ionizing radiation. Washington, DC: National Academy Press.

Berman KF, Zec RF, Weinberger DR (1986): Physiologic dysfunction of dorsolateral prefrontal cortex in schizophrenia. II. Role of neuroleptic treatment, attention, and mental effort. Arch Gen Psychiatry 43:126–135.

Brill AB, Adelstein SJ, et al. (eds) (1982): "Low Level Radiation Effects: A Fact Book." New York: The Society of Nuclear Medicine.

Brownell GL, Budinger TF, Lauterbach PC, McGeer PL (1982): Positron tomography and nuclear magnetic resonance imaging. Science 215:619–626.

Buchsbaum MS, DeLisi LE, Holcomb HH, Cappelletti J, King AC, Johnson J, Hazlett E, Dowling-Zimmerman S, Post RM, Morihisa J, Carpenter W, Cohen R, Pickar D, Weinberger DR, Margolin R, Kessler RM (1984): Anteroposterior gradients in cerebral glucose use in schizophrenia and affective disorders. Arch Gen Psychiatry 41:1159–1166.

Buchsbaum MS, Ingvar DH, Kessler R, Waters RN, Cappelletti J, van Kammen DP, King C, Johnson JL, Manning RG, Flynn RW, Mann LS, Bunney WE, Sokoloff L (1982): Cerebral glucography with positron tomography. Arch Gen Psychiatry 39:251–259.

Buchsbaum MS, Wu J, Haler R, Hazlett E, Ball R, Katz M, Socolski K, Lagunas-Solar M, Langer D (1987): Positron emission tomography assessment of effects of benzodiazepines on regional glucose metabolic rate in patients with anxiety disorder. Life Sci 40:2393–2400.

Carr DG, Sheehan MB (1984): Panic anxiety: A new biological model. J Clin Psychiatry 45:323–330.

Charney DS, Heninger GR, Breier A (1984): Noradrenergic function in panic anxiety: Effects of yohimbine in healthy subjects and patients with agoraphobia and panic disorder. Arch Gen Psychiatry 41(8):751–763.

Charney DS, Heninger GR, Jatlow PI (1985): Increased anxiogenic effects of caffeine in panic disorder. Arch Gen Psychiatry 42:233–243.

Church GA, Kimelberg HK, Sapirstein VS (1980): Stimulation of carbonic anhydrase activity and phosphorylation in primary astroglial cultures by norepinephrine. J Neurochem 34:873–879.

Crowe RR (1985): The genetics of panic disorder and agoraphobia. Psychiatric Dev 2:171–186.

DeLisi LE, Holcomb HH, Cohen RM, Pickar D, Carpenter W, Morihisa HM, King AC, Kessler R, Buchsbaum MS (1985): Positron emission tomography in schizophrenic patients with and without neuroleptic medication. J Cereb Blood Flow Metab 5:201–206.

Early TS, Reiman EM, Raichle ME, Spitznagel EL (1987): Left globus pallidus abnormality in never-medicated patients with schizophrenia. Proc Natl Acad Sci USA 84:561–563.

Economo, C von (1929): "Cytoarchitectonics of the Human Cerebral Cortex." London: Oxford University Press.

Eichling JO, Raichle ME, Grubb RL Jr, et al. (1974): Evidence of the limitations of water as a freely permeable tracer in brain of the rhesus monkey. Circ Res 35:358–384.

Evans AC, Beil C, Marrett S, Thompson CJ, Hakim A (1988): Anatomical-functional correlation using an adjustable MRI-based region of interest atlas with positron emission tomography. J Cereb Blood Flow Metab 8:513–530.

Evens RG, Siegel BA, Welch MJ, et al. (1983): Cost analyses of positron emission tomography for clinical use. AJR 141:1073–1076.

Farde L, Ehrin E, Eriksson L, Greitz L, Hall T, Hedstrom CG, Litton JE, Sedvall G (1985): Substituted benzamides as ligands for visualization of dopamine receptor binding in the human brain by positron emission tomography. Proc Natl Acad Sci USA 82:3863–3867.

Farde L, Wiesel FA, Hall H, Halldin C, Stone-Elander S, Sedvall G (1987): Letter to the Editor: No D2 Receptor Increase in PET study of schizophrenia. Arch Gen Psychiatry 44:671–672.

Farkas T, Wolf AP, Jaeger J, Brodie JD, Christman DR, Fowler JS (1984): Regional brain glucose metabolism in chronic schizophrenia. Arch Gen Psychiatry 41:293–200.

Fink M, Taylor MA, Vocavera J (1971): Anxiety precipitated by lactate. N Engl J Med 289:1429.

Fontaine R (1987): (abstract) Magnetic resonance in panic disorder. Paper presented at 42nd Annual Convention of Society of Biological Psychiatry, Chicago, May, 1987.

Fox PT, Burton H, Raichle ME (1987a): Mapping human somatosensory cortex with positron emission tomography. J Neurosurg 63:34–43.

Fox PT, Fox JM, Raichle ME, et al. (1985a): The role of cerebral cortex in the generation of voluntary saccades: A positron-emission tomographic study. J Neurophysiol 54:348–369.

Fox PT, Miezin FM, Allman JM, Van Essen DC, Raichle ME (1987b): Retinotopic organization of human visual cortex mapped with positron emission tomography. J Neurosci 7:913–922.

Fox PT, Mintun MA (1989): Noninvasive functional brain mapping by change-distribution analysis of averaged PET images of $H_2{}^{15}O$ tissue activity. J Nucl Med 30:141–149.

Fox PT, Mintun MA, Raichle ME, Miezin FM, Allman JM, Van Essen DC (1986): Mapping human visual cortex with positron emission tomography. Nature 323:806–809.

Fox PT, Mintun MA, Reiman, Raichle ME (1988): Enhanced detection of focal brain responses using inter-subject averaging and change-distribution analysis of subtracted PET images. J Cereb Blood Flow Metab 8:642–653.

Fox PT, Perlmutter JS, Raichle ME (1985b): A stereotactic method of anatomical localization for positron emission tomography. J Comput Assist Tomogr 9:141–153.

Fox PT, Raichle ME (1984): Stimulus rate dependence of regional cerebral blood flow in human striate cortex, demonstrated with positron emission tomography. J Neurophysiol 51:1109–1121.

Fox PT, Raichle ME (1986): Focal physiological uncoupling of cerebral blood flow and oxidative metabolism during somatosensory stimulation in man. Proc Natl Acad Sci USA 83:1140–1144.

Fox PT, Raichle ME, Thach WT (1985c): Functional mapping of the human cerebellum with positron emission tomography. Proc Natl Acad Sci USA 82:7462–7466.

Franzen G, Ingvar D (1975): Absence of activation in frontal structures during psychological testing of chronic schizophrenics. J Neurol Neurosurg Psychiatry 38:1027–1032.

Garnett ES, Nahmias C, Firnau F, Cleghorn G (1985): Patterns of local cerebral glucose metabolism in untreated schizophrenics. J Cereb Blood Flow Metab 5 [Suppl 1]:S220.

Ghadirian AM, Gauthier S, Bertrand T (1986): Anxiety attacks in a patient with a right temporal lobe meningioma. J Clin Psychiatry 47:270–271.

Gloor P, Olivier A, Quesney LF, Andermann F, Horowitz S (1982): The role of the limbic system in experimental phenomena of temporal lobe epilepsy. Ann Neurol 12:129–144.

Gorman JM, Askanazi J, Liebowitz MR, Fyer AJ, Stein J, Kinney JM, Klein DL (1984): Response to hyperventilation in a group of patients with panic disorder. Am J Psychiatry 141:857–861.

Gorman JM, Cohen BS, Liebowitz MR, et al. (1983): Effects of acute beta-adrenergic blockade on lactate-induced panic. Arch Gen Psychiatry 40:1079–1082.

Gorman JM, Cohen BS, Liebowitz AJ, Fyer AJ, Ross D, Davies SO, Klein DF (1986): Blood gas changes and hypophosphatemia in lactate-induced panic. Arch Gen Psychiatry 43:1067–1071.

Grubb RL, Raichle ME, Eichling JO, et al. (1974): The effects of changes in $PaCO_2$ on cerebral blood volume, blood flow, and vascular mean transit time. Stroke 5:630–639.

Grubb RL, Raichle ME, Higgins CS, Eichling JO (1978): Measurement of regional cerebral blood volume by emission tomography. Ann Neurol 4:322–328.

Gur RE, Gur RC, Skolnick BE, Caroff S, Obrist WD, Resnick S, Reivich M (1985): Brain function in psychiatric disorders. III. Regional cerebral blood flow in unmedicated schizophrenics. Arch Gen Psychiatry 42:329–334.

Gur RE, Skolnick BE, Gur RC, Caroff S, Rieger W, Obrist WD, Younkin D, Reivich M (1983): Brain function in psychiatric disorders. I. Regional cerebral blood flow in medicated schizophrenics. Arch Gen Psychiatry 40:1250–1254.

Halgren E, Walter R (1978): Mental phenomena evoked by electrical stimulation of the human hippocampal formation of amygdala. Brain 101:83–117.

Hall EJ (1984): "Radiation and Life, 2nd Ed." New York: Pergamon Press.

Harber K, Pollimia R (1984): Absorbed dose estimates from radionuclides. J Clin Nuclear Med 9:210–221.

Hays (1980): "Statistics, 3rd Ed." New York: Holt, Rinehart & Winston.

Herman GT (1985): Reconstruction algorithms. In Reivich M, Alavi A (eds): "Positron Emission Tomography." New York: Alan R. Liss, Inc., pp 103–117.

Herscovitch P, Markham J, Raichle ME (1983): Brain blood flow measured with intravenous $H_2{}^{15}O$,I: Theory and error analysis. J Nuclear Med 24:782–789.

Herscovitch P, Raichle ME, Kilbourne MR et al. (1984): Positron emission tomographic measurement of cerebral blood flow and water permeability with 0–15 water and C-11 butanol. Soc Neurosci Abstr 10:792.

Herscovitch P, Raichle ME, Kilbourn MR, Welch MJ

(1987): Positron emission tomographic measurement of cerebral blood flow and permeability-surface area product of water using ^{15}O-water and ^{11}C-butanol. J Cereb Blood Flow Metab (in press).

Huang S, Barrio JR, Phelps ME (1986): Neuroreceptor assay with positron emission tomography: Equilibrium versus dynamic approaches. J Cereb Blood Flow Metab 6:515–521.

Huang S, Barrio JR, Phelps ME (1987): Letter to the editor: Nonlinearity in modeling receptor-binding ligands. J Cereb Blood Flow Metab 7:520–521.

Huang S, Phelps ME, Hoffman EJ, Kuhl DE (1981): Error sensitivity of fluorodeoxyglucose method for measurement of cerebral metabolic rate of glucose. J Cereb Blood Flow Metab 1:391–401.

Humphrey PR, Du Boulay GH, Marshall J, Pearson RC, Russell RWR, Symon L, Wetherley-Mein G, Zilkha E (1979): Cerebral blood-flow and viscosity in relation to polycythaemia. Lancet ii:873–876.

Ingvar D, Franzen G (1974a): Distribution of cerebral activity in chronic schizophrenia. Lancet ii:1484–1486.

Ingvar D, Franzen G (1974b): Abnormalities of cerebral blood flow distribution in patients with chronic schizophrenia. Acta Psychiatry Scand 50:425–462.

Kaada BR (1960): Cingulate, posterior orbital, anterior insular and temporal pole cortex. In Field J, Magoun HW (eds): "Handbook of Physiology, Section I: Neurophysiology." Washington, DC: Am Physiol Soc, Vol 55, pp 1345–1372.

Kelly D, Mitchell-Heffs N, Sherman D (1971): Anxiety and the effects of sodium lactate assessed clinically and physiologically. Br J Psychiatry 119:129–141.

Klein DF (1967): Importance of psychiatric diagnosis in prediction of clinical drug effects. Arch Gen Psychiatry 16:118–126.

Kling A, Steklis HD (1976): A neural substrate for affiliative behavior in nonhuman primates. Brain Behav Evol 12:216–238.

Kluver H, Bucy PC (1939): Preliminary analysis of functions of the temporal lobe in monkeys. Arch Neurol Psychiatry 42:979–1000.

Lader M (1981): Physiological studies in anxiety. In Burrows GD, Davies B (eds): "Handbook of Studies on Anxiety." New York: Elsevier, pp 59–88.

LeDoux JE (1987): Emotion. In Mountcastle VB, Plum F, Geiger SR (eds): Handbook of Physiology, Section I: The Nervous System. Baltimore: Williams and Wilkins, pp 419–460.

Leusen I (1972): Regulation of cerebrospinal fluid composition with reference to breathing. Physiol Rev 52:1–56.

Liebowitz MR, Fyer AJ, Gorman JM, Dillon D, Appleby I, Levy G, Anderson S, Levitt M, Palij M, Davies SO, Klein DF (1984): Lactate provocation of panic attacks. I. Clinical and behavioral findings. Arch Gen Psychiatry 41:764–770.

Liebowitz MR, Fyer AJ, Gorman JM et al. (1986): Alprazolam in the treatment of panic disorders. J Clin Psychopharmacol 6(1):13–20.

Liebowitz MR, Gorman JM, Fyer AJ, Levitt M, Dillon D, Levy G, Appleby IL, Anderson S, Palij M, Davies SO, Klein DF (1985): Lactate provocation of panic attacks.

II. Biochemical and physiological findings. Arch Gen Psychiatry 42:709–719.

Mathew RJ, Duncan GC, Weinman ML, Barr DL (1982): Regional cerebral blood flow in schizophrenia. Arch Gen Psychiatry 39:1121–1124.

Mathew RJ, Wilson WH, Caniel CG (1985): The effect of nonsedating doses of diazepam on regional cerebral blood flow. Biol Psychiatry 20:1109–1116.

Mazziotta JC, Phelps ME, Plummer D, Kuhl DE (1981): Quantitation in positron emission computed tomography: 5. Physical-anatomical effects. J Comput Assist Tomogr 5:734–743.

Mazzochi F, Vignolo LA (1978): Computer assisted tomography in neuropsychological research: A simple procedure for lesion mapping. Cortex 14:136–144.

McGeer PL (1984): In: "National Conference Biological Imaging II, 181." Washington, DC: National Academy of Science.

McNair DM, Kahn RJ (1981): Imipramine compared with a benzodiazepine for agoraphobia. In Klein DF, Rabkin J (eds): "Anxiety: New Research and Changing Concepts." New York: Raven Press.

Mesulam MM, Mufson EJ (1982): Insula of the old world monkey. I: Architectonics in the insulo-orbito-temporal component of the paralimbic brain. J Comp Neurol 212:1–22.

Mintun MA, Fox PT, Raichle ME (1986): (abstract) Discrimination of functional brain responses beneath image resolution with positron emission tomography. J Nuclear Med 27:1025–1026.

Mintun MA, Fox PT, Raichle ME (1989): A highly accurate method of localizing regions of neuronal activation in the human brain using positron emission tomography. J Cereb Blood Flow Metab 9:96–103.

Mintun MA, Raichle ME, Kilbourn MR, Wooten GF, Welch MJ (1984a): A quantitative model for the in vivo assessment of drug binding sites with positron emission tomography. Ann Neurol 15:217–227.

Mintun MA, Raichle ME, Martin WRW, Herscovitch P (1984b): Brain oxygen utilization measured with 0–15 radiotracers and positron emission tomography. J Nuclear Med 25:177–187.

Moran MA, Mufson EJ, Mesulam MM (1987): Neural inputs into the temporopolar cortex of the rhesus monkey. J Comp Neurol 256:88–103.

Mountz JM, Curtis JM, Modell JG, Wilson M, Myung A, Schmaltz S, Kuhl DE (1989): Positron emission tomographic evaluation of cerebral blood flow during state-anxiety in simple phobia. Arch Gen Psychiatry 46:501–504.

Nieuwenhuys R, Vooad J, van Huitzen C (1981): "The Human Central Nervous System, a Synopsis and Atlas," 2nd Ed." Berlin: Springer Verlag.

Noyes R Jr, Anderson DJ, Clancy J, et al. (1984): Diazepam and propranolol in panic disorder and agoraphobia. Arch Gen Psychiatry 41:287–292.

Palacios JM, Kuhar MJ (1982): Beta-adrenergic receptor localization in rat brain by light microscopic autoradiography. Neurochem Int 4:473–490.

Pappata S, Samson Y, Chavoix C, Hantraye P, Bert C, Crouzel M, Prenant C, Maziere MA, Baron JC (1987): Measurement of specifically bound ^{11}C-R015-1788 in human brain in vivo with PET (abstract). J Cereb Blood Flow Metab 7 [Suppl 1]:S352.

Penfield W, Jasper H (1954): "Epilepsy and the Functional Anatomy of the Human Brain." Boston: Little, Brown and Co, p 444.

Perlmutter JS, Larson KB, Raichle ME, Markham J, Mintun MA, Kilbourn MR, Welch MJ (1986): Strategies for in vivo measurement of receptor binding using positron emission tomography. J Cereb Blood Flow Metab 6:154–169.

Petersen SE, Fox PT, Mintun MA, Posner MI, Raichle ME (1988): Studies of the processing of single words using averaged positron emission tomographic measurements of cerebral blood flow change. Nature 331: 585–589.

Phelps ME, Hoffman EJ, Huang TE, Ter-Pogossian MM (1975): Effect of positron range on spatial resolution. J Nuclear Med 16:649–652.

Pitts FN Jr (1984): Lactate, beta-agonists, beta-blockers, and anxiety. J Clin Psychiatry Monogr 2:25–39.

Pitts JR Jr, McClure JN Jr (1967): Lactate metabolism in anxiety neurosis. N Engl J Med 277:1328–1336.

Preskorn SH, Hartman BK, Raichle ME, et al. (1980): The effects of dibenzepines (tricyclic antidepressants) on cerebral capillary permeability in the rat in vivo. J Pharmacol Exp Ther 213:313–320.

Price HL, Marall DG (1981): An autoradiographic study of the projections of the central nucleus of the monkey amygdala. J Neurosci 1:1242–1259.

Raichle ME (1983a): Positron emission tomography. Annu Rev Neurosci 6:249–267.

Raichle ME (1983b): Neurogenic control of blood-brain barrier permeability. Acta Neuropathol [Suppl 8]:75–79.

Raichle ME (1987): Circulatory and metabolic correlates of brain function in normal humans. In: "Handbook of Physiology, The Nervous System V. Higher Functions of the Brain." Bethesda, MD: The American Physiological Society, pp 643–674.

Raichle ME, Grubb RL, Gado MJ, et al. (1976): Correlations between regional cerebral blood flow and oxidative metabolism. Arch Neurol 33:523–526.

Raichle ME, Martin MRW, Herscovitch P, Mintun MA, Markham J (1983): Brain blood flow measured with intravenous $H_2^{15}O$,II: Implementation and validation. J Nuclear Med 24:790–798.

Rainey JM, Frohman CE, Freedman RR, et al. (1984): Specificity of lactate infusion as a model of anxiety. Psychopharmacol Bull 20:45–49.

Redmond DE Jr, Huang YH (1979): New evidence for a locus coeruleus-norepinephrine connection with anxiety. Life Sci 25:2149–2162.

Reiman EM (1987): The study of panic disorder using positron emission tomography. Psychiatr Dev 1:63–78.

Reiman EM (1988): The quest to establish the neural substrates of anxiety. Psychiatr Clin North Am 11: 295–307.

Reiman EM, Fusselman MS, Fox PT, Raichle ME (1989a): Neuroanatomical correlates of anticipatory anxiety. Science 243:1071–1074.

Reiman EM, Raichle ME, Butler FK, Herscovitch P, Rob-

ins E (1984): A focal brain abnormality in panic disorder, a severe form of anxiety. Nature 310:683–685.

Reiman EM, Raichle ME, Robins E (1986a): PET Studies of Panic Disorder: An Update. Presented at American Psychiatic Association Annual Meeting, Washington, DC.

Reiman EM, Raichle ME, Robins E, Butler FK, Herscovitch P, Fox P, Perlmutter J (1986b): The application of positron emission tomography to the study of panic disorder. Am J Psychiatry 143:469–477.

Reiman EM, Raichle ME, Robins E, Mintun MA, Fusselman MS, Fox PT, Price JL, Hackman KA (1989b): Neuroanatomical correlates of a lactate-induced anxiety attack. Arch Gen Psychiatry 46:493–500.

Reivich M, Alavi A (eds) (1985): "Positron Emission Tomography." New York: Alan R. Liss, Inc.

Reivich M, Gur R, Alavi A (1983): Positron emission tomographic studies of sensory stimuli, cognitive processes and anxiety. Hum Neurobiol 2:25–33.

Schad L, Lott S, Schmitt F, Sturm V, Lorenz WJ (1987): Correction of spatial distortion in MR imaging: A prerequisite for accurate stereotaxy. J Comput Assist Tomogr 11:499–505.

Schwartz WJ, Smith CB, Davidsen L, Savaki H, Sokoloff L, Mata M, Fink DJ, Gainer H (1979): Metabolic mapping of functional activity in the hypothalamic neurophysical system of the rat. Science 205:723–725.

Sedvall G, Farde L, Persson A, et al. (1986): Imaging of neurotransmitter receptors in the living human brain. Arch Gen Psychiatry 43:995–1005.

Sheehan DV, Ballenger J, Jacobsen G (1980): Treatment of endogenous anxiety with phobic, hysterical, and hypochondriacal symptoms. Arch Gen Psychiatry 37: 51–59.

Sheehan DV, Davison J, Manschreck T, et al. (1983): The lack of efficacy of a new antidepressant (bupropion) in the treatment of panic disorder with phobias. J Clin Psychopharmacol 3:28–31.

Sheppard G, Gruzelier J, Manchanda R, Gruzelier J, Hirsch SR, Wise R, Frackowiak R, Jones T (1983): ^{15}O-Positron emission tomographic scanning in predominantly never-treated acute schizophrenic patients. Lancet ii:1448–1451.

Sokoloff L, Reivich M, Kennedy C, Des Rosiers DH, Patlak CS, Pettigrew D, Sakurada O, Shinohara M (1977): The [^{14}C]deoxyglucose method for the measurement of local cerebral glucose utilization: Theory, procedure and normal values in the conscious and anesthetized albino rat. J Neurochem 28:897–916.

Stewart R, Devous MD, Rush AJ, Lane L, Bonte FJ (1988): Cerebral blood flow changes during sodium lactate induced panic attacks. Am J Psychiatry 145:442–449.

Strauss E, Risser A, Jones MW (1982): Fear responses in patients with epilepsy. Arch Neurol 39:626–630.

Talairach J, Szikla G (1967): "Atlas d'Anatomie Stereotaxique due Telencephale." Paris: Masson.

Ter-Pogossian MM (1985a): Positron emission tomography instrumentation. In Reivich M, Alavi A (eds): "Positron Emission Tomography." New York: Alan R. Liss, Inc., pp 43–61.

Ter-Pogossian MM (1985b): PET, SPECT and NMRI: Competing or complementary disciplines? J Nuclear Med 26:1487–1498.

Ter-Pogossian MM, Ficke DC, Hood JT, Yamamoto M, Mullani NA (1982): A positron emission tomograph utilizing cesium fluoride scintillation detectors. J Comput Assist Tomogr 6:125–133.

Thomas DJ, DuBoulay GH, Marshall J, Pearson RC, Russell RWR, Symon L, Wetherley-Mein G, Zilkha E (1977): Cerebral blood-flow in polycythaemia. Lancet ii:161–163.

United States Code of Federal Regulations, Title 21, Food and Drug Administration, PMR 361.

Van Hoesen GW (1982): The parahippocampal gyrus: New observations regarding its cortical connections in the monkey. Trends Neurosci, October, pp 345–350.

Volkow ND, Brodie JD, Wolf AP, Angrist B, Russell J, Cancro R (1986): Brain metabolism in patients with schizophrenia before and after acute neuroleptic administration. J Neurol Neurosurg Psychiatry 49:1199–1202.

Wall M, Mielke D, Luther JS (1986): Panic attacks and psychomotor seizures following right temple lobectomy. J Clin Psychiatry 47:219.

Wall M, Tuchman M, Mielke D (1985): Panic attacks and temporal lobe seizures associated with a right temporal lobe arteriovenous malformation: Case Report. J Clin Psychiatry 46:143–145.

Weinberger DR, Berman KF, Zec RF (1986): Physiologic dysfunction of dorsolateral prefrontal cortex in schizophrenia. I. Regional cerebral blood flow evidence. Arch Gen Psychiatry 43:114–124.

Widen L, Blomqvist G, Greitz T, Litton JE, Bergstrom M, Ehrin E, Ericson K, Eriksson L, Ingvar DH, Johansson L, Nilsson JLG, Stone-Elander S, Sedvall G, Wiesel F, Wiik G (1983): PET studies of glucose metabolism in patients with schizophrenia. Am J Neuroradiol 4:550–552.

Wilson R (1979): Analyzing the daily risks of life. Technol Rev, p 45.

Winsky RL, Preskorn SH, Blotzbach R, et al. (1982): Novel antidepressants and neuroleptics: effect on the central adrenergic system. Soc Neurosci Abstr 8:644.

Wolkin A, Jaeger J, Brodie JD, Wolf AP, Fowler J, Rotrosen J, Gomez-Mont F, Cancro R (1985): Persistence of cerebral metabolic abnormalities in chronic schizophrenia as determined by positron emission tomography. Am J Psychiatry 142:564–571.

Wong DF, Wagner HN, Tune LE, Dannals RF, Pearlson GD, Links JM, Tamminga CA, Broussolle EP, Ravert HT, Wilson AA, Thomas Toung JK, Malat J, Williams JA, O'Tuama LA, Snyder SH, Kuhar MJ, Gjedde A (1986): Positron emission tomography reveals elevated D_2 dopamine receptors in drug-naive schizophrenics. Science 234:1558–1563.

Woods SW, Koster K, Krystal JH, Smith EO, Zubal IG, Hoffer PB, Charney DS (1988): Effects of yohimbine on regional cerebral blood flow in patients with panic disorders. Soc Neurosci Abstr 14:47.

Yamamoto M, Ficke DC, Ter-Pogossian MM (1982): Performance study of PET VI, positron computed tomograph with 288 cesium fluoride detectors. IEEE Trans Nuclear Sci 29:529–533.

Yarowski PJ, Ingvar DH (1981): Neuronal activity and energy metabolism (symposium summary) Fed Proc 40:2353–2362.

Zhu XP, Checkley DR, Hickey DS, Isherwood I (1986): Accuracy of area measurements made from MR images compared with computed tomography. J Comput Assist Tomogr 10:96–102.

16

Computed Tomography and Magnetic Resonance Imaging in Panic Disorder

CHARLES KELLNER, MD, AND PETER P. ROY-BYRNE, MD

Department of Psychiatry and Behavioral Sciences, Medical University of South Carolina, Charleston, South Carolina 29425 (C.K.); Department of Psychiatry and Behavioral Sciences, University of Washington School of Medicine, Seattle, Washington 98195 (P.R.-B.)

INTRODUCTION

Computed tomography (CT) scanning ushered in the modern era of in vivo brain imaging in the early 1970s. Its application to psychiatric research has led to the discovery of structural brain changes such as ventricular enlargement and cerebral atrophy in patients with schizophrenia (Weinberger et al., 1979) and major affective disorder (Jacoby and Levy, 1980). Similar abnormalities have also been demonstrated in patients with anorexia nervosa (Artman et al., 1985) and bulimia (Krieg et al., 1987). Curiously, few studies with CT scanning in panic disorder have been carried out. The recent advent of magnetic resonance imagings (MRI) promises to take the field of brain imaging forward a quantum leap. MRI, with its vastly increased resolution, has many advantages and few disadvantages compared with CT. Individual brain nuclei, cortical gyri, and cranial nerves can now be imaged in exquisite detail. In this chapter, we review the literature on both CT and MRI in panic disorder and discuss the potential research and clinical applications of these techniques to anxiety disorders.

Since CT and MRI are techniques to examine gross brain structure (with the exception of MR spectroscopy, which can provide neurochemical information), we focus our discussion on the likelihood of finding structural abnormalities in patients with panic disorder. However, some spectroscopic applications of MRI may

be relevant to panic disorder, and these will be briefly touched on as potentially interesting avenues of investigation. As recently as 10 years ago, it came as a major breakthrough and a surprise that a substantial percentage of schizophrenic patients had ventricular enlargement and cerebral atrophy. Following the initial paper of Johnstone et al. (1976), a large literature substantiating these abnormalities in schizophrenic patients developed. Although it is tempting to assume that no such major abnormalities could be present in panic disorder, few CT or brain morphologic studies have been carried out. Furthermore, even if gross abnormalities are not present, it remains a reasonable possibility that more subtle, yet still grossly detectable, brain abnormalities are involved in panic disorder. The definitive CT studies have not been done, and now MRI studies likely will be used to investigate this issue.

Several lines of evidence have converged to make it quite clear that there are major biochemical underpinnings to panic disorder. Such biological abnormalities or "markers" that function at a molecular or neurotransmitter level could be associated with macroscopic brain changes. These changes might be 1) intrinsic to the illness; 2) "permissive" primary factors that allow the full expression of the biochemical defects intrinsic to the illness; 3) a downstream result of the effects of the illness (e.g., chronic anxiety causing biochemical changes, which, in turn, cause structural changes); or 4) an effect of the medication used to treat the illness. If ongoing studies do, in

Neurobiology of Panic Disorder, Pages 271–280
© 1990 Alan R. Liss, Inc.

fact, detect significant abnormalities, it should be possible to design studies to clarify whether they are intrinsic to the illness or secondary phenomena.

Brain structural changes could either be diffuse and "nonspecific" (e.g., atrophy or ventricular enlargement) or selectively involve specific brain regions. Reiman's recent positron emission tomography (PET) studies (Reiman et al., 1986) showing asymmetrical metabolic activity in the parahippocampal region of patients with panic disorder suggest that a specific regional abnormality could exist, although this finding was not confirmed by a subsequent study (Harsch et al., 1987) using single photon emission tomography, a method with lower resolution, to measure blood flow. Gloor's studies (Gloor et al., 1982) of epileptic patients in which electrical stimulation of the hippocampus, parahippocampal gyrus, and amygdala elicited a fear response also support the possibility that discrete brain areas are involved in the genesis of panic disorder. Animal studies of the cortical connections of the hippocampal formation (Gray, 1982; Van Hoesen, 1982) lend further support to the notion of a defined system that integrates sensory information and directs responses to noxious environmental cues.

CT SCANNING

CT scanning was introduced in the early 1970s and rapidly changed the practice of neurology and neurosurgery. For the first time it became possible to image the brain in great detail in living patients. Prior to CT, the only neuroimaging techniques available had been skull X-rays, pneumoencephalography, cerebral angiography, cerebral ultrasound, and radioisotope brain scanning. All these techniques were severely limited by either their invasive nature or their lack of sensitivity in imaging the brain. CT scanning is safe and noninvasive. The only risks involved are those of the exposure to a relatively small amount of radiation and the small risk of reaction to contrast dye (Chiu et al., 1986) when it is used.

CT technique involves passing X-rays through body tissues and then detecting the X-rays after their travel through the tissue. Scintillation detectors pick up radiation counts and feed these data to a computer, which constructs an image that is based on tissue density. More radioopaque substances, such as bone, appear white, and more radiolucent substances such as brain or cerebrospinal fluid (CSF) appear gray and black, respectively. Individual units of data of the CT film are called pixels, and the degree of blackness or whiteness (reflecting density) is measured on the scale of "Hounsfield units." CT pictures are axial cross sections ("slices") of the body, and a routine brain examination consists of approximately 12 slices from the base of the skull to the vertex.

Limitations of CT scanning include the fact that posterior fossa structures are not well visualized due to bony artifact and that resolution, at least compared with the MRI technique, is relatively poor. Additionally, ability to reconstruct images in various planes is limited. Finally, as alluded to above, there is the small but definite risk of exposure to radiation. This consideration limits the number of scans that a patient or subject might be allowed to receive for research purposes. On the positive side, a routine CT scan takes only about 15–30 minutes to perform, and patients usually tolerate it without difficulty.

Various methodologies have been developed to use CT scan measurements in psychiatric research. Both linear (Trimble and Kingsley, 1978) and area (Synek and Reuben, 1976) measurements of neuroanatomic structures have been used. Most commonly, the "ventricular-brain ratio" (VBR) is used to compare cerebral ventricular size between scans (Synek and Reuben, 1976; Weinberger et al., 1979). This involves measurement of the area of the lateral ventricles on the CT slice in which the ventricles appear largest, divided by the area of the entire brain on that slice. By custom, this is multipled by 100 to get the VBR. Measurements have been made using hand-held planimeters on either the actual CT film itself or on projected enlargements. A more sophisticated technique involves measuring these areas directly on the CT console using a cursor to enclose areas that are then measured by the CT computer. Alternatively, a pixel density method (Schmauss and Krieg, 1987) to determine VBR has been used in which the CT computer can be made to select all the pixels of a given density in a slice and then measure their area. In such a way, the approximate density of CSF could be chosen, and all CSF spaces in a particular slice are then measured and compared to the total area of brain on that slice.

More sophisticated volume measurements of CSF spaces have been attempted by some investigators. Jernigan et al. (1982) employed a computerized CT scan analysis using a volume-averaging model to estimate CSF content in defined segments of the intracranial space. By summing these segments, they obtained measurements of ventricular fluid volume and sulcal fluid volume in a group of schizophrenic patients and a group of normal volunteers. This technique has not, however, been applied to studies in panic disorder patients.

Direct comparison of absolute VBR data is confounded by differences in CT scanners and differences in the techniques used to make the measurements. It is also recognized that differences in control populations (e.g., healthy volunteers versus medical patients) can account for variability in the mean VBR across studies (Smith and Iacono, 1986). Thus, caution must be used when comparing results from different studies (Jernigan et al., 1982). Despite this, Synek and Reuben (1976) have reported a quantitative method for evaluating the clinical significance of ventricular size and suggest that the VBR is approximately 5 in normals, 7 in borderline cases, and greater than 10 in abnormal conditions.

Various visual scales to rate cortical atrophy and sulcal size have also been devised. However, there is less agreement about the best way accurately to measure cortical atrophy on CT scans (Jernigan et al., 1980; Kreig et al., 1986; Turkheimer et al., 1984).

Studies in alcoholics (Artman et al., 1981), eating disorder patients (Krieg et al., 1986b), and affectively ill patients (Kellner et al., 1982) have addressed the issue of potential reversibility of the brain structural changes seen on CT scans. The possibility that ventricular enlargement and/or cortical atrophy may be either state-dependent changes or changes related to medication is intriguing and requires further investigation. A particularly intriguing hypothesis that we have proposed elsewhere (Kellner et al., 1982) is that chronic or episodic endogenous hypercortisolism associated with affective illness or eating disorders may be the cause of apparent cerebral atrophy on CT scans. The observation that ultimately led to this hypothesis was that the administration of high-dose exogenous steroids for the treatment of collagen-vascular and other illnesses produced cortical atrophy on CT scans that resolved within months after cessation of the drug treatment (Bentson et al., 1978; Lagenstein et al., 1979; Okuno et al., 1980). Since panic disorder patients have been reported to have normal levels of urinary-free cortisol (Uhde et al., 1988) and most demonstrate normal cortisol suppression with dexamethasone (Curtis et al., 1982; Peterson et al., 1985; Roy-Byrne et al., 1985), this may not be a mechanism with particular relevance in panic disorder.

The mechanism by which alcohol could cause cerebral atrophy is unknown, but shifts in brain water have been postulated (Smith et al., 1985). Until the neuropathological correlates of the atrophy observed on CT scans are known (i.e., are changes in cellular protein content or structure involved or merely shifts of fluids from one compartment to another?), it will be difficult to fully understand the mechanism underlying cerebral atrophy.

CT STUDIES IN PANIC DISORDER

Lader et al. (1984) investigated structural brain abnormalities in a group of 20 long-term benzodiazepine users, 18 of whom were described as having an anxiety state (the specific DSM III diagnosis was not provided). The hypothesis that the authors were investigating was whether benzodiazepines taken on a long-term basis could cause CT scan changes. They measured VBR and also rated sulcal, sylvian fissure, and interhemispheric fissure widening. They compared the results of the benzodiazepine user group with those of a group of 19 normal controls and another group of 19 alcoholics. They found that the VBR of the benzodiazepine group was significantly larger than that of the control group (7.09 vs. 5.77) but smaller than that of the alcoholic group (9.22). Among the benzodiazepine users, there was no correlation with length of previous benzodiazepine usage. The measures of cortical atrophy showed a nonsignificant trend for the benzodiazepine group to be larger than the control group. Three of the benzodiazepine users had definite CT scan abnormalities (compared with one of the controls and three of the alcoholics) consisting of ventricular enlargement, sulcal widening, or sylvian or interhemispheric fissure widening. In their discussion, Lader et al. considered several possible explanations for their findings, including 1) that benzodiazepines themselves caused the observed changes, 2) that people with these brain changes due to other causes are prone to develop anxiety disorders that require prolonged sedative use, and 3) that concomitant unreported alcohol use might explain some of the abnormalities. They stressed that, given the widespread use of benzodiazepines, it is "important to establish the nature, extent, and reversibility of functional and structural brain changes." Lader (personal communication) is carrying out a follow-up study in a group of general practice patients and is finding a similar but probably a smaller effect than was seen in the original study.

The next CT study in panic disorder was that of Uhde and Kellner (1987). They studied 25 panic disorder patients from the anxiety clinic at the NIMH. The patients exhibited panic and phobic (agoraphobia subtype) disorders by RDC. Seven of these patients had a history of major melancholic depression, and two had concurrent major depression without melancholia. Lifetime exposure to benzodiazepines to the nearest 6 months was calculated. The mean for the group was 2.6 ± 3.5 years (range 0–12 years) of use. Each patient had a routine brain CT scan and the VBR was measured by planimetry. We found that, overall, patients had normal (or even small, when compared to other control groups) ventricular size (mean VBR 3.4 ± 2.4 SD). In fact, the only scan that was read as clinically abnormal was that of a patient with "abnormally small" ventricles for age. Of particular interest, however, was the finding of a significant association between VBR and duration of benzodiazepine use. This association was not found by Lader et al. (1984), but differences in the patient population might account for this. Lader et al. studied only patients with at least 2.5 years of benzodiazepine therapy; 70% of our sample were subjects with less than 2.5 years of benzodiazepine use. Since those patients in our study

with less than 2.5 years of benzodiazepine treatment had significantly smaller VBR (2.5 ± 1.8) compared to patients with greater than 2.5 years of benzodiazepine use (5.4 ± 2.4), the lack of association between VBR and duration of benzodiazepine use in the study by Lader et al. might be related to exclusion of subjects within the lower range of benzodiazepine exposure.

The nature of changes in VBR in panic disorder patients who take benzodiazepines is unclear. As was discussed above, it remains to be discovered whether apparent changes in brain structure are the result of drug use or are intrinsic to anxiety disorders themselves. It is also possible that concurrent alcohol use (which is notoriously underreported by patients) might account for some of the changes observed in this study.

Schmauss and Krieg (1987) carried out another study to investigate the nature of brain structural changes in patients on benzodiazepines. They studied 17 inpatients who were admitted to the hospital for benzodiazepine withdrawal. Diagnoses included generalized anxiety disorder, agoraphobia with panic attacks, depressive neurosis, and social phobia (Schmauss et al., 1987). They divided their patients into a high-dose benzodiazepine group (daily benzodiazepine dose >50 mg of diazepam equivalents, N = 8) and a low-dose benzodiazepine group (daily benzodiazepine dose <50 mg diazepam equivalents, N = 9). A comparison group of 22 age- and sex-matched patients with no history of drug abuse or neuropsychiatric illness was used. CT scans were used to calculate VBR with a pixel-density method on the computer console. In addition, linear measurements to assess ventricular size and external CSF spaces were performed. The latter included width of the insular cisterns, width of the anterior part of the interhemispheric fissure, and width of the four most prominent cortical sulci. They found significantly higher mean VBRs for both high- and low-dose benzodiazepine-dependent patients (6.81 ± 0.64, 4.47 ± 1.01, respectively) compared to the control group (2.91 ± 0.18). The difference in VBR between the high- and low-dose groups was also significant and could not be accounted for by age or duration of benzodiazepine use. Furthermore, they found a moderate enlargement of "external" CSF spaces in both high- and low-dose benzodiazepine groups compared to the controls.

The authors emphasize their finding that increases in VBR were independent of the *duration* of benzodiazepine use but related to benzodiazepine *dose*. [Interestingly, this is exactly the opposite of what is seen in benzodiazepine dependence, which is much more affected by duration of treatment than by dose (Rickels et al., 1983; Roy-Byrne and Hammer, 1988).] They discuss the fact that similar CT scan changes are seen in anorexia, alcoholism, and benzodiazepine use, raising the question of whether the underlying mechanism of the observed changes is common to all of these entities.

Clearly, longitudinal studies are needed to address the issue of the nature and potential reversibility of the CT scan changes seen in anxiety disorder patients in these few studies. A study design using repeat CT scans in patients on and off benzodiazepines would help clarify the extent to which these diffuse changes are the result of treatment or the disease process itself. It is likely that these questions will be addressed in MR studies rather than CT studies, because of the ability to perform repeated scans without exposing the patient to the risk of radiation.

MRI

MRI has revolutionized the clinical neurosciences with its ability to examine in minute detail the structural anatomy of the central nervous system. It is such a new technique that its full impact on clinical and research efforts in the neurosciences cannot yet be fully evaluated. Early studies (Matthew et al., 1985; Rangel-Guerra et al., 1983; Smith et al., 1984) in psychiatric patient populations suggest that it will have wide applicability in clinical diagnosis and many aspects of psychiatric research.

An explanation of the physics underlying the production of MRI images is beyond the scope of this chapter. In brief, MRI depends on the fact that some atomic nuclei, when placed in a magnetic field, absorb or emit radiofrequency energy of a specific frequency (Bydder, 1988). Only nuclei that have an odd number of protons or neutrons (and therefore produce a net charge) participate in this phenomenon. Several such nuclei that are of medical interest include hydrogen (proton), phosphorus (^{31}P), sodium (^{23}Na), carbon (^{13}C), fluoride (^{19}F), and potassium (^{39}P). Of these, hydrogen is by far the most important, given the abundance of water in the body, and to date has been the focus of most clinical MRI.

In simplified form, the subject to be scanned is placed in a powerful magnetic field into which a radiofrequency is pulsed. This perturbs the hydrogen nuclei (protons) in the tissue, which then give off a detectable signal when they relax to their resting condition. This signal can then be constructed into an image by a computer.

Two time constants, T_1 and T_2, describe different aspects of the relaxation of atomic nuclei to their equilibrium positions. T_1, the longitudinal (spin-lattice) relaxation time represents that part of the energy that is lost to the surrounding tissue (lattice). T_2, the transverse (spin-spin) relaxation time, represents the part of the energy that is lost to adjacent nuclei with the same spin (Buonanno et al., 1983; DeMyer et al., 1985).

The intensity of an MRI signal also depends on the number of atomic nuclei spinning at the frequency being investigated, and this is called spin (or proton) density (DeMyer et al., 1985). MR images are referred to as either "T_1-weighted" or "T_2-weighted" sequences depending on how the pulse sequences are selected (Gerard and Rossi, 1984).

Each bodily tissue has its own characteristic T_1 and T_2 values, which may be altered in disease states. Watery liquids (e.g., CSF) have signal characteristics different from those of proteinaceous liquids, which in turn are different from lipids or solids. In general, T_1-weighted images reveal excellent anatomic detail, with good contrast between white and gray matter. On T_1-weighted images, white matter, fat, and bone marrow appear white, gray matter appears gray, and CSF and bone appear black (DeMyer et al., 1985). T_2-weighted images, in general, are excellent for differentiating pathological from normal tissue. Inflammatory tissue and edema may appear bright, and CSF appears brighter than in T_1-weighted sequences.

The results of this process are images of unparalleled resolution and clarity. Anatomic structures are visualized in exquisite detail. Cortical gyral patterns and even individual brainstem nuclei (e.g., the red nucleus) can be distinguished. Excellent gray-white matter differentiation is obtainable.

Compared with CT scanning, MRI has many advantages and few disadvantages. With MRI, the patient is not exposed to any ionizing radiation. In fact, it is currently believed that there are no ill effects from being subjected to MR scanning (Budinger, 1981). Whether this will be shown to be true over the course of years remains to be seen. The implication of the safety of MRI is that patients could be scanned repeatedly without fear of ill effects. This would enable longitudinal data to be gathered, which will be crucial in determining the natural history of any brain structural changes in panic disorder and in determining whether such changes may be related to treatment and are potentially reversible.

MR images can be reconstructed in multiple planes (sagittal, coronal, axial), giving a much clearer picture of anatomic structures. Posterior fossa structures, which are often obscured by streak artifact from bone on CT scan, are clearly seen with MRI. MRI has some unique abilities such as the measurement of flowing blood (Gerard and Rossi, 1984) or other fluids and also the potential to measure physiological and chemical parameters (when nuclei other than protons are imaged). Finally, it may be possible to repeat accurately measurements of anatomic structures from scans done at different times on the same patient because of the ability to locate internal anatomic landmarks. Such consistency between CT scans is not currently attainable and at best, approximations are made by attempts to position the patient in a similar fashion from one scan to the next. Drawbacks to MRI are few, but include the fact that scan acquisition time is much longer than with CT. A typical MR examination may take 1–2 hr, whereas a CT scan may take 15–30 min. As in CT, movement artifact can seriously degrade the quality of the images.

In addition, the MRI scanner is perceived as an extremely claustrophobic environment by a significant minority of patients (Fishbain et al., 1988; Klonoff et al., 1986). Whether this will prove to be a bigger problem in a population of psychiatric patients remains to be seen. Preliminary observations in a study we are performing on obsessive–compulsive disorder patients indicate that these patients can tolerate the scan procedure as well as normal controls. Among the first eight patients scanned, none required termination of the procedure nor any sedation for completion of the procedure. One would predict that panic disorder patients might have more difficulty tolerating the procedure. Sedation with various agents, including the ultrashort-acting benzodiazepine medazolam, can be used effectively to treat anxiety and minimize movement artifact.

The current cost benefit of CT over MRI is likely to diminish as MRI becomes the scanning procedure of choice. In neurology and neurosurgery, MRI has revolutionized the diagnosis of many illnesses. Multiple sclerosis stands out as the most dramatic example (Lukes et al., 1982). This is because of the particularly exquisite ability of MRI to visualize white matter lesions. Preliminary studies in psychiatric patient populations have focused on both anatomic (Smith et al., 1984) and physiologic parameters (Rangel-Guerra et al., 1983).

Rangel-Guerra et al. (1983) looked at T_1 values in frontal and temporal lobes of manic-depressive patients. (The T_1 relaxation time is related to the state of water in the tissue; T_1 increases with increases in the ratio of free to bound water.) They reported higher T_1 values in the patient group compared to controls before lithium treatment, with a normalization of this parameter following lithium treatment. Besson et al. (1981) as well as other investigators (Smith et al., 1985) have used MRI to study brain water content in alcoholics in the intoxicated and withdrawal states. Andreason et al. (1986) have studied schizophrenic patients with MRI and found significantly smaller skull, brain, and frontal lobe sizes. Other preliminary studies have investigated the size of the corpus callosum (Nasrallah et al., 1986).

MRI STUDIES IN PANIC DISORDER

To our knowledge, the study by Fontine et al. (1987) is the first and only MRI study in panic disorder patients. These authors studied

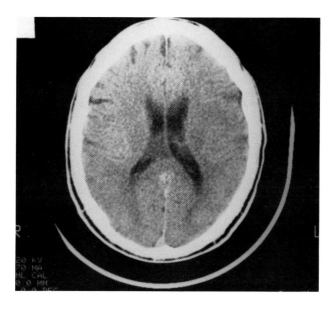

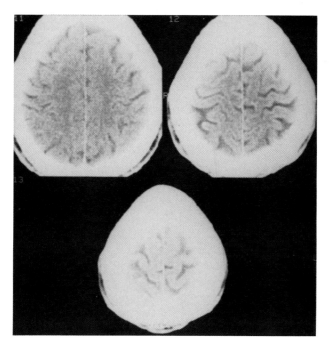

Fig. 16–1. CT scan demonstrating moderate cerebral atrophy in a 39-year-old man with panic disorder.

13 patients with panic disorder who were between 20 and 40 years old (mean 33.3 years). These patients had all been treated with clonazepam, but it is not reported whether they were on medication at the time of the scan. Of interest, two patients had to be excluded from the study, one because of a panic attack 10 min into the scan and one because of last-minute

refusal. In addition, 10 controls (mean of 33.4 years) were scanned.

Several scan abnormalities were found in panic disorder patients as compared to controls. Five of the 13 panic disorder patients showed areas of decreased signal on T_1- weighted images in white matter "mostly in the right temporal lobe." None of the controls demonstrated this abnormality. In one patient, decreased signal on T_1-weighted images was seen in both right frontal and temporal lobes. Furthermore, various measures of atrophy were more frequent in the panic disorder patients. Atrophy of the temporal horns was seen in five patients compared to two controls. "Subcortical atrophy" was seen in two patients and no controls. Overall, 54% of panic disorder patients vs. 20% of controls had some measure of brain atrophy.

This is clearly a very preliminary study; nonetheless its findings are provocative. The significance of decreased T_1 signal in the temporal lobes is unclear but may relate to alterations of brain water concentration. Similarly the finding of atrophy, particularly focal atrophy of the right temporal lobe, is of unclear significance. The authors suggest that old ischemic or infectious insults or developmental abnormalities might underlie these changes. It should also be kept in mind that the possible contribution of concurrent benzodiazepine therapy to any of the observed abnormalities cannot be discounted.

Further studies are underway by various groups that may replicate and further expand the above findings. More detailed studies measuring other neuroanatomic structures with greater precision are clearly needed. In addition, MRI studies using nuclei other than hydrogen will enable researchers to investigate neurophysiological as well as neuroanatomic abnormalities. For example, MRI spectroscopy using phosphorus can provide information about some enzymatic reactions as well as determinations of concentrations of phosphorylated metabolites such as adenosine diphosphate (ADP) and adenosine triphosphate (ATP). In addition, it can provide measurements of intracellular pH (Buonanno et al., 1983). A recent study (Miatto et al., 1986) used ^{31}P MRI spectroscopy to study phospholipid metabolism in autopsy brain samples from Alzheimer's disease patients and found evidence of altered phospholipid metabolism. Neurotransmitter systems may be able to be studied in panic disorder as well as other psychiatric patient populations using MRI spectroscopic techniques. It may also be possible to measure regional brain lactate concentrations in panic disorder after intravenous lactate infusions.

From the CT and MRI work to date, it appears that structural brain abnormalities may be more common in panic disorder than in controls (Fig. 16-1). It remains to be discovered whether these abnormalities are diffuse or focal, whether they are related to the disease process itself or to treatment with medication, whether they are reversible, and what is their specific underlying pathophysiology. With the techniques now at hand it seems likely that these questions are answerable. Hopefully, the answers will eventually help in the diagnosis and treatment of panic disorder.

REFERENCES

Andreasen N, Nasrallah HA, Dunn V, Olson SC, Grove WM, Ehrhardt JC, Coffman JA, Crossett JH (1986): Structural abnormalities in the frontal system in schizophrenia. Arch Gen Psychiatry 43:136–144.

Artman H, Gall MV, Hacke H, Herrlich J (1981): Reversible enlargement of CSF spaces in chronic alcoholics. AJNR 2:23–27.

Artman H, Grau H, Adelmann M, Schleiffer R (1985): Reversible and nonreversible enlargement of cerebrospinal fluid spaces in anorexia nervosa. Neuroradiology 27:304–312.

Bentson JR, Reza M, Winter J, Wilson G (1978): Steroids and apparent cerebral atrophy on computed tomography scans. J Comput Assist Tomogr 2:16.

Besson JAD, Glen AIM, Iljon FE, MacDonald A, Smith FW, Hutchinson JM, Mallard JR, Ashcroft GW (1981): Nuclear magnetic resonance observations in alcoholic cerebral disorder and the role of vasopressin. Lancet ii:923–924.

Budinger TF (1981): Nuclear magnetic resonance in vivo studies: known thresholds for health effects. J Comput Assist Tomogr 5:800–811.

Buonanno FS, Pykett IL, Brady TJ, Pohost GM (1983): Clinical applications of nuclear magnetic resonance (NMR). Disease-a-Month 29(8):8–79.

Bydder GM (1988): NMR imaging of the central nervous system. In Symon L (ed): "Advances and Technical Standards. Neurosurgery, Vol II." New York: Springer-Verlag, pp 7–35.

Chiu LE, Lipcamon JD, Yiu-Chiu VS (1986): "Clinical Computed Tomography." Rockville, MD: Systems Corporation.

Curtis GC, Cameron OG, Nesse RM (1982): The dexamethasone suppression test in panic disorder and agoraphobia. Am J Psychiatry 139:1043–1046.

DeMyer MK, Hendrie HC, Gilmore RL, DeMyer WE (1985): Magnetic resonance imaging in psychiatry. Psychiatr Ann 15(41):262–267.

Fishbain DA, Goldberg M, Labbe E, Zacher D, Rosomoff-Steele R, Rosomoff H (1988): Long-term claustrophobia following magnetic resonance imaging [letter]. Am J Psychiatry 145:1038–1039.

Fontaine R, Breton G, Dery R, Elie R, Fontaine S (1987): MRI in panic disorder: subcortical atrophy and decreased signal in T_1. Paper presented at the Biological Psychiatry Meeting, May, 1987.

Gerard G, Rossi DR (1984): Nuclear magnetic resonance imaging of the brain. Hosp Pract 7:143–156.

Gloor P, Oliver A, Quesney LF, Andermann F, Horowitz S (1982): The role of the limbic system in experimental phenomena of temporal lobe epilepsy. Ann Neurol 12:129–144.

Gray JAC (1982): "The Neuropsychology of Anxiety: An Enquiry Into the Functions of the Septo-Hippocampal System." New York: Oxford University Press.

Harsch HH, Goldstein M, Hellman RS, Lauren S, Young D, Tikofsky R, Collier BD (1987): Regional cerebral blood flow in panic disorder. American Psychiatric Association, 140th Annual Meeting, New Research Abstract 172.

Jacoby RJ, Levy R (1980): Computed tomography in the elderly, Part 3 (affective disorder). Br J Psychiatry 136:270.

Jernigan TL, Zatz LM, Feinberg I, Fein G (1980): Measurement of cerebral atrophy in the aged by computed tomography. In Poon LW (ed): "Aging in the 1980s." Washington, DC. American Psychological Association, pp 86–94.

Jernigan TL, Zatz LM, Moses JA, Cardellino JP (1982): Computed tomography in schizophrenics and normal volunteers. Arch Gen Psychiatry 39:765–777.

Johnstone EC, Crow TJ, Frith CS, Husband J, Kreel L (1976): Cerebral ventricular size and cognitive impairment in chronic schizophrenia. Lancet ii:294.

Kellner CH, Rubinow DR, Gold PW, Post RM (1982): Relationship of cortisol hypersecretion to brain CAT scan alterations in depressed patients. Psychiatry Res 8:191–197.

Klonoff EA, Jeffrey JW, Kaufman B (1986): The use of systematic desensitization to overcome resistance to magnetic resonance imaging (MRI) scanning. Behav Ther Exp Psychiatry 17:189–192.

Krieg JC, Backmund H, Pirke, KM (1987): Cranial computed tomography findings in bulimia. Acta Psychiatr Scand 75:144–149.

Kreig JC, Emrich HM, Backmun H, Pirke KM, Herholz K, Pawlik G, Heiss WD (1986): Brain morphology (CT) and cerebral metabolism (PET) in anorexia nervosa. In Ferrari E, Brambilla F (eds): "Disorders of Eating Behaviors. A Psychoneuroendocrine Approach." Oxford: Pergamon Press.

Lader MH, Ron M, Petursson H (1984): Computed axial brain tomography in long-term benzodiazepine users. Psychol Med 14:203–206.

Lagenstein I, Willy RP, Kuhne D (1979): Cranial computed tomography (CCT) findings in children treated with ACTH and dexamethasone: First results. Neuropaediatrics 10:370.

Lukes SA, Aminoff MJ, Mills C, Norman D, Crooks L, Panitch HS (1982): Nuclear magnetic resonance imaging in patients with definite multiple sclerosis. Ann Neurol 12:76.

Mathew RJ, Partain CL, Prakash R, Kulkarni MV, Logan TP, Wilson WH (1985): A study of the septum pellucidum and corpus callosum in schizophrenia with MR imaging. Acta Psychiatrica Scand 72:414–421.

Miatto O, Gonzalez TG, Buonanno F, Growdon JH (1986): In vitro ^{31}PNMR spectroscopy detects altered phospholipid metabolism in Alzheimer's disease. Can J Neurol Sci 13:535–539.

Nasrallah HA, Andreason NC, Coffman JA, Olson SC, Dunn VD, Ehrhardt JC, Chapman SM (1986): A controlled magnetic resonance imaging study of corpus callosum thickness in schizophrenia. Biol Psychiatry 21:274–282.

Okuno T, Ito M, Konishi Y, Yoshioka M, Nakano Y (1980): Cerebral atrophy following ACTH therapy. J Comput Assisted Tomogr 4:20.

Peterson GA, Ballenger JC, Cox DP, Hucek A, Lydiard RB, Laraia MT, Trockman C (1985): The dexamethasone suppression test in agoraphobia. J Clin Psychopharmacol 5:100–102.

Rangel-Guerra RA, Perez-Payan H, Minkoff L, Todd LE (1983): Nuclear magnetic resonance in bipolar affective disorders. AJNR 4:229–231.

Reiman EM, Raichle ME, Robin EL, Butler FK, Herscovitch P, Fox P, Perlmutter J (1986): The application of positron emission tomography to the study of panic disorder. Am J Psychiatry 143:4.

Rickels K, Case WG, Downing RW, Winokur A (1983): Long-term diazepam therapy and clinical outcome. JAMA 250:767–771.

Roy-Byrne PP, Bierer LM, Uhde TW (1985): The dexamethasone suppression test in panic disorder: Comparison with normal controls. Biol Psychiatry 20:1237–1240.

Roy-Byrne P, Hommer D (1988): Benzodiazepine withdrawal syndromes: Overview and implications for the treatment of anxiety. Am J Med 84:1041–1051.

Schmauss C, Apelt S, Emrich HM (1987): Characterization of benzodiazepine withdrawal in high and low-dose dependent psychiatric inpatients. Brain Res Bull 19:393–400.

Schmauss C, Krieg JC (1987): Enlargement of cerebrospinal fluid spaces in long-term benzodiazepine abusers. Psychol Med 17:869–873.

Smith GN, Iacono WG (1986): Lateral ventricular size in schizophrenia and choice of control group. Lancet i:1450.

Smith MA, Chick J, Kean DM, Douglas RH, Singer A, Kendell R, Best JJ (1985): Brain water in chronic alcoholic patients measured by magnetic resonance imaging. Lancet i:1273–1274.

Smith RC, Calderon M, Ravichandran GK, Largen J, Vroulis G, Shvartsburd A, Gordon J, Schoolar JC (1984): Nuclear magnetic resonance in schizophrenia: A preliminary study. Psychiatry Res 12:137–147.

Synek V, Reuben JR (1976): The ventricular-brain ratio

using planimetric measurement of EMI scans. Br J Radiology 49:233–237.

Trimble M, Kingsley D (1978): Cerebral ventricular size in chronic schizophrenia. Lancet i:278–279.

Turkheimer E, Cullum C, Munro H, Donn WM, Hubler DW, Paver SW, Yeo RA, Bigler ED (1984): Quantifying cortical atrophy. J Neurol Neurosurg Psychiatry 47:1314–1318.

Uhde TW, Kellner CH (1987): Cerebral ventricular size in panic disorder. J Affect Disord 12:175–178.

Van Hoesen GW (1982): The parahippocampal gyrus: New observations regarding its cortical connections in the monkey. Trends Neurosci 10:345–350.

Weinberger DR, Torrey EF, Neophytides AN, Wyatt J (1979): Lateral cerebral ventricular enlargement in chronic schizophrenia. Arch Gen Psychiatry 36:735.

17

Cerebral Blood Flow in Anxiety and Panic

ROY J. MATHEW, MD, AND **WILLIAM H. WILSON**, PhD

Department of Psychiatry, Duke University Medical Center, Durham, North Carolina 27710

INTRODUCTION

Acute attacks of anxiety and panic are associated with profound, widespread physiological changes. Some of these changes are circulatory, and others influence circulation through indirect mechanisms, such as autonomic activation. Both general circulation and blood flow to specific vascular beds are usually effected; blood flow to the skin is reduced, and flow to muscle is increased (Lader, 1975). Although brain blood flow is of considerable clinical significance, the effect of anxiety on cerebral circulation is only poorly understood. In this chapter, we examine ways in which physiological changes known to accompany anxiety might influence cerebral blood flow (CBF), describe the results of the available studies on this topic, and discuss the possible clinical implications of anxiety-related CBF changes.

NEUROPHYSIOLOGY OF ANXIETY

The Brainstem Reticular Formation

The concept of arousal is central to the neurophysiology of anxiety. In simple terms, "arousal" refers to levels of generalized, diffuse activation of the brain. The concept had its origins in the learning theorist's search for a nonspecific component of drive that energized behavior. The concept was largely supported by electroencephalographic (EEG) and neurophysiologic experiments and physiological studies of "behavioral energetics" (Lader, 1982; Malmo, 1959; Duffy, 1972). Studies of

Neurobiology of Panic Disorder, Pages 281–309
© 1990 Alan R. Liss, Inc.

the EEG changes induced by stimulation of different parts of the brain enabled Moruzzi and Magoun (1949) to identify the brainstem reticular formation as the brain region responsible for arousal. The reticular formation is composed of an extensive network of neurons, outside of the major nuclear groups of the brainstem. Caudally, it is continuous with the less extensive interneuronal network in the spinal cord and rostrally with the medullary nucleus of the thalamus, the zona incerta, and the lateral region of the hypothalamus. The reticular formation was originally thought to be diffuse and nonspecific, but more recent studies have identified ascending and descending pathways, facilitatory and inhibitory components, and groups of neurons (based on their anatomic location and chemical characteristics) within the network of reticular neurons (Kandel and Schwartz, 1981; Siegel, 1979). Groups of reticular neurons such as the norepinephrine-containing locus ceruleus and the serotonin-containing raphe nuclei are well known for their neuropsychiatric significance. Although these neuron groupings have been ascribed other functions, there is general agreement that the brainstem reticular core is intimately related to arousal.

The Limbic System

The involvement of brain regions other than the reticular formation in the arousal mechanism is more complex. The role played by various parts of the limbic system, to which the reticular formation is connected, is a highly controversial topic. The limbic system is closely related to autonomic activity and arousal, and it has both facilitatory and inhibitory components. It subserves several other physiological functions (hunger, thirst, sex drive, aggression, memory) that would seem to be related to arousal. An extensive body of information is available on the anatomy and physiology of the limbic system (Isaacson, 1982). Several complex arousal systems, which incorporate reticular formation and limbic system, have been postulated (Routtenberg, 1968; Fowles, 1980).

The Cerebral Cortex

The nature of involvement of cerebral cortex in the arousal mechanism would seem less controversial. Frontal lobe has been identified as the cortical region with the most intimate connections with such parts of the subcortical arousal system as the thalamus and upper parts of the brainstem. Frontal lobes also have dense connections with other cortical regions (Nauta, 1971; Kelly, 1976). Thus it would seem highly likely that frontal lobes constitute the cortical apparatus responsible for maintaining levels of activation of the brain. This possibility is supported by a large body of clinical and experimental evidence, especially those provided by Luria (Luria, 1973; Fuster, 1980; Pribram, 1973). The well known EEG pattern of the predominant wave forms of higher frequency over the frontal lobe during wakefulness supports this hypothesis. It should also be noted that the cortical gray matter is thicker on cross section over the frontal regions compared with the occipital pole (Noback, 1975; Carpenter, 1976). In addition to arousal, more complicated functions closely related to wakefulness, such as abstract thought, synthetic reasoning, and organization of independent behaviors in time and space toward future goals have also been ascribed to the frontal lobes (Goldman-Rakic, 1984).

The Two Hemispheres

A growing body of literature suggests hemispheric differences in the mediation of emotions, and a greater role has been ascribed to the right hemisphere (Galin, 1974; Prohovnik, 1978; Ross, 1984). This may be an oversimplification in the case of anxiety. Studies conducted by Tucker and associates indicate that differing levels of anxiety may be associated with asymmetrical hemispheric activation and

performance. Mild situational stress was found to be associated with greater right hemispheric contribution to cognition (Tucker et al., 1977). However, later studies involving highly anxious subjects showed an excessive reliance on left hemispheric cognitive processing (Tucker et al., 1978; Tyler and Tucker, 1982). Since the few studies conducted in this area relied on indirect techniques for assessing brain function, no firm conclusions are warranted.

AROUSAL AND CBF

Global CBF

Under normal conditions, cerebral function is closely coupled with brain blood flow and metabolism (Raichle et al., 1976; Mazziotta, 1985). Increases and decreases in arousal should therefore be associated with parallel changes in CBF. Conditions characterized by an increase in arousal, such as rapid eye movement (REM) sleep, mental activation, and epileptic seizures, are indeed associated with CBF increases (Gur et al., 1982; Risberg et al., 1981; Sakai et al., 1980; Townsend et al., 1973; Larsen et al., 1973; Broderson et al., 1973; Meyer et al., 1978), and conditions characterized by hypoarousal, such as drug-induced narcosis, slow-wave sleep, and coma are associated with global decreases in CBF (Vernheit et al., 1978; Forster et al., 1982; Rockoff et al., 1980; Obrist et al., 1979; Frewen et al., 1985). Additional support for the association between global CBF and arousal is provided by the close relationship between EEG (which has been extensively utilized in arousal research) and CBF (Ingvar and Soderberg, 1956; Menon et al., 1980).

Blood Flow to the Brainstem

Two lines of evidence support an association between global CBF and levels of activity within the brainstem that, as was pointed out earlier, is believed to mediate arousal. Juge and associates (1979) demonstrated correlations between blood flow to the brainstem and cerebellar regions and state of awareness as judged by clinical and EEG evaluations in semicoma, stupor, slow-wave sleep, drowsiness, rest, activation, REM sleep, and epileptic seizures. Ingvar and associates (1964) measured CBF with two different measurement techniques in a 60-year-old patient in a coma-

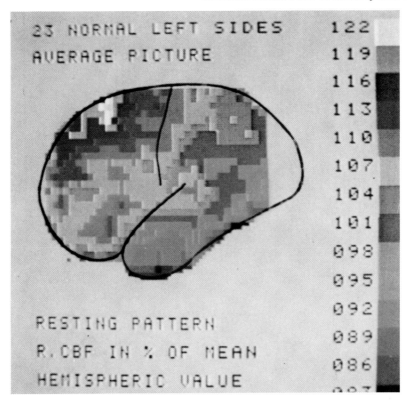

Fig. 17–1. Normal pattern of regional cerebral blood flow distribution as found with a two-dimensional measurement technique, [133]xenon intracarotid injection. Courtesy of Dr. N.A. Lassen, Department of Neuromedicine, Rigs Hospitalet, Copenhagen, Denmark. (Reproduced in color in Color Figure Section.)

tose state following an acute vascular lesion of the brainstem. Air encephalography revealed only moderate degrees of cerebral atrophy. EEG showed severe depression with low-voltage slow waves. Cortical biopsy taken from the left frontal lobe showed normal findings with no evidence of neuronal loss or gliosis. CBF and cerebral oxygen consumption were found to be significantly reduced. This would seem to suggest that the upper brainstem lesion was responsible for the coma and the associated reduction in CBF. Ingvar and Soderberg (1958) also demonstrated cortical blood flow increase related to EEG patterns evoked by stimulation of the brainstem.

Blood Flow to the Frontal Cortex

CBF research also supports the involvement of the frontal lobe in the arousal mechanism.

Ingvar (1979) first reported a 20–40% increase in blood flow to the frontal regions in comparison to occipital and temporal regions in 11 patients undergoing carotid angiography while they were awake but resting. He ascribed this CBF increase to the activity of the frontal lobe in maintaining wakefulness. This "hyperfrontal" pattern of CBF distribution (Figs. 17–1, 17–2) was found to become more pronounced when arousal was increased through stimulation (Ingvar and Lassen, 1976). During slow-wave sleep, the hyperfrontal pattern of flow distribution was found to become less significant (Townsend et al., 1973). Risberg and associates (1977) studied the CBF changes associated with the administration of a problem-solving test on 2 consecutive days. During the first test, both frontal and posterior flow increased. However, during the second test, only

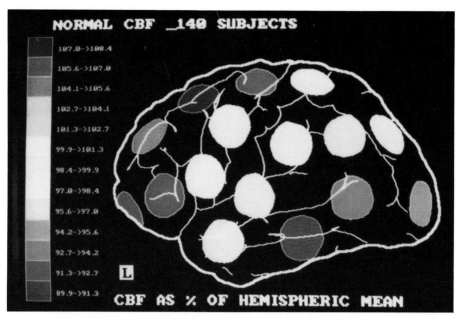

Fig. 17–2.   Normal pattern of regional cerebral blood flow distribution as found with another two-dimensional measurement technique, [133]xenon inhalation. (Reproduced in color in Color Figure Section.)

the posterior flow increased; frontal flow remained the same. The frontal flow increase was attributed to the apprehension associated with the novelty of the test, which was absent during the second session. (In experiments involving repeated CBF measurements under resting conditions, the second set of values tend to be lower than the first. This also may be due to habituation to the measurement technique (unpublished observation). Thus degrees of hyperfrontality would seem to be related to degrees of brain activation supporting the association between the frontal lobe and arousal.

Tranquilization and CBF

We conducted a small-scale study on the effects of nonsedating doses of diazepam, a commonly used tranquilizer, on regional CBF in normal human subjects (Mathew et al., 1985). Twenty right-handed volunteers, free of significant medical and psychiatric disorders, participated in the project. Regional CBF was measured twice in each participant, at an interval of 30 min. Five minutes before the second CBF, one-half of the subjects (mean age 23

years, SD 10; five males and five females) were given an iv injection of diazepam (0.1 mg/kg; mean 7, SD 1.6 mg) and the other 10 subjects (mean age 22 years, SD 4; five males and five females) an iv injection of saline. The subjects were assigned to the two groups on a random basis, and injections were given under double-blind conditions. The subjects were specifically instructed to stay awake with their eyes open, and they were questioned about levels of wakefulness during the postmeasurement debriefing. During the CBF measurement, respiratory rate, end-tital CO_2 levels ($PECO_2$), and a one-channel EEG were continuously recorded. None of the subjects became drowsy during the experiment. The CBF values obtained during the second measurement for each participant were adjusted for differences in $PECO_2$ (Maximilian et al., 1980) ($PECO_2$ levels in mm Hg: Diazepam group, first CBF 38, SD 5; second CBF 39, SD 3 mm Hg. Placebo group, first CBF 39, SD 4; second CBF 39, SD 3 mm Hg).

The CBF data were analyzed with a two-step process. The first step consisted of an overall analysis of variance that compared group × hemisphere × region, using a split-plot re-

TABLE 17–1.
Posthoc (Newman-Keuls) Comparisons Between Diazepam and Placebo Groups on rCBF (ml/100 g/min)*

	Right				Left			
	Pre-	Post-	Change	P	Pre-	Post-	Change	P
Diazepam group								
Frontal								
Mean	88.3	79.5	−8.8	<0.01	87.4	82.1	−5.3	<0.01
SD	11	12			11	14		
Central								
Mean	84.1	77.9	−6.2	<0.01	83.8	79.3	−4.5	<0.01
SD	10	11			10	13		
Temporal								
Mean	77.7	71.6	−6.1	<0.01	76.7	72.7	−4.0	<0.01
SD	11	11			9	11		
Parietal								
Mean	78.4	72.5	−5.9	<0.01	78.5	72.8	−5.7	<0.01
SD	9	10			10	10		
Occipital								
Mean	75.7	69.7	−6.0	<0.01	77.1	70.9	−6.2	<0.01
SD	9	10			11	9		
Placebo group								
Frontal								
Mean	84.9	83.9	−1.0	NS	83.1	83.6	+0.5	NS
SD	12	11			12	12		
Central								
Mean	83.1	81.2	−1.0	NS	80.5	82.6	+2.1	NS
SD	13	12			12	12		
Temporal								
Mean	75.4	73.7	−1.7	NS	74.2	75.7	+1.5	NS
SD	10	11			11	8		
Parietal								
Mean	76.4	77.8	+1.4	NS	78.0	77.0	−1.0	NS
SD	14	12			12	12		
Occipital								
Mean	72.8	73.9	+1.1	NS	74.1	73.5	−0.6	NS
SD	13	10			10	12		

*The rCBF values were corrected for pre/post differences in $PECO_2$.

peated measures model followed by posthoc Newman-Keuls. This analysis revealed a significant group × period interaction (F = 4.45; $P < 0.05$), a significant period × hemisphere interaction (F = 6.25; $P < 0.03$), a significant region main effect (F = 94.11; $P < 0.001$), and a significant period × hemisphere × region interaction (F = 2.95; $P < 0.03$). Posthoc Newman-Keuls indicated a significant change for diazepam in all regions in both left and right hemispheres, whereas none of the regions in the placebo group revealed significant changes (Table 17–1, Fig. 17–3).

The period × hemisphere × region interaction suggested differences between brain regions in both hemispheres on the post-diazepam blood flow changes. The maximum regional CBF reduction was seen in the right frontal area (−8.8). To examine the regional differences in blood flow changes in greater detail, a second repeated measure analysis of variance was performed with each of the 32 detector channels (Fig. 17–2) using a group × period model. The post hoc analysis found significant regional CBF decreases in the right hemisphere, especially the frontal lobe.

The findings indicate that iv administration of small, nonsedating doses of diazepam is ac-

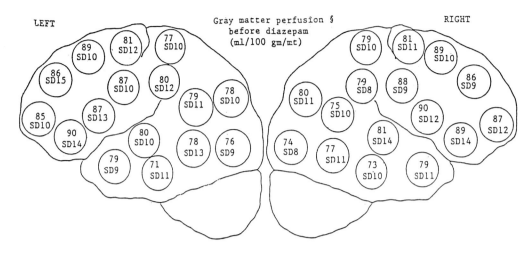

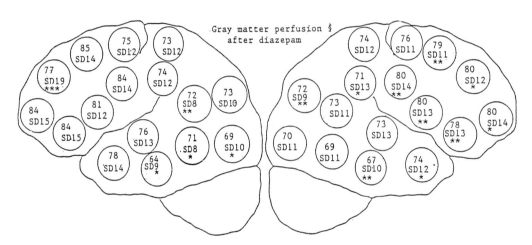

Fig. 17–3. Changes in regional cerebral blood flow after diazepam and placebo. §, Gray matter flow after correction for within PECO$_2$ changes. The diazepam and placebo groups were compared for between and within group CBF differences via analysis of variance with repeated measures. *, Significantly lower CBF ($P < 0.05$) after diazepam with no changes after placebo (posthoc Newman-Keuls). **, Significantly lower CBF ($P < 0.01$) after diazepam with no changes after placebo. ***, Significantly lower CBF ($P < 0.01$) after diazepam and significantly higher CBF ($<.05$) after placebo.

companied by marked right hemispheric CBF reduction, especially that of the frontal lobe. Milder CBF changes in the same direction were seen in the left hemisphere. These findings thus support the hypothesis that the frontal lobe is involved in the mediation of levels of arousal.

The "Hyperfrontality Controversy"

Increased frontal perfusion in normal subjects during wakefulness has been reported by all laboratories that utilize two-dimensional CBF measurement techniques (^{133}xenon intracarotid injection and inhalation techniques; Fig. 17–1, 17–2) (Wilkinson et al., 1969; Meyer et al., 1978; Blauenstein et al., 1977; Prohovnik et al., 1980; Mathew et al., 1986; Weinberger et al., 1986; Gur et al., 1985; Mamo et al., 1983). However, this could not be replicated by the majority of laboratories that utilize three-dimensional CBF and cerebral metabolism (CMR) measurement techniques (Devous et al., 1986; Rapoport et al., 1985), with a few exceptions. Buchsbaum and associates (1982) have consistently reported higher glucose metabolism (measured with positron emission tomography; PET) in the frontal gray matter as compared with the posterior brain regions. Metter and associates (1984) found only partial support for hyperfrontality with PET scan measurements of glucose metabolism. They found negative correlations between the frontal and posterior regions. However, the frontal value was higher only when the superior frontal region was compared with posterior temporal regions; the occipital and Wernicke regions had values that were on the average higher than frontal measures. Similar findings were reported by Meyer and associates (1981), who measured CBF with another three-dimensional technique: CT scanning during stable xenon inhalation. They found higher frontal flow in comparison to temporal and parietal areas; occipital (cortical) flow was, in general, higher than the frontal values. The differences between various regional flow values were small and insignificant in comparison to the two-dimensional studies. Devous and associates (1986) could not find hyperfrontality in their study with yet another three-dimensional technique—single photon emission computed tomography (with [133]xenon).

Since anxiety and arousal are closely related, CBF changes related to arousal such as hyperfrontality are of considerable relevance. The inconsistent replication of the earlier finding of hyperfrontality with two-dimensional measurement techniques by more recent three-dimensional techniques needs to be examined closely. Both techniques are based on the rate of accumulation and/or clearance of radioactive tracers by the brain. In two-dimensional techniques, rate of clearance is estimated by recording a progressive decline in radioactivity by stationary scintillation detectors applied to the scalp, and they measure only cortical perfusion. The scalp scintillation detectors will not "see" blood flow to deeper brain structures and the medial part of the hemispheres. Three-dimensional techniques, on the other hand, take tomographic slices with a rotating gantry of scintillation detectors that depict cortical and subcortical flow. Thus the two types of measurement techniques differ in the nature of information they provide.

Contamination of the frontal flow values measured with the two-dimensional techniques by the isotope trapped in the frontal sinuses has been offered as an explanation for hyperfrontality (Devous et al., 1986). This would seem to be inadequate since hyperfrontality is most obvious over the superior frontal areas (Figs. 17–1, 17–2), which is away from the frontal sinuses in most subjects. [133]Xenon is the tracer used for all currently available two-dimensional CBF measurement techniques. Separation of different regional flow values based on these techniques rests upon the assumption that the relative solubility of xenon in the brain tissue compared with blood is the same in different parts of the brain. It is possible that the blood brain partition coefficient for xenon is higher over the frontal lobe compared with the rest of the brain. However, it should be noted that CBF measurements with three-dimensional techniques (SPECT) with [133]xenon as a tracer could not detect hyperfrontality (Devous et al., 1986).

Differences between the two types of techniques in the accuracy of gray matter measurements is another possible explanation. Cortical gray matter, while large in surface area, is relatively thin on cross section; in most regions it is much less than 5 mm (Carpenter, 1976). The three-dimensional techniques used for CBF measurement have a spatial resolution well above 5 mm. The problem is made worse by technical difficulties in separating cerebrospinal fluid and white matter (low radioactivity areas) from the undulating cortical gray (high radioactivity areas; partial volume artifact) (Powers and Raichle, 1986). Two-dimensional techniques, on the other hand, do not depend on their spatial resolution to separate cortical gray matter flow from white matter flow. The separation is made by the analysis of the clearance curves recorded over the scalp with a two-compartmental model (Obrist et al., 1975).

Gray matter flow is calculated from the fast clearing compartment.

Extensive literature implicating the frontal lobe's association with the arousal mechanism, EEG findings indicative of high frontal activity during wakefulness, and increases and decreases in the hyperfrontal pattern of CBF distribution with parallel changes in arousal add validity to the concept of hyperfrontality of CBF distribution.

ANXIETY AND AROUSAL

The majority of psychophysiological studies support the idea that anxiety is a hyperarousal state (Duffy, 1972; Lader, 1975). For example, electroencephalography, which probably is a direct measure of arousal, shows fairly consistent and predictable changes in anxiety: less alpha- than normal and more beta-frequency than at rest. Peripheral physiological changes, mostly involving the autonomic nervous system, also show evidence of overactivity. However, it should be noted that these changes also occur in such emotional states as anger and excitement (Duffy, 1972). Anxiety and these emotions have been hypothesized to have the same physiologic substrate, i.e., increased arousal. The precise nature of the emotion depends on the subject's perception and interpretation of the environment (Schachter and Singer, 1962; Lader, 1982; Sarason, 1984). However, since the subjective experience of these emotions is different, one would expect neurobiological differences between them. Even the peripheral neurophysiologic factors that differentiate different emotions are controversial and poorly understood (Ax, 1953). Very little is known about the associated brain mechanisms.

CBF AS AN INDEX OF BRAIN FUNCTION IN ANXIETY

CBF and brain function are coupled, and CBF has been used as an index of brain function in studies of arousal. Thus it would seem to be of use in identifying the neuroanatomic substrates of anxiety. Unfortunately, CBF is influenced by factors other than brain function, and these factors need to be taken into account. As was pointed out earlier, anxiety is associated with a variety of physiologic and biochemical changes, some of which may be relevant to CBF.

Catecholamines and CBF

Stress and acute anxiety are very well known to increase epinephrine and norepinephrine in the periphery (Levi, 1972; Frankenhaeuser, 1971; Mathew et al., 1982a). The possible effects of these substances on brain blood flow may, therefore, be important.

Intravenous epinephrine infusions have been found to increase CBF and cerebral metabolism by over 200% in animals (Abdul-Rahman et al., 1979; Dahlgren et al., 1980). Gibbs and associates (1935) reported increased CBF following intravenous epinephrine infusion in man. They measured CBF with a thermoelectric flow meter inserted into the internal jugular vein. Kety (1952) investigated the effect of epinephrine and norepinephrine infusions on CBF and cerebral oxygen consumption with the nitrous oxide inhalation technique. This technique involves inhalation of a mixture of nitrous oxide and oxygen for 10 min with serial blood sample withdrawals from the femoral artery and superior jugular bulb. CBF and cerebral metabolism are calculated based on the arteriovenous differences in nitrous oxide, glucose, carbon dioxide, oxygen, and pyruvate. While norepinephrine infusions were not associated with any significant changes, epinephrine increased CBF by 21% and cerebral oxygen consumption by 22%. King and associates (1952), with the same measurement technique, showed that the increases in CBF and cerebral oxygen consumption following epinephrine infusion were not associated with changes in cerebrovascular resistance. This would seem to argue against the possibility of CBF increases being secondary to a direct vascular effect of epinephrine. Norepinephrine, on the other hand, was found to increase cerebrovascular resistance and reduce CBF. Sensenbach and associates (1953) could not replicate these findings. They found no changes in CBF, cerebrovascular resistance, or cerebral oxygen utilization following epinephrine injections; norepinephrine injections, on the other hand, reduced CBF. All of the studies mentioned above were conducted with the nitrous oxide inhalation technique.

Olesen injected epinephrine and isoproterenol into the internal carotid artery in human subjects and measured CBF via the [133]xenon intracarotid injection technique (Olesen et al., 1971; Olesen, 1975). This measurement technique, similar to the other two-dimensional techniques, measures CBF to cortical gray matter only. Intracarotid isoprenaline and epinephrine were not associated with any CBF changes.

In summary, several animal experiments and human studies found increases in CBF following intravenous epinephrine infusions. Intracarotid epinephrine and isoproterenol, on the other hand, do not affect CBF. Thus, in all probability, the epinephrine-induced CBF changes are secondary to the behavioral manifestations of the drug and not due to the direct vascular effects of the drug. The latter is important since adrenergic receptors (alpha and beta) have been demonstrated on cerebral microvasculature (Harik et al., 1981). Norepinephrine may reduce CBF, but it is unclear whether this is due to the direct effect of the drug on cerebral blood vessels.

Recent years have seen an upsurge of interest in the central nervous system biochemistry of anxiety. Evidence suggesting the involvement of such neurotransmitters as norepinephrine, serotonin, and gamma-aminobutyric acid (GABA) have been reported (Hoehn-Saric, 1982). Large numbers of norepinephrine- and serotonin-containing neurons in the brainstem centers have been shown to innervate cerebral capillaries (intraparenchymal innervation) and form varicosities from which neurotransmitters are released. These fibers have also been shown to make synaptic contacts with other neurons. An extensive body of literature is available on the effects of intravenous, intracarotid, and intraventricular infusions and cortical applications of these neurotransmitters on CBF. Cerebral blood vessels are also known to contain appreciable quantities of enzymes relevant to the synthesis and destruction of these neurotransmitters. This would include tyrosine hydroxylase, monoamine oxidase, dopamine beta-hydroxylase, and tryptophan hydroxylase. The influence of these neurotransmitters on CBF is a complicated and controversial matter, and a detailed discussion of this is beyond the scope of this chapter. Interested readers should consult the review by Edvinsson and MacKenzie (1977). Much less is known about the influence of these substances on anxiety-related changes in CBF and CMR.

Sympathetic Nervous System and CBF

Activation of the autonomic nervous system, especially the sympathetic division, is an integral part of acute anxiety. Sympathetic stimulation is believed to be responsible for anxiety-related circulatory changes in such peripheral vascular beds as the muscle and skin; anxiety increases blood flow to the muscle and decreases that to the skin (Kelly and Walter, 1969; Ackner, 1956). Sympathetic fibers also innervate cerebral blood vessels in man and other animals, and adrenergic receptors have been demonstrated on cerebral microvasculature (Busija and Heistad, 1984a). Nerve fibers containing neurotransmitters, epinephrine and norepinephrine, are present in the walls of pial and cerebral parenchymal capillaries. The sympathetic fibers originate from the ipsilateral superior cervical ganglion. Nerve endings on cerebral blood vessels contain considerable amounts of norepinephrine and have an active, specific uptake mechanism. Adrenergic agonists, such as phentolamine and yohimbine release tritiated norepinephrine from brain blood vessels, preloaded with the labeled neurotransmitter, and this efflux is reduced by clonidine. For additional details, the reader should consult the review articles by Edvinsson and MacKenzie (1977), Edvinsson (1982), and Busija and Heistad (1984b).

CBF response to sympathetic stimulation varies across different species; in man, a 5–15% CBF reduction is seen (Edvinsson, 1982). There is general consensus that brain blood vessels are less responsive to sympathetic stimulation in comparison to peripheral vessels. Thus in normal individuals the autonomic nervous system may have only an insignificant role in the control of CBF, even during anxiety. However, it is quite likely that the cerebral vasculature in anxious patients is much more sensitive to sympathetic activation than in normals; patients with panic disorders have been shown to be oversensitive to sympathetic stimulation in the periphery (Nesse et al., 1984).

Hemorrheology and CBF

Several investigators have reported an increase in hematocrit and blood viscosity secondary to stress (Lawrence and Berlin, 1951; Wilson and Boyle, 1952; Dameshek, 1953; Russell and Conley, 1964; Benitone and Kling, 1970; Dintenfass and Zador, 1976, 1977). Hematocrit of 50–56% and hemoglobin levels between 16 and 18 g% are the commonly accepted criteria for this syndrome, known as stress *polycytosis* (Dameshek, 1953; Benitone and Kling, 1970). Blood viscosity is known to influence CBF; CBF is increased in conditions associated with low blood viscosity (anemias) and reduced in high blood viscosity conditions (polycythemia) (Thomas, 1982). There is some uncertainty as to whether this inverse relationship between blood viscosity and CBF is dependent on alterations in blood rheology or that of the associated changes in oxygen delivery to the brain (Marshall, 1982). Anxiety-related changes in blood viscosity can thus be very important to CBF.

Upon careful examination of the literature on stress polycytosis, it became apparent that none of the studies established a positive association between stress and increased blood viscosity. Most investigators measured hematocrit in subjects with vague symptoms of anxiety, in patients referred to hematology clinics with elevated hematocrit for which no other explanations could be found, in patients with a wide variety of ill-defined psychiatric disorders, and in patients with hypertension. Few investigators used standard criteria for making psychiatric diagnoses, and no attempt was made to correlate degrees of distress, anxiety, or depression with the hematocrit elevations. Stress polycytosis is believed to be more common in males compared with females (Dameshek, 1953; Russell and Conley, 1964): Hematocrit is normally higher in males (Kelly and Munan, 1977). The assumption that males may be more stressed than females is questionable in view of the higher incidence of anxiety and depression in the latter.

We examined the possibility of an anxiety-related increase in hematocrit in a group of patients with a DSM III diagnosis of generalized anxiety disorder. All participants were physically healthy and medication free for a minimum of 2 weeks. Blood samples were drawn twice: 3 min after venipuncture and 10 min later. During these 10 min, 12 patients received an iv infusion of epinephrine (0.2 µg/kgm/min)

while the remaining 12 patients received saline infusions. There were six males and six females in both groups of patients. The patients were assigned to epinephrine and saline groups on a random basis, and the infusions were given under double-blind conditions. Pulse rate and blood pressure were taken before each blood sample, and levels of anxiety at the time of blood sample withdrawal were quantified with the State Anxiety Scale of the State Trait Anxiety Inventory (STAI) (Spielberger et al., 1970). Degrees of anxiety proneness and depression were measured with the Trait Anxiety Scale of the STAI (Spielberger et al., 1970) and Beck Depression Inventory (Beck and Beck, 1972). In a group of control subjects carefully screened for psychiatric disorders and matched for age and sex, the physiological and rating scale measurements were obtained just once. The three groups of subjects were compared on state anxiety, trait anxiety, depression, and hematocrit (Table 17–2).

There were no differences between anxiety patients and normal controls concerning hematocrits obtained under resting conditions. The two groups of anxiety patients were examined for changes following epinephrine/saline infusions via repeated measure analysis of variance and posthoc Scheffe. Epinephrine infusions were associated with significant increases in state anxiety, pulse, and systolic blood pressure (Table 17–3) but not in hematocrit (Table 17–4). Pearson correlations were calculated between hematocrit, trait anxiety, state anxiety, depression, pulse rate, and blood pressure under resting conditions and after epinephrine infusions. Hematocrit level did not correlate significantly with any index (Mathew and Wilson, 1986).

It should be noted that the state anxiety scale, with which an increase in postepinephrine anxiety was demonstrated, does not contain any item related to the peripheral sympathetic-adrenal activation, and it measures psychic anxiety, exclusively.

Other experiments conducted in our laboratory involving anxiety induction with carbon dioxide inhalation and marijuana smoking (unpublished data; see below) did not reveal any anxiety-related changes in hematocrit. In addition, we have not found hematocrit to be a significant predictor of CBF in any of our stud-

TABLE 17–2.
Comparisons Between Anxious Patients and Controls on Rating Scale and Physiological Indices (Analysis of Variance)

	Anxious patients, epinephrine		Anxious patients, saline		Normal controls		F	P
	Mean	SD	Mean	SD	Mean	SD		
State anxiety	39.1	10	41.4	10	29.7	6	3.9	<0.02
Trait anxiety	43.3	11	58.7	9	32.1	5	23.18	<0.001
Depression (BDI)	3.9	5	9.3	5	1.4	2	9.32	<0.001
Pulse (per min)	76.3	16	79.3	15	76.2	9		NS
Systolic BP (mm Hg)	115	13	117	16	114	15		NS
Diastolic BP (mm Hg)	72.7	10	73.1	7	69.2	10		NS
Age (years)	37.8	17	38.8	13	39.5	12		NS

TABLE 17–3.
Rating Scales and Physiological Indices Before and After Epinephrine and Saline*

	Epinephrine				Saline				F	P
	Pre-		Post-		Pre-		Post-			
	Mean	SD	Mean	SD	Mean	SD	Mean	SD		
State anxiety	39	10	53	12	41	10	42	10	7.72	<0.01
Pulse (per min)	76	16	88	17	79	15	73	12	35.58	<0.001
Systolic BP (mm Hg)	115	13	124	14	117	16	116	14	16.30	<0.001
Diastolic BP (mm Hg)	73	10	72	9	73	7	72	7		NS

*The comparisons were made with analysis of variance with repeated measures.

TABLE 17–4.
Hematocrit in Anxious Patients and Controls

	Patients						Controls	
	Epinephrine			Placebo				
Subject	Pre-	Post-	Subject	Pre-	Post-	Subject	Pre-
Male	44	41	Male	43	42	Male	42.5
Male	47.5	47	Male	39.5	40	Male	42
Male	41	38	Male	44.5	44	Male	46
Male	43	43	Male	43	42	Male	44
Male	42.5	43.5	Male	38	38	Male	41
Male	40	42	Male	38	40	Male	44
Female	37	35	Female	40	38	Female	38.5
Female	35	33.5	Female	38	39	Female	40.5
Female	35	35	Female	35	34	Female	38
Female	35.5	38	Female	40	40.5	Female	36
Female	42	40	Female	37	38	Female	38
Female	37	38	Female	41	42	Female	38
Mean	39.5	39.5		39.75	39.79		40.7
SD	4	4		3	3		3

ies (Mathew et al., 1986). It may be that modest hematocrit changes, within the normal physiological range, exert only a minimal influence on CBF. Thus hematocrit does not seem to be a significant factor in the determination of anxiety-related CBF changes.

CO$_2$ AND CBF

Carbon dioxide is a potent cerebral vasodilator (Purves, 1972; Maximilian et al., 1980; Busija and Heistad, 1984b). Even modest changes in arterial concentrations of CO$_2$ are accompanied by marked alterations in CBF in a parallel direction. Anxiety is often associated with an increase in the rate of respiration and a reduction in carbon dioxide levels (Lader, 1975; Fried, 1987). Hyperventilation and the resultant hypocapnia have been repeatedly shown to be associated with significant reductions in CBF (Gotoh et al., 1965). The decrease in CO$_2$ causes alkalosis, leading to reduction in oxyhemoglobin dissociation (Bohr effect), which may reduce cerebral oxygen metabolism (Fried, 1987).

Pulse Rate, Perfusion Pressure, and CBF

Increases in pulse rate and blood pressure are the most common physiological changes associated with anxiety. However, this will have only limited relevance to CBF. Cerebral autoregulation ensures a constant blood supply to the brain in spite of moderate changes in perfusion pressure (Strandgaard and Paulson, 1984). However, CBF can be impaired by profound increases or decreases in blood pressure. In addition, acute changes in blood pressure can damage the blood–brain barrier, which may cause extravasation of vasoactive substances into the brain (Abdul-Rahman et al., 1979; Dahlgren et al., 1980). Lack of clarity concerning the degree of blood pressure increases needed to trigger such mechanisms and the wide differences between individuals on anxiety-related blood pressure changes make the evaluation of these factors difficult.

Stress and CBF

A fair number of studies have been performed on the effect of stress on CBF. Stress induced in animals by immobilization for 5–10 min was found to increase CBF and cerebral metabolism (CMR) by up to twofold (Carlsson et al., 1975, 1977). However, a few investigators have reported reduced CBF in association with immobilization (Ohata et al., 1984; Rapoport et al., 1981). The CBF reduction may have been induced by hyperventilation and hypocapnia. The mechanism responsible for the CBF increase, on the other hand, is unclear.

The direct effect of epinephrine on CBF and CMR was considered responsible by some investigators, since prior adrenalectomy and/or administration of propranolol abolished this stress-induced change in CBF and CMR. Under normal conditions, epinephrine present in the peripheral blood does not cross the blood–brain barrier (Schildkraut and Kety, 1967). However, the anxiety-related increase in blood pressure might disrupt the blood–brain barrier, with subsequent extravasation of epinephrine into the brain (Abdul-Rahman et al., 1979; Dahlgren et al., 1980). Sharma and Dey (1986) found increased blood–brain barrier permeability after 8 hr of immobilization. However, in their study, CBF was diminished by 2–37% in 12 of 14 regions. Dahlgren and associates (1980) demonstrated regional variations in the CBF response to immobilization stress. They found increased blood flow to cortical structures such as frontal and parietal lobes and reduced flow in other brain regions such as inferior colliculus, superior olive, hippocampus, and septal nuclei.

Lasvennes and associates (1986) compared freely moving rats and mildly restrained rats. The restrained rats showed more evidence of stress as indicated by elevated heart rate, blood pressure, and corticosterone level. Frontal and parietal cortical CBF were more elevated in the freely moving rats compared with the stressed ones. Absence of greater differences in CBF between the two groups of animals were explained on the basis of the mutually antagonistic effects of two anxiety-related factors on CBF: cerebral vasoconstriction secondary to increased blood catecholamine levels and arousal-related increases in CBF.

LeDoux and associates (1983) measured local CBF in rats during the processing of environmental stimuli. Presentation of a tone increased CBF in the auditory pathways. However, when the animal was previously conditioned to fear the tone, blood flow additionally increased in the hypothalamus and amygdala. The increase in CBF was explained on the basis of local increases in neuronal activity.

Animal studies on the effect of stress on CBF have not yielded consistent results. Both CBF decreases and increases and regional differences have been reported. When hyperventilation and reduced blood carbon dioxide levels were controlled for, the CBF change seemed to be one of increase. It is unclear to what extent these results can be extrapolated to anxiety. The concept of stress is rather diffuse and vague, and its relationship with anxiety unclear. The term *stress* has been defined as the "nonspecific response of the body to any demand made upon it," regardless of whether the demand is of a pleasant or unpleasant nature (Selye, 1956). It is also uncertain whether anxiety and associated physiological changes can be subsumed under "nonspecific responses" (Lader, 1982).

STUDIES OF ANXIETY AND CBF

Resting Cerebral Blood Flow in Patients With Anxiety Disorders

We measured CBF via the ^{133}xenon inhalation technique (a two-dimensional technique) in nine right-handed subjects who met the criteria for generalized anxiety disorder according to DSM III and in nine controls matched for age, sex, and hand preference (Mathew et al., 1982b). The participants underwent a drug washout period of 4 weeks and were required to avoid coffee, tea, and tobacco for 2 hr before the CBF measurements. The STAI was utilized to quantify levels of anxiety. CBF measurements were obtained under resting conditions after the subjects acclimated to the laboratory. The laboratory was kept quiet and semidark during the measurements. PECO$_2$, pulse rate, and blood pressure were monitored. Special care was taken to make sure that the subjects did not become drowsy during the experiment, since sleep has been reported to influence CBF. The anxious patients and controls were compared on global and regional CBF, PECO$_2$, pulse rate, and blood pressure. There were no differences between the two groups of subjects on any of these indices. Pearson correlations were computed between trait anxiety, state anxiety, and rCBF values in patients. Left and right hemispheric CBF (left hemisphere r = -0.63, $P < 0.03$; right hemisphere r = 0.67, $P < 0.02$) and most brain regions on both sides showed significant inverse correlations with state anxiety. Trait anxiety did not show any significant correlations.

Reiman and associates (1984) studied resting CBF with PET in ten patients with a history of panic attacks (DSM III) and in six normal controls (see Chapter 15, this volume). Subsequently, all patients and two controls received an iv infusion of sodium lactate (10 mg/kg 500 mM sodium DL) given over 20–30 min. Panic disorder patients who had a panic attack following lactate infusion and patients who did not develop panic following the infusion and the normal controls were compared on resting CBF values. The three groups of subjects did not differ significantly in CBF to the whole brain, left or right hemisphere, or in the left/right ratio of hemispheric CBF. The subjects were compared on left to right ratios for CBF in seven preselected regions (parahippocampal gyrus, hippocampus, hypothalamus, orbito-insular gyri, anterior cingulate gyrus, amygdala, and inferior parietal lobule). Patients who developed panic following lactate showed a significantly lower right to left ratio in the parahippocampal gyrus compared with the other two groups. The investigators were not able to determine whether this asymmetry was due to decreased left or increased right CBF values in the parahippocampal gyrus, since the absolute CBF values in both regions were within the normal range. The investigators reanalyzed the data with 20 additional neurologically normal volunteers, 19 of whom showed ratios of parahippocampal blood flow identical with those of the original normal control group. One patient who had a high ratio comparable to that of the lactate-sensitive panic disorder patients was found to suffer from panic disorder, and she responded to lactate infusions with panic.

Reiman and associates (1986) extended the findings of their first study with a larger number of subjects. In the second study, they included 16 patients with panic disorder; eight were vulnerable to lactate-induced panic, and eight were not. Twenty-five normal controls were recruited for this project. The subjects included the patients and controls from the previously mentioned lactate studies. All subjects were physically well, and none had any other psychiatric disorders. Twelve patients were right-handed and the rest left-handed. At the time of the study, four were receiving medications including tricyclic antidepressants and alprazolam. In addition to CBF, information concerning cerebral blood volume, cerebral oxygen extraction ratio, and metabolic rate for oxygen were obtained with PET. Once again, all measurements were made under resting conditions with eyes closed. Lactate sensitivity was verified in all patients and 11 controls with a lactate infusion after the initial PET scan. PET scanning was repeated during the lactate infusion. The CBF and cerebral blood volumes were adjusted for intersubject differences in $PECO_2$. Again, lactate-sensitive panic disorder patients, lactate-insensitive panic disorder patients, and the controls were compared on CBF and CMR indices using whole brain and regional values. The second study replicated the original finding of asymmetry of parahippocampal blood flow in patients with panic disorder who were vulnerable to lactate infusions. However, in this study, the demarcation between the three groups of subjects on this index was not as sharp as it was in the first report. Lactate-sensitive panic disorder patients also had abnormal asymmetries of parahippocampal blood volume and metabolic rate for oxygen, with significantly lower ratios. Analysis of parahippocampal measurements on each side suggested an abnormal increase in right parahippocampal measures in the lactate-sensitive panic disorder patients. There were no significant differences between the groups in left parahippocampal indices of blood flow or metabolism; as a matter of fact, the left hemispheric values were somewhat higher for the lactate-sensitive panic disorder group compared with the others. Lactate-sensitive panic disorder patients also showed significantly higher whole brain metabolic rates for oxygen. This group of subjects, however, did not differ from the second group of patients on degrees of anxiety experienced during the PET scan. Correlations between anxiety levels and blood flow were not calculated.

The results of our study and those of Reiman and associates are not comparable because of the substantial differences in methodology and CBF measurement technique. We measured CBF with the [133]xenon inhalation technique in patients with generalized anxiety disorder, while Reiman and associates utilized PET scan to measure CBF in lactate-sensitive and insensitive panic disorder patients. In our study, no differences were found between anxiety disorder patients and controls. The only positive finding was a significant inverse correlation

between state anxiety and CBF. This will be discussed in greater detail together with the results of other studies involving anxiety induction in the following section. The studies done by Reimen and associates provide results of considerable heuristic significance. The hippocampal area has been implicated in the control of anxiety (Gray, 1982). However, the physiological differences between lactate-sensitive and lactate-insensitive panic disorder are difficult to explain. The problem is further complicated by the uncertainty concerning the mechanism through which lactate induces panic. This study would need to be replicated by other laboratories with larger sample sizes.

CBF Changes Associated With Anxiety Induction

CBF is influenced by a variety of factors, and therefore it shows a significant degree of variation among subjects (Mathew et al., 1986). On the other hand, CBF within the same individual tends to be more stable over time, and therefore measurements made before and after anxiety induction would seem to be a useful approach. The effects of a variety of agents and techniques known to increase anxiety on CBF have been examined.

Caffeine is one of the most widely used psychotropic agents, and it is known to induce anxiety in normal subjects and in patients with anxiety disorders (Veleber and Templer, 1984; Charney et al., 1985). We examined the effect of orally administered caffeine on CBF and anxiety (Mathew and Wilson, 1985). Twenty-four physically and mentally healthy normal volunteers, who were medication-free for a period of 2 weeks, participated in the study. The subjects abstained from all caffeine-containing substances for a minimum of 2 hr before the experiment. CBF measurements were obtained with the [133]xenon inhalation technique three times in each subject, under identical laboratory conditions. Immediately after the first measurement, the subjects received either 250 mg of caffeine or a placebo, with lemonade, under double-blind conditions. The drug/placebo administrations were completed in less than 5 min. Subjects were assigned to the caffeine or placebo group on a random basis. Fourteen subjects received caffeine, and ten, placebo. CBF measurements were repeated twice more, 30 and 90 min after the administration of the drug/placebo. During the CBF measurements, blood pressure, respiratory rate, PECO$_2$, and a one-channel EEG recording were monitored. After each CBF measurement, levels of anxiety were quantified with the State Anxiety Scale of the STAI (Spielberger et al., 1970).

Subjects who received caffeine and placebo were compared on the three sets of CBF values (each set consisted of right and left hemispheric and 32 regional flow values) (Fig. 17–4), physiological indices, and state anxiety scores via analysis of variance with repeated measures and posthoc Newman-Keuls. There was a statistically significant decrease in CBF for the caffeine group after both 30 and 90 min, which were not present in the placebo group (Fig. 17–4) (left hemisphere: F = 15.4; p < .001; right hemisphere: F = 12.8; p < .001.) There were no regional differences. These findings were substantiated by posthoc testing, which indicated no differences between the two groups on resting CBF and between the three sets of CBF in the placebo group. PECO$_2$, blood pressure, respiratory rate, and state anxiety did not differentiate between the three groups, and they were stable across the three measurements in both groups.

Cerebral vasoconstriction induced by caffeine is in keeping with previous reports (Mathew et al., 1983). However, this CBF change was independent of changes in state anxiety and indices of sympathetic activity. As a matter of fact, in spite of the significant reduction in CBF following caffeine, there were no changes in state anxiety, blood pressure, pulse rate, or respiratory rate. However, it should be noted that other investigators have reported significant elevations in anxiety following the administration of caffeine in comparable and even lower doses (Veleber and Templer, 1984). The most important finding of the study is that caffeine, which can induce anxiety, also induces cerebral vasoconstriction. However, the study does not warrant any conclusions about the relationship between the cerebral vasoconstrictive and anxiogenic properties of caffeine. Perhaps caffeine given in much higher doses might have induced both anxiety and cerebral vasoconstriction.

Epinephrine is well known to induce anxiety in predisposed people (Pitts and Allen, 1982). We measured CBF before and 2 min after iv infusions of epinephrine or saline, given under double-blind conditions, in 40 patients with generalized anxiety disorder. Twenty patients received epinephrine (0.2 µg/kgm), and 20 others received saline. The subjects were assigned to the two groups on a random basis, and the infusions were given under double-blind conditions. Trait anxiety and depression were measured with State Trait Anxiety Inventory and Beck Depression Inventory (Beck and Beck, 1972). The demographic and clinical characteristics of the two groups are given in Table 17–5. CBF measurements were obtained with the [133]xenon inhalation technique with the other routine quantifications and precautions. Anxiety experienced during the CBF measurements was measured with the State Anxiety Scale of the STAI (Spielberger et al., 1970).

Epinephrine infusions were followed by significant increases in state anxiety, respiration, and pulse rate and nonsignificant decreases in PECO$_2$ (repeated measure analysis of variance; Table 17–6). Saline infusions, on the other hand, were not associated with any changes. There were no significant differences between the epinephrine and saline groups on hemispheric or regional CBF before or after the infusions (repeated measure analysis of variance—group × hemisphere × region). Correction for differences in PECO$_2$ did not alter the results (Maximilian et al., 1980). The relationship between changes in state anxiety, the physiological indices, and CBF were examined with Pearson correlations in both groups of subjects. In the epinephrine group, inverse correlations were found between state anxiety and CBF (right hemisphere, r = 0.51, P < 0.05; left hemisphere, r = 0.52, P < 0.05), while in the saline group the relationship was positive (right hemisphere, r = 0.50, P < 0.05; left hemisphere, r = 0.44, P < 0.05). PECO$_2$ correlated significantly with global CBF in the saline group (r = 0.42, P < 0.05) but not in the epinephrine group (r = 0.14).

The findings in the saline group are more straightforward and easy to explain. As was pointed out earlier, PECO$_2$ changes are well known to be associated with parallel CBF changes (Maximilian et al., 1980). Similarly,

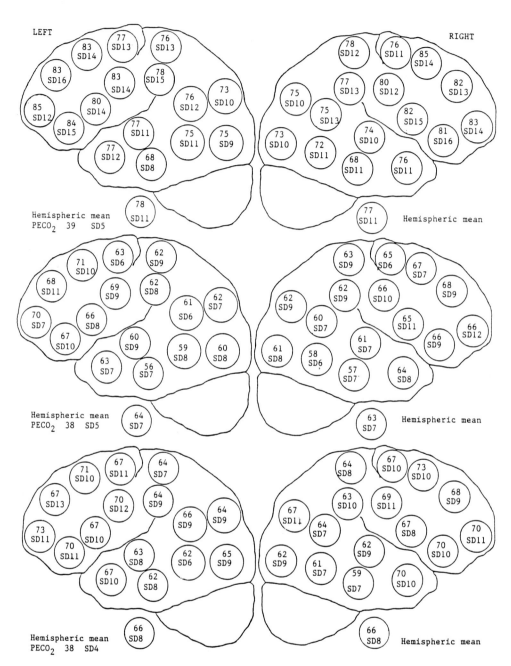

Fig. 17–4. Upper: Resting CBF for the caffeine group (Fg in ml/100 g/mt). **Middle:** CBF 30 min after caffeine (250 mg po). **Lower:** CBF 90 min after caffeine (250 mg po).

an anxiety-related increase in arousal can account for the CBF increase. The situation is much more complicated in the epinephrine group. In that group, which showed significant increases in state anxiety, there was an inverse correlation between anxiety and CBF. The nor-

TABLE 17–5.
Demographic and Psychopathological Characteristics of the Epinephrine and Placebo Groups

	Epinephrine group	Control group
Age	42 years, SD 10	46 years, SD 18
Sex	12 males, 8 females	12 males, 8 females
Trait Anxiety	53, SD 8	53, SD 11
BDI	9, SD 6	8, SD 6

TABLE 17–6.
Changes Associated With Epinephrine and Placebo*

	Epinephrine				Placebo				F	
	Pre-		Post-		Pre-		Post-		(group ×	
Variable	Mean	SD	Mean	SD	Mean	SD	Mean	SD	period)	P
State anxiety	45.8	12	54.9	12	44.1	12	40.4	13	10.5	<.003
CBF										
Right hemisphere	75.2	12	74.1	13	69.7	11	66.4	9		NS
Left hemisphere	75.9	11	74.8	13	71.1	12	66.6	9		NS
PECO$_2$	37.7	5	35.6	8	37.4	5	36.1	5		NS
Respiration	10.7	3	15.7	8	11.7	3	11.9	4	7.33	<.02
Pulse	79.2	14	84.4	24	75.9	14	70.1	14	4.2	<.05
Hematocrit	40.8	4	40.6	5	39.7	3	39.5	3		NS

*Gray matter flow given as ml/100 g/unit uncorrected for PECO$_2$. PECO$_2$ is given as mm Hg and respiratory and pulse rates as per minute. The comparisons were made with repeated measure analysis of variance.

mal close association between CBF and PECO$_2$ was distorted. The results of the study would seem to suggest that mild increases in state anxiety tend to increase CBF (placebo group) while marked elevation in anxiety is associated with CBF decrease (epinephrine group). The factor or factors responsible for such a CBF decrease might also account for the distorted relationship between CO$_2$ and CBF (Mathew and Wilson, 1988a). As was pointed out earlier, sympathetic activation may be this anxiety-related vasoconstrictive factor.

Carbon dioxide inhalation is another technique utilized by several investigators to induce anxiety in patients with anxiety disorders (van den Haut and Griez, 1984; Gorman et al., 1984; Woods et al., 1986). We examined CBF and mood changes induced by inhalation of 5% CO$_2$ in anxiety disorder patients and normals. (Mathew and Wilson, 1988b) Nine males and females with a DSM III diagnosis of generalized anxiety disorder (age mean 31.1, SD 6.1) and normal controls of matched sex distribution and comparable age (mean 26.5 years, SD 7.3) participated in this study. All

subjects were right-handed and in good physical health. They were medication-free for a minimum of 2 weeks and avoided coffee and tobacco for 3 hr before the experiment.

CBF was measured twice at an interval of 30 min with the standard measurement technique and usual precautions in all subjects. All subjects inhaled a mixture of 5% carbon dioxide in room air for 2 min before and during the second CBF measurement. Anxiety experienced by the subjects during the CBF measurements were quantified with the STAI (Spielberger et al., 1970), and a short rating scale was utilized to measure somatic symptoms of anxiety (Tyrer, 1976).

The two groups were compared on blood pressure, pulse, respiratory rate, hematocrit, and PECO$_2$ by a two factor (group × period) analysis of variance on each variable. No between-group differences were noted. However, as would be expected, significant increases in PECO$_2$, which were equivalent for both groups, were found. No group × period interactions were revealed. When state anxiety and somatic symptoms were also analyzed with the

TABLE 17–7.
Mean Change in CBF as a Function of State Anxiety Change*

Subjects	Direction of change in state anxiety	Mean CBF increase	SD
Patients	Decrease	16.9	7.4
	Increase	10.0	7.2
Controls	Decrease	16.0	2.6
	Increase	7.2	8.2
Combined	Decrease	16.2	5.6
	Increase	8.7	7.8

*Total state anxiety decrease, 8 ± 4.9; increase, 7.2 ± 4.9; $t = 7.86$, $P < 0.001$. Analysis of variance with prepost CBF (group $\times$ hemisphere $\times$ region), $F = 6.61$, $P < 0.05$.

same technique, no significant difference between the two groups on state anxiety emerged. However, anxious patients had significantly higher state anxiety during both measurements (before: CO_2, 47.3, SD 9.8; after: 48.2, SD 12.4) compared with controls (before: 38.0, SD 6.8; after: 36.3, SD 10.8, $F = 8.0$, $P < 0.009$). Both groups reported difficulty in breathing. The two groups were compared on regional CBF in a single overall analysis of variance with a group $\times$ period $\times$ hemisphere $\times$ region repeated measures model. This model revealed significant pre- and post-CBF increases to both hemispheres; however, there were no differences between the two groups and no significant interactions.

Inspection of the data indicated that approximately one-half of the subjects (patients and controls) had a decrease in anxiety scores (-8.0 units of STAI, SD 4.9) while the other one-half had an increase ($+7.2$ units, SD 4.9) from the first to the second CBF measurement. This difference was statistically significant ($t = 7.86$, $P < 0.001$). The latter also showed a significant increase in somatic symptoms of anxiety during the second run ($t = 2.1$, $P < 0.05$). There were no differences between the two groups according to age or $PECO_2$ during the second measurement. Further examination showed that there was a consistent pattern of CBF change (Table 17–7). For both patients and controls, those who had a decrease in anxiety scores had a greater CBF increase than those who had an increase in state anxiety. An analysis of variance using change scores (group $\times$ hemisphere $\times$ region repeated measures model) confirmed the observation with a

significant between-group difference ($F = 6.61$, $P < 0.05$). There were no significant hemispheric or regional CBF differences between or within groups.

A significant Pearson correlation between CBF and $PECO_2$ for the total sample was found ($r = 0.43$, $P < 0.05$). This relationship approached significance in those who had a decrease in state anxiety ($r = 0.54$, $P < 0.1$), but not for those who had a state anxiety increase. There was a significant negative relationship between CBF and state anxiety for the entire group ($r = -0.40$, $P < 0.05$).

Lack of an anxiety response to carbon dioxide inhalation was surprising. Although CO_2 inhalation has been reported to increase anxiety (van den Hout and Griez, 1984), it has also been reported to relieve anxiety (Ley and Walker, 1973). Subjects who reported anxiety also reported significantly more somatic symptoms, especially difficulty in breathing, confirming the previous observation that peripheral symptoms induced by CO_2 trigger central feelings of anxiety in predisposed people (Griez and van den Hout, 1982). CO_2 increased CBF in both anxious patients and control subjects in an identical manner. However, when patients and controls who became anxious were separated from those who did not, significant differences emerged. Those who reported anxiety showed a less marked CBF increase compared with those who did not. Similarly, changes in CBF and CO_2 showed near significant correlations in subjects who did not become anxious, but not in those who became anxious.

Once again, there seems to be a cerebral vasoconstrictive factor related to anxiety, and the

TABLE 17–8.
Demographic and Physiologic Characteristics of the Three Groups*

	Experienced marijuana smokers	Inexperienced marijuana smokers	Controls	
Sex				
M	7	10	9	$x^2 =$ NS
F	2	7	6	
Age (years)				
Mean	25.9	28.3	26.9	F = NS
SD	3.9	8.3	7.5	
Trait anxiety				
Mean	28.2	37.1	32.1	F = NS
SD	7.3	10.5	5.9	
State anxiety				
Mean	27.2	31.4	30.0	F = NS
SD	4.5	9.6	7.5	
Beck depression				
Mean	0.9	2.8	1.2	F = NS
SD	1.0	4.8	1.5	
BP/systolic (mm Hg)				
Mean	115.8	121.4	117.5	F = NS
SD	9.2	6.5	9.5	
BP/diastolic (mm Hg)				
Mean	69.9	70.4	70.0	F = NS
SD	7.4	9.9	16.4	
Pulse (per min)				
Mean	68.9	71.0	69.9	F = NS
SD	8.1	9.5	8.9	
Respiration (per min)				
Mean	9.8	11.3	10.4	F = NS
SD	2.1	1.8	3.0	
$PECO_2$ (mm Hg)				
Mean	38.2	37.9	38.0	F = NS
SD	3.9	3.8	3.9	
Hematocrit				
Mean	41.5	42.5	43.4	F = NS
SD	4.1	3.1	4.0	

*Comparisons were made with analyses of variance.

factor also seems to distort the relationship between CBF and CO_2 in subjects who become anxious. Busija and Heistad (1984a) recently showed that electric and reflex activation of the sympathetic nervous system reduces CBF and increases cerebral vascular resistance during hypercarbia in anesthetized cats and awake dogs. The same mechanism might be responsible for the limited CBF response to CO_2 in subjects who became anxious.

Marijuana has sympathomimetic properties, and it often induces anxiety and panic in inexperienced users (Nahas et al., 1984; Benedikt et al., 1986; Weil, 1970). We measured CBF be-

fore and after marijuana smoking in experienced (a minimum of 10 "joints" per week for 3 years) and inexperienced subjects (no marijuana for a minimum of 3 years). The subjects were physically and mentally healthy and medication-free for a minimum of 1 month. They avoided alcohol and marijuana for 12 hr (experienced smokers) and coffee and tobacco for 3 hr before the experiments. Demographic characteristics of the 17 experienced smokers and 24 inexperienced smokers are given in Table 17–8.

CBF measurements were made with the [133]xenon inhalation technique using the standard procedure with usual precautions. Anxiety experienced during CBF measurements was quantified with the STAI (Spielberger et al., 1970). A high-potency marijuana cigarette (THC 2.2%) was administered 60 min before the second CBF. CBF was measured twice at an interval of 60 min in 15 inexperienced smokers under resting conditions. The remaining 26 subjects (9 experienced and 17 inexperienced smokers) smoked a high-potency marijuana cigarette (THC 2.2%) 60 min before the second CBF. Mood changes during CBF measurements were quantified with the Profile of Mood States (McNair et al., 1971).

CBF before and after marijuana in experienced and inexperienced smokers were compared with the two resting CBF runs using multivariate analysis of variance (group × period × hemisphere × region model). The second CBF was corrected for pre to post changes in $PECO_2$ with a 3% correction factor (Maximilian et al., 1980). This analysis indicated a group × period interaction ($F = 15.7$, $P < 0.001$) and a group × region interaction ($F = 2.53$, $P < 0.02$). To examine these interactions, analysis of variance was conducted on each group using a period × hemisphere × region repeated measure model, and, when appropriate, the change was examined with posthoc Scheffe test on each region (before and after). Inexperienced smokers showed significant CBF decreases in all regions after marijuana; there were no significant regional differences. The experienced smokers, on the other hand, showed a CBF increase in both hemispheres (Table 17–9). However, regional CBF reached significance only in the right and left frontal regions and left temporal region. Covarying out the baseline differences on CBF between the experienced and inexperienced smokers and controls did not alter the results.

A similar set of analyses were employed to examine changes in the physiological variables and state anxiety. Inexperienced smokers had significant increases in blood pressure, pulse rate, respiration, and state anxiety, and the experienced smokers had increases in diastolic blood pressure and pulse rate. Changes in mood as quantified with the Profile of Mood States (POMS) are given in Table 17–11. Pearson correlations were computed between CBF, physiologic, and rating scale data. Pulse rate showed a significant inverse correlation with all regions except left frontal. Changes in state anxiety correlated negatively with all regions. Correlations between POMS factor scores and CBF are given in Table 17–12.

The results of this study indicate an increase in state anxiety following marijuana smoking in inexperienced smokers. This finding is further validated by the significant postmarijuana increases in pulse rate, blood pressure, and respiration in this group. State anxiety, as quantified by STAI and POMS, showed significant inverse correlations with CBF. However, vigor, which is also considered to be a hyperarousal state, showed positive correlations. It should be noted that such indices of sympathetic activity as pulse rate, blood pressure, and respiratory rate showed less pronounced increases in the experienced smokers compared with the inexperienced ones. The results of this study are in keeping with the other CBF/anxiety induction studies described above: All indicated the existence of an anxiety-related cerebral vasoconstrictive factor.

Studies on stress and CBF conducted by two groups of investigators also suggest similar conclusions. Sokoloff and associates (1955) reported no CBF changes following mental arithmetic tasks that induced peripheral sympathetic activation. They utilized the nitrous oxide inhalation technique for CBF measurement. Under normal conditions, changes in brain function associated with the tasks should cause a CBF increase. Its absence suggests that sympathetic activation overshadowed this cerebral vasodilation. Shakhnovich and associates (1980) studied CBF changes induced by mental activity (speaking and counting) with the hydrogen polarographic method. The test induced diffuse CBF increases in subjects who showed no increase in pulse rate and muscle blood flow. The CBF increase was, however, absent in those who showed increased pulse rate and peripheral circulation. These findings support our hypothesis that a cerebral vasoconstrictive factor, probably sympathetic activation, limits the CBF increase induced by behavioral tasks.

Reivich and associates (1983) examined the association between anxiety and cerebral metabolic rate for glucose in 18 right-handed males. Anxiety levels were measured with the

TABLE 17–9.
Comparisons Between the Three Groups on Regional CBF Before and After Marijuana (Right Hemisphere)*

	Inexperienced marijuana smokers	Experienced marijuana smokers	Controls
Frontal			
Pre-			
Mean	87.4	72.1	87.0
SD	13.4	9.1	9.5
Post-			
Mean	75.4	77.5	88.4
SD	16.0	10.3	11.0
Central			
Pre-			
Mean	83.7	72.3	84.5
SD	13.3	10.6	10.2
Post-			
Mean	73.9	76.7	86.9
SD	12.9	11.7	11.5
Temporal			
Pre-			
Mean	78.5	66.4	75.7
SD	11.7	7.2	7.4
Post-			
Mean	68.4	71.2	78.5
SD	11.6	11.1	10.6
Parietal			
Pre-			
Mean	79.6	69.4	79.9
SD	9.8	8.4	8.8
Post-			
Mean	70.1	71.3	79.7
SD	13.8	7.7	11.0
Occipital			
Pre-			
Mean	76.8	66.0	73.9
SD	10.9	6.6	7.2
Post-			
Mean	68.7	69.6	77.4
SD	12.5	11.1	10.9

*Gray matter flow is in ml/100 g/min. Analysis of variance (group × period × hemisphere × region): group × period interaction, $F = 15.68$, $P \leq 0.001$; group × region interaction, $F = 2.53$, $P \leq 0.02$.

STAI (Spielberger et al., 1970). They found a curvilinear relationship between anxiety and frontocortical metabolic rates. A quadratic function fit the data for the state anxiety significantly better than a linear function ($F = 11.05$, $P < 0.001$). Frontal metabolism seemed to increase as a function of anxiety up to a point after which greater anxiety was associated with decreased metabolic activity. This pattern was not seen in other brain regions. When the subjects were divided into high anxious and low anxious groups, an interaction between anxiety and the metabolic rates in the two hemispheres was found ($F = 6.64$, $P < 0.02$).

STUDIES OF CLINICAL RELEVANCE

Cerebral Ischemic Symptoms in Anxiety Disorder

We studied the incidence of symptoms suggestive of cerebral ischemia in 16 patients who

TABLE 17–10.
Comparisons Between the Three Groups on Regional CBF Before and After Marijuana (Left Hemisphere)*

	Inexperienced marijuana smokers	Experienced marijuana smokers	Controls
Frontal			
Pre-			
Mean	85.5	72.0	87.5
SD	12.4	8.5	11.5
Post-			
Mean	77.0	76.8	81.1
SD	15.0	10.0	13.7
Central			
Pre-			
Mean	84.1	75.0	85.4
SD	11.6	12.7	9.3
Post-			
Mean	77.0	76.3	88.2
SD	13.7	12.1	13.4
Temporal			
Pre-			
Mean	78.3	65.6	76.5
SD	8.5	6.4	8.8
Post-			
Mean	69.4	72.5	78.9
SD	12.6	9.0	11.4
Parietal			
Pre-			
Mean	78.4	67.5	78.6
SD	12.0	8.9	8.9
Post-			
Mean	69.8	70.8	81.1
SD	12.4	8.6	10.2
Occipital			
Pre-			
Mean	79.9	66.0	75.4
SD	12.9	8.3	8.7
Post-			
Mean	67.5	69.4	78.3
SD	11.6	8.6	10.0

*Gray matter flow is in ml/100 g/min. Analysis of variance (group $\times$ period $\times$ hemisphere $\times$ region): group $\times$ period interaction, F = 15.68, $P \leq 0.001$; group $\times$ region interaction, F = 2.53, $P \leq 0.02$.

met the DSM III criteria for agoraphobia with panic, 26 patients with generalized anxiety disorder, and normal volunteers of comparable age and sex distribution (both patients and controls, 19 males and 23 females; male patients, 43 years, SD 15.2; male controls, 44.7 years, SD 15.1; female patients, 42.8 years, SD 15; female controls, 39.4 years, SD 15.9). Both patients and controls were physically healthy and free of all medication for 2 weeks. Anxiety was quantified with the STAI (Spielberger et al., 1970) and Beck Depression Inventory (Beck and Beck, 1972). Cerebral ischemic events were evaluated with a questionnaire developed for use in a neurology clinic to identify patients with transient ischemic attacks (TIAs). It provided information on the frequency, duration, and nature of such symptoms of TIA as loss of speech and vision, tingling and numbness, weakness and paralysis, and dizziness and fainting. Symptoms induced by postural changes, head movements, and

TABLE 17–11.
Profile of Mood States Before and After Smoking Marijuana (Analysis of Variance)

	Inexperienced smokers		Experienced smokers	
Anxiety				
Mean	6.5	18.2	9.8	6.9
SD	2.6	10.2	3.3	2.7
P	<0.001		<0.05	
Anger				
Mean	1.0	2.4	5.7	5.5
SD	1.1	4.3	8.3	10.6
P	NS		NS	
Fatigue				
Mean	4.6	7.2	5.6	6.2
SD	4.9	5.6	5.5	7.2
P	NS		NS	
Confusion				
Mean	4.7	11.6	6.4	9.4
SD	2.2	6.5	1.7	4.4
P	<0.002		<0.05	
Depression				
Mean	1.9	8.1	6.1	6.6
SD	1.9	7.7	6.6	7.5
P	<0.016		NS	
Vigor				
Mean	19.1	9.5	18.3	15.8
SD	4.7	8.3	6.9	6.4
P	<0.003		NS	

TABLE 17–12.
Pearson Correlations Between Profile of Mood States and rCBF Based on Change Scores Before and After Marijuana

	POMS factors					
	Anxiety	Anger	Fatigue	Confusion	Depression	Vigor
Right						
Frontal	−0.7458†	−0.2858	−0.4703	−0.7201†	−0.5334*	0.5737*
Central	−0.5265*	−0.2919	−0.3944	−0.5304*	−0.4554	0.3063
Temporal	−0.6415*	−0.0599	−0.3624	−0.5271*	−0.2739	0.1964
Parietal	0.8080†	−0.2161	−0.2815	−0.7196†	−0.5843*	0.7269†
Occipital	−0.6981†	−0.5123*	−0.3683	−0.7162†	−0.5072*	0.6138*
Left						
Frontal	−0.4872*	0.0118	−0.2002	−0.4933*	−0.2889	0.3021
Central	−0.3929	−0.3036	−0.3784	−0.3325	−0.3768	0.2366
Temporal	−0.5802*	0.0009	−0.5108*	−0.6543*	−0.2302	0.2976
Parietal	−0.6022*	−0.1423	−0.2160	−0.6123*	−0.3475	0.3624
Occipital	−0.7867†	−0.2588	−0.4032	−0.6885*	−0.3295	0.4874*

*$P \leq 0.05$.
†$P \leq 0.01$.

keeping limbs in a fixed position for long periods were not counted as ischemic symptoms. When the two groups were compared with analysis of variance, the patients had a significantly higher ($P < 0.001$) incidence of all cerebral ischemic symptoms except loss of vision (dizziness, 47%; tingling, 37%; loss of speech, 32%; weakness and paralysis, 16%). There were no differences between patients with agoraphobia with panic and generalized anxiety disorder. Multiple regression analysis with the ischemic symptoms total as the criterion variable and depression, state anxiety, and trait anxiety scores as predictor variables identified state anxiety as the factor that explained the largest percentage of variance (semipartial r^2 = 0.239, partial r^2 = 0.339).

The symptoms reported by patients differed from classic TIAs in several ways. TIAs, by definition, last from 5 to 15 min, while the anxious patients' symptoms lasted less than 2 min. Unlike TIAs, these symptoms were not related to age, and even patients who gave a long history of such symptoms (more than 10 years) did not have any demonstrable neurological deficits. TIA patients often suffer from a variety of physical disorders, unlike anxious patients, who were physically healthy. Forty-seven percent of the patients reported dizziness, and three subjects reported fainting spells. Dizziness and fainting in the absence of other symptoms are not indicative of focal ischemia and are not accepted as typical transient ischemic symptoms. These are probably caused by diffuse cerebral ischemia secondary to a sudden drop in perfusion pressure. In our patients, these symptoms were precipitated by acute elevations in the state anxiety (Mathew et al., 1987).

Coyle and Sterman (1986) also reported that 5% of the patients referred to their neurology service had panic attacks manifesting as focal neurologic symptoms. The symptoms these patients often complained of consisted of unilateral numbness, transient bilateral blindness, visual blurring, and diffuse headache. They attributed the symptoms to hypocapnia resulting from hyperventilation and consequent CBF reduction.

The foregoing discussion concerning an anxiety-related CBF reduction raises questions about anxiety and stroke. Indeed, stress is considered to be a risk factor by clinicians (Leonberg and Elliot, 1978). Several case reports and small-scale epidemiological studies suggest such a possibility, but firm evidence in this regard is lacking (Adler et al., 1971). This obviously is an area that needs to be researched more extensively.

SUMMARY

Nonspecific arousal mediated by the reticular formation is paralleled by changes in blood flow, since the two are closely coupled. Conditions associated with increases and decreases in arousal are associated with parallel changes in global CBF. Stimulation and destruction of the brainstem region that houses the reticular formation are associated with increases and decreases in CBF, respectively. Frontal lobe is the cortical apparatus responsible for the maintenance of arousal. Under resting conditions, frontal regions show higher perfusion than either cortical regions; degree of this hyperfrontal pattern of flow distribution varies with levels of arousal.

The relationship between CBF and anxiety is complicated by the multiple factors that influence the former and the widespread physiological changes that accompany the latter. Such anxiety-related factors (other than arousal) as plasma catecholamines, sympathetic nervous system, blood viscosity, and CO_2 levels can influence CBF. Previous investigators have reported CBF increases following the administration of epinephrine. This effect does not appear to be due to the vasoactive properties of the drug: The precise mechanism for this change is unknown. Cerebral blood vessels receive sympathetic innervation from the superior cervical ganglion. Stimulation of these fibers causes cerebral vasoconstriction. Thus the anxiety-related increases in sympathetic activity might result in reduced cerebral perfusion. CBF has an inverse relationship with blood viscosity. However, studies conducted in our laboratory have thus far failed to confirm previous reports of stress-induced polycytosis. Anxious patients and controls showed similar hematocrit levels under resting conditions, and anxiety induced by epinephrine infusions, caffeine infusions, CO_2 inhalation, and marijuana smoking did not alter the hematocrit. Furthermore, mild changes in hematocrit level did not appear to affect CBF. CO_2 is a potent cerebral vasodilator, and acute anxiety is often associated with rapid breathing and hypocapnia.

Normal subjects and anxious patients do not show any significant differences on global CBF under resting conditions. However, patients with panic disorder, prone to develop panic attacks during lactate infusions, show asymmetry of blood flow to the parahippocampal regions.

The effect of acute anxiety on CBF is complex. Mild anxiety might increase CBF and CMR, while severe anxiety, especially in anxious patients, seems to have the opposite effect. This is compatible with the concept that mild to moderate degrees of arousal improve performance, with more marked increases having the opposite effect (Eason, 1963). Mild increases in arousal associated with problem solving, sensory motor stimulation, and stress related to the first CBF and CMR measurement increase CBF and CMR (Risberg et al., 1977). However, experiments involving epinephrine infusions, marijuana smoking, and carbon dioxide inhalations suggest an association between acute anxiety and CBF reduction. This CBF decrease seems to be associated with the anxiety-related increase in sympathetic cerebral vasoconstrictive tone. However, any conclusions in this regard would be premature.

Anxious patients frequently report symptoms suggestive of cerebral ischemia. However, the degree of CBF reduction found to accompany induced anxiety is not substantial enough to produce cerebral ischemia (Frackowiak, 1985). It is possible that certain anxiety disorder patients may develop severe cerebral vasospasm and cerebral ischemia. Oversensitivity to sympathetic stimulation has been implicated in the causation of cerebral vasospasm (Bevan et al., 1987), and anxious patients have been shown to have heightened sensitivity to sympathetic activation.

CBF during acute anxiety will depend on the interplay of the central (arousal) and peripheral (sympathetic tone, CO_2) factors. The extensive volume of literature on the psychophysiology of anxiety indicates wide variations between and within subjects. In all probability, this will be true also of cerebral circulation. The CBF changes associated with anxiety are likely to depend on a number of factors, some of which were discussed in this chapter. There are others about which much is not known (the effects of neurotransmitters, intraparanchymal blood vessel innervation, and so forth).

CBF changes might vary between psychic or somatic subtypes of anxiety (Tyrer, 1976; Morrow and Labrum, 1978), since the central and peripheral changes influence CBF in different directions. Furthermore, perception of the bodily symptoms of anxiety (Tyrer, 1976) should increase CBF and CMR in the brain regions that mediate this function. Facilitatory and inhibitory brain regions may show blood flow changes in opposite directions, and, at the moment, little is known about regional differences in CBF during anxiety. All this points to the need to study large numbers of subjects with careful consideration not only of the behavioral aspects of anxiety but also of relevant physiological variables. A great deal of work needs to be done in this area before any firm conclusions can be drawn.

REFERENCES

Abdul-Rahman A, Dahlgren N, Johansson BB, Siesjo BK (1979): Increase in local cerebral blood flow induced by circulating adrenalin: Involvement of blood–brain barrier dysfunction. Acta Physiol Scand 107:227–232.

Ackner B (1956): The relationship between anxiety and the level of peripheral vasomotor activity. J Psychosom Res 1:21–48.

Adler R, MacRitchie K, Engel GL (1971): Psychological processes and ischemic stroke. Psychosom Med 33: 1–29.

Ax AF (1953): The physiological differentiation between fear and anger. Psychosom Med 15:433–442.

Beck AT, Beck RW (1972): Screening depressed patients in family practice. Postgrad Med 52:81–85.

Benedikt RA, Cristofaro P, Mendelson JH (1986): Effects of acute marijuana smoking in post-menopausal women. Psychopharmacology 90:14–17.

Benitone J, Kling A (1970): Polycythemia of stress in psychiatric hospital populations. J Psychosom Res 14: 105–108.

Bevan JA, Bevan RD, Frazer JG (1987): Functional arterial changes in a chronic cerebrospasm in monkeys: An in vitro assessment of the contribution to arterial narrowing. Stroke 18:472–481.

Blauenstein UW, Halsey JH, Wilson EM, Willis EL, Risberg J (1977): ^{133}Xenon inhalation method, analysis of reproducibility: Some of its physiological implications. Stroke 8:92–102.

Broderson P, Paulson OB, Bolgic TC, Rogon ZE, Rafaelsen OJ, Larsen NA (1973): Cerebral hyperemia during epileptic seizures in man. Arch Neurol 28:334–338.

Buchsbaum MS, Ingvar DH, Kessler R, Walters RN, Cappeletti J, Van Kammen DP, King AC, Johnson JL, Manning RG, Flynn RW, Mann LS, Bunney WE, Sokoloff L (1982): Cerebral glucography with positron tomography: Use in normal subjects and in patients with schizophrenia. Arch Gen Psychiatry 39:251–259.

Busija DW, Heistad DD (1984a): Effects of activation of the sympathetic nerves on cerebral blood flow during hypercarbia in cats and rabbits. J Physiol 347:35–45.

Busija DW, Heistad DD (1984b): Factors involved in the

physiological regulation of the cerebral circulation. Rev Physiol Biochem Pharmacol 101:161–211.

Carlsson C, Hagerdal M, Kaasik AE, Siesjo BK (1977): A catecholamine mediated increase in cerebral oxygen uptake during immobilization stress in rats. Brain Res 119:223–231.

Carlsson C, Hagerdal M, Siesjo BK (1975): Increase in cerebral oxygen uptake and blood flow in immobilization stress. Acta Physiol Scand 95:206–208.

Carpenter MB (1976): "Human Neuroanatomy," 7th ed. Baltimore: Williams & Wilkins, pp 547–599.

Charney DS, Heninger GR, Jatlow PI (1985): Increased anxiogenic effects of caffeine in panic disorders. Arch Gen Psychiatry 42:233–243.

Coyle PK, Sterman AB (1986): Focal neurologic symptoms in panic attacks. Am J Psychiatry 143:648–649.

Dahlgren N, Rosen I, Sakabe T, Siesjo BK (1980): Cerebral functional, metabolic and circulatory effects of intravenous infusion of adrenalin in the rat. Brain Res 184:143–152.

Dameshek W (1953): Stress erythrocytosis. Blood 8:282–289.

Dintenfass L, Zador I (1976): Blood rheology in patients with depressive and schizoid anxiety. Biorheology 13:33–36.

Dintenfass L, Zador I (1977): Hemorheology, chronic anxiety and psychosomatic pain: An apparent link. Lex Sci 13:154–162.

Devous MD, Stokely EM, Chehabi HH, Bonte FJ (1986): Normal distribution of regional cerebral blood flow measured by dynamic single-photon emission tomography. J Cerebral Blood Flow Metab 6:95–104.

Duffy E (1972): Activation. In Greenfield NS, Sternbach RA (eds): "Handbook of Psychophysiology." New York; Holt, Rinehart and Winston, pp 577–622.

Eason RG (1963): Relation between effort, tension level, skill and performance efficiency in a perceptual-motor task. Percept Motor Skills 16:297–317.

Edvinsson L (1982): Sympathetic control of cerebral circulation. Trends Neurosci 5:425–429.

Edvinsson L, MacKenzie ET (1977): Amine mechanisms in the cerebral circulation. Pharmacol Rev 28:275–353.

Forster A, Juge O, Morel D (1982): Effects of midazolam on cerebral blood flow in human subjects. Anesthesiology 56:453–455.

Fowles DC (1980): The three arousal model: Implications of Gray's two factor learning theory for heart rate electrodermal activity and psychopathy. Psychophysiology 17:87–104.

Frackowiak RSJ (1985): The pathophysiology of human cerebral ischemia: A new perspective obtained with positron tomography. Q J Med 57:713–727.

Frankenhaeuser M (1971): Brain and circulating catecholamines. Brain Res 31:241–262.

Fried R (1987): "The Hyperventilation Syndrome: Research and Clinical Treatment." Baltimore: The Johns Hopkins University Press, pp 58–87.

Frewen TC, Sumabat WO, Del Maestro RF (1985): Cerebral blood flow, metabolic rate and cross-brain oxygen consumption in brain injury. J Pediatr 107:510–513.

Fuster JM (1980): The prefrontal cortex. In Fuster JM (ed): "Anatomy, Physiology and Neuropsychology of the Frontal Lobe." New York: Raven Press, pp 125–145.

Galin D (1974): Implications for psychiatry of left and right hemispheric specialization. Arch Gen Psychiatry 31:572–583.

Gibbs FA, Gibbs EL, Lennox WG (1935): The cerebral blood flow in man as influenced by adrenalin, caffeine, amyl nitrite and histamine. Am Heart J 10:916–924.

Goldman-Rakic PS (1984): The frontal lobes: Uncharted provinces of the brain. Trends Neurosci 7:425–429.

Gorman JM, Askanaz J, Liebowitz MR, Fyer AJ, Stein J, Kinney JM, Klein DF (1984): Response to hyperventilation in a group of patients with panic disorder. Am J Psychiatry 141:857–861.

Gotoh F, Meyer JS, Takagi Y (1965): Cerebral effects of hyperventilation in man. Arch Neurol 12:410–423.

Gray JAC (1982): "The Neuropsychology of Anxiety: An Enquiry Into the Functions of the Septo-Hippocampal System." New York: Oxford University Press.

Griez E, van den Hout MA (1982): Effects of carbon dioxide inhalation on subjective anxiety and some investigative parameters. J Behav Ther Exp Psychiatry 13:27–32.

Gur RC, Gur RE, Obrist WD, Hungerbuhler JP, Younkin D, Rosen AD, Skolnick BE, Reivich M (1982): Sex and handedness differences in cerebral blood flow during rest and cognitive activity. Science 217:659–661.

Gur RE, Gur RC, Skolnick BE, Caroff S, Obrist WD, Resnick S, Reivich M (1985): Brain function in psychiatric disorders. III. Regional cerebral blood flow in unmedicated schizophrenics. Arch Gen Psychiatry 42:329–334.

Harik SI, Sharma VK, Wetherbee JR, Warren RH, Banergee SP (1981): Adrenergic and cholinergic receptors of cerebral microvessels. J Cerebral Blood Flow Metab 1:329–338.

Hoehn-Saric R (1982): Neurotransmitters in anxiety. Arch Gen Psychiatry 39:735–742.

Ingvar DH (1979): "Hyperfrontal" distribution of the cerebral gray matter flow in resting wakefulness; on the functional anatomy of the conscious state. Acta Neurol Scand 60:12–25.

Ingvar DH, Haggendal E, Nilsson NJ, Sourander P, Wickbom I, Lassen NA (1964): Cerebral circulation and metabolism in an unconscious patient. Arch Neurol 11:13–21.

Ingvar DH, Lassen NA (1976): Regulation of cerebral blood flow. In Himwich HE (ed): "Brain Metabolism and Cerebral Disorders." New York: Spectrum Publications. pp 181–206.

Ingvar DH, Soderberg UMK (1956): A new method for measuring cerebral blood flow in relation to the electroencephalogram. Electroencephalogr Clin Neurophysiol 3:403–412.

Ingvar DH, Soderberg U (1958): Cortical blood flow related to EEG patterns evoked by stimulation of the brain stem. Acta Physiol Scand 42:130–143.

Isaacson RL (1982): "The Limbic System." New York: Plenum Press.

Juge O, Meyer JS, Sakai F, Yamaguchi F, Yamamoto M, Shaw T (1979): Critical appraisal of cerebral blood flow measured from brain stem and cerebellar regions after ^{133}xenon inhalation in humans. Stroke 10:428–437.

Kandel ER, Schwartz JH (1981): "Principles of Neurological Science." Amsterdam: Elsevier, pp 359–382.

Kelly A, Munan L (1977): Hematologic profile of natural populations: Red cell parameters. Br J Haematol 35: 153–160.

Kelly D (1976): Neurosurgical treatment of psychiatric disorders. In Granville-Grossman K (ed): "Recent Advances in Clinical Psychiatry Number Two." London: Churchill Livingstone 1976, pp 227–261.

Kelly DHW, Walter CJS (1969): The relationship between clinical diagnosis and anxiety, assessed by forearm blood flow and other measurements. Br J Psychiatry 112:871–882.

Kety SS (1952): Consciousness and the metabolism of the brain. In Abramson HA (ed): "Conference on Problems of Consciousness (Third Conference)." New York: Josiah Macey Foundation, pp 11–75.

King BD, Sokoloff L, Wechsler RL (1952): The effects of l-epinephrine and l-norepinephrine upon cerebral circulation and metabolism in man. J Clin Invest 31:273–279.

Lader M (1975): "The Psychophysiology of Mental Illness." London: Routledge & Kegan Paul, pp 103–104.

Lader M (1982): Biological differentiation of anxiety, arousal and stress. In Mathew RJ (ed): "The Biology of Anxiety." New York: Brunner/Mazel, 1982, pp 11–22.

Lasvennes F, Lestage P, Bobillier P, Seylaz J (1986): Stress and local cerebral blood flow: Studies on restrained and unrestrained rats. Exp Brain Res 63:163–168.

Lawrence JH, Berlin NI (1951): Relative polycythemia— The polycythemia of stress. Yale J Biol Med 24:498–505.

Levi L (1972): Stress and distress in response to psychosocial stimuli. Acta Med Scand [Suppl] 528:1–157.

LeDoux JE, Thompson ME, Iadecola C, Tucker LW, Reis DJ (1983): Local cerebral blood flow increases during auditory and visual processing in the conscious rat. Science 221:576–578.

Leonberg SC, Elliott FA (1978): Preventing stroke after TIA. Am Fam Physician 17:179–183.

Ley R, Walker H (1973): Effects of carbon dioxide-oxygen inhalation on heart rate, blood pressure and subjective anxiety. J Behav Ther Exp Psychiatry 4:223–228.

Luria AR (1973): "The Working Brain: An Introduction to Neuropsychology." New York: Basic Books, pp 187–226.

Malmo RB (1959): Activation: A neuropsychological dimension. Psych Rev 66:367–386.

Mamo H, Meric P, Luft A, Seylaz J (1983): Hyperfrontal pattern of human cerebral circulation. Variations with age and atherosclerotic state. Arch Neurol 40: 626–632.

Marshall J (1982): The viscosity factor in cerebral ischaemia. J Cereb Blood Flow Metabol (Suppl 1) 2:S47–S47.

Mathew RJ, Barr DL, Weinman ML (1983): Caffeine and cerebral blood flow. Br J Psychiatry 143:604–608.

Mathew RJ, Ho BT, Francis DJ, Taylor DL, Weinman ML (1982a): Catecholamines and anxiety. Acta Psychiatr Scand 65:142–147.

Mathew RJ, Weinman ML, Claghorn JL (1982b): Anxiety and cerebral blood flow. In Mathew RJ (ed): "The Biology of Anxiety." New York: Brunner/Majel, pp 23–33.

Mathew RJ, Wilson WH (1985): Caffeine induced changes in cerebral circulation. Stroke 16:814–817.

Mathew RJ, Wilson WH (1986): Hematocrit and anxiety. J Proychosom Res 30:307–311.

Mathew RJ, Wilson WH (1988a): Epinephrine-induced anxiety and regional cerebral blood flow in anxious patients. In Lerer B, Gershon S (eds): "New Directions in Affective Disorders." New York: Springer-Verlag (in press).

Mathew RJ, Wilson WH (1988b): Carbon dioxide-induced cerebral blood flow changes in anxiety. Psychiatry Res (in press).

Mathew RJ, Wilson WH, Daniel DG (1985): The effect of nonsedating doses of diazepam on regional cerebral blood flow. Biol Psychiatry 20;1109–1116.

Mathew RJ, Wilson WH, Nicassio PM (1987): Cerebral ischemic symptoms in anxiety disorders. Am J Psychiatry 144:265.

Mathew RJ, Wilson WH, Tant SR (1986): Determinants of resting regional cerebral blood flow in normal subjects. Biol Psychiatry 21:907–914.

Maximilian VA, Prohovnik I, Risberg J (1980): Cerebral hemodynamic response to mental activation in normo- and hypercapnia. Stroke 11:342–347.

Mazziotta JC (1985): PET scanning: Principles and applications. Discussions Neurosci 11:9–47.

McNair DM, Lorr M, Doppleman LF (1971): "Manual for Profile of Mood States." San Diego: Educational and Industrial Testing Service.

Metter EJ, Riege WH, Kuhl DE, Phelps ME (1984): Cerebral metabolic relationships for selected brain regions in healthy adults. J Cerebral Blood Flow Metab 4:1–7.

Menon D, Koles Z, Dobbs A (1980): The relationship between cerebral blood flow and the EEG in normals. Cnd J Neurol Sci 7:195–198.

Meyer JS, Heyman A, Amano T, Nakajima S, Shat T, Lauzon P, Derman S, Karacan I, Harati Y (1981): Mapping local blood flow of human brain by CT scanning during stable xenon inhalation. Stroke 12:426–436.

Meyer JS, Ishihara N, Deshmukh VD, Naritomi H, Sakai F, Hsu M-C, Pollack P (1978): Improved method for noninvasive measurement of regional cerebral blood flow by ^{133}xenon inhalation. Part I: Description of method and normal values obtained in healthy volunteers. Stroke 9:195–205.

Morrow GR, Labrum AH (1978): The relationship between psychological and physiological measures of anxiety. Psychol Med 8:95–101.

Moruzzi G, Magoun HW (1949): Brain stem reticular formation and activation of the EEG. Electroencephalogr Clin Neurophysiol 1:455–473.

Nahas GG, Harvey DJ, Paris M, Brill H (1984): "Marihuana in Science and Medicine." New York: Raven Press, pp 160–246.

Nauta WJH (1971): The problem of frontal lobe: A reinterpretation. J Psychiatr Res 8:167–187.

Nesse RM, Cameron OG, Curtis GC, McCann DS, Huber-Smith MJ (1984): Adrenergic function in patients with panic anxiety. Arch Gen Psychiatry 41:771–776.

Noback CR (1975): "The Human Nervous System: Basic Principles of Neurobiology, 2nd ed." New York; McGraw-Hill, pp 443–480.

Obrist WD, Gennarelli TA, Segawa H, Dolinskas CA, Langfitt TW (1979): Relation of cerebral blood flow to neurological status and outcome in head-injured patients. J Neurosurg 51:292–300.

Obrist WD, Thompson HK, Wang HS, Wilkinson WE (1975): Regional cerebral blood flow estimated by [133]xenon inhalation. Stroke 6:245–256.

Ohata M, Fredericks WR, Sunderan U, Rapoport SI (1984): Effects of immobilization stress on regional cerebral blood flow in the conscious rat. J Cereb Blood Flow Metabol 1:187–194.

Olesen J (1975): Effect of intercarotid isoprenaline, propranolol, and prostaglandin E on regional cerebral blood flow in man. In Harper M, Jennett B, Miller D, Rowan J (eds): "Blood Flow and Metabolism in the Brain." London: Churchill Livingstone, pp 4.10–4.11.

Olesen J, Paulson B, Lassen NA (1971): Regional cerebral blood flow in man determined by the initial slope of the clearance of intra-arterially injected [133]xenon. Stroke 2:519–540.

Pitts FN, Allen RE (1982): Beta-adrenergic blockade in the treatment of anxiety. In Mathew RJ (ed): "The Biology of Anxiety." New York: Brunner/Mazel, pp 162–186.

Powers WJ, Raichle ME (1986): Positron emission tomography and its application to the study of cerebrovascular disease in man. Stroke 16:361–376.

Pribam KH (1973): The primate frontal cortex—Executive of the brain. In Pribram KH, Luria AR (eds): "Psychophysiology of the Frontal Lobes." New York: Academic Press, pp 293–314.

Prohovnik I (1978): Cerebral lateralization of psychologic processes. A literature review. Arch Psychol (Frankfurt) 130:161–211.

Prohovnik I, Hakansson K, Risberg J (1980): Observations on the functional significance of regional cerebral blood flow in resting normal subjects. Neuropsychologia 18:203–217.

Purves MJ (1972): "The Physiology of Cerebral Circulation." Cambridge: Cambridge University Press, pp 173–199.

Raichle M, Grubb RL, Gado MH, Eichling JO, Ter-Pogossian MM (1976): Correlation between regional cerebral blood flow and oxidative metabolism: In vivo studies in man. Arch Neurol 33:523–526.

Rapoport SI, Duara D, Grady CL, Culter NR (1985): Cerebral glucose utilization in relation to age in man. In Greitz T, Ingvar DH, Widen L (eds): "The Metabolism of the Human Brain Studies With Positron Emission Tomography." New York: Raven Press, pp 339–350.

Rapoport SI, Ohata M, Sundaram U, Fredericks WR (1981): Regional cerebral blood flow following immo-

bilization stress in the conscious rat. J Cerebral Blood Flow Metab 1:477–478.

Reiman EM, Raichle ME, Butler FK, Herscovitch P, Robins E (1984): A focal brain abnormality in panic disorder, a severe form of anxiety. Nature 310:683–685.

Reiman EM, Raichle RE, Robins E, Butler FK, Herscovitch P, Fox P, Perlmeitter J (1986): The application of positron emission tomography to the study of panic disorder. Am J Psychiatry 143:469–477.

Reivich M, Gur R, Alavi A (1983): Positron emission tomographic studies of sensory stimuli, cogniture processes and anxiety. Hum Neurobiol 2:25–33.

Risberg J, Maximilian AV, Prohovnik I (1977): Changes in cortical activity patterns during habituation to a reasoning test. Neuropsychologia 15:793–798.

Risberg J, Gustafson L, Prohovnik I (1981): rCBF measurements by [133]xenon inhalation: Applications in neuropsychology and psychiatry. Prog Nucl Med 7:82–94.

Rockoff MA, Naughton KVH, Shapiro HM, Ingvar M, Ray KF, Gagnon RL, Marshall LF (1980): Cerebral circulatory and metabolic responses to intravenously administered lorazepam. Anesthesiology 53:215–218.

Ross ED (1984): Right hemisphere's role in language, affectate behavior and emotion. Trends Neurosci 7:342–346.

Routtenberg A (1968): The two arousal hypothesis: Reticular formation and the limbic systems. Psych Rev 75:51–80.

Russell RP, Conley CL (1964): Benign polycythemia: Gaisbock's syndrome. Arch Intern Med 114:734–740.

Sakai F, Meyer JS, Karacan I, Derman S, Yamamoto M (1980): Normal human sleep: Regional cerebral hemodynamics. Ann Neurol 7:471–478.

Sarason IG (1984): Stress, anxiety and cognitive interference: Reaction to tests. J Pers Soc Psychol 46:929–938.

Schachter S, Singer JE (1962): Cognitive social and physiological determinants of emotional state. Psychol Rev 69:379–399.

Schildkraut JJ, Kety SS (1967): Biogenic amines and emotion. Science 156:21–30.

Selye H (1956): "The Stress of Life." New York: McGraw-Hill.

Sensenbach W, Madison L, Ochs L (1953): A comparison of the effects of l-norepinephrine, synthetic l-epinephrine, and USP-epinephrine upon cerebral blood flow and metabolism in man. J Clin Invest 32:226–232.

Shakhnovich AR, Serbinenko FA, Razumovsky AY, Radionov IM, Oskolok LN (1980): The dependence of cerebral blood flow on mental activity and on emotional state in man. Neuropsychologia 18:465–476.

Sharma HS, Dey PK (1986): Influence of long term immobilization stress on regional blood–brain barrier permeability cerebral blood flow and 5 HT level in conscious normotensive young rats. J Neurol Sci 72:61–76.

Siegel JM (1979): Behavioral functions of the reticular formation. Brain Res Rev 1:69–105.

Sokoloff L, Mangold R, Wechsler R, Kennedy C, Kety S

(1955): The effect of mental arithmetic on cerebral blood flow and metabolism. J Clin Invest 34:1101–1108.

Spielberger CD, Gorsuch RL, Lushene RD (1970): "STAI Manual." Palo Alto, CA: Consulting Psychologists Press.

Strandgaard S, Paulson OB (1984): Cerebral autoregulation. Stroke 15:413–416.

Thomas DJ (1982): Whole blood viscosity and cerebral blood flow. Stroke 13:285–287.

Townsend RE, Prinz PN, Obrist WD (1973): Human cerebral blood flow during sleep and waking. J Appl Physiol 35:620–625.

Tucker DM, Antes JR, Stenslie CE, Barnhardt TN (1978): Anxiety and lateral cerebral function. J Abnorm Psychol 87:380–383, 1978.

Tucker DM, Roth RS, Arneson BA, Buckingham V (1977): Right hemispheric activation during stress. Neuropsychologia 15:697–700.

Tyler SK, Tucker DM (1982): Anxiety and perceptual structure: Individual differences in neuropsychological function. J Abnorm Psychol 91:210–220.

Tyrer P (1976): "The Role of Bodily Feelings in Anxiety." London: Oxford University Press, p 32.

van den Hout MA, Griez E (1984): Panic symptoms after the inhalation of carbon dioxide. Br J Psychiatry 144:503–507.

Veleber DM, Templer DI (1984): Effects of caffeine on anxiety and depression. J Abnorm Psychol 93:120–122.

Vernheit J, Renou AM, Orgogozo JM, Constant P, Caille JM (1978): Effects of a diazepam-fentanyl mixture on cerebral blood flow and oxygen consumption in man. Br J Anaesthesiol 50:165–169.

Weil AT (1970): Adverse reactions to marijuana. N Engl J Med 282:997–1000.

Weinberger DR, Berman KF, Zec RF (1986): Physiologic dysfunction of dorsolateral prefrontal cortex in schizophrenia. I. Regional cerebral blood flow evidence. Arch Gen Psychiatry 43:114–124.

Wilkinson IMS, Bull JWD, Du Boulay GH, Marshall J, Ross Russell RW, Symon L (1969): Regional blood flow in normal cerebral hemisphere. J Neurol Neurosurg Psychiatry 32:367–378.

Wilson SJ, Boyle P (1952): Erroneous anaemea and polycythemia. Arch Intern Med 90:602–609.

Woods SW, Charney DS, Goodman WK, Redmond DE, Heninger GR (1986): Carbon dioxide sensitivity in panic anxiety, ventilatory and anxiogenic response to carbon dioxide in healthy subjects and patients with panic anxiety before and after alprazolam treatment. Arch Gen Psychiatry 43:900–909.

Anxiety and Depression

18

Hypothalamic–Pituitary–Adrenal Axis in Panic Disorder

PHILIP W. GOLD, MD, TERESA A. PIGOTT, MD, MITCHEL A. KLING, MD,
HARRY A. BRANDT, MD, KONSTANTINE KALOGERAS, MD,
MARK A. DEMITRACK, MD, AND THOMAS D. GERACIOTI, MD

Clinical Neuroendocrinology Branch (P.W.G., M.A.K., H.A.B., K.K., M.A.D., T.D.C.), and Section on Clinical Neuropharmacology (T.A.P.), Laboratory of Clinical Sciences, National Institute of Mental Health, Bethesda, Maryland 20892

INTRODUCTION

Because of the paroxysmal nature of the anxiety and associated physical symptoms that are characteristic of panic disorder, the principal central effectors of the stress response have often been implicated. The stress response involves both the sympathetic nervous system and the hypothalamic–pituitary–adrenal (HPA) axis. Of these two systems, the locus ceruleus–norepinephrine (LC-NE) and corticotropin-releasing factor (CRF) components are two of the best-described central effectors of the acute generalized stress response. Yet while panic disorder can be conceptualized as a syndrome of at least episodic dysregulation of the stress response based on its symptom presentation and the large volume of evidence showing that experimental activation of the LC–NE and CRF systems in experimental animals produces symptoms of intense anxiety, panic disorder patients often lack evidence of substantial sympathetic nervous system or pituitary adrenal activation even in the midst of acute panic attacks (Liebowitz et al., 1986).

In this chapter, we present some of the clinical data concerning the level of activation of the HPA axis in panic disorder and attempt to summarize current preclinical and clinical data suggesting a possible role for the CRF system in the development and perpetuation of panic disorder. We will also include potential explanations for the relative absence of HPA activation in the setting of putative activation of the CRF system in panic disorder. In this regard, we will also include some of our previous data suggesting that CRF plays an integral role in the symptom complex of major depressive disorder, which has often been hypothesized to share important genetic and pathophysiological features with panic disorder (Breier et al., 1987; Weissman and Merikangas, 1986).

HISTORICAL CONSIDERATIONS

The discovery of the neuropeptides has contributed much to the growing field of neuroendocrinology and the neurosciences; it is now evident that neuropeptides act as putative neurotransmitters, as well as generalized modulators of neuronal activities. While neuropeptides have only been recently extensively localized outside the brain, the idea of the brain as the source of multiple neurohormones is far from new. In fact, Hippocrates in 400 BC conceptualized the brain as a functioning gland: "The flesh of the glands is different from the rest of the body, being spongy and full of veins; they are found in the moist part of body where they receive humidity . . . and the brain is a gland as well as the mammae . . ." (Iason, 1946; Zuingerus, 1669). However, it was not until 500 years later that further endocrine functions of the brain were mentioned and at that time Galen (Medvei, 1984) identified one of the primary targets of the neurohor-

Neurobiology of Panic Disorder, Pages 313–320
Published 1990 by Alan R. Liss, Inc.

mones inadvertently as a "mucous (pituita) secretion of the brain." The hypothalamic–pituitary system of portal veins was described 200 years later (Lieutaud, 1742), but not functionally clarified for another 200 years. At that time, Scharrer and Scharrer (1940) pioneered the concept of hypothalamic neurosecretion in the supraopticohypophyseal system, and Harris (1948) then hypothesized that the pituitary was regulated by hypothalamic nerve cells via chemicals secreted into the portal vasculature. Through the development of immunocytochemistry and radioimmunoassay, peptide hormones in the brain have been precisely localized not only in the hypothalamus but also in several extrahypothalamic brain regions where they have considerable neuromodulatory functions (Dodd and Kelly, 1978; Henry, 1977).

In 1955, hypothalamic fragments were found to possess remarkable corticotropin (ACTH) releasing properties when incubated with pituicytes in vitro (Saffran et al., 1955). The 41 amino acid peptide CRF was only isolated from ovine hypothalamus in 1981 (Vale et al., 1981). This delay reflects the fact that CRF is a relatively large peptide, is easily oxidized, loses its biological activity, and, in fact, must be largely intact structurally for full biological activity. Shortly after the sequencing of ovine CRF, the structures of porcine CRF (Schally et al., 1981) and rat CRF (Rivier et al., 1983) were described. Interestingly, although differences exist in the sequences of ovine and rat CRF, recent studies have shown CRF in rats and humans to be immunologically identical, as well as structurally (Furatani et al., 1983; Shibahara et al., 1983).

CRF is now known to be produced in the paraventricular nucleus of the hypothalamus and carried from the median eminence to the basophilic cells of the anterior pituitary by the hypophyseal portal blood supply. This hormone then connects the complex neurophysiological reactions that occur during the stress response. CRF directly controls corticotropin (ACTH) synthesis and release from the anterior pituitary, and ACTH in turn regulates cortisol synthesis and release from the zona fasciculata and zona reticularis of the human adrenal cortex. The control of cortisol by ACTH occurs in a reciprocal fashion and is modulated by a complex negative-feedback system on the hypothalamic receptors and higher neural centers.

CRF is also of interest to psychiatrists and neurobiologists for reasons other than its putative role in regulating the HPA axis. CRF is synthesized not only by the hypothalamus for transport by hypophyseal portal blood but, like other hypothalamic hormones, CRF is widely distributed and/or synthesized beyond the boundaries of the hypothalamus to play an important role in coordinating complex behavioral and/or physiological processes of survival value. Neuroanatomically, it has been shown that there are extensive aggregations of CRF cell bodies and terminal fields in the limbic system, cortex, and in close association with the central autonomic system and the locus ceruleus (Bloom et al., 1982; Olschowka et al., 1982). This distribution of CRF within and beyond the hypothalamus provides an anatomical context for the observation that CRF can simultaneously activate and modulate metabolic, circulatory (Brown et al., 1982), and behavioral (Britton et al., 1982; Sirinathsinghji et al., 1983; Sutton et al., 1982) responses that are adaptive in stressful situations.

In animals, intracerebroventricular (icv) administration of CRF leads to a number of behaviors considered consistent with a response to anxiogenic or stressful stimuli, including decreased feeding (Britton et al., 1982), decreased sexual behavior (Sirinathsinghji et al., 1983), assumption of a freeze posture in a foreign environment, and increased exploration in familiar surroundings (Sutton et al., 1982). These behaviors are coupled with activation of both the HPA axis and the sympathetic nervous system. This "anxiogenic effect" of CRF is particularly interesting in light of recent data suggesting that control of the HPA axis is much more complicated than originally surmised. As previously mentioned, in the resting state, ACTH and cortisol bear a reciprocal control relationship to one another, but during stressful situations this control is much less well understood. It appears that complex central nervous system responses can stimulate CRF secretion even in the presence of high circulating plasma concentrations of cortisol and that, furthermore, the CRF and LC–NE systems may participate in a mutually reinforcing positive-feedback loop. Hence, the direct application of CRF onto locus ceruleus neurons markedly increases the LC firing rate, and norepinephrine is a potent stimulus to the in vitro release of CRF. Additional data from our group (Freo V, Perini GI, Kling MA, Gold PW, unpublished observations) and others (Sharkey et al., 1989) show that the icv administration of CRF markedly increases the LC glucose utilization rate.

The sequencing, precise localization, and eventual synthesis of CRF has greatly enhanced the capacity for clinical neuroendocrinologists to explore the hypothalamic–pituitary components of Cushing's disease and adrenal insufficiency. Interest in CRF by psychoneuroendocrinologists has also been heightened by the persistent finding of evidence of HPA axis activation in a number of psychiatric disorders. First, many patients with depression (Carroll et al., 1976; Sachar et al., 1970), anorexia nervosa (Gerner and Gwirtsman, 1981), alcoholism (Stokes, 1973), generalized anxiety disorder (Schweizer et al., 1986), and obsessive–compulsive disorder (Insel et al., 1982; Jenike et al., 1987) manifest evidence of a hyperactive HPA axis. In fact, the hypercortisolism seen in depressive illness, particularly with psychotic features, can be so severe that it is difficult to distinguish it from Cushing's disease. Moreover, CRF has integral connections with the opioid system that have become increasingly implicated as a potential crucial component in the development, pathogenesis, and perpetuation of many psychiatric disorders. Indeed it has been shown that ACTH is secreted synchronously with beta-endorphin, one of the principal endogenous opioid peptides (Guillemin et al., 1977). Both beta-endorphin and ACTH are contained within the sequence of a common precursor molecule, pro-opiomelanocortin (POMC) (Mains et al., 1977), and CRF is the principal central signal for the cleavage of pituitary POMC into biologically active peptides.

Our recent observation that the icv administration of CRF produces limbic seizures that cross-sensitize with electrically kindled seizures (Weiss et al., 1986) may also provide further support for CRF as a possible component in the pathophysiology of psychiatric illnesses such as depression and panic disorder. The kindling of limbic substrates, as proposed by Post et al. (1981) has been hypothesized to be crucial in the development and eventual perpetuation of certain forms of periodic psychiatric disorders such as rapid-cycling bipolar affective disorder and panic disorder. Additional work from our group of possible interest to this role in kindling includes data that procaine, which promotes limbic kindling in rats, produces a dose-dependent activation of pituitary–adrenal function in humans (Kling et al., 1987) and increases in vitro CRF release from rat hypothalami. Interestingly, this effect is blocked by carbamazepine (Calogero AE, Kling, MA, unpublished observation).

HPA AXIS MEASURES IN PANIC DISORDER

As noted previously, the clinical presentation and associated physical symptoms of panic disorder suggest activation of the generalized stress response, presumably with both adrenergic and HPA axis components. Consequently, both the peripheral and central adrenergic systems and HPA axis have been extensively studied in panic disorder patients. While the locus ceruleus and noradrenergic systems are presumed to play a central role in the pathogenesis and perpetuation of anxiety in animals (Redmond, 1977), biochemical indices of adrenergic activation in the basal state and during panic attacks in humans have failed to exhibit consistent evidence of catecholaminergic activation. However, there have been several reports suggesting that high noradrenergic neuronal activity exists and contributes to the pathophysiology of panic attacks in at least a subgroup of panic disorder patients (Charney et al., 1987).

A similar controversy exists concerning the level of activation of the HPA axis in panic disorder and in agoraphobia with panic attacks. There have been a number of reports of normal plasma cortisol suppression after dexamethasone administration in such patients (Grunhaus et al., 1987; Lieberman et al., 1983; Peterson et al., 1985; Sheehan et al., 1983). Conversely, there have also been reports of a high incidence of DST nonsuppression in panic disorder patients (Faludi et al., 1986). This controversy may be resolved in the future by measurement of dexamethasone levels and further standardization of DSTs. Perhaps more intriguing has been the recent observation that the mean basal cortisol level and postdexamethasone cortisol concentration of patients with panic disorder may be significantly higher than controls, despite considerable suppression following the DST (Judd et al., 1987; Goldstein et al., 1987). A compilation of these various investigations does at least suggest that cortisol hypersecretion occurs in many, if not the majority, of panic patients. Additionally, Halbreich et al. (unpublished observations) and Ballenger et al. (unpublished observations) have noted that patients with panic disorder exhibit higher than normal 24 hr urinary free cortisol excretion, again supporting HPA activation in panic disorder.

Our group has shown that patients with panic disorder have also been shown to have blunted ACTH and cortisol responses to corticotropin-releasing hormone (Roy-Byrne et al., 1986). This blunted result resembles those we previously reported for depressed patients, except that in the depressed patients they occurred in the face of significantly elevated basal cortisol and ACTH levels. These results also support the premise that patients with panic disorder have an element of chronic hypercortisolemia, like depressed patients, but probably exhibit a more acute pertubation in ACTH secretion not previously seen in depressed patients. Moreover, this suggests that the hypercortisolemia in patients with panic disorder reflects a defect at or above the hypothalamus that results in hypersecretion of endogenous CRF. These multiple observations have led to the implication of CRF as an important component in the pathophysiology of panic disorder.

CRF HYPOTHESIS IN THE PATHOPHYSIOLOGY OF PANIC DISORDER

We currently have data showing that alprazolam, one of the most effective pharmacological agents in the treatment of panic disorder, produces a profound dose-dependent suppression of in vitro CRF release, with a maximally suppressive dose of 10^{-9} M (Calogero et al., 1987). This CRF suppressive effect of alprazolam is at least ten times more potent than that of diazepam, and may account for the more pronounced clinical efficacy of alprazolam in acute panic attacks. We have also shown that alprazolam produces a dose-dependent decrease in ACTH and cortisol secretion in non-

restrained primates (Kalogeras et al., unpublished observation) despite associated data that alprazolam has no effect on ACTH release by in vitro pituitary organ culture (Luger et al., unpublished data). Thus the pituitary–adrenal suppression of alprazolam in primates most likely occurs via suppression of the CRF neuron, compatible with the data obtained exploring alprazolam's effects on hypothalamic CRF release.

Expanding these observations to clinical research, we studied volunteer subjects exploring the effects of a physical stress (exercise) on HPA function (Luger et al., 1987) at 50, 70, and 90% of their maximal oxygen utilization capacity. We noted a dose-dependent increase in plasma ACTH and cortisol responses during exercise. Moreover, we noted a concomitant dose-dependent increase in plasma lactate concentrations, which correlated with both the plasma ACTH and cortisol concentrations during each of the three exposures to graded levels of exercise. In an additional study (Calogero et al., unpublished data), we noted that lactate produced a dose-dependent increase in CRF release from in vitro rat hypothalamic organ culture, with the maximally stimulatory dose similar to the lactate concentrations achieved by volunteers during exercise at 90% of maximal oxygen utilization. While there has been considerable controversy concerning the specificity of iv sodium lactate as an anxiogenic agent, sodium lactate has been repeatedly demonstrated to provoke panic attacks in panic disorder patients (Cowley et al., 1987). In this regard, while lactate-induced panic has been shown to be associated with decreased hippocampal blood flow, we have shown, as noted, that the icv administration of CRF to the rat hypothalami markedly increases LC glucose utilization in association with decreased glucose utilization in LC terminal fields, e.g., the hippocampus (Perini et al., unpublished observations).

This model of panic disorder, suggesting a role of the CRF system, is not incompatible with other models of the pathophysiology of this disorder. In particular, the data suggesting that panic disorder is associated with an activation of the LC–NE system in the brain fits nicely with a possible concomitant defect in the inhibition of the CRF system. For example, our group has shown that norepinephrine stimulates CRF release from in vitro rat hypothalamic organ culture (Calogero et al., 1988), while other investigators (Valentino et al., 1986) have shown that CRF markedly enhances the LC firing rate in experimental animals. Taken together, these data suggest that the CRF and LC–NE systems may act in a positive-feedback loop to produce some of the clinical and biochemical manifestations of panic disorder.

We have recently advanced several lines of data suggesting that hypercortisolism in major depression reflects a defect at or above the hypothalamus resulting in the hypersecretion of endogenous CRF. Hence, like the panic disorder patients, hypercortisolemic depressed patients showed reduced ACTH responses to ovine CRF (Gold et al., 1984, 1986), suggesting that the pituitary corticotroph cell is appropriately restrained by cortisol negative feedback. We also have shown that depressed patients have cerebrospinal (CSF) CRF levels that correlate positively with postdexamethasone cortisol levels (Roy et al., 1987) and that volunteers given a continuous infusion of CRF show circadian cortisol responses whose pattern and magnitude closely resemble those seen in depression (Schulte et al., 1985). In light of this hypothetical common defect in CRF dysregulation, which we propose for both major depression and panic disorder, the question arises as to why the two disorders clearly manifest themselves as distinct clinical entities. One speculation is that in contrast to depression, where activation of the CRF neuron seems to occur more or less in a chronic, unremitting pattern, panic disorder may represent a disorder in which there is intermittent, explosive activation of the CRF system. Thus, in depressive illness, the greater relative exposure of the CRF system to hypercortisolism could sufficiently restrain the system via negative feedback, such that it is incapable of exhibiting the kind of eruptive activation postulated for panic disorder. On the other hand, the intermittence of panic disorder may provide the context for its explosive nature. For example, it would be during times of eucortisolism, when glucocorticoid restraint upon the CRF system is minimal, that periodic, explosive upward excursions of the CRF system are most

possible. This possibility is strengthened by clinical observations that panic attacks may occur at rest, during relaxation, and soon after the onset of sleep, when cortisol negative feedback is at a minimum.

As previously discussed, although several lines of circumstantial evidence support a role for CRF in some components of the symptom complex of panic disorder, other lines of data, e.g., the dexamethasone investigations, raise important questions that have not yet been resolved. It should be noted, however, that if panic disorder were, in fact, associated with episodic explosive activation of the CRF neuron and the pituitary–adrenal axis, such patients may already be showing some suppression in pituitary–adrenal function because of the possible long-term negative feedback effects of a sporadic outpouring of glucocorticoids upon the HPA axis. Hence, if dexamethasone were administered sufficiently close to a panic attack, one could expect normal postdexamethasone cortisol levels. Also, these feedback effects may be cumulative in patients having more frequent panic attacks, when the HPA axis does not have sufficient time to reopen completely.

A second experimental observation calling into question the possibility of CRF activation in panic disorder are data showing that lactate-induced panic is not associated with evidence of HPA axis activation. Although this information has been cited as powerful evidence against the involvement of CRF in panic disorder, the following data should be taken into account in interpreting the lactate data: 1) Sodium lactate infusions represent a significant osmotic and volume load, which could lead to secondary changes that could affect the pituitary corticotroph cell. For instance, a volume load of the magnitude of a lactate infusion would clearly lead to release of atrial natriuretic factor, which has been shown to inhibit significantly the response of the pituitary corticotroph cell to CRF and vasopressin. In this instance, activation of the CRF neuron by lactate would not be associated with HPA axis activation, leading to an even further enhancement of CRF release, which could proceed without the ordinary restraining influence of glucocorticoid negative feedback. 2) The activating effects of CRF on the central nervous system may occur via either hypothalamic CRF, which conveys this peptide to such key areas as the arcuate nucleus and the locus ceruleus, or extrahypothalamic CRF located in disparate areas such as the limbic system and cerebral cortex. Recent data suggest that there is an inverse correlation between pituitary–adrenal function and the secretion of CRF into the CSF. This suggests that hypothalamic CRF is not the source for CRF in the CSF, which some hypothesize is the relevant communication pathway for mediating putative CRF effects on behavioral and physiological responses associated with the stress response. In this regard, activation of the extrahypothalamic CRF system would not only occur without apparent activation of the hypothalamic CRF neuron but also, in fact, would be facilitated by low tonic pituitary–adrenal function. Moreover, such an activation of the extrahypothalamic CRF system could conceivably occur without evidence of HPA activation.

In summary, we have presented an overview of the HPA axis in panic disorder, including the continuing inability to clarify the level of activation of the axis despite circumstantial evidence suggesting that the stress response is integrally involved in the pathogenesis of anxiety states. In an attempt to understand this discrepancy, we have presented several lines of evidence suggesting a possible role for CRF in the panic disorder syndrome. Such a role has by no means been demonstrated and is indeed challenged by several lines of contradictory data. Therefore critical evaluation of this hypothesis must await further basic research on the role of hypothalamic and extrahypothalamic CRF in stress-mediated phenomena and on their interrelationships. Moreover, additional clinical research will be required to delineate further the landscape of HPA function in patients with panic disorder both during and between acute panic episodes; it is hoped that such investigations will result in further elucidation of the presumed complex interplay that results in the development and maintenance of this intriguing disorder.

REFERENCES

Bloom FE, Battenberg EL, Rivier J, Vale W (1982): Corticotropin releasing factor (CRF): Immunoreactive neurons and fiber in rat hypothalamus. Regul Peptides 4:43–48.

Breier A, Charney DS, Henninger GR (1987): The diagnostic validity of anxiety disorders and their relationship to depressive illness. Am J Psychiatry 142:787–797.

Britton DR, Koob GF, Rivier J (1982): Intraventricular corticotropin releasing factor enhances behavioral effects of novelty. Life Sci 31:363–367.

Brown MR, Fisher LA, Speiss J, Rivier C, Vale W (1982): Corticotropin releasing factor: Actions on the sympathetic nervous system and metabolism. Endocrinology 111:928–931.

Calogero AE, Galluci WT, Chrousos GP, Kling MA, Gold PW (1987): Interactions between GABAergic neurotransmission and rat hypothalamic corticotropin-releasing hormone secretion in vitro. Brain Res (in press).

Calogero AE, Gallucci WT, Chrousos GP, Gold PW (1988): Catecholamine effects upon rat hypothalamic corticotropin-releasing hormone secretion in vitro. J Clin Invest 82:839–846.

Carroll BJ, Curtis GC, Mendels J (1976): Neuroendocrine regulation in depression. Arch Gen Psychiatry 33:1039–1058.

Charney DS, Woods SW, Goodman WK, Heninger GR (1987): Neurobiological mechanisms of panic anxiety: Biochemical and behavioral correlates of yohimbine-induced panic attacks. Am J Psychiatry 144:1030–1036.

Cowley DS, Dager SR, Dunner DL (1987): Lactate infusions in major depression without panic attacks. J Psychiatr Res 21:243–248.

Dodd J, Kelly JS (1978): Is somatostatin an excitatory transmitter in the hippocampus? Nature 273:674–675.

Faludi G, Kasko M, Perenyi A, Arato M, Frecska E (1986): The dexamethasone suppression test in panic disorder and major depressive episodes. Biol Psychiatry 21:1008–1014.

Furatani M, Morimoto Y, Shibahara S, Noda M, Takahasho H, Hirose T, Asai M, Inayama S, Hayashida H, Miyata T, Numa S (1983): Cloning and sequence analysis of cDNA for ovine corticotropin-releasing factor precursor. Nature 301:537–540.

Gerner GH, Gwirtsman HE (1981): Abnormalities of dexamethasone suppression test and urinary MHPG in anorexia nervosa. Am J Psychiatry 138:650–653.

Gold PW, Chrousos GP, Kellner CH, Post R, Roy A, Augerinos P, Schulte H, Oldfield EH, Loriaux DL (1984): Overview: Psychiatric implications of basic and clinical studies with corticotropin releasing factor. Am J Psychiatry 141:619–627.

Gold PW, Loriaux DL, Roy A, Calabrese JR, Kellner CH, Nieman LK, Post RM, Pickar D, Gallucci WT, Avgerinos PC, Paul S, Oldfield EH, Cutler GB, Chrousos GP (1986): Responses to corticotropin releasing hormone in the hypercortisolism of depression and Cushing's disease: Pathophysiologic and diagnostic implications. N Engl J Med 314:1329–1335.

Goldstein S, Halbreich U, Asnis G, Endicott J, Alvir J (1987): The hypothalamic–pituitary–adrenal system in panic disorder. Am J Psychiatry 144:1320–1323.

Grunhaus L, Flegel P, Haskett RF, Greden JF (1987): Serial dexamethasone suppression tests in simultaneous panic and depressive disorders. Biol Psychiatry 22:332–338.

Guillemin R, Vargo T, Rossier J, Minick S, Ling N, Rivier C, Vale W, Bloom F (1977): Beta-endorphin and adrenocorticotropin are secreted concomitantly by the pituitary gland. Science 197:1367–1368.

Harris GW (1948): Neural control of the pituitary gland. Physiol Rev 28:134–179.

Henry JL (1977): Substance P and pain: A possible relation in afferent transmission. In von Euler US, Pernow B (eds): "Substance P." New York: Raven Press, pp 231–240.

Iason AH (1946): "The Thyroid Gland in Medical History." New York: Froben Press.

Insel TR, Kalin WH, Guttmacher, Cohen RM, Murphy DL (1982): The dexamethasone suppression test in obsessive–compulsive disorder. Psychiatry Res 6:153–160.

Jenike MA, Baer L, Brotman A, Goff DC, Minichiello WE, Regan NJ (1987): Obsessive-compulsive disorder, depression, and the dexamethasone suppression test. J Clin Psychopharmacol 7(3):182–184.

Judd FK, Norman TR, Burrows GD, McIntyre IM (1987): The dexamethasone suppression test in panic disorder. Pharmacopsychiatry 20:99–101.

Kling MA, Kellner CH, Post RM, Cowdry RW, Gardner D, Coppola R, Putnam F, Gold PW (1987): Neuroendocrine effects of limbic activation by electrical, spontaneous and pharmacological modes: relevance to the pathophysiology of affective dysregulation in psychiatric disorders. Prog Neuropsychopharmacol Biol Psychiatry 11:459–481.

Lieberman JA, Brenner R, Lesser M, Coccaro E, Borenstein M, Kane JM (1983): Dexamethasone suppression tests in patients with panic disorder. Am J Psychiatry 140:917–919.

Liebowitz MR, Gorman JM, Fyer A, Dillon D, Levitt M, Klein DF (1986): Possible mechanisms for lactate induction of panic. Am J Psychiatry 140:917–919.

Lieutaud J (1742): "Essais Anatomiques, Contenant L'Histoire Exact de Toutes les Parties qui Composent le Corps de L'Homme, Avec la Manier de Dissequer." Paris: Huart.

Luger A, Deuster PA, Kyle SB, Gallucci WT, Montgomery LC, Gold PW, Loriaux DL, Chrousos GP (1987): Acute hypothalamic–pituitary–adrenal responses to stress of treadmill exercise: Physiologic adaptations to physical training. N Engl J Med 316:1309–1315.

Mains R, Eipper E, Ling N (1977): Common precursors to corticotropin and endorphins. Proc Natl Acad Sci USA 74:3014–3018.

Medvei VC (1984): "A History of Endocrinology." Boston: MTP Press.

Olschowka JA, O'Donhue TL, Mueller GP (1982): The distribution of corticotropin releasing factor-like immunoreactive neurons in rat brain. Neuroendocrinology 35:305–308.

Peterson GA, Ballenger JC, Cox DP, Hucek A, Lydiard RB, Laraia MT, Trockman C (1985): The dexamethasone suppression test in agoraphobia. J Clin Psychopharmacol 5:100–102.

Post RM, Ballenger JC, Uhde TW (1981): Kindling and drug sensitization: Implications for the progressive development of psychopathology and treatment with CBZ. In Sandler M (ed): "The Psychopharmacology of the Anticonvulsants." Oxford: Oxford University Press.

Redmond DE (1977): Alterations in the function of the nucleus locus coeruleus: A possible model for studies of anxiety. In Hanin I, Usdin E (eds): "Animal Models in Psychiatry and Neurology." Oxford: Pergamon Press.

Rivier J, Speiss J, Vale W (1983): Characterization of rat hypothalamic corticotropin releasing factor. Proc Natl Acad Sci USA 80:4851–4855.

Roy A, Pickar D, Paul S, Doran A, Chrousos GP, Gold PW (1987): CSF corticotropin-releasing hormone in depressed patients and normal control subjects. Am J Psychiatry 144:641–645.

Roy-Byrne PP, Uhde TW, Post RM, Gallucci W, Chrousos GP, Gold PW (1986): The corticotropin-releasing hormone stimulation test in patients with panic disorder. Am J Psychiatry 143:896–899.

Sachar EJ, Hellman L, Fukushima DK, Gallagher TF (1970): Cortisol production in depressive illness: A clinical and biochemical classification. Arch Gen Psychiatry 23:289–298.

Saffran M, Schally AV, Bentey BG (1955): Stimulation of the release of corticotropin from the adenohypophysis by a neurohypophyseal factor. Endocrinology 57:439–444.

Schally AV, Chang RC, Arimura A (1981): High molecular weight peptide with corticotropin-releasing factor activity from porcine hypothalami. Proc Natl Acad Sci USA 78:5197–5201.

Scharrer E, Scharrer B (1940): Secretory cells within the hypothalamus. Res Public Assoc Nervous Mental Dis 20:170–194.

Schulte HM, Chrousos GP, Gold PW, Booth JD, Oldfield EH, Cutler GB, Loriaux DL (1985): Continuous administration of synthetic ovine corticotropin-releasing factor in man: Physiological and pathophysiological implications. Clin Invest 75:1781–1785.

Schweizer EE, Swenson CM, Winokur A, Rickels K, Maislin G (1986): The dexamethasone suppression test in generalized anxiety disorder. Br J Psychiatry 149:320–322.

Sharkey J, Appel NM, DeSouza EB (1989): Alterations in local cerebral glucose utilization following central administration of corticotropin-releasing factor in rats. Synapse 4:80–87.

Sheehan DV, Claycomb JB, Surnam OS, Baer L, Coleman J, Gelles L (1983): Panic attacks and the dexamethasone suppression test. Am J Psychiatry 140:1063–1064.

Shibahara S, Morimoto Y, Furatani Y, Notake M, Takahashi H, Shimizu S, Horikawa S, Numa S (1983): Isolation and sequence analysis of the human corticotropin-releasing factor precursor gene. Embro J 2:775–779, 1983.

Sirinathsinghji DJS, Rees LH, Rivier J, Vale W (1983): Corticotropin releasing factor is a potent inhibitor of sexual receptivity in the female rat. Nature 305:232–235.

Stokes PE (1973): Adrenocortical activation in alcoholics during chronic drinking. Ann NY Acad Sci 215:77–81.

Sutton RE, Koob GF, Le Moal M, Rivier J, Vale W (1982): Corticotropin releasing factor produces behavioral activation in rats. Nature 297:331–333.

Vale W, Spiess J, Rivier C, Rivier J (1981): Characterization of a 41-residue ovine hypothalamic peptide that stimulates secretion of corticotropin and beta-endorphin. Science 213:5197–5201.

Valentino RJ, Foote SL, Aston-Jones G (1986): Corticotropin releasing factor activates noradrenergic neurons of the locus coeruleus. Brain Res 270:363–367.

Weiss SRB, Post RM, Gold PW, Chrousos G, Sullivan TL, Walker D, Pert A (1986): CRF-induced seizures and behavior: Interaction with amygdala kindling. Brain Res 372:345–351.

Weissman MM, Merikangas KR (1986): The epidemiology of anxiety and panic disorders: An update. J Clin Psychiatry 47[suppl]:11–17.

Zuingerus T (1669): "Commentarii Hippocratis." Basileae: Episcorium Opera.

Color Figure Section

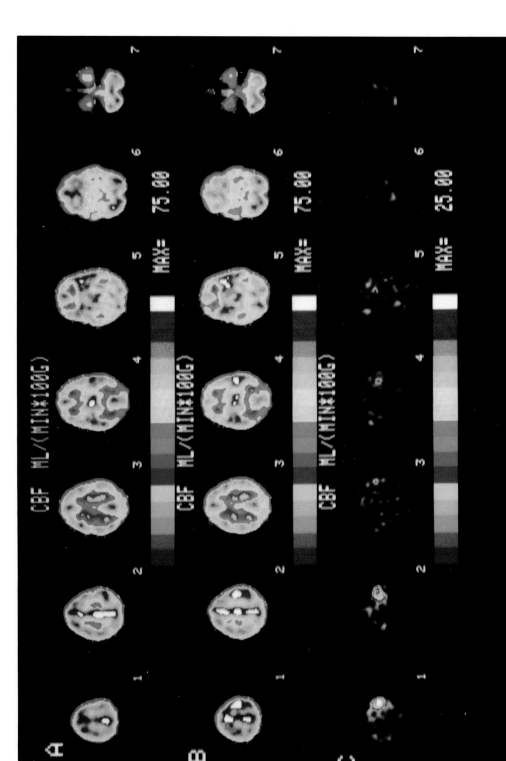

CBF ML/(MIN*100G)

MAX= 75.00

MAX= 75.00

MAX= 25.00

IMAGE C = B - A

15

PET, Panic Disorder, and Normal Anticipatory Anxiety

ERIC M. REIMAN, MD

Pages 245–270

Fig. 15–4. Application of image subtraction to functional brain mapping. Row A is a seven-slice image of cerebral blood flow (CBF), which was obtained in a normal volunteer who was resting quietly with eyes closed and with minimal sensory stimulation. Row B is a CBF image from the same volunteer, which was obtained in the identical head position during left hand vibration. Row C is a "subtraction image," derived from the pixel-by-pixel subtraction of image A from image B. The subtraction image indicates the regional increases in CBF due to left hand vibration. The white area in slice 1 of this row indicates a large CBF increase in a region of right somatosensorycortex (as determined by our stereotactic method of anatomical localization). Each row of color-coded slices corresponds to the scale below it. In each row, the horizontal slices proceed from higher to lower sections of the brain. In each slice, the subject's left is to the reader's left, and anterior is at 12 o'clock. Image subtraction improves our ability to detect and localize functionally activated brain regions. Unfortunately, more subtle state-dependent changes in CBF may be difficult to distinguish from noise in an individual subtraction image. (Reproduced courtesy of Peter Fox.)

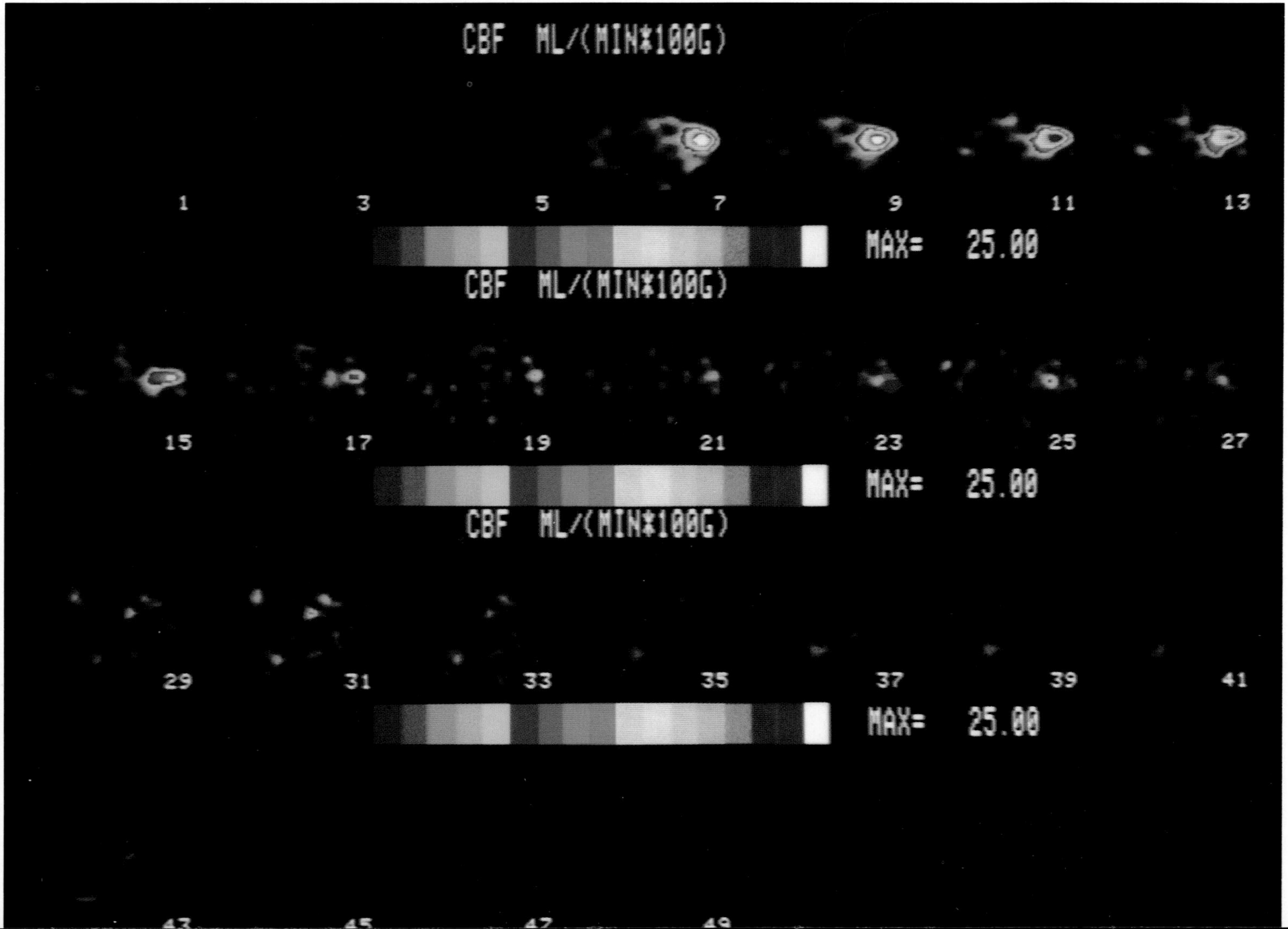
CBF ML/(MIN*100G)
1
3
5
7
9
11
13
MAX= 25.00
CBF ML/(MIN*100G)
15
17
19
21
23
25
27
MAX= 25.00
CBF ML/(MIN*100G)
29
31
33
35
37
39
41
MAX= 25.00
43
45
47
49

Fig. 15–5. Transformation of a subtraction image into standard spatial coordinates. Figure shows every other slice of a 49-slice subtraction image, corresponding to coordinates from an atlas of the brain (Talairach and Szilka, 1967), and representing the regional increase in CBF induced by left hand vibration. This image was derived from the subtraction image in Figure 15–4, row C, but depicts only CBF increases. The maximal change in CBF was localized to right somatosensory cortex utilizing an automated search routine; this maximal change is located in slice 10. Once transformed into the standard spatial coordinates, the data from each subject can be averaged. Image averaging reduces noise and improves our ability to detect small changes in regional blood flow. This strategy was employed to identify neuroanatomical correlates of lactate-induced panic and normal anticipatory anxiety.

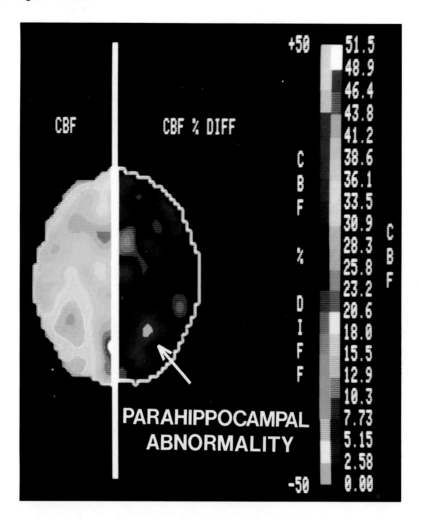

Fig. 15–6.   Illustration of the abnormal parahippocampal asymmetry in a patient with panic disorder who was vulnerable to a lactate-induced anxiety attack. This is a horizontal PET slice obtained in the nonpanic state prior to lactate infusion. The patient's left is to the reader's left and anterior is at 12 o'clock. The left side of the image is a color-coded map of cerebral blood flow (ml/min per 100g). The right side of the image is a color-coded map of the percent difference in blood flow between homologous regions on the left and right sides. Areas with no difference appear black. Areas of increase on the right appear red to white. Areas of decrease on the right appear green and blue. The arrow points to a bright yellow area, which corresponds to the abnormal parahippocampal region. The abnormal asymmetry was identified in the resting, nonpanic state and was demonstrated independent of the visual inspection of the image. Other asymmetries analyzed in the image varied randomly from subject to subject. The abnormality was identified independent of the visual inspection of the image. (Reprinted by permission from *Nature*, Volume 310:683–685, © 1984, Macmillan Magazines Limited.)

17

Cerebral Blood Flow in Anxiety and Panic

ROY J. MATHEW, MD, AND WILLIAM H. WILSON, PhD

Pages 281–309

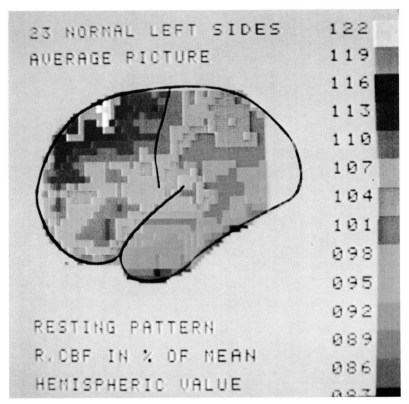

Fig. 17–1.   Normal pattern of regional cerebral blood flow distribution as found with a two-dimensional measurement technique, [133]xenon intracarotid injection.   Courtesy of Dr. N.A. Lassen, Department of Neuromedicine, Rigs Hospitalet, Copenhagen, Denmark.

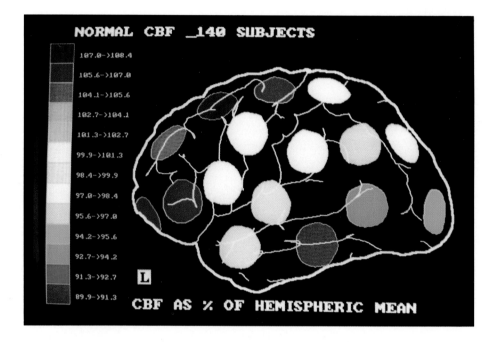

Fig. 17–2.   Normal pattern of regional cerebral blood flow distribution as found with another two-dimensional measurement technique, [133]xenon inhalation.

Biological Discrimination Between Anxiety and Depression

ALAN F. SCHATZBERG, MD, DAVID V. SHEEHAN, MD, AND JAN LERBINGER, BS

McLean Hospital, Harvard University School of Medicine (A.F.S.), Belmont, Massachusetts 02178 (A.F.S., J.L.); Department of Psychiatry, University of South Florida School of Medicine, Tampa, Florida 33612 (D.V.S.)

INTRODUCTION

For many years, investigators and clinicians alike have debated whether patients with depressive disorders could be differentiated from those with anxiety. Earlier attempts at demarcating the two groups of illnesses were aimed at comparing specific symptoms in the two groups (Costello and Comrey, 1967; Derogatis et al., 1972; Roth et al., 1972; Zung, 1971). These approaches produced varying results, in part dependent on populations studied, rating scales used, and the statistical methods applied (McNair and Fisher, 1978). In one major study, Roth and colleagues (1972) reported two major symptom factors that emerged in a large group of hospitalized patients with anxiety or depression. One was highly akin to agoraphobia/panic disorder and the other to endogenous depression. In addition, a variety of symptoms of anxiety and depression did not separate the two disorders, but could be present in either or both. These data suggested that endogenous depression and panic disorder are indeed distinct syndromes. In their major review of this and other attempts to separate the two disorders, McNair and Fisher (1978) came to a similar conclusion, but also noted that data from a variety of studies pointed to a mixed anxiety/depression syndrome that was not easily classified as either an anxiety or a depressive disorder.

Other approaches have explored differences in family history and course. Here, too, a variety of studies point to differences between the disorders (Coryell et al., 1983; Gurney et al., 1972;

Schapira et al., 1972), particularly in anxious patients showing poorer outcomes. However, one recent study pointed to possible common underpinnings in the two, with patients who met criteria for both panic and depression having higher incidences in first-degree relatives of both disorders than did patients with major depression alone (Leckman et al., 1983).

Interest in this area has recently been rekindled with the observations that certain medications with antidepressant properties and that act on catecholamine systems were also extremely effective in decreasing various primary symptoms of anxiety, particularly in preventing panic attacks (Klein and Fink, 1962; Sheehan et al., 1980, 1984; Zitrin et al., 1980). These observations have again suggested that in spite of symptomatic differences, common biochemical processes may underlie both panic and depression. In this report, we review recent studies on the application of biochemical measures to separate anxious and depressed patients, with particular emphasis placed on the hypothalamic–pituitary–adrenal (HPA) axis and catecholamine systems. These studies indicate that the debate on separating these disorders is still alive, although progress has been made in biologically separating a depressive subtype from panic/agoraphobia.

HPA ACTIVITY

Depressive Disorders

In recent years, a great deal of attention has been paid to HPA activity in depression. Early on, various researchers reported that HPA activity was markedly abnormal in depressed patients, with increased 24 hr excretion of

Neurobiology of Panic Disorder, Pages 321–330

urinary corticoids and disruption of the normal HPA diurnal architecture. Subsequently, depressed patients with melancholia were reported to show a marked resistance to suppression of cortisol after dexamethasone administration (Carroll et al., 1982). However, the dexamethasone suppression test (DST) has become a source of much debate, with various studies reporting that DST nonsuppression was also more prevalent in patients with mania, Alzheimer disease, and so forth, than it was in normal control subjects (Arana et al., 1983, 1985). In addition, a variety of disease "nonspecific" factors (e.g., weight loss, dexamethasone metabolism, and so forth) have been reported to affect DST results, bringing the diagnostic significance of nonsuppression into further question. Of particular note is that anxiety has generally not been found to be a major determinant of nonsuppression in depressed patients (Saleem, 1984; Sangal et al., 1984), although not all studies agree (Kocsis et al., 1985). Although the importance of various factors needs to be evaluated further, Arana et al. (1985) in their extensive review argued that the DST could be useful in separating depressed patients in some instances (particularly those with psychosis) from normal control subjects, schizophrenic patients, and those with anxiety disorders, even though other nondepressed patients may also show nonsuppression.

Anxiety Disorders

In the past, interest in HPA activity in anxiety was primarily spurred by observations that stress increases cortisol levels in normal subjects. Such effects have been observed in subjects of all ages, including young children taking school examinations (Tennes and Kreye, 1985). In recent years, increased cortisol levels have been reported in a variety of other populations, e.g., individuals living close to the Three Mile Island nuclear facility, adults about to undergo surgery, and even those in a sailboat for an extended period (Ceulemans et al., 1986; Jeffcoate et al., 1986; Schaeffer and Baum, 1984).

Moreover, in recent years, a number of studies on the effects of corticotropin-releasing factor (CRF) in lower animals have pointed to HPA activity as playing a key role in stress responses. In this regard, several investigators have reported that intracerebroventricular CRF induces stress-like or "anxiety" responses in rats, responses that are blocked by a CRF antagonist and chlordiazepoxide but not by dexamethasone (Britton et al., 1986; Swerdlow et al., 1986). These studies in lower animals have lent further support to studying HPA activity in anxious patients.

However, a review of data on cortisol responses in anxious patients suggests that their HPA activity is not markedly abnormal and appears less pronounced than that seen in depression. For example, our group failed to find significant differences in 24 hr urinary free cortisol in patients with generalized anxiety disorder (GAD) when compared with normal control subjects (Rosenbaum et al., 1983b). Of interest was that the mean 24 hr urinary free cortisol level in patients who also met Research Diagnostic Criteria (RDC) for major depression was higher than that in control subjects. This difference was not statistically significant in part because of the large variance in the major depression subgroup, with only two of the six subjects showing markedly elevated levels.

Another approach has involved studying cortisol responses to lactate infusion in patients with panic disorder. Two major studies on this subject have appeared in the literature (Carr et al., 1986; Liebowitz et al., 1986). Neither demonstrated a marked cortisol increase (over baseline) in response to lactate, even in patients who had frank panic attacks. In one study, panic patients did demonstrate significantly higher cortisol levels (10 min after the lactate infusion) compared with patients who failed to have a panic attack (Liebowitz et al., 1986). In a somewhat related study, Woods and colleagues (1987) reported that phobics exposed to their environmental phobic situations do not demonstrate large cortisol responses, although again a small peak in cortisol over baseline was found at the midpoint of exposure.

In contrast, a number of recent studies suggest increased cortisol activity does occur in panic patients. A recent study by Goldstein and colleagues (1987) on integrated measures of afternoon (1–4 PM) cortisol, which may more accurately reflect 24 hr cortisol production than single measures, reported higher val-

TABLE 19–1.
DST Nonsuppression Rates* in Anxious Patients, Depressed Patients and Normal Controls

References	Panic	Generalized anxiety disorder	Major depressive disorder	Normals
Curtis et al. (1982)	0/13			
Sheehan et al. (1983)	6/51			
Lieberman et al. (1983)	0/10		9/22[b]	
Bueno et al. (1984)	7/15[a]			
Whiteford and Evans (1984)	2/21			
Avery et al. (1985)	5/35	6/26	5/60	
Coryell et al. (1985)	9/50		6/37	1/23
Peterson et al. (1985)	12/97			
Roy-Byrne et al. (1985)	4/15			3/22
Schweizer et al. (1986)		19/79		
Bridges et al. (1986)	2/15			2/8
Faludi et al. (1986)	5/30		17/30[b]	
Goldstein et al. (1987)	3/24		5/38	3/59
Totals	55/376	25/105	42/187	9/112
Percent nonsuppression	15	24	23	8

*$\geq$ 5 μg/dl.
[a]Panic patients with secondary depression.
[b]Includes hospitalized and primarily endogenously depressed patients.

ues in panic patients than in normal control subjects. Moreover, Mellman and Uhde (1986) reported that withdrawal from alprazolam in a group of primarily panic patients was associated with increases in plasma cortisol, and Roy-Byrne and colleagues (1986) found that adrenocorticotropic hormone (ACTH) responses to CRF were blunted in panic patients, a pattern of response reported in depressed patients (Gold et al., 1984). Further studies will be required to reconcile these various results. It is conceivable that some panic patients demonstrate abnormal HPA activity that is missed in certain paradigms that may decrease the signal to noise ratio. For example, panic patients undergoing lactate infusion might show baseline cortisol increases merely caused by intravenous catheterization or anticipating possible discomfort, and such increases could blur the panic-induced surge in cortisol. Also, hemodilution secondary to the infusion could have an effect on cortisol levels, and AM studies might be less useful than PM or evening studies when the cortisol axis is at relative rest. However, at this point in time, the various studies on baseline function and response to lactate challenges, when taken together, do not support a *robust* or *major* HPA abnormality in patients

with anxiety disorders, although recent data do suggest some increase in HPA activity.

Of particular clinical importance has been the observation that patients with agoraphobia/panic demonstrate low rates of DST nonsuppression, suggesting that the DST, which is but one measure of HPA activity, could be useful in separating anxious and depressed patients. We reviewed all reports comparing DST results in patients with agoraphobia/panic, generalized anxiety, depression, or normal control subjects (Table 19–1). Emphasis was placed on 4 PM postdexamethasone cortisol values. As can be seen, patients with panic disorders showed a relatively low rate (15%) of nonsuppression (defined as $\geq$ 5 μg/dl), comparable with, but slightly higher than, that seen in normal control subjects. The DST nonsuppression rate in the five studies that included patients with major depression was 25%, comparable to that reported in patients with generalized anxiety disorder and higher than that seen in panic. Of the five studies that included patients with major depressive disorder, only two included inpatients or patients with endogenous depression (Faludi et al., 1986; Lieberman et al., 1983); one study included symptomatic volunteers (Avery et al.,

TABLE 19–2.
Test Confidence Measures (%) for Separating Depression From Panic

	Sensitivity	Specificity	Positive predictive power	Negative predictive power
5 Studies (N = 336)	23	85	66	47
4 Studies (N = 274)[a]	25	85	66	49
2 Studies (N = 92)[b]	50	88	84	58

[a]Excludes study using symptomatic volunteers.
[b]Excludes symptomatic volunteer and outpatient depressive studies.

1985). The DST nonsuppression rate in the two studies with more severely ill patients was 50%.

We calculated test confidence measures for applying the DST to separate depressed patients from those with panic. As seen in Table 19–2, low sensitivity (23%) was observed in the five studies, but specificity for a positive test result was considerably higher. Positive and negative predictive values were relatively low. Similar values were calculated for four studies, excluding the study on symptomatic volunteers. Sensitivity and positive predictive values were similar. In contrast, in the two studies that included clearly endogenous patients and inpatients, sensitivity and specificity rose to 50% and 88%, respectively. Positive predictive value increased to 84%. These data suggest that panic and depressed patients could be discriminated using the DST if more severely depressed patients were included in the comparison group but that the demarcation between panic and less severely depressed patients using the test is less likely.

CATECHOLAMINE ACTIVITY

Response to Clonidine Challenge

One approach to studying catecholamine activity in patients with either depression or panic has involved responses to challenge with clonidine, an alpha-2-adrenoceptor agonist. Interestingly patients with panic/agoraphobia and depression share some common responses to clonidine challenges while differing on others. For example, both demonstrate blunted growth hormone (GH) responses and greater decreases in cortisol compared with healthy control subjects (Charney and Heninger, 1986; Siever and Uhde, 1984). In contrast, clonidine produced greater decreases in plasma 3-methoxy-4-hydroxyphenylglycol

(MHPG) and blood pressure in panic patients than it did in healthy control subjects (Charney and Heninger, 1986), but produced smaller decreases in plasma MHPG and no change in blood pressure in depressives in comparison to controls. These data suggest some common alpha-2-adrenergic mechanisms in both disorders but also point to major differences in some aspects of adrenergic function, perhaps related to the effect of another neurotransmitter system on adrenergic function. Interestingly, depressed patients showed significantly higher cortisol levels than did controls (Siever and Uhde, 1984), whereas anxious patients showed slightly lower cortisol levels (Charney and Heninger, 1986).

Siever and Uhde (1984) reported a wide variance of responses to clonidine in depression, suggesting possible biological heterogeneity of depressive disorders. Indeed, our group has argued that catecholamine and cortisol measures could help to identify subtypes of unipolar depressions (Schatzberg et al., 1982). These data would suggest that separating anxious and depressed patients could be hindered by the inclusion of multiple subtypes of depressive disorders that might blur clearer differences between specific subtypes of depressive and anxiety disorders.

Catecholamine/HPA Activity

As noted above, the simultaneous determination of HPA and catecholamine activity has become an increasingly common approach to developing biochemical profiles of depressive disorders. The earliest studies in this area revolved around measurement of MHPG and cortisol in depressed patients. MHPG has been measured in various tissues, including plasma and urine. Significant positive correlations between MHPG and cortisol have been reported in severely depressed patients (Jimerson et al., 1983; Rosenbaum et al., 1983a; Stokes et al., 1981). In our hands, these correlations are most robust in endogenous depressed patients (Schatzberg et al., unpublished data). Recently, Stokes and colleagues (1987) and our group (Schatzberg et al., 1987) also reported positive correlations between measures of epinephrine and cortisol in depressed patients.

Another approach has been to explore relationships between platelet monoamine oxidase (MAO) activity and HPA activity. Platelet MAO contains mainly MAO B, which acts primarily on dopamine and serotonin. Several years ago, Agren and Oreland (1982) reported a significant positive correlation between platelet MAO and urinary free cortisol in unipolar depressed patients. Subsequently, we reported a relationship between high platelet MAO activity and dexamethasone nonsuppression in a sample consisting mainly of unipolar patients (Schatzberg et al., 1983a, 1985). This finding has been replicated by others (Georgotas et al., 1986; Hartong et al., 1985), although some investigators have failed to find this relationship in bipolar patients (Maj et al., 1984).

We compared platelet MAO and DST results in a group of panic patients (included in Table 19–1) (Sheehan et al., 1983, 1984) with those of a matched subsample of the depressed patients that we had reported on previously (Schatzberg et al., 1985). Platelet MAO activity and plasma cortisol levels were determined using the same assays. The overall age range in the two samples were matched (age range: 20–61 years panic, and 23–61 years depressed; mean $\pm$ SD age: 38 $\pm$ 11 years panic, and 39 $\pm$ 11 years depressed). The panic group included some patients with depression but in all cases these were secondary to the panic and none of the patients were melancholic. In the depressed comparison group, patients met RDC criteria for the following diagnoses: major depression (unipolar), 31; minor depression, 2; bipolar II, 9; bipolar I, 2; and schizoaffective, 2.

The DST nonsuppression rate using a cut-off of 5 μg/dl in the depressed group was 39% (17 of 46 patients) in contrast to 11% panic patients (5 of 45) (χ^2 = 6.96, P = 0.008). A relationship between high platelet MAO and DST nonsuppression was observed in the depressed group but not in the panic group. Thirteen of

22 depressed patients with high MAO activity failed to suppress in contrast to 4 of 24 low MAO patients (χ^2 = 7.14, P < 0.01). In the panic group, 1 of 18 high MAO patients failed to suppress in contrast to 4 of 27 low MAO patients (χ^2 = 0.23, P = NS).

The two groups were compared using analysis of variance (ANOVA). Cortisol values were log corrected prior to analyses. Covarying for age and sex, depressed patients demonstrated higher platelet MAO and higher 4 PM postdexamethasone cortisol levels than did those with panic (Table 19–3). In addition, total Hamilton Depression Rating Scale (HDRS) scores were higher in depressed patients, as were scores using an endogenous subscale of the HDRS (Thase et al., 1983).

To explore more carefully the effects of hospital status (inpatient vs. outpatient) and degree of endogenous symptoms, ANOVAs were computed comparing the panic patients with depressed outpatients, all major (unipolar) definite endogenous patients, and major (unipolar) definite endogenous outpatients. As indicated in Table 19–3, differences in postdexamethasone cortisol measures between the panic and depressed patients were found only when inpatients were included (i.e., when all depressed and all major (unipolar) definite endogenous groups were the comparison groups). There were no differences when the depressed outpatients or the major (unipolar) definite endogenous depressed outpatients were compared with the panic patients. We also compared 4 PM postdexamethasone cortisol levels in the depressed inpatients, depressed outpatients, panic subjects, and a group of healthy control subjects (Rosenbaum et al., 1984; Schatzberg et al., 1983b). A significant effect for group was observed (F = 4.2, P < 0.01), with inpatient/depressed patients showing the highest values. Posthoc Neuman-Keuls revealed that the mean 4 PM postdexamethasone cortisol level was significantly greater in the inpatient group than in all remaining groups. The remaining groups did not differ from one another. These data again indicate that panic patients and healthy controls do not differ dramatically in their DST responses.

In contrast to cortisol, differences in platelet MAO activity were noted when the major def-

TABLE 19–3.
ANOVA Comparing Depressive (D) Subgroups With Panic (P), Age and Sex Covaried*

Measure	Comparison group	F	P	Comments
Cortisol	All depressed (N = 46)	4.0	0.05	D > P
	Depressed outpatients (N = 28)	0.79	NS	No difference
	All uni def end (N = 23)	3.6	0.06	D > P
	Uni def end outpatients (N = 13)	1.0	NS	No difference
MAO	All depressed	3.2	0.08	D > P
	Depressed outpatients	0.94	NS	No difference
	All uni def end	5.2	0.03	D > P
	Uni def end outpatients	7.7	0.008	D > P
HDRS	All depressed	12.5	0.001	D > P
	Depressed outpatients	10.6	0.002	D > P
	All uni def end	13.4	0.001	D > P
	Uni def end outpatients	7.7	0.008	D > P
HES	All depressed	35.8	<0.001	D > P
	Depressed outpatients	30.6	<0.001	D > P
	All uni def end	27.6	<0.001	D > P
	Uni def end outpatients	14.6	<0.001	D > P

*HDRS, Hamilton depression rating scale total score. HES, endogenous subscale score of the HDRS; uni def end, nonbipolar (i.e., unipolar) definite endogenous.

inite endogenous outpatients were compared with the panic subjects. Total HDRS scores and total scores on the Hamilton Endogenous Subscale score (HES) were significantly higher in all depressed vs. panic comparisons. These data suggest that hospital status may play a major role in depressed vs. panic cortisol comparisons. In contrast, degree of endogenous symptoms and unipolar vs. bipolar status appear to exert a greater effect on MAO activity differences in depressed vs. panic comparisons than does hospital status.

We calculated test confidence measures for separating panic patients from depressed inpatients and outpatients. As indicated in Table 19–4, sensitivity values for the DST and high MAO activity were higher for separating depressed inpatients from panic patients than they were for separating outpatients from panic. Sensitivity of combining high platelet MAO and DST results was considerably higher in separating the depressed inpatients from the panic subjects (44%) than was seen for separating the outpatients from the panic subjects (14%). Specificity and positive predictive power were enhanced in both comparisons when combined high MAO and DST-positive results were used. These data support the idea that combining the two measures can provide higher specificity and positive predictive power than that obtained using the DST alone.

DISCUSSION

Data from our group point to HPA and catecholamine measures as separating some depressed patients from those with panic, although some depressed and panic patients are not easily discriminated. Panic patients demonstrate low rates of dexamethasone nonsuppression, although baseline cortisol measures may be elevated in some patients. DST nonsuppression is more common in depressed patients as a whole, although in the previous studies that directly compared panic and depressed patients, DST nonsuppression rates in depressed patients were relatively low (mean rate = 25%). A closer look at our data and those of others points to hospital status exerting significant effects on DST results in depressed patients. In earlier studies, better separation of panic from depression had been reported in studies that included inpatients or endogenously depressed patients, in line with other investigators who have reported higher rates of nonsuppression in recently hospitalized depressed patients than in other depressed groups (Roy-Byrne et al., 1984). Differences in diagnosis, severity, and suicidality may account for these observations, as could the stress of initially coming into a hospital and the subsequent relief of continued hospitalization. In our data, depressed vs. panic cor-

TABLE 19–4.
Test Confidence Measures (%) in Separating Depressed From Agoraphobic/Panic Patients

	Sensitivity	Specificity	Positive predictive power	Negative predictive power
Depressed outpatients vs. panic				
DST (+)	29	89	62	62
High MAO	36	60	38	60
Both	14	98	80	65
Depressed inpatients vs. panic				
DST (+)	50	89	64	82
High MAO	61	60	40	79
Both	44	98	89	81

tisol differences were more closely related to hospital than to endogenous status. Indeed, unipolar endogenous outpatients did not demonstrate higher postdexamethasone cortisol levels than did those with panic. Since the nonsuppression rates in depressed outpatients in this and other studies have been relatively low, it is at best unclear whether unipolar endogenous outpatients and panic patients can be easily separated using the DST, although a positive DST appears to be relatively specific for depression (i.e., sensitivity may be low, specificity may be high).

Previously, Roth and colleagues (1972) had reported that certain endogenous depressive symptoms and panic symptoms appeared to separate panic from depressed patients. Symptoms more common in the depression factor included psychomotor retardation, early morning awakening, diurnal mood variation, and suicidal ideation. In contrast, reactive depressive symptoms appeared to occur in panic patients. Further studies are required to determine if a particular, more severe, form of depression—defined in ways other than meeting specific RDC definite endogenous criteria—can be easily separated from panic or other forms of depression. One approach would be to define those clinical characteristics that appear to aggregate with DST nonsuppression (e.g., weight loss, sleep disturbance, and so forth) and to compare this subtype with panic patients. Another approach may be to use other biological measures, e.g., urinary MHPG, to subtype depressive disorders further and to compare those biological subtypes of anxiety disorders. At any rate, DST data suggest that differences do exist between certain depressed and panic patients, although there are many depressed and panic patients who are not easily separated by the DST alone.

One biochemical explanation of DST nonsuppression in some depressed patients but not in panic patients might rest with cholinergic supersensitivity in some depressed but not panic patients. Rapid eye movement (REM) sleep latency has been reported to be shortened by arecoline (a procholinergic agent) in euthymic depressed patients (Sitaram et al., 1980) and to be shorter in depressed patients than in normal control subjects (Kupfer and Foster, 1972). Moreover, physostigmine has been reported to increase cortisol in healthy controls, to increase dysphoria in healthy controls and depressives, and to increase cerebrospinal fluid MHPG (Davis et al., 1977; Risch et al., 1980). The data suggest that acetylcholine could be a key clue in understanding the biology of some depressed patients and separating them from panic patients (Schatzberg et al., 1982). Moreover, since serotonin affects cortisol and has been implicated in some depressive disorders, it too could prove a useful dimension for comparing the two groups, but a discussion of this neurotransmitter is beyond the scope of this chapter.

Platelet MAO activity did appear to be more closely related to endogenous symptoms than did DST results. In a separate sample of depressed patients, we have reported that platelet MAO activity correlated with severity and specific symptoms and that unipolar endogenous patients demonstrated significantly higher platelet MAO activity than did patients with nonendogenous or probable endogenous depressions (Samson et al., 1986). Platelet MAO activity has also been reported to correlate with severity of anxious symptoms

(Sheehan et al., 1984) and to decrease with behavioral therapy (Mathew et al., 1981). However, Khan et al. (1986) failed to find significant differences when depressed patients, anxious patients, and healthy controls were compared. That study did not control for degree of endogenous symptoms in depressed patients. In our study, platelet MAO was higher in depressed patients (particularly those with unipolar definite endogenous symptoms) than in panic patients. Moreover, it appeared that platelet MAO activity when combined with DST results did enhance specificity and positive predictive power. These data suggest that platelet MAO activity could prove of use in aiding panic vs. depression separation.

Platelet MAO activity has been largely thought to be a trait-dependent marker, although a variety of psychotropic agents can either increase or decrease platelet MAO activity (Huang and Bowden, 1984). Moreover, infusions of catecholamines can also increase platelet MAO activity (Gentil et al., 1976; Zis et al., 1981), and MAO, particularly type A, can be affected by glucocorticoids (Edelstein and Breakefield, 1981). Thus the relationship of elevated platelet MAO activity to DST nonsuppression may reflect the internal milieu of the individual as well as his or her genetic constitution. This issue can only be determined with prospective studies that include follow-up evaluations. At any rate, platelet MAO activity may help to identify those depressive patients who can be separated from panic subjects, although, again, there is some overlap between these two groups.

ACKNOWLEDGMENTS

This work was supported in part by NIMH grants MH15413 and MH38671 and by a grant from the Upjohn Company. The manuscript was prepared by Linda Messier Dent.

REFERENCES

Agren H, Oreland L (1982): Early morning awakening in unipolar depressives with higher levels of platelet MAO activity. Psychiatry Res 7:245–254.

Arana GW, Baldessaini RJ, Ornsteen M (1985): The dexamethasone suppression test for diagnosis and prognosis in psychiatry. Arch Gen Psychiatry 42:1193–1204.

Arana GW, Barreira PJ, Cohen BM, Lipinski JF, Fogelson

D (1983): The dexamethasone suppression test in mania. Am J Psychiatry 140:1521–1523.

Avery DH, Osgood TB, Ishiki DM, Wilson LG, Kenny M, Dunner DL (1985): The DST in psychiatric outpatients with generalized anxiety disorder, panic disorder, or primary affective disorder. Am J Psychiatry 142:844–848.

Bridges M, Yeragani VK, Rainey JM, Pohl R (1986): Dexamethasone suppression test in patients with panic attacks. Biol Psychiatry 21:853–855.

Britton KT, Lee G, Vale W, Rivier J, Koob GF (1986): Corticotropin releasing factor (CRF) receptor antagonist blocks activating and "anxiogenic" actions of CRF in the rat. Brain Res 369:303–306.

Bueno JA, Sabenes F, Gascon J, Gasto C, Salomero M (1984): Dexamethasone suppression test in patients with panic disorder and secondary depression. Arch Gen Psychiatry 41:723–724.

Carr DB, Sheehan DV, Surman DS, Coleman JH, Greenblatt DJ, Heninger GR, Jones KJ, Levine PH, Watkins WD (1986): Neuroendocrine correlates of lactate-induced anxiety and their response to chronic alprazolam therapy. Am J Psychiatry 143:483–494.

Carroll BJ (1982): The dexamethasone suppression test for melancholia. Br J Psychiatry 140:292–304.

Ceulemans DLS, Westenberg HGM, van Praag HM (1986): The effect of stress on the dexamethasone suppression test. Psychiatry Res 14:189–195.

Charney DS, Heninger GR (1986): Abnormal regulation of noradrenergic function in panic disorders. Arch Gen Psychiatry 43:1042–1054.

Coryell W, Noyes R, Clancy J (1983): Panic disorder and primary unipolar depression: A comparison of background and outcome. J Affective Disord 5:311–317.

Coryell W, Noyes R, Clancy J, Crowe R, Chandhry D (1985): Abnormal escape from dexamethasone in agoraphobia with panic attacks. Psychiatry Res 15:301–311.

Costello CG, Comrey AL (1967): Scales for measuring depression and anxiety. J Psychol 66:303–313.

Curtis GC, Cameron OG, Nesse RM (1982): The dexamethasone suppression test in panic disorder and agoraphobia. Am J Psychiatry 139:1043–1046.

Davis KL, Hollister LE, Goodwin FK (1977): Neurotransmitter metabolites in cerebrospinal fluid of man following physostigmine. Life Sci 21:933–936.

Derogatis LR, Klerman GL, Lipman RS (1972): Anxiety states and depressive neuroses. J Nervous Mental Dis 155:392–403.

Edelstein SB, Breakefield XO (1981): Dexamethasone selectively increases monoamine oxidase type A in human skin fibroblasts. Biochem Biophys Res Commun 98:836–843.

Faludi G, Kasko M, Perenyi A, Arato M, Frecska E (1986): The dexamethasone suppression test in panic disorder and major depressive episodes. Biol Psychiatry 21:1008–1014.

Gentil V, McCurdy RL, Alenizos B, Lader MH (1976): The effects of adrenaline injections on human platelet monoamine oxidase and related measures. Psychopharmacology 50:187–192.

Goergotas A, McCue RE, Friedman E, Hapworth WE,

Kim M, Cooper TB, Chang I, Stokes PE (1986): Relationship of platelet MAO activity to characteristics of major depressive illness. Psychiatry Res 19:247–256.

Gold PW, Chrousos G, Kellner C, Post R, Roy A, Augerinos P, Schutte H, Oldfield E, Loriaux DL (1984): Psychiatric implications of basic and clinical studies with corticotropin-releasing factor. Am J Psychiatry 141: 619–627.

Goldstein S, Halbreich U, Asnis G, Endicott J, Alvir J (1987): The hypothalamic-pituitary-adrenal system in panic disorder. Am J Psychiatry 144:1320–1323.

Gurney C, Roth M, Garside RF, Kerr TA, Schapira K (1972): Studies in the classification of affective disorders: The relationship between anxiety states and depressive illnesses—II. Br J Psychiatry 121:162–166.

Hartong EGTM, Goekoop JG, Penning EJM, Van Kampen GMJ (1985): DST results and platelet MAO activity. Br J Psychiatry 147:730–731.

Huang LG, Bowden CL (1984): Platelet monoamine oxidase response to lithium treatment in psychiatric patients. J Clin Psychopharmacol 4:326–331.

Jeffcoate WJ, Lincoln NB, Selby C, Herbert M (1986): Correlation between anxiety and serum prolactin in humans. J Psychosom Res 30:217–222.

Jimerson DC, Insel TR, Reus VI, Kopin IJ (1983): Increased plasma MHPG in dexamethasone-resistant depressed patients. Arch Gen Psychiatry 40:173–176.

Khan A, Lee E, Dager S, Hyde T, Raisys V, Avery D, Dunner D (1986): Platelet MAO-B activity in anxiety and depression. Biol Psychiatry 847–849.

Klein DF, Fink M (1962): Psychiatric reaction patterns to imipramine. Am J Psychiatry 119:432–438.

Kocsis JH, Davis JM, Katz MM, Koslow SH, Stokes PE, Casper R, Redmond DE (1985): Depressive behavior and hyperactive adrenocortical function. Am J Psychiatry 142:1291–1298.

Kupfer DJ, Foster FG (1972): Interval between onset of sleep and rapid-eye movement as an indication of depression. Lancet 2:684–686.

Leckman JF, Weissman MM, Merikangas KR, Pauls PL, Prusoff BA (1983): Panic disorder and depression: Increased risk for depression, alcoholism, panic and phobic disorders in families of depressed probands with panic disorder. Arch Gen Psychiatry 40:1055–1060.

Lieberman JA, Brenner R, Lesser M, Coccaro E, Borenstein M, Kane TM (1983): Dexamethasone suppression tests in patients with panic disorder. Am J Psychiatry 140:917–919.

Liebowitz MR, Gorman JM, Fyer A, Dillon D, Levitt M, Klein DF (1986): Possible mechanisms for lactate's induction of panic. Am J Psychiatry 143:495–502.

Maj M, Ariano MG, Arena F, Kemoli D (1984): Plasma cortisol, catecholamine and cyclic AMP levels, response to dexamethasone suppression test and platelet MAO activity in manic-depressive patients. Neuropsychobiology 11:168–173.

Mathew RJ, Ho BT, Kralik P, Weinman M, Claghorn JL (1981): Anxiety and platelet MAO levels after relaxation training. Am J Psychiatry 138:371–373.

McNair DM, Fisher S (1978): Separating anxiety from depression. In Lipton MA, DiMascio A, Killam KF (eds): "Psychopharmacology: A Generation of Progress." New York: Raven Press, pp 1411–1418.

Mellman TA, Uhde TW (1986): Withdrawal syndrome with gradual tapering of alprazolam. Am J Psychiatry 143:1464–1466.

Peterson GA, Ballenger JC, Cox DP, Hacek A, Lydiard RB, LaRaia MT, Trockman C (1985): The dexamethasone suppression test in agoraphobia. J Clin Psychopharmacol 5:100–101.

Risch SC, Cohen RM, Janowski DS, Kalin NH, Murphy DL (1980): Mood and behavioral effects of physostigmine on humans are accompanied by elevations in plasma β-endorphin and cortisol. Science 209:1545–1546.

Rosenbaum AH, Maruta T, Schatzberg AF, Orsulak PJ, Jiang N-S, Cole JO, Schildkraut JJ (1983a): Toward a biochemical classification of depressive disorders VII: Urinary free cortisol and urinary MHPG in depressions. Am J Psychiatry 140:314–318.

Rosenbaum AH, Schatzberg AF, Jost FA, Cross PD, Wells LA, Jiang N-S, Maruta T (1983b): Urinary free cortisol levels in anxiety. Psychosomatics 24:835–837.

Rosenbaum AH, Schatzberg AF, MacLaughlin RA, Snyder K, Jiang N-S, Ilstrup D, Rothschild AJ, Klineman B (1984): The dexamethasone suppression test in normal control subjects: Comparison of two assays and effect of age. Am J Psychiatry 141:1550–1555.

Roth M, Gurney C, Garside RF, Kerr TA (1972): Studies in the classification of affective disorders: The relationship between anxiety states and depressive illnesses—I. Br J Psychiatry 121:147–161.

Roy-Byrne P, Bierer IM, Uhde TW (1985): The dexamethasone suppression test in panic disorder: Comparison with normal controls. Biol Psychiatry 20: 1237–1240.

Roy-Byrne P, Gwirtsman H, Sternbach H, Gerner RH (1984): Effects of acute hospitalization on the dexamethasone suppression and TRH stimulation test. Biol Psychiatry 19:607–612.

Roy-Byrne P, Uhde TW, Post RM, Gallucci W, Chrousos GP, Gold PW (1986): The corticotropin-releasing hormone stimulation test in patients with panic disorder. Am J Psychiatry 143:896–899.

Saleem PT (1984): Dexamethasone suppression test in depressive illness: Its relation to anxiety symptoms. Br J Psychiatry 144:181–184.

Samson JA, Gudeman JE, Schatzberg AF, Kizuka PP, Orsulak PJ, Cole JO, Schildraut JJ (1986): Toward a biochemical classification of depressive disorders VIII: Platelet MAO activity in subtypes of depression. J Psychiatric Res 19:547–555.

Sangal R, Correa EI, DePaul JR (1984): Depression and anxiety inventories, and the dexamethasone suppression test. Biol Psychiatry 19:1207–1213.

Schaeffer MA, Baum A (1984): Adrenal cortical response to stress at Three Mile Island. Psychosom Med 46:227–237.

Schapira K, Roth M, Kerr TA, Gurney C (1972): The prognosis of affective disorders: The differentiation of anxiety states from depressive illness. Br J Psychiatry 121:175–181.

Schatzberg AF, Orsulak PJ, Rosenbaum AH, Maruta T,

Kruger ER, Cole JO, Schildkraut JJ (1982): Toward a biochemical classification of depressive disorders V: Heterogeneity of unipolar depressions. Am J Psychiatry 139:417–475.

Schatzberg AF, Orsulak PJ, Rothschild AJ, Salomon MS, Lerbinger J, Kizuka PP, Cole JO, Schildkraut JJ (1983a): Platelet MAO activity and the dexamethasone suppression test in depressed patients. Am J Psychiatry 140:1231–1233.

Schatzberg AF, Rothschild AJ, Gerson B, Lerbinger JE, Schildkraut JJ (1985): Toward a biochemical classification of depressive disorders IX: DST results and platelet MAO activity. Br J Psychiatry 146:633–637.

Schatzberg AF, Rothschild AJ, Langlais PJ, Lerbinger JE, Schildkraut JJ, Cole JO (1987): Psychotic and nonpsychotic depressions, II: Relationships among platelet MAO activity, plasma catecholamines, cortisol, and specific symptoms. Psychiatry Res 20:155–164.

Schatzberg AF, Rothschild AJ, Stahl JB, Bond TC, Rosenbaum AH, Lofgren SB, MacLaughlin RA, Sullivan MA, Cole JO (1983b): The dexamethasone suppression test: Identification of subtypes of depression. Am J Psychiatry 140:88–91.

Schweizer EE, Swenson CM, Winokur A, Rickels K, Maislin G (1986): The dexamethasone suppression test in generalized anxiety disorder. Br J Psychiatry 149:320–322.

Sheehan DV, Ballenger J, Jacobson G (1980): The treatment of endogenous anxiety with phobic, hysterical and hypochondriacal symptoms. Arch Gen Psychiatry 37:51–59.

Sheehan DV, Claycomb JB, Surman OS, Baer L, Coleman J, Gelles L (1983): Panic attacks and the dexamethasone suppression test. Am J Psychiatry 140:1063–1064.

Sheehan DV, Coleman JH, Greenblatt DJ, Jones KJ, Levine PH, Orsulak PJ, Peterson M, Schildkraut JJ, Uzogara E, Watkins D (1984): Some biochemical correlates of panic attacks with agoraphobia and their response to a new treatment. J Clin Psychopharmacol 4:66–75.

Siever LJ, Uhde TW (1984): New studies and perspectives on the noradrenergic receptor system in depression: Effects of the α_2-adrenergic agonist clonidine. Biol Psychiatry 19:131–156.

Sitaram N, Nurnberger JI, Gershon ES, Gillin JC (1980): Faster cholinergic REM sleep induction on euthymic patients with primary affective illness. Science 208:200–202.

Stokes PE, Frazer A, Casper R (1981): Unexpected neuroendocrine-transmitter relationships. Psychopharmacol Bull 17:72–75.

Stokes PE, Maas JW, Davis JM, Koslow SH, Casper RC, Stoll PM (1987): Biogenic amine and metabolite levels in depressed patients with high versus normal hypothalamic–pituitary–adrenocortical activity. Am J Psychiatry 144:868–872.

Swerdlow NR, Geyer MA, Vale WW, Koob GF (1986): Corticotropin-releasing factor potentiates acoustic startle in rats: Blockade by chlordiazepoxide. Psychopharmacology 88:147–152.

Tennes K, Kreye M (1985): Children's adrenocortical responses to classroom activities and tests in elementary school. Psychosom Med 47:451–460.

Thase ME, Hersen M, Bellack AS, Himmelhoch JM, Kupfer DJ (1983): Validation of a Hamilton subscale for endogenomorphic depression. J Affective Disord 5:267–278.

Whiteford HA, Evans L (1984): Agoraphobia and the dexamethasone suppression test: Atypical depression? Aust NZ J Psychiatry 18:374–377.

Zis AP, Gold PW, Paul SW, Goodwin FK, Murphy DL (1981): Elevation of human plasma and platelet amine oxidase activity in response to intravenous dopamine. Life Sci 28:371–376.

Zitrin CM, Klein DF, Woerner MG (1980): Treatment of agoraphobia with group exposure in vivo and imipramine. Arch Gen Psychiatry 37:63–72.

Zung WWK (1971): The differentiation of anxiety and depressive disorders: A biometric approach. Psychosomatics 12:380–384.

Immunology and Sleep Abnormalities

20

Anxiety and the Immune System

MARVIN STEIN, MD, AND ROBERT L. TRESTMAN, PhD, MD

Department of Psychiatry, Mount Sinai School of Medicine, City University of New York, New York, New York 10029-6574

INTRODUCTION

The central nervous system (CNS) and immune system are major integrative networks concerned with homeostasis. Converging knowledge from a variety of areas utilizing findings and techniques derived from the neurosciences and immunology provides evidence of reciprocal interactions between the CNS and the immune system. The demonstration that behavioral states and perturbations of the CNS are associated with immune function suggests that alterations in the immune system may be found in patients with anxiety disorders. Many of the neurobiologic manifestations associated with anxiety disorders are known to influence the immune system. There are, however, relatively few studies concerned with immune function and anxiety disorders.

We review CNS and immune system interactions; behavioral influences on immune function, with an emphasis on the effect of stress on the immune system; and the association between depression and immune processes. A consideration of each of these areas may provide a general understanding of the influence of brain and behavior on the immune system and further understanding of the biology of anxiety. It is worth emphasizing that the investigation of the immune system in psychiatric conditions, including anxiety disorders, may be considered from several different frames of reference. Immune function may be relevant in terms of its role in the maintenance of health and the development of physical disease. Stress, depression, and anxiety may be associated with alterations in immunocompetence and may serve as salient factors in the pathogenesis of immune-related conditions such as infections, cancer, and autoimmune disorders. Since lymphocytes and neurons share surface receptors for multiple molecules, including neurotransmitters, peptides, and hormones, it may be that lymphocyte function reflects central neuronal processes, and the lymphocyte may serve as a readily available peripheral model for CNS alterations in psychiatric disorders and in response to stressors. Both of these considerations of immune function in relation to brain and behavior are discussed.

CNS AND IMMUNE SYSTEM INTERACTIONS

Evidence for interactions between the CNS and the immune system is derived from a wide range of studies concerned with the effect of lesions of the hypothalamus and other areas of the brain on immune responses; the presence of receptors on lymphocytes for hormones and neurotransmitters; the influence on hormones, neurotransmitters, and peptides on immune function; neuroanatomic and neurochemical evidence of direct innervation of lymphoid tissue; and the effect of immune responses on the CNS.

Effects of the Hypothalamus on Immunity

Some of the earliest reports linking the central nervous and immune systems utilized the investigation of the effect of destructive lesions of specific areas of the brain on immune function. Systematic investigation of the relationship between the brain and immune function was initiated in a series of studies concerned with the effects of lesions on lethal anaphy-

Neurobiology of Panic Disorder, Pages 333–348
© 1990 Alan R. Liss, Inc.

laxis. Anaphylaxis is a humoral immune response related to severe allergic and asthmatic reactions in humans. In experimental models of anaphylaxis, animals are sensitized to an antigen that induces a specific antibody, usually IgE or IgG, that attaches to cells such as mast cells in the lung. On reexposure to the antigen, an immune reaction between the antigen and tissue-fixed antibody occurs. This reaction results in the release of a variety of chemical mediators from the mast cell that, in guinea pigs and in humans, induce bronchiolar obstruction, resulting in dyspnea, wheezing, asphyxiation, and death.

In 1958, Freedman and Fenichel reported that bilateral midbrain lesions in the guinea pig inhibited anaphylactic death. Following that report, attention was directed primarily to the effect of lesions of the hypothalamus on anaphylaxis. The hypothalamus is involved in the regulation of endocrine and neurotransmitter processes, and both of these systems participate in the modulation of humoral and cell-mediated immunity. Szentivanyi and Filipp (1958) were among the first to study the role of the hypothalamus in anaphylaxis. They demonstrated that lethal anaphylactic shock in the guinea pig and rabbit could be prevented by bilateral focal lesions in the tuberal region of the hypothalamus.

In the initial studies conducted in our laboratory, we found that anterior but not posterior hypothalamic lesions inhibited the development of lethal anaphylaxis in the rat (Luparello et al., 1964). Similarly, we found that there was significant protection against lethal anaphylaxis in guinea pigs with electrolytic lesions in the anterior hypothalamus. Median and posterior hypothalamic lesions had no significant effect on lethal anaphylaxis (Macris et al., 1970). The effect of hypothalamic lesions on anaphylaxis could be explained by both antigen-specific and -nonspecific changes in the immune system, as well as by changes in tissue factors and target organ responsivity (Stein et al., 1981).

Brain lesions have also been shown to have an effect on cell-mediated immunity. In 1970, our laboratory (Macris et al., 1970) reported that anterior hypothalamic lesions in the guinea pig suppressed the delayed cutaneous hypersensitivity response to picryl chloride and to tuberculin. Median and posterior hypothalamic lesions did not alter the response. Our laboratory has also found that hypothalamic lesions in the guinea pig alter in vitro lymphocyte functions (Keller et al., 1980). Animals with hypothalamic lesions had significantly smaller cutaneous tuberculin reactions than nonoperated or sham-operated controls. Anterior hypothalamic lesions suppressed in vitro lymphocyte stimulation by the antigen purified protein derivative (PPD) and by the mitogen phytohemagglutinin (PHA) in whole blood cultures, demonstrating that the hypothalamus can directly influence lymphocyte function.

Cross and coworkers (1980, 1982) have demonstrated short-term effects of brain lesions on cell-mediated immune function in the rat. Animals with bilateral anterior hypothalamic lesions had lower spleen and lymphocyte numbers than controls 4 days following the placement of lesions, but did not differ from controls at 14 days following the procedure. The response of spleen cells to the mitogen conconavalin A (Con A) was suppressed 4 days after hypothalamic lesioning but not at 7 or 14 days after lesion placement. In contrast, lesions in the amygdaloid complex or hippocampus were found to increase mitogen responses. Roszman and coworkers (1982), in an effort to explain the immunologic mechanisms by which brain lesions alter immunity, investigated the role of splenic macrophage suppressor function following anterior hypothalamic lesions. Although no increase in the number of splenic macrophages occurred following the placement of lesions, macrophages from anterior hypothalamic-lesioned animals had more suppressor activity than those from control rats. It thus appears that anterior hypothalamic lesions may produce functional changes in macrophages and thereby influence lymphocyte function.

Anterior hypothalamic lesions in rats also result in decreased splenic natural killer (NK) activity, which returns to normal activity by 14 days following lesion placement (Cross et al., 1984). The effect of hypothalamic lesions on NK activity was not related to cytotoxic macrophages, and the altered NK function was not due to macrophage suppression. Different mechanisms therefore appear to be involved in the effect of CNS perturbations on various aspects of the immune system.

Neuroendocrine and Neurotransmitter Regulation

The hypothalamus is at the interface between the brain and a range of critical regulatory peripheral mechanisms that may alter the immune response. It is rich in neurotransmitters and neurohormones and is involved in the integration of endocrine secretion, autonomic processes, and behavior. A number of studies have examined some of the mechanisms whereby the hypothalamus may alter immune and, in particular, lymphocyte activity. There is considerable evidence that changes in endocrine activity may be related, at least in part, to the effect of hypothalamic lesions on immune function (Stein et al., 1981).

In an effort to determine whether neuroimmunomodulation is mediated solely by the neuroendocrine system, Cross and colleagues (1982) investigated lymphocyte function in brain-lesioned animals prior to and following hypophysectomy. The suppression of splenic mitogenic lymphocyte stimulation in anterior hypothalamic-lesioned rats was abolished by hypophysectomy, as was the increase in splenic cell reactivity following hippocampal and amygdaloid lesions. However, hypophysectomy did not alter the suppression of thymocyte mitogenic responses following hypothalamic lesions. It is of note that hypophysectomy decreased NK activity in both intact and hypothalamic-lesioned animals (Cross et al., 1984). Taken together, these findings suggest that some alterations in immunity following lesions of the brain involve an intact endocrine system and that multiple mechanisms appear to be involved in the CNS modulation of immune function.

There is considerable experimental evidence in support of the concept that neurotransmitters are involved in the modulation of immune function (Hall and Goldstein, 1985). The demonstration of receptors for neurotransmitters on surface membranes of lymphocytes (Hohlfield et al., 1984; Singh and Fudenberg, 1986; Williams et al., 1976) are in keeping with the possibility that neurotransmitters play a major role in the regulation of immunity. It has been shown that pharmacologic manipulation of norepinephrine in postganglionic sympathetic nerve fibers innervating lymphoid tissue results in alterations in immune function (Felten et al., 1985). It has also been demonstrated that serotonin has enhancing and inhibitory effects on immunity (Jackson et al., 1984).

Most of the research concerned with neurotransmitter regulation of immune function has involved peripheral or systemic manipulation of lymphoid tissues and has not investigated the effect of central neurotransmitter processes on immune reactivity. Recently, Cross and colleagues (1986) showed that humoral immune responsiveness is impaired by the injection of 6-hydroxydopamine (6-OHDA) into the cisterna magna. 6-OHDA significantly reduced norepinephrine in the hypothalamaus, midbrain, and pons medulla. The treatment with 6-OHDA decreased the primary antibody response to sheep red blood cells and also impaired the development of immunological memory. If 6-OHDA was administered prior to immunization, it did not have an effect on the antibody response. These findings suggest that norepinephrine may play a role in the modulation of the afferent limb of the immune response and provide further evidence for CNS influences on immune function.

Direct Noradrenergic Innervation of Lymphoid Tissue

Considerable evidence has accumulated demonstrating direct autonomic innervation of parenchymal lymphoid tissue in the spleen, lymph nodes, thymus, appendix, and bone marrow (Bulloch and Pomerantz, 1984; Felten et al., 1985; Livnat et al., 1987). Noradrenergic fibers innervate both the vasculature and parenchyma in lymphoid organs. This structural link between the nervous and immune systems provides another possible route for the neuromodulation of immunity. The effect may be related to catecholamine neurotransmitters altering blood flow and regulating humoral factors entering lymphoid tissue. Direct interaction on lymphocytes is also possible in view of the availability of noradrenergic and peptide receptors on the cell surface of lymphocytes and could thus have a direct effect on lymphocyte function. Further in vitro and in vivo studies are required to investigate the effects of neurotransmitters on lymphoid tissue; however, the demonstration of direct sympathetic innervation of lymphoid tissue supports the concept of CNS modulation of immunity.

Immune System–CNS Interactions

Recently, a series of observations suggested that the relationship of the CNS and the neuroendocrine system with the immune system is not unidirectional and that immune processes can modulate CNS function and neuroendocrine activity. In 1975, Besedovsky and coworkers found that rats with a primary immune response to sheep red blood cells had increased levels of corticosterone and decreased levels of thyroxine in temporal relationship with the development of the antibody response. These findings suggest that the primary immune response can influence the neuroendocrine system, perhaps by means of effects on the CNS. In further studies, Besedovsky and Sorkin (1977) found an increase in the firing rate of neurons in the ventromedial nucleus of the hypothalamus during the course of an immune response in rats as well as altered hypothalamic noradrenergic activity (Besedovsky et al., 1983) concurrent with the immunization process. Others (Dafny et al., 1985) have shown that alpha-interferon (IFN) applied microiontophoretically into the rat brain increased the firing of neurons of the cortex and hippocampus in a dose-related manner, while in the ventromedial hypothalamus low doses of interferon tended to suppress firing while high doses enhanced the firing rate. In contrast, IFN did not alter the activity of thalamic neurons, and gamma-IFN had no effect on any of the neuronal systems. These results suggest the presence of a feedback loop between specific components of the immune reponse and specific structures in the CNS.

Besedovsky and coworkers (1985) have demonstrated a possible mechanism of immune system–neuroendocrine feedback. They found that mitogen-stimulated lymphocytes produce a factor that increases glucocorticoid levels and have suggested (Besedovsky et al., 1986) that the factor that stimulates corticosterone in rats following the onset of an immune response is interleukin-1 (IL-1). IL-1 is a monokine produced by monocytes and has a role in the regulation of immune, metabolic, and nervous system functions. IL-1 was first described in the 1940s and initially designated as an endogenous pyrogen for its role in the production of fever. IL-1 is derived primarily from activated phagocytic cells but is produced by other cells, including other immunocytes and astrocytes and microglia of the CNA (Dinarello, 1988). It is the principal activator of lymphocytes and in general increases intracellular metabolism. CNS effects of IL-1 stem from its actions on the hypothalamus and pituitary and include fever production, increased slow-wave sleep, and increases in neuropeptides, e.g., endorphins (Besedovsky et al., 1986). It has been demonstrated that IL-1 also increases plasma levels of corticosterone (Berkenbosch et al., 1987; Sapolsky et al., 1987; Bernton et al., 1987) and elevates plasma adrenocorticotropic hormone (ACTH) concentrations. It is not clear, however, if the site of action of IL-1 is in the hypothalamus with the release of CRF or in the pituitary with the release of ACTH. IL-1 produced by cells of the immune system thus may be mediating between the immune, central nervous, and endocrine systems.

Another area of research has suggested that the immune system may also influence neuroendocrine activity by mechanisms not involving the classical hypothalamic–pituitary axis. Blalock and coworkers reported that lymphocytes can secrete an ACTH-like substance following viral infection (Smith et al., 1983). Hypophysectomized mice infected with Newcastle disease virus had increased corticosterone and IFN production. Furthermore, splenic cells from infected animals showed positive immunofluorescence with antibodies to ACTH, suggesting that the lymphocytes were secreting an ACTH-like substance along with the lymphokine IFN. The viral-induced increase in corticosterone but not IFN was blocked by dexamethasone.

It has also recently been shown, utilizing molecular cloning techniques, that mitogen activation of T-helper cells of mice induces the preproenkephalin gene in T cells (Zurawski et al., 1986). The production of a peptide neurotransmitter from activated T cells may provide a means by which T cells may be involved in the modulation of the CNS. Furthermore, the neurohypophyseal peptides oxytocin and neurophysin have been identified in human thymus, providing additional support for the idea of integrated neuroendocrine functions and immune processes (Geenen et al., 1986). These findings, taken together, suggest a regulatory feedback system involving the CNS, the neuroendocrine system, and the immune system.

Many of the neurobiological processes involved in CNS and immune system interactions, which have been reviewed in this section, are known to be associated with anxiety disorders. The possible biological or clinical significance of these relationships is unknown and remains to be determined.

BEHAVIORAL INFLUENCES ON IMMUNE FUNCTION

A range of behavioral influences have been considered in relation to immune function. These include developmental processes, conditioning of immune responses, and the effect of life and experimental stressors on the immune system. Each of these areas of research will be considered as they may relate to further understanding of the psychobiology of anxiety disorders.

Development and the Immune System

Hofer (1981) described many of the ways in which early life events can have subtle yet enduring consequences on the organism. Neonatal experiences may produce persisting patterns of behavior on the one hand and altered CNS cytoarchitecture on the other (Greenough and Schwark, 1986). Density and distribution of cortical and subcortical dendritic and axonal synapses are affected, as is the level of arousal and response tendency to conflict situations (Meaney et al., 1988).

Several studies have begun to consider the ways in which immune alterations may follow neonatal events. For example, Solomon and colleagues (1968) studied the effect of daily handling from birth to weaning in rats and found a persisting enhancement of both primary and secondary humoral immune responses 6 weeks later. The effects of early maternal deprivation on B-cell function in mice has been studied (Michaut et al., 1981) using temporary maternal deprivation during the first weeks of life followed by premature permanent separation at 2 weeks of age. At 8

weeks, prematurely separated and control animals were immunized with sheep red blood cells (SRBC). Specific anti-SRBC antibody and total IgM and IgG titers were significantly lower in the prematurely weaned animals.

Our laboratory has investigated the effects of permanent premature maternal separation on cell-mediated immune processes in the rat (Keller et al., 1983a). Premature separation was associated with a significant decrease in the number of peripheral blood lymphocytes in both male and female rats. PHA stimulation of peripheral blood lymphocytes was also significantly lower in the early separated animals. Consistent with previous studies (Ackerman et al, 1977), prematurely separated animals weighed less than normally weaned controls. Nutritional factors must be considered among the mechanisms that contribute to the effects of premature separation on peripheral blood lymphocytes, since nutritional deprivation has been associated with suppressed mitogen responses (Bistrian et al, 1975). However, a significant effect of weaning on lymphocyte responsivity remained when weight was taken into account in the analysis of the data. Effects of premature maternal separation on the immune system could be related to a generalized defect in the maturation of hypothalamic functions. Ackerman and coworkers (1977; Ackerman, 1981) and Hofer (1980, 1981) demonstrated immature patterns of temperature and sleep regulation as well as altered maturation of adrenergic and cholinergic systems in prematurely weaned rats. The effects of premature separation on the immune system may therefore be mediated by altered hypothalamic function manifested in altered neuroendocrine activity. Premature maternal separation may also affect the immune system by mechanisms similar to those found following exposure to stressful stimuli.

Preliminary evidence for effects of early life deprivation on immune function in primates has also been reported. Laudenslager and coworkers (1982) reported a decrease in PHA- and Con A-induced lymphocyte stimulation in bonnet monkeys during a 2 week period of maternal separation. Lymphocyte activity returned to baseline after mother–infant reunion. In another study, maternal or peer separation in a group of pigtail monkeys during the first year of life was associated with significantly lower mitogen responses in adulthood compared with those of control animals (Laudenslager et al., 1985). It is of note that separation experiences are frequently associated with anxiety disorders and panic attacks (Cowley and Roy-Byrne, 1988).

These studies suggest that developmental experiences, such as maternal separation, may alter some aspects of immune function. It is well known that early experiences in animal models influence the onset, course, and outcome of a variety of tumors and infections (Ader and Friedman, 1965; Levine and Cohen, 1959; Riley, 1981); however, it has not been demonstrated that these various disorders are due to immune alterations.

Conditioning of Immune Processes

An association between CNS and immune processes is further suggested by a series of studies concerned with behavioral conditioning of immune responses. This research is of considerable importance in that it concerns a behavioral effect involving higher cortical function. Studies from Eastern Europe over the past 50 years based on pavlovian concepts have attempted to condition a variety of immune responses with variable results (Ader, 1981). Ader and Cohen (1975) pursued the investigation of conditioning effects on the immune system and demonstrated that antibody responses can be suppresssed by conditioned stimuli that have been paired previously with a pharmacologic immunosuppressant. The paradigm employed used taste aversion learning, a passive avoidance paradigm in which saccharin, the conditioned stimulus (CS), was paired with cyclophosphamide, an immunosuppressive agent (the unconditioned stimulus [US]). Three days after the conditioning procedure, which can be accomplished by a single pairing of the CS and US, the animals were immunized with SRBC and then exposed to the CS, US, or placebo. Six days later, hemagglutinating antibodies to SRBC were measured and were found to be significantly lower in the conditioned animals than in controls, although not as low as in animals injected with cyclophosphamide. These findings have been replicated by Rogers et al. (1976) and by Wayner et al. (1978).

Since the humoral immune response to SRBC involves T-helper cell function, Ader and coworkers undertook a study to determine whether B-cell function is subject to conditioning effects independent of effects on T cells (Cohen et al., 1979). Using the saccharin/cyclophosphamide conditioning paradigm, they found that the antibody response to the T cell-independent antigen TNP-LPS was attenuated by exposure to the CS, although the findings were less consistent than those obtained with SRBC in rats. Since Wayner and associates (1978) found no significant conditioning effect in rats on the response to Brucella, a T cell-independent antigen, further investigation of conditioning effects on the B cell is required.

Two other models of immune responsivity have also been found to be subject to conditioning effects. The graft versus host response, a function of cellular immunity, was found to be lower in conditioned rats than in controls (Bovbjerg et al., 1982). This response was assessed by measuring the size of draining lymph nodes after injection of splenic leukocytes from donor rats. Ader and Cohen (1982) also reported conditioning effects in relation to cyclophosphamide-induced suppression of autoimmune glomerulonephritis in mice, an animal model of systemic lupus erythematosus. Both proteinuria and mortality were significantly reduced by conditioning.

Smith and McDaniel (1983) reported an experiment suggesting that cell-mediated immune responses in humans may be subject to conditioning effects. Subjects were skin tested with tuberculin monthly, with antigen placed on one arm and saline on the other. At the sixth trial, however, the placement of tuberculin and saline was reversed without the knowledge of the subject or of the nurse who applied the antigen. A markedly diminished or absent delayed cutaneous response was found for the tuberculin placed on the arm where saline was expected. When the subjects were then informed of the identity of the test substances and the tuberculin again applied to the "saline" arm, a brisk response comparable to that of the first five trials was obtained. These findings may represent conditioning effects in which the skin testing protocol was the CS and the tuberculin response to the US. Alternatively, as suggested by the investigators, the

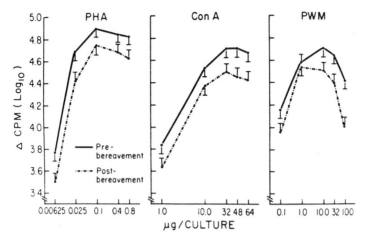

Fig. 20–1. Mitogen-induced lymphocyte stimulation before and after (1–2 months) bereavement. Each point represents group mean ± SEM (n = 15) of each subject's mean log △CPM for each period. (Adapted from Schleifer et al., 1983, *Journal of the American Medical Association* 250:374–377, with permission of the publisher.)

effects may have been related to the subjects' cognitive state of expectation unrelated to conditioning effects per se. Black and associates (1963), for example, reported inhibition of the tuberculin reaction by hypnotic suggestion. According to either hypothesis, the data demonstrate an association between high cortical function and an immune response. While findings of conditioning of various immune responses and measures have been replicated and extended (e.g., Ader et al., 1987; Irwin and Livnat, 1987), the mechanisms mediating these changes are still largely unexplained, and further investigation is required.

Stress and the Immune System

The major neurobiologic processes associated with stress have been observed in anxiety states, and a consideration of the effect of stress on the immune system may provide further understanding of the biology of anxiety. A variety of stressors have been found to alter humoral and cell-mediated immunity in animals and man and have been described in detail elsewhere (Stein et al., 1987). Attention in this chapter will be directed primarily to studies of stress and immune function, which may further our knowledge of the biologic processes that may be involved in anxiety disorders.

Bereavement and Lymphocyte Function

Conjugal bereavement is among the most potentially stressful of commonly occurring life events and has been associated with increased medical mortality (Helsing et al., 1981) and with onset of panic attacks in susceptible individuals (Uhde et al., 1985). A link between bereavement and altered immunity was suggested by the report of Bartrop and coworkers (1977), who found that group of bereaved individuals had decreased lympohcyte function compared with controls.

Our laboratory has investigated the effects of bereavement on immune measures in a prospective longitudinal study of spouses of women with advanced breast carcinoma (Schleifer et al., 1983). Lympohcyte stimulation was meausured in 15 men before and after the deaths of their wives. Lymphocyte stimulation responses to the mitogens PHA, Con A, and pokeweed mitogen (PWM) were significantly lower during the first 2 months following bereavement compared with prebereavement responses (Fig. 20–1). The number of peripheral blood lymphocytes and the percentage and absolute numbers of T and B cells during the prebereavement period were not significantly different from those in the postbereavement period. Follow-up during the remainder of the postbereavement year revealed that lymphocyte stimulation responses had returned to prebereavement levels for the majority but not for all of the subjects. Moreover, prebereavement mitogen responses did not differ from those of age- and sex-matched controls. These findings demonstrate that suppression of mitogen-induced lymphocyte stimulation is a direct consequence of the bereavement event and that a preexisting suppressed immune state does not account for the depressed lymphocyte responses in the bereaved. Furthermore, the long-term stress of the spouse's illness does not appear to result in a habituation of lymphocyte stress responses following bereavement. The long-term stress may in fact have sensitized the subject to the effects of bereavement.

It is important to emphasize that the immune findings associated with bereavement do not adequately explain the epidemiologic findings of increased morbidity and mortality following bereavement. It remains to be determined whether stress-induced immune changes such as decreased mitogen responses are related to the onset or course of physical illness following life stress.

The processes linking the experience of bereavement with effects of lymphocyte activity are complex and require further investigation. Changes in nutrition, activity and exercise levels, sleep, and drug use, which are often found in the widowed, could influence lymphocyte function. Our subjects, however, did not report major or persistent changes in diet or activity levels or in the use of medication, alcohol, tobacco, or other drugs, and no significant changes in weight were noted. Further study is required to determine if subtle changes in these variables are related to the effects of bereavement on lymphocyte function.

The effects of death of spouse on lymphocyte function could result from centrally mediated stress effects. Stressful life experiences may be related to changes in CNS activity associated with psychologic states such as depression and anxiety. Bereaved subjects have been characteristically described as manifesting depressed mood (Clayton et al., 1972; Parkes, 1972), and a subgroup of bereaved individuals has been reported to have symptom patterns consistent with the presence of major depressive disorder (Clayton et al., 1972). The literature also suggests that the widowed have

more anxiety symptoms than married controls (Parks and Brown, 1972; Parkes and Weiss, 1983).

Life Stress and Immune Function

The effects of life stress on various biologic systems and on health vary with the nature and intensity of the stressor, and individual characteristics such as age, sex, and psychologic responses to an event may modulate the impact of the stressful life event. Our laboratory has undertaken a series of studies to consider some of these factors in relation to life stress and the immune system. A broad battery of immune measures were determined for a group of women whose husbands were hospitalized acutely in a cornary care unit (CCU) and for their age- and sex-matched controls studies on the same day. There were no significant differences between the spouses of the hospitalized men and their controls in the number of lymphocytes or lymphocyte subtypes, mitogen responses, or natural killer cell function. The previous investigation of bereavement and immunity studied men who had experienced a relatively homogenous major life stress—death of a spouse following a chronic progressive terminal illness of approximately 3 years duration. The differential immune responses to a stressful life event in the studies of the effect of bereavement or admission to a CCU on the spouse's immune system may be related to the acute or chronic nature of the event. Monjan and Collector (1977) have shown different immune response patterns to an acute or a chronic stressor. The role of sex must also be considered in relation to stressful life events and immune function studies.

The psychologic responses to life stress are often varied, depending on a range of factors, including biologic, personal, and social processes. In the study of female spouses of CCU patients studied within 10 days of their husbands' hospitalization, 24% of the spouses met the criteria for major or minor depressive disorder, 24% had depressed mood states, 24% manifested significant anxiety, and 28% showed no persistent mood disturbance. The sample was not large enough to determine if the immune responses were associated with these diagnostic classifications, and further research is required to clarify the stress-depression and stress-anxiety effects on immunity. Attention should also be directed to the comorbidity of depression and anxiety as well as personality disorders in the investigation of stress, psychiatric disorders, and immune function. It appears that a variety of factors, including the nature and intensity of a stressful life event, the sex of the subject, and the psychologic responses to the event, need to be considered and studied in the investigation of the effect of life events on immunity.

Mediation of Stress Effects on Immune Function

A variety of biologic factors may be involved in mediating the association among the brain, behavioral states, and the immune system. The endocrine system is highly responsive to both life experiences and psychologic state and has a significant although complicated effect on immune processes. The most widely studied hormones are those of the hypothalamic–pituitary–adrenal (HPA) axis. A wide range of stressful experiences is capable of inducing the release of corticosteroids (Rose, 1984), and corticosteroids have extensive and complex effects on the immune system. Of particular interest is the demonstration that glucocorticosteroids can suppress mitogen-induced lymphocyte stimulation (Cupps and Fauci, 1982) and induce a redistribution of T cells and T-helper cells from the circulating pool to the bone marrow (Clayman, 1972; Cupps et al., 1984). Several reports have demonstrated that the recirculating lymphocyte traffic in humans is sensitive to endogenous corticosteroids and varies in relation to endogenous cortisol levels (Abo et al., 1981; Thomson et al., 1980) as does the response to PHA stimulation (Abo et al., 1981; Tavadia et al., 1975).

Secretion of corticosteroids has long been considered to be the mechanism of stress-induced modulation of immunity and related disease processes (Riley, 1981; Selye, 1976). The regulation of immune function in response to stress, however, may not be limited to corticosteroids. In our laboratory it has been shown in rats that unpredictable, unavoidable electric tail shock suppressed immune function, as measured by the number of circulating lymphocytes and PHA stimulation (Keller et

al., 1981). In an effort to determine if the adrenal is required for stress-induced suppression of lymphocyte function in the rat, our laboratory investigated the effect of stressors in adrenalectomized animals (Keller et al., 1983b). Four groups of rats were studied, including nonoperated, adrenalectomized, sham-adrenalectomized, and adrenalectomized animals with a corticosterone pellet. Four behavioral conditions were used: home-cage control, apparatus control, and low-shock and high-shock animals. There was a progressive increase in corticosterone with increasing stress in both of the groups with adrenals, no corticosterone was detected in the adrenalectomized group, and the concentration of corticosterone in the adrenalectomized group that received the corticosterone pellets was constant. A progressive stress-induced lymphopenia was found in the nonoperated and sham-operated groups, but no stress-related changes in lymphocyte number were found in the adrenalectomized groups. Lymphopenia following exposure to stress was described as early as 1937 (Harlow and Selye, 1937) and has been associated with adrenal hypertrophy and involution of the thymus and spleen (Marsh and Rasmussen, 1960). It has been shown that stress-induced leukopenia can be prevented by adrenalectomy in mice (Jensen, 1969). The findings of the study from our laboratory demonstrate that stress-induced lymphopenia in the rat occurs in association with stress-induced secretion of corticosteroids and can be prevented by adrenalectomy.

The stressful conditions suppressed the stimulation of lymphocytes by PHA in the adrenalectomized animals (Fig. 20–2). The stressors similarly suppressed PHA responses in nonoperated animals, in sham-adrenalectomized rats, and in adrenalectomized animals with steroid replacement. These findings demonstrate that stress-related adrenal secretion of corticosteroids and catecholamines is not required for the stress-induced suppression of lymphocyte stimulation by the T-cell mitogen PHA in the rat. It may well be that there is an adrenal-independent stress-induced depletion of functional subpopulations of T cells or a selective redistribution of lymphoid tissues. A variety of other hormonal and neurosecretory systems may be involved in the adrenal-inde-

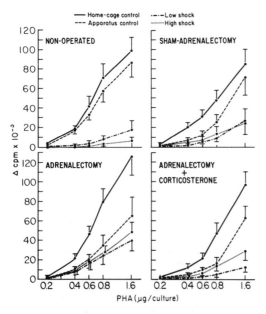

Fig. 20–2. Stimulation of isolated peripheral blood lymphocytes by PHA for each of the four operative groups and four treatment procedures. Means ± SEM are presented as △CPM. (Reproduced from Keller et al., 1983b, with permission of the publisher. Copyright 1983 by the AAAS.)

pendent stress-induced modulation of T-cell function. Because corticosteroids have been reported to have differential effects on T- and B-cell populations (Meyer et al,. 1980; Roess et al., 1982), further studies are required to investigate the role of adrenal hormones in stress effects on B-cell functions.

These findings of adrenal-dependent stress-induced lymphopenia and of adrenal-independent effects on lymphocyte stimulation indicate that stress-induced modulation of immunity is a complex phenomenon involving several, if not multiple, mechanisms. Changes in thyroid hormones, growth hormones, and sex steroids have been associated with exposure to stressors, and all have been reported to modulate immune function (Stein et al., 1981). Further, this laboratory (Keller et al., 1980; Stein et al., 1982), as previously noted, and others (Cross et al., 1982) have shown that the hypothalamus, which plays a central role in neuroendocrine function, modulates both humoral and cell-mediated immunity. These findings suggest that a range of neuroendo-

crine processes may be involved in stress-induced altered immunity.

Since a variety of hormones under pituitary control have been associated with immunoregulatory processes, our research program investigated the role of the pituitary in mediating stress-induced alterations of immunity. Our laboratory studied the effects of a stressor on immune function in hypophysectomized rats (Keller et al., 1988). Three groups of rats were studied, including nonoperated, sham-hypophysectomized, and hypophysectomized. Two treatments, home-cage controls and tail-shocked animals, were similar to those in previous studies. Plasma ACTH and corticosterone were increased in the stressed groups with pituitaries and were below detectable levels in the hypophysectomized animals.

In both the nonoperated and sham-hypophysectomized groups a stress-induced peripheral blood lymphopenia was found, as well as a stress-related decrease in the number of T cells and T-helper cells, but not in the number of T-suppressor cells. The number of B cells was not altered by the stressful condition. No stress-related changes were found in the absolute numbers of lymphocytes or lymphocyte subpopulations in the hypophysectomized animals. These findings indicate that the stress-induced lymphopenia in the rat is selective for T cells and specifically T-helper cells and that stress-induced lymphopenia is pituitary-dependent and associated with increased levels of plasma ACTH and corticosterone, consistent with the observation that the number of circulating immunocompetent cells in response to a stressor is regulated by the HPA axis. The stress-related decrease in lymphocyte numbers from the peripheral blood may be related to vascular margination or migration into the interstitial compartment, the lymphatics, or lymph nodes.

The stressful condition suppressed PHA-induced stimulation of peripheral blood lymphocytes in the hypophysectomized animals as well as in both control groups. These findings demonstrate that factors of other than pituitary origin mediate the stress-induced suppression of peripheral blood lymphocyte proliferation. In addition to the hypothalamic–pituitary axis, the autonomic nervous system is another major stress-activated system, and stress-induced modulation of lymphocyte function may be related to neurotransmitter alterations. Utilizing a stressor similar to that employed in the hypophysectomy study, Weiss and Simson (1986) found marked depletion of norepinephrine in various regions of the rat brain, including the hypothalamus and locus ceruleus. It may well be that the present findings of a pituitary-independent stress-induced suppression of peripheral blood lymphocyte proliferation is related to the involvement of central and peripheral catecholamine systems, which, as previously discussed, have been shown to regulate immune processes.

It is of note that in the study of stress-induced alterations of the immune system in hypophysectomized rats, the magnitude of the stress-induced suppression of lymphocyte function in the hypophysectomized animals was significantly greater than in animals with pituitaries. These findings demonstrate that pituitary processes are involved in countering stress-induced immunosuppressive mechanisms. While the specific pituitary-dependent mitigating or compensating processes are not known, the findings suggest that there is a regulatory network of hormonal and nonhormonal systems involved in the maintenance of immunologic capacity following exposure to stressors. The restraining influence of the pituitary on stress responses may be of relevance to the understanding of homeostatic maintenance of critical body functions.

The findings of a stress-induced pituitary-dependent lymphopenia, of pituitary-independent stress effects on peripheral blood lymphocyte stimulation, and of a pituitary-restraining influence on the stress-induced suppression of peripheral blood lymphocyte proliferation indicate that stress-induced modulation of immunity is complex and involves a range of mechanisms. Interactions between the nervous system and the immune system are extensive and are known to include hormones, catecholamines, monoamines, neuropeptides, and opioids. Each of these systems requires consideration in the elucidation of the processes involved in stress-induced modulation of immunity.

The various neuroendocrine and neurotransmitter interactions that may be involved in mediating stress and immune function have been associated with anxiety and panic disorders. The behavioral and biologic effects of stress, however, are multifaceted, and it would be important and of value to study anxiety and measures of the immune system in clearly defined diagnostic categories of anxiety states and disorders.

DEPRESSION AND IMMUNITY

Depression and immunity have been studied more extensively than anxiety and immunity. It may be useful in the context of this chapter to review the association between depression and immunity, since there appear to be some similar underlying critical neurobiologic processes in depression and anxiety that may influence immunity.

An association between depression and altered immunity has been suggested by a number of studies but has not been consistently demonstrated. Cappel and coworkers (1978) reported that lymphocyte stimulation responses to the mitogen PHA were lower in hospitalized depressed patients during the acute phase of their illness than following clinical remission. Other investigators found decreased lymphocyte responses to mitogens (Kronfol et al., 1983) and decreased circulating lymphocytes (Murphy et al., 1987) in patients with major depressive disorders. Albrecht et al. (1985), however, did not find immune changes in patients with major depression.

This laboratory has conducted a series of studies to determine if depressive disorders are associated with altered immunity. In the initial studies (Schleifer et al., 1984), significantly lower PHA, Con A, and PWM responses were found in 18 drug-free hospitalized depressed patients compared with age- and sex-matched controls. These findings were not confirmed in a sample of 15 ambulatory patients with major depressive disorder who did not differ from controls in mitogen response (Schleifer et al., 1985). These observations suggest that some but not all patients with major depressive disorder may show immune changes. Since the depressed patients in whom decreased lymphocyte responses were found were hospitalized, more severely depressed, older, and predominantly male, these factors may be related to immune changes in depressed patients. Studies with nonde-pressed hospitalized patients suggested that hospitalization itself does not result in altered immunity (Schleifer et al., 1985).

In a recent investigation immune function was studied in 91 drug-free hospitalized and ambulatory patients with major depressive disorder representative of a range of ages, illness severity, and sex (Schleifer et al., 1989). There were no significant mean differences between the depressed patients and age- and sex-matched controls in the number of peripheral blood lymphocytes, T and B lymphocytes, or T4 or T8 cells. Mitogen-induced lymphocyte stimulation responses to PHA, Con A, and PWM for the depressed patients were similar to those of the matched controls, with no significant mean differences between the depressed and control groups. NK cell activity did not differ between the depressed patients and control subjects.

To investigate the contribution of age, sex, severity of depression, and hospitalization status to altered immunity in depressed patients and in controls, multiple regression analyses were undertaken. There were significant age-related differences between the depressed patients and controls in mitogen responses and in the number of T4 lymphocytes. In contrast to age-related increases in mitogen responses and in T4 cells in controls, depressed patients did not show increased lymphocyte responses or T4 numbers with advancing age. Severity of depression and hospitalization status were also significantly associated with immune changes.

Altered immune system measures do not appear to be a specific biologic correlate of major depressive disorder but may occur in subgroups of depressed patients. These recent findings suggest that alterations in the immune system in major depressive disorder may be present in elderly, severely depressed patients, and age and severity of depression should be considered in the investigation of the immune system in depression. The age-related differences between depressed patients and controls, however, must be interpreted with caution because of the small number of patients and controls over 60 years of age in the study. The investigation of specific alterations in the immune system of older and more severely depressed patients and their behavioral and neu-robiologic correlates may provide a biologic basis for the investigation and identification of subtypes of affective disorder.

It is important to note that the measures of the immune system used in the depression studies assess in vitro correlates of immune system activity. It has not been established, however, that the level of mitogen-induced lymphocyte stimulation is related to in vivo immune responses. Altered peripheral blood lymphocyte responses to mitogens may indicate that biologically important systemic events are occurring, and reduced lymphocyte proliferative activity could have a variety of consequences for the organism. Whether these will include changes in the ability to respond to infections or other in vivo challenges affecting the health outcome of elderly severely depressed patients is unknown.

ANXIETY AND THE IMMUNE SYSTEM

As previously noted, there have been relatively few studies investigating anxiety disorders and the immune system. There are, however, several paradigms in humans and animals that may be related to anxiety. For example, Kiecolt-Glaser et al. (1984) and Glaser et al. (1985) have conducted a series of life stress studies with medical students. In a prospective paradigm, they followed medical students for a 6 week period of time spanning examinations. Significant correlations were found between state anxiety and the total number of T lymphocytes, T-helper cells, and T-suppressor cells and the proliferative response to PHA and Con A. These findings occurred during the examination period, with recovery to baseline levels of anxiety and immune measures after the examinations.

Breier et al. (1987) administered 2-deoxy-D-glucose to human subjects to create an acute experimental stress situation of biological significance. This metabolic stressor inhibits intracellular glucose utilization and produces signs and symptoms mimicking certain aspects of a panic attack, e.g., fatigue, diaphoresis, tachycardia, increased cortisol output, and hypersympathetic tone. The findings in a preliminary study revealed a rapid decrease in lymphocyte responsiveness to PHA and Con A (Brier et al., 1987). In another study insulin-induced hypoglycemia was used to achieve a similar biological state in healthy adult men (Melmed et al., 1987). A biphasic response pattern of peripheral lymphocytes to the acute stress was found, with an early increase in numbers of cells followed by a decrease. These studies suggest that experimentally induced states similar to the autonomic arousal seen with panic attacks is associated with measurable changes in immune function and cellular distribution.

Animal models of anxiety have been utilized in the investigation of anxiolytics. Teshima et al. (1987) recently explored the effect of diazepam on the immune response of mice to immobilization stress. They found that diazepam, when administered during the 17 hr period of immobilization stress, blocked a stress-induced decrement of T-cell subsets 24–48 hr later. Further investigation utilizing acute experimental models of anxiety in humans and animals may provide further understanding of immune alterations in anxiety disorders.

SUMMARY

There are relatively few studies of anxiety and the immune system. The demonstration that behavioral states and CNS processes are associated with immune function suggests that there may be a relationship between anxiety and the immune system. Many of the neurobiologic processes associated with stress and with depression have been observed in anxiety and are known to influence the immune system. A review of the immune response to stress and of immune alterations in depression has been presented in an effort to provide further understanding of the biology of anxiety. It appears that a variety of factors such as age; sex; nature, intensity, and chronicity of a stressful life event; and psychologic response to life stress need to be considered in the investigation of behavior and measures of the immune system. The biologic effects of stress on the immune system are multifaceted, including complex neuroendocrine and neurotransmitter interactions. Further investigation is required of anxiety and the immune system in clearly delineated and diagnosed anxiety states and disorders. Such studies may help to elucidate the pathophysiology of anxiety disorders manifested in patterns of dysregulation of neuroendocrine, neurotransmitter, and immune systems and may help to identify risk factors and subtypes of anxiety for the ultimate development of intervention strategies.

REFERENCES

Abo T, Kawate T, Itko K, Kumagai K (1981): Studies on the bioperiodicity of the immune response. I: Circadian rhythms of human T, B, and K cell traffic in the peripheral blood. J Immunol 126:1360–1363.

Ackerman SH (1981): Premature weaning, thermoregulation, and the occurrence of gastric pathology. In Weiner H, Hofer MA, Stunkard AJ (eds): "Brain, Behavior, and Bodily Disease." New York: Raven Press, pp 67–86.

Ackerman SH, Hofer MA, Weiner H (1977): Some effects of a split litter cross foster design applied to 15-day-old pups. Physiol Behav 19:433–436.

Ader R (1981): A historical account of conditioned immunobiologic responses. In Ader R (ed): "Psychoneuroimmunology." New York: Academic press, pp 321–354.

Ader R, Cohen N (1975): Behaviorally conditioned immunosuppression. Psychosom Med 37:333–340.

Ader R, Cohen N (1982): Behaviorally conditioned immunosuppression and murine systemic lupus erythematosus. Science 215:1534–1536.

Ader R, Friedman SB (1965): Differential early experiences and susceptibility to transplanted tumor in the rat. J Comp Physiol Psychol 59:361–364.

Ader R, Grota LJ, Cohen N (1987): Conditioning phenomena and immune function. Ann NY Acad Sci 496:532–544.

Albrecht J, Helderman J, Schlesser M, Rush AJ (1985): A controlled study of cellular immune function in affective disorders before and during somatic therapy. Psychiatry Res 15:185–193.

Bartrop RW, Lazarus L, Luckherst E, Kiloh LG, Penny R (1977): Depressed lymphocyte function after bereavement. Lancet 1:834–836.

Berkenbosch F, VanOers J, delRey A, Tilders F, Besedovsky H (1987): Corticotropin-releasing factor-producing neurons in the rat activated by Interleukin-1. Science 238:524–526.

Bernton EW, Beach JE, Holaday JW, Smallridge RC, Fein HG (1987): Release of multiple hormones by a direct action of interleukin-1 on pituitary cells. Science 238:519–521.

Besedovsky H, del Ray A, Sorkin E, DePrada M, Burri R, Honegger C (1983): The immune response provokes changes in brain noradrenergic neurons. Science 221:564–566.

Besedovsky H, del Rey A, Sorkin E, Dinarello CA (1986): Immunoregulatory feedback between interleukin-1 and glucocorticoid hormones. 233:652–654.

Besedovsky H, del Rey AE, Sorkin E, Lotz W, Schwulera U (1985): Lymphoid cells produce an immunoregulatory glucocorticoid increasing factor (GIF) acting through the pituitary gland. Clin Exp Immunol 59:622–628.

Besedovsky H, Sorkin E (1977): Network of immune–neuroendocrine interactions. Clin Immunol 27:1–12.

Besedovsky H, Sorkin E, Keller M, Muller J (1975): Changes in blood hormone levels during the immune response. Proc Soc Exp Biol Medicine 150:466.

Bistrian BR, Blackburn GL, Serimshaw NS (1975): Cellular immunity in semistarved states in hospitalized adults. Am J Psychiatry 28:1148–1155.

Black S, Humphrey JH, Niven JS (1963): Inhibition of Mantoux reaction by direct suggestion under hypnosis. Bri Med J 1:1649–1652.

Bovbjerg DM, Ader R, Cohen N (1982): Behaviorally conditioned suppression of a graft-versus-host response. Proc Nat Acad Sci USA 79:583–585.

Breier A, Albus M, Pickar D, Zahn TP, Wolkowitz OM, Paul SM (1987): Controllable and uncontrollable stress in humans: Alterations in mood and neuroendocrine and psychosysiological function. Am J Psychiatry 144:1419–1425.

Bulloch K, Pomerantz W (1984): Autonomic nervous system innervation of thymic-related lymphoid tissue in wild-type and nude mice. J Comp Neurol 228:57–68.

Cappel R, Gregoire F, Thiry L, Spreches S (1978): Antibody and cell mediated immunity to herpes simplex virus in psychotic depression. J Clin Psychiatry 39:266–268.

Claman HN (1972): Corticosteroids and lymphoid cells. N Engl J Med 287:388–397.

Clayton PJ, Halikes JA, Maurice WL (1972): The depression of widowhood. Br J Psychiatry 120:71–78.

Cohen N, Ader R, Green N, Bovbjerg D (1979): Conditioned suppression of a thymus independent antibody response. Psychosom Med 41:487–491.

Cowley DS, Roy-Byrne PP (1988): Panic disorder: Psychosocial aspects. Psychiatr Ann 18:464–467.

Cross RJ, Brook WH, Roszman TL, Markesbery WR (1982): Hypothalamic–immune interactions: Effect of hypophysectomy on neuroimmunomodulation. J Neurol Sci 53:557–566.

Cross RJ, Jackson JC, Brooks WH, Roszman TL, Markesbery WR (1986): Neuroimmunomodulation: Impairment of humoral immune responsiveness by 6-hydroxydopamine treatment. Immunology 57:145–152.

Cross RJ, Markesbery WR, Brooks WH, Roszman TL (1980): Hypothalamic–immune interactions: The acute effect of anterior hypothalamic lesions on the immune response. Brain Res 196:79–87.

Cross RJ, Markesbery WR, Brooks WH, Roszman TL (1984): Hypothalamic–immune interactions. Neuromodulation of natural killer activity by lesioning of the anterior hypothalamus. Immunology 51:399–405.

Cupps TR, Edgar LC, Thomas CA, Fauci AS (1984): Multiple mechanisms of B cell immunoregulation in man after administration of in vivo corticosteroids. J Immunol 132:170–175.

Cupps TR, Fauci AS (1982): Corticosteroid-mediated immunoregulation in man. Immunol Rev 65:134–155.

Dafny N, Prieto-Gomez B, Reyes-Vasquez C (1985): Does the immune system communicate with the central nervous system? Interferon modifies central nervous activity. J Neuroimmunol 9:1–12.

Dinarello C (1988): Biology of interleukin 1. FASEB J 2:108–115.

Felten DL, Felten SY, Carlson SL, Olschawka J, Livnat S (1985): Noradrenergic and peptidergic innervation of lymphoid tissue. J Immunol 135s:755s–765s.

Freedman DX, Fenichel G (1958): Effect of midbrain lesion on experimental allergy. Arch Neurol Psychiatry 79:164–169.

Geenen V, Legros JJ, Franchimont P, Baudrihaye M, Defresne MP, Boniver J (1986): The neuroendocrine thymus: Coexistence of oxytocin and neurophysin in the human thymus. Science 232:508–511.

Glaser R, Kiecolt-Glaser JK, Speicher CE, Holiday JE (1985): Stress, loneliness and changes in herpes virus latency. J Behav Med 8:249–260.

Greenough WT, Schwark HD (1986): Age-related aspects of experience: Effects upon brain structure. In Emde RN, Harmon RJ (eds): "Continuities and Discontinuities in Development." New York: Raven Press, pp 69–91.

Hall NR, Goldstein AL (1985): Neurotransmitters and host defense. In Guillemin R, Cohn M, Melnechuk T (eds): "Neural Modulation of Immunity." New York: Raven Press, pp 143–156.

Harlow CM, Selye H (1937): The blood picture in the alarm reaction. Proc Soc Exp Biol Med 104:180.

Helsing KJ, Szklo M, Comstock GW (1981): Factors associated with mortality after widowhood. Am J Public Health 71:802–809.

Hofer MA (1980): Effects of reserpine and amphetamine on the development of hyperactivity in maternally deprived rat pups. Psychosom Med 42:513–520.

Hofer MA (1981): Toward a developmental basis for disease predisposition. In Hofer A, Stunkard J (eds): "Brain, Behavior, and Bodily Disease." New York: Raven Press, pp 209–228.

Hohlfield R, Toyka KV, Heininger K, et al. (1984): Autoimmune T lymphocytes specific for acetylcholine receptors. Nature 310:244.

Irwin J, Livnat S (1987): Behavioral influences on the immune system: Stress and conditioning. Prog Neuropsychopharmacol Biol Psychiatry 11:137–143.

Jackson JC, Cross RJ, Walker RF (1984): Neuroimmunomodulation: Influence of serotonin on the immune response. Immunology 54:505.

Jensen MM (1969): Changes in leukocyte counts associated with various stressors. J Reticuloendothel Soc 6:457–465.

Keller S, Weiss J, Schleifer S, Miller NE and Stein M (1981): Suppression of immunity by stress: effect of a graded series of stressors on lymphocyte stimulation in the rat. Science 213:1397–1400.

Keller SE, Ackerman SH, Schleifer SJ, Shindeldecker RD, Camerino MS, Hofer MA, Weiner H, Stein M (1983a): Effect of premature weaning on lymphocyte stimulation in the rat. Psychosom Med 45:75.

Keller SE, Schleifer SJ, Liotta AS, Bond RN, Farhoody N, Stein M (1988): Stress-induced alterations of immunity in hypophysectomized rats. Proc Nat Acad Sci USA 85:9297–9301.

Keller SE, Stein M, Camerino MS, Schleifer SJ, Sherman J (1980): Suppression of lymphocyte stimulation by anterior hypothalamic lesions in the guinea pig. Cell Immunol 52:334–340.

Keller SE, Weiss JM, Schleifer SJ, Miller NE, Stein M (1983b): Stress-induced suppression of immunity in adrenalectomized rats. Science 221:1301–1304.

Kiecolt-Glaser JK, Garner W, Speicher C, Penn GM, Holliday J, Glaser R (1984): Psychosocial modifiers of immunocompetence in medical students. Psychosom Med 46:7–14.

Kronfol Z, Silva JJR, Greden J, Dembinski S, Gardner R, Carroll B (1983): Impaired lymphocyte function in depressive illness. Life Sci 33:241–247.

Laudenslager ML, Capitanio JP, Reite M (1985): Possible effects of early separation experiences on subsequent immune function in adult macaque monkeys. Am J Psychiatry 142:862–864.

Laudenslager ML, Reite M, Harbeck R (1982): Immune status during mother–infant separation. Psychosom Med 44:303.

Levine S, Cohen C (1959): Differential survival to leukemia as a function of infantile stimulation in DBA/Z mice. Proc Soc Exp Biol Med 102:53–54.

Livnat S, Madden KS, Felten DL, Felten SY (1987): Regulation of the immune system by sympathetic neural mechanisms. Prog Neuropsychopharmacol Biol Psychiatry 11:145–152.

Luparello TJ, Stein M, Park CD (1964): Effect of hypothalamic lesions on rat anaphylaxis. Amer J Physiol 207:911–914.

Macris NT, Schiavi RC, Camerino MS, Stein M (1970): Effect of hypothalamic lesions on immune processes in the guinea pig. Am J Physiol 219:1205–1209.

Marsh JT, Rasmussen AF (1960): Response of adrenal, thymus, spleen, and leukocytes to shuttle box and confinement stress. Proc Soc Exp Biol Med 104:180.

Meaney MJ, Aitken DH, VanBerkel C, Bhatnagar S, Sapolsky RM (1988): Effect of neonatal handling on age-related impairments associated with the hippocampus. Science 239:766–768.

Melmed RN, Roth D, Weinstock-Rosin M, Edelstein EL (1987): The influence of emotional state on the mobilization of marginal pool leukocytes after insulin-induced hypoglycemia. Ann NY Acad Sci 496:467–476.

Meyer EM, Meyer G, Niehaus W, Schlake W, Grundmann E (1980): Divergence of cortisol-induced involution of T and B cell areas in mouse lymph nodes and spleen. A histomorphometrical, enzyme histochemical, and immunohistochemical study. Invest Cell Pathol 3:175–185.

Michaut RJ, Dechambre RP, Doumerc S, Lesourd B, Devillechabrolle A, Moulias R (1981): Influence of early maternal deprivation on adult humoral immune response in mice. Physiol Behav 26:189–191.

Monjan AA, Collector MI (1977): Stress-induced modulation of the immune response. Science 196:307–308.

Murphy D, Gardner R, Greden J, Carroll B (1987): Lymphocyte numbers in endogenous depression. Psychol Med 17:381.

Parkes CM (1972): "Bereavement: Studies of Grief in Adult Life." New York: University Press.

Parkes CM, Brown R (1972): Health after bereavement: A controlled study of young Boston widows and widowers. Psychosom Med 34:449–461.

Parkes CM, Weiss RS (1983): "Recovery From Bereavement." New York: Basic Books.

Riley V (1981): Psychoneuroendocrine influences on immunocompetence and neoplasia. Science 212:1100–1109.

Roess DA, Bellone MF, Ruh MF, Nadel EM, Ruh TS (1982): The effect of glucocorticoids on mitogen-stimulated B-lymphocytes. Thymidine incorporation and Ab secretion. Endocrinology 110:169–175.

Rogers MP, Reich P, Strom TB, and C. Carpenter (1976): Behaviorally conditioned immunosuppression: replication of a recent study. Psychosom Med 38:447–452.

Rose RM (1984): Overview of endocrinology of stress, in Neuroendocrinology and Psychiatric Disorder. Edited by Brown GM, Koslow SH, Reichlin S. New York: Raven Press, pp 95–122.

Roszman TL, Cross RJ, Brooks WJ, Markesberry W (1982): Hypothalamic–immune interactions, II: The effect of hypothalamic lesions on the ability of adherent spleen cells to limit lymphocyte blastogenesis. Immunology 45:737–742.

Sapolsky R, Rivier C, Yamamoto G, Plotsky P, Vale W (1987): Corticotropin-releasing factor-producing neurons in the rat activated by interleukin-1. Science 238:522–524.

Schleifer SJ, Keller SE, Bond RN, Cohen J, Stein M (1989): Major depressive disorder: Role of age, sex, severity, and hospitalization. Arch Gen Psychiatry 46:81–87.

Schleifer SJ, Keller SE, Camerino M, Thornton JC, Stein M (1983): Suppression of lymphocyte stimulation following bereavement. JAMA 250:374–377.

Schleifer SJ, Keller SE, Meyerson AT, Reskin MJ, Davis KL, Stein M (1984): Lymphocyte function in major depressive disorder. Arch Gen Psychiatry 41:484–486.

Schleifer SJ, Keller SE, Siris SG, Davis KL, Stein M (1985): Depression and immunity. Lymphocyte function in ambulatory depressed patients, hospitalized schizophrenic patients, and patients hospitalized for herniorrhaphy. Arch Gen Psychiatry 42:129.

Selye H (1976): Stress in Health and Disease. Boston: Butterworth's.

Singh VK, Fudenberg HH (1986): Can blood immunocytes be used to study neuropsychiatric disorders? J Clin Psychiatry 47:592–595.

Smith EM, Phan M, Kruger TE, Coppenhaver DH, Blalock JE (1983): Human lymphocyte production of immunoreactive thyrotropin. Proc Natl Acad Sci USA 80:6010–6013.

Smith RG, McDaniel SM (1983): Psychologically mediated effect on the delayed hypersensitivity reaction to tuberculin in humans. Psychosom Med 45:65–70.

Solomon GF, Levine S, Kraft JK (1968): Early experience and immunity. Nature 220:821–822.

Stein M, Keller S, Schleifer S (1981): The hypothalamus and the immune response. In Weiner H, Hofer MA, Stunkard AJ (eds): "Brain, Behavior and Bodily Disease." New York: Raven Press, pp 45–65.

Stein M, Schleifer S, Keller S (1982): The role of the brain and neuroendocrine system and immune regulation: Potential links to neoplastic disease. In Levy S (ed): "Biological Mediators of Behavior and Disease." New York: Elsevier/North Holland, pp 147–174.

Stein M, Schleifer SJ, Keller SE (1987): Psychoimmunology in Clinical Psychiatry. In Hales RE, Frances AJ (eds): "Annual Review of Psychiatry: Neuroscience Techniques in Clinical Psychiatry." Washington, DC: American Psychiatric Press, pp 210–234.

Szentivanyi A, Filipp G (1958): Anaphylaxis and the nervous system, Part II. Ann Allergy 16:143–151.

Tavadia HB, Fleming KA, Hume RD, Simpson HW (1975): Circadian rhythmicity of human plasma cortisol and PHA-induced lymphocyte transformation. Clin Exp Immunol 22:190.

Teshima H, Sogawa H, Kihara H, Nagata S, Ago Y, Nakagawa T (1987): Changes in populations of T-cell subsets due to stress. Ann NY Acad Sci 496:459.

Thomson SP, McMahon LJ, Mugent CA (1980): Endogenous cortisol: A regulator of lymphocytes in peripheral blood. Clin Immunol Immunopathol 17:506.

Uhde TW, Boulenger JP, Roy-Byrne PP (1985): Longitudinal course of panic disorder: Clinical and biological considerations. Prog Neuropsychopharmacol Biol Psychiatry 9:39–51.

Wayner EA, Flannery GR, Singer G (1978): The effects of taste aversion conditioning on the primary antibody response to sheep red blood cells and Brucella abortus in the albino rat. Physiol Behav 21:995–1000.

Weiss JM, Simson PG (1986): "Antidepressants and Receptor Function." Chichester: Ciba Foundation Symposium 123, p 191.

Williams LT, Synderman R, Lefkowitz RJ (1976): Identification of β-adrenergic receptors on human lymphocytes by [^{3}H]-alprenolol binding. J Clin Invest 57:149–155.

Zurawski G, Benedik M, Kamb BJ, Abrams JS, Zurawski SM, Lee FD (1986): Activation of mouse T-helper cells induces abundant preproenkephalin mRNA synthesis. Science 232:772–775.

21

Prostaglandins: Relationship to the Central Nervous System and the Platelet in Panic Disorder

RAYMOND F. ANTON, MD

Department of Psychiatry and Behavioral Sciences, Medical University of South Carolina, Charleston, South Carolina 29425

INTRODUCTION

Although prostaglandins (PGs) have been shown to be ubiquitous and to play functional roles in a variety of mammalian tissues, it has only been over the last decade that their presence in brain and cerebrospinal fluid (CSF) has been recognized. Although understanding of their function in nervous tissue is still in evolution (Chiu and Richardson, 1985), hypotheses have been formulated regarding how abnormalities in this system may relate to psychopathologic states (Gross et al., 1977; Horrobin, 1979; Horrobin and Manku, 1980; Ragheb and Ban, 1982; Rotrosen et al., 1980). However, it has been only in the last few years that attention has been paid to the PG system in relationship to panic disorder (Anton et al., 1989; Carr et al., 1986; Sheehan et al., 1984). This chapter reviews the biochemistry and the neurobehavioral function of central nervous system (CNS) PGs, examines how the platelet relates to PG function, and, finally, details what is known about PGs in psychopathologic states, in general, and in panic disorder, in particular.

CNS PGs

PGs are the functional derivatives of the 20 carbon chain fatty acid arachidonic acid, which is present in large amounts in three phospholipid moieties of cellular membranes (phos-phatidylcholine, phosphatidylethanolamine, and phosphatidylinositol). Arachidonic acid is released from these phospholipids by enzymatic cleavage during both receptor-linked and ionically mediated stimulation. After the release of arachidonic acid, an enzymatic cascade initiated either by cyclooxygenase or lipoxygenase leads to the formation of PGs or leukotrienes, respectively. A diagrammatic representation of the synthetic pathway of PG production is provided in Figure 21–1. As can be seen, a variety of PG derivatives can be synthesized depending on the tissue, cell type, and perhaps type of stimulation.

The predominant PG in the brain depends on the species, but in human cerebral cortex the predominant types are $PGF_{2\alpha}$ and PGE_2 (Abdel-Halim et al., 1980b; Wolfe et al., 1976). These subtypes are prominent in neuronal tissue, whereas the CNS blood vascular and platelets (as they do in the periphery) produce mainly prostacyclin (PGI_2) and thromboxane (TXA_2), respectively (Abdel-Halim et al., 1980a). The neuronal production of PGs was confirmed by cell culture techniques. Five distinct neuroblastoma cell lines have been shown to produce predominantly $PGF_{2\alpha}$ and PGE_2 from their exogenously supplied precursor arachidonic acid (Tansik and White, 1979). In man, the predominant PG type measured in the CSF was $PGF_{2\alpha}$ (Latorre et al., 1974; Wolfe and Mamer, 1975) and PGE_2 (Abdel-Halim et al., 1979). Since it is generally accepted that the brain does not possess the capacity to degrade PGs, it is thought that they are actively

Neurobiology of Panic Disorder, Pages 349–363

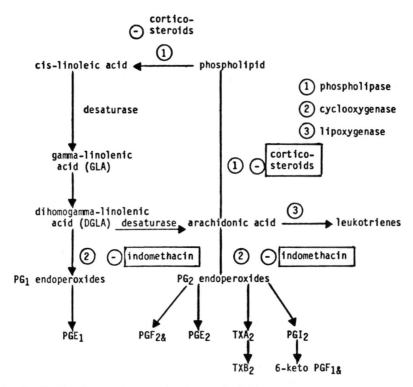

Fig. 21–1. Synthetic scheme of prostaglandins and leukotrienes. Corticosteroids block the release of arachidonic acid from membrane phospholipid stores, and indomethacin and other aspirin-like drugs block cyclooxygenase (PG synthetic enzyme complex).

transported across the blood–brain barrier, and, as animal studies suggest (Bito and Davson, 1974; Bito et al., 1976), this transport may be probenecid-sensitive. The half-life of PGs in plasma is very short, since most of the PGs are degraded in one pass through the lungs. Peripheral PG levels, therefore, are very unlikely to reflect CNS production. It is clear from animal brain studies (Anton et al., 1983) and postcerebrovascular human CSF studies (Fagan et al., 1986) that ischemia and/or anoxia caused a rapid rise in PG production.

Although it is clear that CNS tissue and, in particular, neuronal cells have the capacity to produce PGs, the physiologic significance of this production continues to be studied. The functional role of PGs has been examined in receptor, electrophysiologic, biochemical, pharmacologic, and behavioral studies. A general review of this area is available (Chiu and Richardson, 1985).

One of the more important findings was the discovery of both a PGE$_2$ (Malet et al., 1982) and a PGD$_2$ (Yamashita et al., 1983) receptor in rat brain. These receptors met most of the requirements for receptors found on synaptosomal membranes and exhibited an anatomical distribution coincident with many of the previously reported pharmacologic effects of PGs in the CNS. These findings extended our knowledge; we now know that neuronal cells can sense the PGs that they, or other neuronal projections, produce in a manner similar to most of the known neurotransmitters.

Most investigators, however, believe that PGs act more like neuromodulators than neurotransmitters (i.e., they modify, either by transduction or amplification, the primary signal created by neurotransmitters). In some very elegant experiments, it was shown that microiontophoretically placed PGE could modify the inhibitory effect of norepinephrine on the firing of the cerebellar Purkinje cell (Siggins et al., 1971). The functional role of PGs on cere-

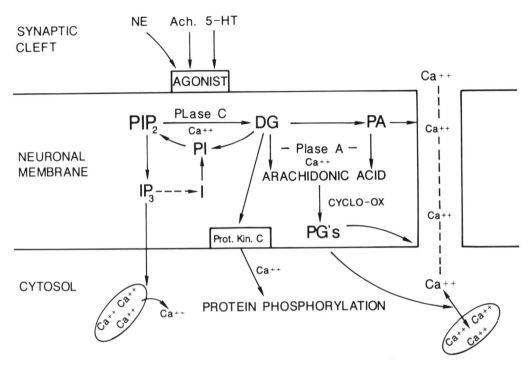

Fig. 21–2. Relationship between receptor stimulation and signal transduction through the phosphatidylinositol (PI) pathway with associated diacylglycerol (DG) formation and prostaglandin (PG) production. Plase C, phospholipase C; Plase A, phospholipase A; I, inositol; PIP$_2$, inositol 4–5-bisphosphate; IP$_3$, inositol 1,4,5-triphosphate; cyclo-ox, cyclooxygenase; Prot. Kin. C, protein kinase C; PA, phosphatidic acid.

bellar Purkinje cells is supported by the discovery of a PG receptor in the Purkinje cell layer of pig cerebellum (Watanabe et al., 1983). Additionally, a number of investigators have observed that the neurally active catecholamines (norepinephrine, epinephrine, and dopamine) are capable of stimulating PG (PGE$_2$ and PGF$_2$) production in whole brain homogenates (Hillier et al., 1976), cerebral cortical slices (Wolfe et al., 1976), brain microsomes (Schaefer et al., 1978), and brain synaptosomes (Hillier et al., 1979; Schaefer et al., 1978). Indeed, both the alpha-1-adrenoceptor (Schoepp et al., 1984) and the beta-adrenoceptor (Hillier and Templeton, 1982) have been specifically implicated in stimulation of the release of PG precursors or synthesis of PGE$_2$ and PGF$_{2\alpha}$ themselves.

Figure 21–2 illustrates the putative receptor-linked events by which PGs may be formed by neuronal synapses. An excellent review of this subject is available (Fisher and Agranoff, 1987), but, because research progress is rapid, the hypothetical interrelationships between these neuronal events is bound to be modified or clarified over time.

Since catecholamine levels (Cameron et al., 1984; Nesse et al., 1984) and receptors (Cameron et al., 1984; Charney and Henninger, 1986) have been reported to be abnormal in panic disorder, the subsequent discussion focuses on the relationship between norepinephrine (NE) and PGs only, although similar, and perhaps more convincing, evidence is available for the role of acetylcholine (muscarinic) and to a lesser extent serotonin (5-HT$_2$ receptor ligands) in the possible stimulation of PG production.

The NE receptor shown in Figure 21–2 is most likely an alpha-1-receptor (Johnson and Minneman, 1985). When NE binds to its alpha-1-receptor, a G-protein-linked activation of phospholipase C is thought to occur, leading to a cleavage of inositol 4,5-bisphosphate (PIP_2) to both diacylglycerol (DG) and inositol 1,4,5-triphosphate (IP_3). DG can directly stimulate protein kinase C, which can phosphorylate several neuronal proteins. IP_3, on the other hand, can directly affect intraneuronal calcium release, which may be the primary ingredient of instantaneous receptor-effector coupling. Germane to the purpose of this chapter, however, is that DG can be further metabolized by phospholipase A, in the presence of calcium, to arachidonic acid, which in turn can be converted into PGs through the action of cyclooxygenase. Through this mechanism, norepinephrine-stimulated alpha-1-receptors may stimulate intraneuronal protein phosphorylation, calcium release, and prostaglandin formation. Stimulation of the beta-receptor in rat cerebral cortex also has been implicated in PG production (Hillier and Templeton, 1982); however, since inositol lipid turnover has not been documented with beta-receptor agonists, the mechanism of this reported stimulation is unclear.

Does the stimulation or release of PGs by catecholamines have a functional importance or is it just an epiphenomenon? There are two lines of evidence that suggest PGs, and particularly PGE_2, do play a functional role in the CNS at a biochemical/physiologic level. First, it appears that PGE_2 antagonizes NE release from brain cortical slices (Reimann et al., 1981), hypothalamic slices (Dray and Heaulme, 1984), and synaptosomes (Wendel and Strandhoy, 1978). Dopamine release also was antagonized (Bergstrom et al., 1973). The PGE_2 antagonism of NE release was thought to work through a mechanism utilizing its own receptor site (Dray and Heaulme, 1984). In a behavioral paradigm, PGE_2 and to a lesser extent PGD_2 and $PGF_{2\alpha}$ were able to antagonize amphetamine-induced circling in unilaterally 6-hydroxydopamine lesioned mice, supporting an inhibitory role for the PGs on dopamine release (Schwarz et al., 1982). These data suggest that PGE_2 acts as a neuromodulator.

A second line of thought suggests that PGs may play a role in receptor-effector transduction. There is evidence that some brain regions and certain receptors (alpha-adrenergic) utilize PGE_2 as a transducer for cyclic adenosine

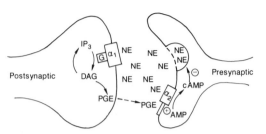

Fig. 21–3. Hypothetical model of how NE and PGE_2 may interact in neuronal transmission. DAG = Diacylglycerol; G = G Protein (see text for explanation).

monophosphate (cAMP) stimulation (Cardinali and Ritta, 1983; Partington et al., 1980). Prostaglandin synthetase (cyclooxygenase) inhibitors "uncouple" the alpha-adrenoceptor stimulation of cAMP. However, PGE_2 and PGD_2 may directly stimulate cAMP production in cultured neuronal cells (Howlett, 1982; Shimizu et al., 1979), indicating that other neurotransmitters need not be involved for PGs to have cellular effects. PGs may also have a direct effect on the neuronal membrane since PGD_2 has a depolarizing effect on neuronal cells in culture, which may be related to calcium permeability (Kondo et al., 1981).

Both a direct neuromodulator role and a transducer role may have functional importance in synaptic transmission. One effect may be important presynaptically and the other postsynaptically. It seems we now know that catecholamines and in particular NE stimulate PG (especially PGE_2) production, which in turn may inhibit NE release. PGs also directly stimulate cAMP production, which plays a direct role either in presynaptic NE release inhibition or in postsynaptic effector transduction.

A hypothetical model of how NE and PGs (particularly PGE_2) may interact is shown in Figure 21–3. In essence, when NE is released presynaptically, it crosses and binds to an alpha-1-receptor. This causes turnover of inositol phosphates and subsequent PGE_2 formation. Then, the PGE_2 may be released into the synaptic cleft, raising the local concentration and thereby increasing its binding to a presynaptic regulatory site near the alpha-2-receptor. Occupancy at this binding site increase the efficiency of NE binding (Kitamura and Nomura, 1986) or cAMP production (Partington et al.,

1980), which, in turn, decreases the release of presynaptic NE. This model seems to fit the data now available and provides a mechanistic explanation of how PGs may act as neuromodulators. The NE-producing presynaptic cell not only would get immediate feedback about the concentration of NE within the synaptic cleft but also would get feedback about the effectiveness of this concentration from the postsynaptic receptor-effector coupling. In essence, therefore, the concentration of NE in the cleft may be reduced or amplified depending on its effectiveness postsynaptically. This would imply that only by simultaneously measuring both PGE_2 and NE could the effectiveness of the NE concentration (which may be high or low) be determined. Additionally, if there is some dysregulation in the production of PGE_2, adequate feedback may not be immediately available to the presynaptic alpha-2-receptor, and, in essence, it would become dysregulated (either reduce or amplify its response).

The other neurotransmitter implicated in anxiety states and benzodiazepine actions is gamma-aminobutyric acid (GABA). It is of interest that membrane lipids, and the enzymes that affect these lipids, recently have been implicated in GABA mediated events. Specifically, arachidonic acid, the PG precursor, has been shown to block the uptake of GABA in neuronal cultures (Yu et al., 1986). Phospholipase A_2, the enzyme that cleaves arachidonic acid from its membrane precursor diacylglycerol, appears to be crucial in the process of both alpha-adrenergic and $GABA_B$ receptor cAMP activation (Duman et al., 1986). Although the $GABA_B$ receptor has been studied less than the $GABA_A$ (or bicuculline-sensitive) receptor in relationship to the anxiolytic action of benzodiazepines (e.g., Paul et al., 1981; Tallman and Gallager, 1985), the fact that fatty acids affect more than one receptor type implies a wider role of this system in neuronal modulation.

PGs AND THE HYPOTHALAMIC-PITUITARY-ARENAL (HPA) AXIS

The HPA axis has received intense study in various psychopathologic states including panic disorder (Bridges et al., 1986; Grunhaus

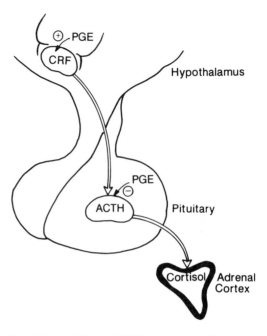

Fig. 21–4. Effect of PGE on the hypothalamic-pituitary-adrenal axis.

et al., 1987). Of interest for this discussion is evidence that PGE_2 plays a role in the regulation of this axis. The data that bear on this regulation come from animal in vivo and in vitro studies and are summarized in Figure 21–4. Essentially, indomethacin, an inhibitor of PG synthesis when given systemically (Weidenfeld et al., 1981) or injected directly into the anterior pituitary (Hedge, 1977a,b), increased adrenocorticotropin (ACTH) secretion. These studies imply that inhibition of PG production leads to an increase in ACTH and that this effect occurs at the pituitary level. When injected into the anterior pituitary after indomethacin, PGs inhibited corticotropin (CRF)-stimulated ACTH release (Hedge, 1977a,b). CRF stimulation of ACTH from rat anterior pituitary hindquarters in vitro was enhanced by indomethacin, whereas CRF alone stimulated the production of PGE_2 (Vlaskovska et al., 1984). Overall, its is hypothesized that PGE_2 is produced by the pituitary in response to CRF and that it acts as a local negative feedback inhibitor of CRF-stimulated ACTH production. However, when PGs are injected into the systemic circulation or directly into the hypothalamic median emminence, there is an increase in ACTH production (Hedge, 1972). This suggests that PGs may directly stimulate CRF which, in turn, stimulates ACTH secretion.

Similar to neuronal synaptic transmission, PGs may act as regulators or modulators that have both stimulatory (CRF) and inhibitory (ACTH) roles on the same system. Although this is speculative, it is conceivable that a dysregulation of PG production is involved with the dysregulated HPA axis observed in affective and panic disorders. Some information bearing on this speculation is presented later in this chapter.

PGs AND THE PLATELET

The platelet has been extensively utilized as a model for biochemical events purported to occur in an analagous fashion in the brain. The platelet is easily accessible, has receptors, processes an uptake and transport mechanism, and utilizes second messenger systems (phosphatidylinositol turnover and cAMP production) as transducers (for review, see Longenecker, 1985, especially the chapter by Stahl). However, platelet functioning may be important in its own right, since platelet abnormalities have been implicated in atherosclerosis, thrombosis (coronary and cerebral), and perhaps hypertension. These pathological processes are easily recognizable as being responsible for great morbidity and mortality. Therefore, any impact of specific psychopathological states or psychotropic drugs on the platelet could have immense importance. A review of the meager data in regard to panic disorder and platelet function is given later in this chapter. For now, let us examine how PGs and the platelet interact as a basis for this later discussion.

Figure 21–5 illustrates in schematic form the rudiments of platelet physiology. Since the platelet is so accessible to study, much as been learned about its structure, function, and pharmacology. The following is only the briefest of reviews.

There are four main ingredients to platelet physiology: 1) the presence of *specific receptors* to a variety of compounds (i.e., proteins, lipids, amines, and various pharmaceuticals such as imipramine, verapamil, etc.); 2) *trans-*ducer (second messenger) *systems,* such as PI turnover, cAMP production, and Ca^{2+} transport are all present and important; 3) intracellular *amplification mechanisms,* of which Ca^{2++} release and PG (thromboxane) synthesis are important; 4) *release of intracellular contents* (serotonin, platelet factor 4, beta-thromboglobulin, and thromboxane), which affect surrounding cells (other platelets, vessel walls, blood elements). For the sake of compactness and focus, the role of amines (especially epinephrine) is highlighted, since this is most germane to this chapter. There is now much evidence that the receptor for epinephrine in the platelet is an alpha-2-receptor (Kerry and Scrutton, 1985). Epinephrine (1–20 μM) will cause the aggregation of platelets in platelet-rich plasma (PRP), with the production of thromboxane (TXB_2) as the aggregation progresses. Epinephrine will also enhance the aggregation of platelets to suboptimal concentrations of other aggregating agents (a proaggregatory response) such as adenosine diphosphate (ADP). The responsiveness of platelets to epinephrine can be blocked by the selective alpha-2-adrenergic antagonist yohimbine. Of specific interest for this chapter is that epinephrine has been shown to block the increase in intracellular cAMP induced by the antiaggregatory agent PGE_1. Since an increase in intracellular cAMP inhibits aggregation and epinephrine suppresses cAMP production, it has been postulated that epinephrine's aggregatory effect occurs through this mechanism. However, a role for a direct effect of epinephrine on phospholipase C activation and calcium release cannot be completely ruled out. In any case, there are three practical ways of measuring the effect of epinephrine on platelets in vitro: 1) by directly measuring aggregation using standard optical turbidity techniques, 2) by measuring TXB_2 production after the addition of epinephrine to platelet-rich plasma or washed platelets, 3) by measuring stimulated (PGE_1) cAMP production in the presence and absence of epinephrine.

One can indirectly assess in vivo platelet function (aggregation) by measuring serum levels of specific platelet release products such as platelet factor 4 and beta-thromboglobulin. However, no direct conclusion can be drawn about the alpha-2-receptor or epinephrine lev-

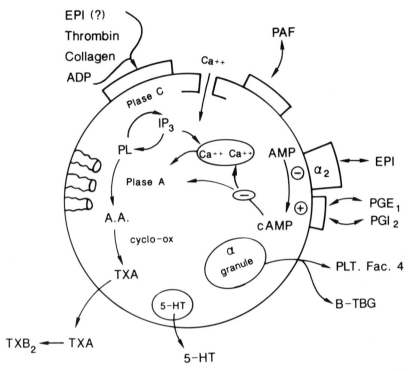

Fig. 21–5. Diagrammatic representation of normal platelet physiology. Epinephrine (EPI), thrombin, collagen, adenosine diphosphate (ADP), and platelet activating factor (PAF) can all cause platelet aggregation either through stimulation of phospholipase C and subsequent PI turnover, calcium release, and thromboxane (TXA) production. Epinephrine inhibits cAMP production, which causes aggregation. During platelet stimulation and aggregation, release of serotonin (5-HT), platelet factor 4 (PLT. Fac. 4), and beta-thromboglobulin (β-TBG) occurs.

els from the measurement of these release products, since they can give only a gross measurement of platelet functioning. Later in this chapter, results of studies employing some of the above techniques with panic disorder patients will be examined.

PGs IN PSYCHIATRIC DISORDERS

From the data presented above, it is clear that enough evidence exists from basic studies that PGs most likely play a physiologic role in the CNS. This has led a number of investigators to hypothesize that these compounds might be abnormal in certain psychopathological states (Gross et al., 1977; Horrobin and Manku, 1980; Ragheb and Ban, 1982). However, relatively little investigation of the role of PGs in psychiatric illness has occurred. There are several possible explanations for this pau-

city of research findings. First, PGs and thromboxane are relatively hard to measure reliably because of the small amounts present in both CSF (pg/ml) and blood (pg–ng/ml). Second, many of these compounds can be synthesized by blood cells and vessel wall endothelium such that local production during blood drawing procedures or during in vitro incubation complicates interpretation of results. Third, the compounds themselves are not very stable, so care must be taken in sample preparation and treatment to minimize autooxidation and loss during extraction/separation procedures. Fourth, since most PGs are metabolized quickly in the periphery during passage through the lung, their half-life is short, with most measured peripheral levels not reflecting neuronal tissue production. Theoretically, CSF PG levels should more accurately reflect neu-

TABLE 21–1.
Prostaglandin Levels (pg/ml) in Patients With Affective Disorders

Study	Site	Type	Control	Mania	Depression (U/B)*	Panic disorder
Gross et al., 1977	CSF	PGF	—	—	50	—
	Plasma	PGF	—	—	148/105	—
Lieb et al., 1983	Plasma	PGE_2	68	—	492/431	—
		TXB_2	64	—	1,217/1,101	—
Linnoila et al., 1983	CSF	PGE	—	—	1,000–4,000	—
Gerner and Merrill, 1983	CSF	PGE	65	149	56	—
Calabrese et al., 1986	Plasma	PGE	9,000	—	40,000	—
Sheehan et al., 1984	Plasma	TXB_2	—	—	—	270
	Plasma	6-Keto $PGF_{1\alpha}$	—	—	—	177
Carr et al., 1986	Plasma	TXB_2	133	—	—	149
	Plasma	6-Keto $PGF_{1\alpha}$	44	—	—	49

*U = Unipolar; B = Bipolar

ronal production and not be metabolized as readily, since the CNS does not process degradive enzymes.

Despite these difficulties, some attempts to examine basal (nonstimulated) levels of PGs and thromboxane in affective disorders have been made. The results of these studies are summarized in Table 21–1. It is readily apparent in review of the data that there is wide variation in reported levels of PGE between the several studies that have examined this PG moiety. Particular difficulty arises when control populations are not utilized as a reference or comparison, both within a single study and across several studies. Despite these caveats, several authors report results that tend in a similar direction. Specifically, Lieb et al. (1983) and Calabrese et al. (1986) suggest that plasma PGE is elevated in depressive states compared to control. Although no normal controls are available for comparison, Linnoila et al. (1983) reported higher levels of CSF PGE in a few depressed patients as compared to schizophrenics. On the other hand, Gerner and Merrill (1983) reported no difference in CSF PGE levels between depressed patients and controls, but an increase of CSF PGE in manic patients.

Only future studies can resolve the discrepancies in both measured levels of PGE and difference between diagnostic groups raised by these initial reports. Improvement in measurement techniques (more specific antibodies for radioimmunoassay (RIA), wider availability of gas chromatography-mass spectrometry) and attention to sample collection, preservation procedures (inhibiting in vitro production with cyclooxygenase inhibitors, quick freezing, correcting for recovery during extraction), and patient preparation (withholding cyclooxygenase inhibitors such as aspirin) prior to sample collection should all lead to more valid and reliable PG measurement.

PGs AND ANXIETY DISORDERS
Circulatory PGs and the Platelet

The available information relating PG dysregulation to anxiety disorders is even more meager than that for major affective disorders. Presently, there are two studies published by the same research group that measured peripheral PG products in panic disorder patients (Carr et al., 1986; Sheehan et al., 1984). The results of these studies are summarized at the bottom of Table 21–1. Additional data on CSF PGE are available from research on patients at our institution, and these are presented subsequently.

Sheehan et al. (1984), in their initial study, examined the platelet proaggregatory substance thromboxane (TXB_2) the vasodilatory PG, prostacyclin (measured as 6-keto $PGF_{1\alpha}$), and platelet-derived platelet factor 4 and beta-thromboglobulin in venous blood of panic disorder patients. They reported that both TXB_2 and 6-keto $PGF_{1\alpha}$ were elevated well above the normal range for historical controls established in their laboratory. These elevated levels of TXB_2 and 6-keto $PGF_{1\alpha}$ tended to normalize upon treatment with alprazolam. However, it is a theoretical problem that a comparison group of patients treated with ibuprofen (a potent PG synthesis inhibitor) showed no decrease in production of either compound, a finding that leaves open to question the soundness of the PG measurement techniques. Perhaps a somewhat more important finding was the report of higher platelet factor 4 and beta-thromboglobulin levels in patient blood compared to controls. The levels of these substances normalized during treatment with either alprazolam or ibuprofen. Taken together, these initial results point to a state of increased platelet reactivity (possibly aggregation) in the panic disorder patients. This finding could have immense theoretical and practical significance considering that the platelet is both a possible model of CNS cellular activity and a crucial element in vascular pathogenesis. Platelet pathophysiology is particularly important in anxiety disorders in general, and in panic disorder in particular, since these illnesses may be associated with increased hypertensive, cardiovascular, and cerebrovascular morbidity (Coryell et al., 1982; Noyes et al., 1978).

In an attempt to replicate and extend the above findings, this group (Carr et al., 1986) again measured TXB_2, 6-keto $PGF_{1\alpha}$, and platelet factor 4 in 25 panic disorder patients and ten concurrent controls before and after a lactate infusion. In addition, they also examined the effect of alprazolam treatment on these parameters. In this study, the previous findings of elevated levels of these factors in panic disorder patients could not be confirmed, although there was a suggestion (at the trend level $P = 0.12$) that platelet factor 4 was higher in the patient group. However, there was no effect of treatment with the triazolodiazepine alprazolam on either TXB_2 or platelet factor 4. Of interest in this regard is a recent finding that triazolodiazepines antagonize the platelet aggregation induced by platelet activating factor, but not other proaggregatory substances, both in vitro and in vivo (Casals-Stenzel, 1987). This would suggest that in certain people or under certain circumstances a drug known for its antipanic effects may decrease platelet aggregation.

It could be argued that measuring whole blood levels of thromboxane and beta-thromboglobulin is, at best, an indirect measure of in vivo platelet function. It is generally accepted that in vitro measurement of platelet aggregation with optical techniques and measurement of release reactions of either serotonin, platelet factor 4, or thromboxane are more likely to reflect the state of platelet function in vivo (Longenecker, 1985). Various in vitro stimulatory factors could be utilized as depicted above in Figure 21–4. Thrombin, collagen, ADP, and platelet activating factor all work through either a direct stimulation of phospholipase C or indirectly through a calcium-mediated channel. Epinephrine, on the other hand, may work through the above mechanism but more likely works by inhibiting the production of cAMP, which is itself an inhibitor of platelet aggregation. Therefore, epinephrine would stimulate platelet aggregation by decreasing cAMP. This effect appears to be mediated by epinephrine's binding to an alpha-2-adrenoceptor (as discussed in the previous section).

Plasma levels of epinephrine have been found to be elevated in panic disorder patients (Ballenger et al., 1984; Nesse et al., 1984). We hypothesized that if the platelets of panic disorder patients were exposed to higher levels of epinephrine over a prolonged period that some change (down-regulation) in the alpha-2-adrenoceptor on the platelet might occur and thereby lead to decreased platelet aggregation on exogenous epinephrine challenge. Therefore, in a pilot study in our laboratory, the sensitivity of platelets to an in vitro epinephrine challenge was compared between panic disorder patients and age- and sex-matched controls run simultaneously. PRP samples from the same patient or control were exposed to various concentrations of epinephrine over a 4 min incubation period at 37°C. The amount of thromboxane produced during that time was measured in aliquots of PRP in duplicate by an RIA procedure. The results are shown in Figure 21–6. The patients produced significantly less TXB_2 than controls at every concentration of epinephrine tested. These results suggest the following possibilities.

1. The epinephrine was more quickly metabolized by monoamine oxidase (MAO). At least one well controlled study (Gorman et al.,

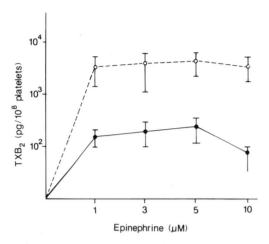

Fig. 21–6. Thromboxane production from PRP after various concentrations of in vitro epinephrine. Solid lines are patients (N = 4); dashed lines are controls (N = 4).

1985) found elevated platelet MAO in panic disorder patients, but platelet MAO did not correlate with plasma epinephrine levels.

2. The alpha-2 receptors on patient platelets were less sensitive to epinephrine. This suggestion is supported by one report (Cameron et al., 1984) showing that the binding (Bmax) of tritiated yohimbine was less on platelets of panic disorder patients than controls. However, a more recent report (Nutt and Fraser, 1987) using a slightly different technique did not confirm this finding.

3. The receptor-effector coupling mechanism between epinephrine and either cAMP inhibition or, possibly, phospholipase C stimulation was less efficient in patient platelets.

4. Other antiaggregating factors (see Fig. 21–5), such as PGE_1 or PGI_2, could be hyperfunctional in patient platelets, thereby negating the epinephrine aggregatory effect.

Only future studies that simultaneously measure several of these parameters in the same patient platelet preparation can directly point to the most valid explanation. Obviously, a greater number of patients and controls must be examined in this regard. It is intriguing, however, to note the findings of Charney and Henninger (1986), which suggest a dysregulation of CNS alpha-2-receptors in panic disorder patients. How platelet function may be related to this CNS phenomenon is worthy of further study.

CNS PGE

In an earlier section of this chapter, data were reviewed suggesting that PGs, particularly of the E type, have a physiologic role in the CNS. It is generally thought that they play a modulatory function on amine systems (NE, dopamine) and on hormonal peptide systems (CRF and ACTH). Therefore, an examination of PGE levels in the CSF of panic disorder patients, particularly in conjunction with measurement of neurotransmitter metabolites and hormonal peptide levels, appeared worthy of pursuit. In this section, data are presented that, in at least a preliminary fashion, may begin to shed some light on what role, if any, is played by the PG system in this and perhaps other psychiatric disorders.

In collaboration with colleagues at our institution, we attempted to measure CSF PGE in 20 patients (age 36 ± 11 years) who met DSM III criteria for agoraphobia with panic attacks and in ten control patients (age 30 ± 9 years). Within the patient group, 35% met the DSM III criteria for past or current major depressive disorder.

CSF PGE was measured in the 33–35th cc of CSF obtained from a patient in a drug-free state (100% of patients >2 days, 75% >1 wk) by a standard RIA procedure utilizing PGE_2 as standard after lyophilization, extraction, and correction for recovery. CSF CRF and CSF ACTH were also measured in a subgroup of patients and controls by colleagues at the NIMH (Philip Gold and colleagues) utilizing standard RIA techniques. Additionally, CSF 3-methoxy-4-hydroxyphenylglycol (MHPG), homovanillic acid (HVA), and 5-hydroxyindole acetic acid (5-HIAA) were measured by C. Ray Lake and colleagues (Uniformed Services University of the Health Services) utilizing high-performance liquid chromatography (HPLC) with electrochemical detection techniques.

The main finding of this study is (Fig. 21–7) that there was no significant difference between CSF PGE levels of patients or controls (164 ± 92 vs 160 ± 88 pg/ml). This was true even if patients with a history of past or current depression were analyzed separately from

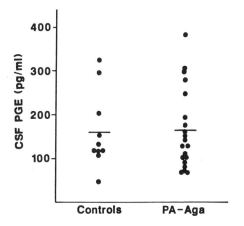

Fig. 21–7. CSF PGE levels in agoraphobia with panic attack patients and controls.

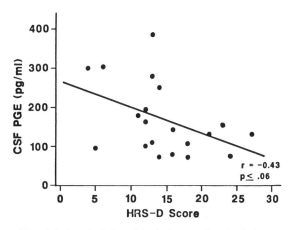

Fig. 21–8. Relationship between level of depression and CSF PGE in patients with agoraphobia and panic attacks.

the nondepressed patients or controls (160 ± 105, 166 ± 87, and 160 ± 88 pg/ml, respectively).

Of interest, particularly in relationship to past reports of increased PGE in the CSF (Linnoila et al., 1983) and serum (Calabrese et al., 1986; Lieb et al., 1983) of depressed patients was the finding in our panic disorder patients of a negative correlation between CSF PGE and depressive symptom level (Fig. 21–8). This was even more significant if the CSF PGE levels were compared in low vs. high Hamilton Depression Score (HRSD) groups utilizing a median split procedure. In the high HRSD group, CSF PGE was 119 ± 55 pg/ml; in the low HRSD group, CSF PGE was 209 ± 100 pg/ml (t = 2.47, P < 0.05). Therefore, contrary to reports in major depression, high depression scores in our agoraphobic panic disorder group were associated with lower CSF PGE levels.

Other preliminary, but nonetheless intriguing, findings from this study lie in the area of associations or correlations between PGE and central neurotransmitter and peptide systems. These data are summarized in Table 21–2. The correlations given in Table 21–2 are a preliminary attempt to explore any relationships between PGE and other central systems. A priori, there is reason to believe that some association exists between ACTH, CRF, and PGE based on the animal work previously summarized in this chapter. Additionally, there is reason to hypothesize a relationship between PGE and

noradrenergic function from both animal and in vitro work also reviewed above. Of note, therefore, is the suggestive positive relationship between CSF PGE and ACTH in patients, but not in controls (which is in fact in the negative direction). Additionally interesting is the stronger positive relationship between CSF PGE and MHPG in the controls but not in the patient group. When the data are reviewed in toto, it is especially intriguing to see the correlations between the controls and the patients on almost every parameter to have an opposite sign. That is, when PGE is positively correlated with a variable in the control group, it is negatively correlated in the patient group and vice versa. The meaning of this is elusive at this time, and only more study can shed light on the validity of this observation. However, one might speculate that if a modulatory system (which affects a number of different systems) is somehow defective, or perhaps is overcompensating, then a situation of this type may arise. That is, a dysregulation or lack of homeostasis and uncoupling of systems may become evident.

Let us examine more closely how this might occur in the relationship between PGE and the CRF stimulation of ACTH first and then PGE modulation of noradrenergic tone. In the former case, evidence exists that PGE stimulates CRF but inhibits ACTH, presumably in a local feedback loop after CRF stimulation (see Fig.

TABLE 21–2.
Association Between CSF PGE and Other CSF Peptides and Neurotransmitter Metabolites
(Correlations are Pearson's R)

	Total subjects		Patients		Controls	
	N	R	N	R	N	R
ACTH	19	0.33	13	0.51*	6	−0.63
CRF	18	0.00	12	−0.19	6	0.56
MHPG	30	0.28	20	0.09	10	0.70**
HVA	28	0.01	18	−0.31	10	0.54
5-HIAA	29	0.01	20	−0.26	9	0.61*

*$P < 0.1$.
**$P < 0.05$.

21–4). In controls, PGE is positively correlated with CRF but negatively with ACTH. This could mean that, when CRF stimulates pituitary corticotrophs, PGE is produced when ACTH is produced but that PGE tonically decreases ACTH. However, in the patient group, the opposite is seen, in that PGE is positively correlated with ACTH and negatively with CRF. This could suggest that the linkage between the systems has broken down and that perhaps less PGE is produced per unit of CRF stimulation and that PGE has lost its effectiveness to inhibit ACTH. This will reverse the association between PGE and ACTH from a negative one to a positive one.

In the case of PGE and MHPG, we will have to assume that MHPG level provides some index of NE release or turnover, although admittedly this may be an incomplete assumption. In any case, it appears that in controls the association between PGE and MHPG (noradrenergic release) is the strongest of any examined. If MHPG is reflective of free NE in the synaptic cleft, then the positive relationship may be reflective of postsynaptic phosphatidylinositol turnover and subsequent arachidonic acid conversion to PGE (see Fig. 21–3) and subsequent release into the synaptic cleft. PGE would provide the neuromodulatory influence on the presynaptic alpha-2-receptor to amplify the feedback inhibition and provide for homeostasis. However, in the panic disorder patient group, this correlation is lacking, suggesting an uncoupling of these two systems. PGE may not be produced to the same degree when the postsynaptic receptor is stimulated and, thereby, not provide the presynaptic amplification necessary for alpha-2-receptor-mediated presynaptic inhibition, functionally down-regulating this receptor.

Although these speculations are heuristically appealing, further study and data collection (possibly including stimulatory paradigms) will be necessary before extension of these ideas is realistic. Nevertheless, they may provide some direction for future research regarding the role of regulatory/modulatory systems in explaining the coupling between major neurotransmitter systems and hormones.

SUMMARY

This chapter provides a brief overview of the PG system as a functional component of both the CNS and the peripheral vasculature. Much is yet to be learned about how the modulatory system functions both during normal physiology and in psychopathological states, such as during a panic attack.

Perhaps even more so than many of the systems (amine and hormonal) that biological psychiatrists study, the PG system may be of central importance in the connection between mind and body. Much knowledge has been gained in the past 10–20 years on the importance of this system for immunological, renal, cardiovascular, intestinal, and hormonal function. It appears that the brain is the next frontier.

More attention is being paid to dysregulation hypotheses (Charney and Henninger, 1986; Siever and Davis, 1985) in relationship to psychiatric illness. This would imply that modulatory systems and mechanisms could be of immense importance in our understanding of psychopathology. The PG system, either as a primary constituent or as a measureable epiphenomenon (e.g., as a marker of phosphatidylinositol turnover) of modulation or regulation, seems worthy of more intensive study. As a putative modulator, it would seem necessary to assess the PG system in relationship to more primary systems such as amines, peptides, hormones, etc. Only in this manner could some light be shed on regulatory mechanisms.

In the periphery, however, direct examination of receptor-effector coupling effects may be examined utilizing the well understood physiology of the platelet. Even if results are not directly generalizable to central neuronal tissue, whatever is learned might have direct applicability to the prevention of physical morbidity and mortality in psychiatric states such as panic disorder. As technological skills in this area advance, more valid and reliable measurements of the prostaglandin system will provide new insights into the etiology of psychiatric pathology, in general, and panic disorder, in particular.

REFERENCES

Abdel-Halim MS, Ekstedt J, Anggard E (1979): Determination of prostaglandin $F_{2\alpha}$, E_2, D_2 and 6-keto-$F_{1\alpha}$ in human cerebrospinal fluid. Prostaglandins 17: 405–409.

Abdel-Halim MS, Lunden I, Cseh G, Anggard E (1980a): Prostaglandin profiles in nervous tissue and blood vessels of the brain of various animals. Prostaglandins 19:249–259.

Abdel-Halim MS, von Kolst H, Meyerson B, Sachs C, Anggard E (1980b): Prostaglandin profiles in tissue and blood vessels from human brain. J Neurochem 34:1331–1333.

Anton RF, Ballenger JC, Lydiard RB, Maraia MT, Howell EF, Gold PW (1989): CSF prostaglandin E in agoraphobia with panic attacks. Biol Psychiatry 26: 257–264.

Anton RF, Wallis C, Randall CL (1983): In vivo regional levels of PGE and thromboxane in mouse brain: Effect of decapitation, focused microwave fixation, and indomethacin. Prostaglandins 26:421–429.

Ballenger JC, et al. (1984): A study of plasma catecholamines in agoraphobia and the relationship of serum tricyclic levels to treatment response. In Ballenger JC (ed): "Biology of Agoraphobia." Washington, DC: American Psychiatric Press, Inc.

Bergstrom S, Farnebo L-O, Fuxe K (1973): Effect of prostaglandin E_2 on central and peripheral catecholamine neurons. Eur J Pharmacol 21:362–368.

Bito LZ, Davson H (1974): Carrier-mediated removal of prostaglandins from cerebrospinal fluid. J Physiol 236:39P.

Bito LZ, Davson H, Hollingsworth JR (1976): Facilitated transport of prostaglandins across the blood-cerebrospinal fluid and blood–brain barriers. J Physiol 256:273–285.

Bridges M, Yeregani VK, Rainey JM, Pohl R (1986): Dexamethasone Suppression Test in patients with panic attacks. Biol Psychiatry 21:849–853.

Calabrese JR, Skwerer RG, Barna B, Gulledge AD, Valenzuela R, Butkus A, Subichin S, Krupp NE (1986): Depression, immunocompetence, and prostaglandins of the E series. Psychiatry Res 17:41–47.

Cameron OG, Smith CB, Hollingsworth PJ, Nesse RM, Curtis GC (1984): Platelet α_2-adrenergic receptor binding and plasma catecholamines. Arch Gen Psychiatry 41-1144–1148.

Cardinali DP, Ritta MN (1983): The role of prostaglandins in neuroendocrine junctions: Studies in the pineal gland and the hypothalamus. Neuroendocrinology 36:152–160.

Carr DB, Sheehan DV, Surman OS, Coleman JH, Greenblatt DJ, Heninger GR, Jones KJ, Levine PH, Watkins WD (1986): Neuroendocrine correlates of lactate-induced anxiety and their response to chronic alprazolam therapy. Am J Psychiatry 143:483–494.

Casals-Stenzel J (1987): Triazolodiazepines are potent antagonists of platelet activating factor (PAF) in vitro and in vivo. Acta Pharmacol 335:351–355.

Charney DS, Henninger GR (1986): Abnormal regulation of noradrenergic function in panic disorders. Arch Gen Psychiatry 43:1042–1054.

Chiu EKY, Richardson JS (1985): Behavioral and neurochemical aspects of prostaglandins in brain function. Gen Pharmacol 16:163–175.

Coryell W, Noyes R, Clancy J (1982): Excess mortality in panic disorder. A comparison with primary unipolar depression. Arch Gen Psychiatry 39:701–703.

Dray F, Heaulme M (1984): Prostaglandins of the E series inhibit release of noradrenaline in rat hypothalamus by a mechanism unrelated to classical α_2 adrenergic presynaptic inhibition. Neuropharmacology 23:457–462.

Duman RS, Karbon EW, Harrington C, Enna SJ (1986): An examination of the involvement of phospholipases A_2 and C in the α-adrenergic and gamma-aminobutyric acid receptor modulation of cyclic AMP accumulation in rat brain slices. J Neurochem 47:800–810.

Fagan SC, Castellani D, Gengo FM (1986): Prostanoid concentrations in human CSF following acute ischaemic brain infarction. Clin Exp Pharmacol Physiol 13:629–632.

Fisher SK, Agranoff BW (1987): Receptor activation and inositol lipid hydrolysis in neural tissues. J Neurochem 48:999–1017.

Gerner RH, Merrill JE (1983): Cerebrospinal fluid prostaglandin E in depression, mania, and schizophrenia compared to normals. Biol Psychiatry 18:565–569.

Gorman J, Liebowitz MR, Fyer AJ, Levitt M, Baron M, Davies S, Klein DF (1985): Platelet monoamine oxidase activity in patients with panic disorder. Biol Psychiatry 20:852–857.

Gross HA, Dunner DL, Lafleur D, Meltzer HL, Muhlbauer HL, Fieve DR (1977): Prostaglandins. A review of neurophysiology and psychiatric implications. Arch Gen Psychiatry 34:1189–1196.

Grunhaus L, Flegel P, Haskett RF, Greden JF (1987): Serial dexamethasone suppression tests in simultaneous panic and depressive disorders. Biol Psychiatry 22:332–338.

Hedge GA (1972): The effects of prostaglandins on ACTH secretion. Endocrinology 91:925–933.

Hedge GA (1977a): Roles for the prostaglandins in the regulation of anterior pituitary secretion. Life Sci 20:17–34.

Hedge GA (1977b): Stimulation of ACTH secretion by indomethacin and reversal by exogenous prostaglandins. Prostaglandins 14:145–150.

Hillier K, Roberts PJ, Templeton WW (1979): Prostaglandin and noradrenaline interactions in rat brain synaptosomes. Br J Pharmacol 66:102–103.

Hillier K, Roberts PJ, Woolard P (1976): Catecholamine stimulated prostaglandin synthesis in rat brain synaptosomes. Br J Pharmacol 58:426–427.

Hillier K, Templeton WW (1982): Stimulation of prostaglandin synthesis in rat cerebral cortex via a β-adrenoceptor. Gen Pharmacol 13:21–25.

Horrobin DF (1979): Schizophrenia: Reconciliation of the dopamine, prostaglandin, and opioid concepts and the role of the pineal. Lancet i:529–530.

Horrobin DF, Manku MS (1980): Possible role of prostaglandin E₁ in the affective disorders and in alcoholism. Br Med J 280:1363–1366.

Howlett AC (1982): Stimulation of neuroblastoma adenylate cyclase by arachidonic acid metabolites. Mol Pharmacol 21:664–670.

Johnson RD, Minneman KP (1985): α₁-Adrenergic receptors and stimulation of [H³]inositol metabolism in rat brain: Regional distribution and parallel inactivation. Brain Res 341:7–15.

Kerry R, Scrutton MC (1985): Platelet adrenoceptors. In Longenecker GL (ed): "The Platelets: Physiology and Pharmacology." Orlando: Academic Press, Inc., pp 113–157.

Kitamura Y, Nomura Y (1986): Enhancement of [³H]clonidine binding to rat cerebral synaptic membranes by treatment with arachidonic acid, prostaglandin (PG) D₂, PGE₂ and PGF₂α. Jpn J Pharmacol 42:321–324.

Kondo K, Shimizu T, Hayaishi O (1981): Effects of prostaglandin D₂ on membrane potential in neuroblastoma × glioma hybrid cells as determined with a cyanine dye. Biochem Biophys Res Commun 98:648–655.

Latorre E, Patrono C, Fortuna A, et al. (1974): Role of prostaglandin F₂α in human cerebral vasospasm. J Neurosurg 41:293–299.

Lieb J, Karmali R, Horrobin, D (1983): Elevated levels of prostaglandin E₂ and thromboxane B₂ in depression. Prostaglandins Leukotreine Med 10:361–367.

Linnoila M, Whorton AR, Rubinow DR, Cowdry RW, Ninan PT, Waters RN (1983): CSF prostaglandin levels in depressed and schizophrenic patients. Arch Gen Psychiatry 40:405–406.

Longenecker GL (1985): "The Platelets: Physiology and Pharmacology." Orlando: Academic Press, Inc.

Malet C, Scherrer H, Saavedra JM, Dray F (1982): Specific binding of [³H]prostaglandin E₂ to rat brain membranes and synaptosomes. Brain Res 236:227–233.

Nesse RM, Cameron OG, Curtis GC, McCann DS, Huber-Smith MJ (1984): Adrenergic function in patients with panic anxiety. Arch Gen Psychiatry 41:771–776.

Noyes R, Clancy J, Hoenk PR, Slymen DJ (1978): Anxiety neurosis and physical illness. Comp Psychiatry 19:407–413.

Nutt DJ, Fraser S (1987): Platelet binding studies in panic disorder. J Affect Disorders 12:7–11.

Partington CR, Edwards MW, Daly JW (1980): Regulation of cyclic AMP formation in brain tissue by α-adrenergic receptors: Requisite intermediacy of prostaglandins of the E series. Proc Natl Acad Sci USA 77:3024–3028.

Paul SM, Marangos PJ, Skolnick P (1981): The benzodiazepine—GABA—chloride ionophore receptor complex: Common site of minor tranquilizer action. Biol Psychiatry 16:213–229.

Ragheb M, Ban TA (1982): Prostaglandins and schizophrenia: A review. Prog Neuropsychopharmacol Biol Psychiatry 6:87–93.

Reimann W, Steinhauer HB, Hedler L, Starke K, Hertting G (1981): Effect of prostaglandins D₂, E₂ and F₂α on catecholamine release from slices of rat and rabbit brain. Eur J Pharmacol 69:421–427.

Rotrosen J, Miller AD, Mandio D, Tarficante LJ, Gershon S (1980): Prostaglandins, platelets, and schizophrenia. Arch Gen Psychiatry 37:1047–1054.

Schaefer A, Komlos M, Seregi A (1978): Effects of biogenic amines and psychotropic drugs on endogenous prostaglandin biosynthesis in the rat brain homogenates. Biochem Pharmacol 27:213–218.

Schoepp DD, Knepper SM, Rutledge CO (1984): Norepinephrine stimulation of phosphoinositide hydrolysis in rat cerebral cortex is associated with the alpha₁-adrenoceptor. J Neurochem 43:1758–1761.

Schwarz RD, Uretsky NJ, Bianchine JR (1982): Prostaglandin inhibition of amphetamine-induced circling in mice. Psychopharmacol 78:317–321.

Sheehan DV, Coleman JH, Greenblatt DJ, Jones KJ, Levine PH, Orsulak PJ, Peterson M, Schildkraut JJ, Uzogara E, Watkins D (1984): Some biochemical correlates of panic attacks with agoraphobia and their response to a new treatment. J Clin Psychopharmacol 4:66–75.

Shimizu T, Mizuno N, Amano T, Hayaishi O (1979): Prostaglandin D₂, a neuromodulator. Proc Natl Acad Sci USA 76:6231–6234.

Siever LJ, Davis KL (1985): Overview: Toward a dysregulation hypothesis of depression. Am J Psychiatry 142:1017–1031.

Siggins G, Hoffer B, Bloom F (1971): Prostaglandin–norepinephrine interactions in brain: Microelectrophoretic and histochemical correlates. Ann NY Acad Sci 180:302–323.

Tallman JF, Gallagher DW (1985): The GABA-ergic system: A locus of benzodiazepine action. Annu Rev Neurosci 8:21–44.

Tansik RL, White HL (1979): Prostaglandin synthesis in homogenates of cultured neuroblastoma cells. Prostaglandins Med 2:225–234.

Vlaskovska M, Hertting G, Knepel W (1984): Adrenocorticotropin and β-endorphin release from rat adenohypophysis in vitro: Inhibition by prostaglandin E_2 formed locally in response to vasopressin and corticotropin-releasing factor. Endocrinology 115:895–903.

Watanabe Y, Yamashita A, Tokumoto H, Hayaishi O (1983): Localization of prostaglandin D_2 binding protein and NADP-linked 15-hydroxyprostaglandin D_2 dehydrogenase in the Purkinje cells of miniature pig cerebellum. Proc Natl Acad Sci USA 80:4542–4545.

Weidenfeld J, Siegel RA, Conforti N, Feldman S, Chowers I (1981): Site and mode of action of indomethacin on the hypothalamo-hypophyseal-adrenal axis: A temporal study in intact, hypothalamic-deafferentated, and hypothalamic-lesioned male rats. Endocrinology 109:205–209.

Wendel OT, Strandhoy (1978): The effects of prostaglandins E_2 and $F_{2\alpha}$ on synaptosomal accumulation and

release of ^{3}H-norepinephrine. Prostaglandins 16:441–449.

Wolfe LS, Mamer D (1975): Measurement of prostaglandin $F_{2\alpha}$ leels in human cerebrospinal fluid in normal and pathological conditions. Prostaglandins 9:183–192.

Wolfe LS, Rostworowski K, Pappius HM (1976): The endogenous biosynthesis of prostaglandins by brain tissue in vitro. Can J Biochem 54:629–640.

Yamashita A, Watanabe Y, Hayaishi O (1983): Autoradiographic localization of a binding protein(s) specific for prostaglandin D_2 in rat brain. Proc Natl Acad Sci USA 80:6114–6118.

Yu ACH, Chan PH, Fishman RA (1986): Effects of arachidonic acid on glutamate and gamma-aminobutyric acid uptake in primary cultures of rat cerebral cortical astrocytes and neurons. J Neurochem 47:1181–1189.

22

Sleep in Panic and Generalized Anxiety Disorders

THOMAS A. MELLMAN, MD, AND THOMAS W. UHDE, MD

Section on Anxiety and Affective Disorders, Biological Psychiatry Branch, National Institute of Mental Health, Bethesda, Maryland 20892

INTRODUCTION

During the past several years, there has been much interest in and a burgeoning amount of research on panic and generalized anxiety disorders. The recent literature on panic disorder has focused on clinical phenomenology, epidemiology, biological "markers," and behavioral and biochemical responses to treatment. Much uncertainty remains, however, regarding the fundamental nature of panic and generalized anxiety disorders. In the large body of recently generated knowledge, sleep physiology has been underrepresented, yet this might improve our understanding of the phenomenology and neurophysiology of these disabling anxiety disorders. The rationale for investigating the sleep physiology of primary anxiety disorders, particularly panic disorder, is threefold.

First, insomnia is commonly believed to result from anxiety or other states of increased autonomic arousal. In accordance with this widely held notion, many clinicians have utilized relaxation techniques, biofeedback, systematic desensitization, and antianxiety pharmacotherapy in the treatment of insomnia. Although anxiety is a frequent concomitant of primary insomnia, the nature, prevalence, and electroencephalographic correlates of insomnia in both panic and generalized anxiety disorders remain poorly understood. Thus, the study of the sleep physiology of patients with primary anxiety disorders will provide direct information regarding the relationship between insomnia and anxiety in patients with pathological anxiety states and offer indirect but valuable information regarding the specificity vs. nonspecificity of selective abnormalities [e.g., shortened rapid eye movement sleep (REM) latency] in the diagnosis of major depressive disorder.

Second, since the DSM III-R proposes that panic attacks are the core symptoms of panic disorder and related agoraphobic syndromes, an improved understanding of the prevalence, phenomenology, and physiology of sleep-related panic attacks would be of both practical and theoretical interest. In fact, the study of sleep panic attacks provides a method for investigating spontaneous panic attacks that are less encumbered by the influence of immediately juxtaposed external variables and psychological mood states, such as anticipatory anxiety.

Third, studies of clinical phenomenology, epidemiology, and neuroendocrinology suggest a partial overlap between panic and major depressive disorders. Although few experts would argue that generalized anxiety disorder and major depressive disorder have common genetic or neuroendocrine underpinnings, the validity of a diagnostic distinction between generalized anxiety disorder and panic disorder remains an area of significant controversy. Since a large body of data suggests some specificity of certain sleep abnormalities in depression (i.e., shortened REM latency, increased early REM activity), the investigation of these same electroencephalographic (EEG) features in panic and generalized anxiety disorders

Neurobiology of Panic Disorder, Pages 365–376
Published 1990 by Alan R. Liss, Inc.

would provide data relevant to questions regarding the utility of sleep EEG parameters in the diagnosis of major depression and the nature of the neurophysiologic overlap among panic, generalized anxiety, and major depressive disorders.

ANXIETY DISORDERS AND SLEEP DISTURBANCE

As heightened arousal is intimately linked to anxiety states, one would predict some increased prevalence of insomnia or other sleep disturbances in the anxiety disorders. In this section, we review sleep disturbances in panic and generalized anxiety disorders from the perspective of initiating and maintaining sleep. In this chapter, disturbances in initiating and maintaining sleep are referred to as "insomnia." We also introduce the concept of sleep panic as a special type of sleep disturbance. Panic attacks occurring in relation to sleep may be of particular relevance in understanding the neurobiology and physiology of panic disorder. Sleep architecture in panic disorder, i.e., the specific distribution and frequency of EEG-defined sleep stages, is discussed in the section on major affective vs. anxiety disorders.

Insomnia in Panic and Generalized Anxiety Disorders

Anecdotal reports and clinical observation suggest that insomnia is a common feature of the anxiety disorders. Sheehan et al. (1980) reported a 68% prevalence of difficulty falling asleep and a 77% prevalence of "restless and disturbed sleep" in a large treatment study of panic-phobic patients. Fifty-two percent of the total group characterized their difficulty falling asleep as moderate or extreme. Fifty-eight percent reported moderate to extreme degrees of restless or disturbed sleep.

Insomnia also appears to be a common feature of generalized anxiety disorder. Anderson et al. (1984) found that 56% of patients with generalized anxiety disorder report "trouble sleeping" compared to 44% of patients with panic disorder. Hoehn-Saric (1981) reported some sleep disturbance in 70% of chronic generalized anxiety disorder patients, with 30% noting moderate to severe symptoms. The incidence was somewhat higher in a comparison group of patients with mixed "anxiety" symptoms, including some patients suffering panic attacks.

We recently conducted a self-report sleep survey in 45 panic disorder patients seeking treatment from three separate clinics specializing in the treatment of anxiety disorders. This survey was also administered to a control group of 26 healthy normal volunteers. Since almost everyone has experienced disturbed sleep, evaluating the lifetime prevalence of insomnia (e.g., "Have you ever had problems falling asleep?") would probably be of little value in discriminating between anxious patients and normal controls. Of greater clinical relevance than the statistic of "lifetime prevalence" is the characterization of insomnia in terms of its regular and pervasive impact on the individual. We assessed, therefore, how frequently various parameters of insomnia (e.g., initiating and maintaining sleep) were "commonly" experienced by the subjects. The following self-report data represent the percentage of panic disorder patients and normal controls who stated that a particular type of sleep problem "commonly" and significantly interfered with their sleep.

Sixty-seven percent of the patients vs. 35% of the controls reported "general insomnia" as a "common" occurrence. The two groups did not differ with regard to experiencing difficulty falling asleep, which was reported by 53% of the patients and 42% of controls. Significantly more of the panic disorder patients, however, reported middle (awakening in the middle of the night) insomnia (67% vs. 23%, $P < 0.001$) and late insomnia (early morning awakening) (76% vs. 31%, $P < 0.001$). These observations are consistent with the other reports that insomnia is a common symptom among anxiety disorder patients. What was an unexpected finding in our data was the pattern of insomnia. Subjective complaints of middle and late insomnia, which are often associated with major depression and melancholia, also appear to occur frequently in panic disorder patients. These findings are interesting in relation to recent findings from our laboratory indicating that symptoms of generalized anxiety and panic attacks also occur more frequently in the morning than in the evening in panic disorder, a pattern reminiscent of early morning exacerbation of depressive symptoms in patients with major melancholia. Difficulty falling asleep, which has traditionally been associated with "neurotic" disorders, however, did not distinguish panic disorder patients from controls. These findings support both the phenomenological relationship of panic disorder and depression and the distinctiveness of panic disorder from the more typical spectra of anxiety-related experiences.

Some studies of insomnia indicate that individuals often substantially overestimate the degree of their sleep disturbance. To verify the character, severity, and frequency of sleep disturbance associated with panic and generalized disorders, it is, therefore, necessary to employ sleep polysomnographic techniques. Sleep polysomnography, also referred to as sleep EEG techniques, generally employs, as a minimum, EEG, electrooculographic (EOG), and electromyographic (EMG) leads. Such monitoring enables investigators to document reliably whether sleep is occurring and additionally to separate sleep into distinct stages. Normal sleep begins with stage 1, progresses into stage 2 and later into stages 3 and 4 (delta sleep). Delta sleep is characterized by increased voltage and slow-wave EEG activity. Delta is considered a "deep" stage of sleep in that it is more difficult to arouse subjects from this sleep stage. These stages make up the first non-REM cycle, typically lasting 70–100 min, and are followed by a period of REM sleep. REM sleep is characterized by relatively fast, low-voltage EEG activity, rapid eye movements, and suppression of peripheral muscle activity. REM sleep is associated with active and vivid dreaming. There are usually three to five non- REM–REM cycles occurring in the course of a night's sleep, with a tendency for REM length and activity to increase as sleep progresses through the night.

Although few sleep EEG studies have been conducted in homogeneous groups of anxiety disorder patients, the limited existing literature does generally support the presence of insomnia, as reflected by objective physiological criteria, in panic and generalized anxiety disorders. Reynolds et al. (1983) reported increased sleep latencies and intermittent wakefulness, and reduced delta sleep among the patients with generalized anxiety in comparison to depressed outpatients with sleep EEG

techniques. This insomnia pattern persisted in the anxious patients from the first to the second night of the study. Akiskal et al. (1984) also found difficulties initiating and maintaining sleep in a mixed sample of anxious patients, including some patients with panic or generalized anxiety. This feature was not characteristic of a dysthymic comparison group and was most pronounced on the initial adaptation night. Because of this first night effect, Akiskal proposed that adaptation difficulties were a characteristic of this anxious group. Sitaram et al. (1984) found increased time awake in an anxiety group with panic and generalized anxiety disorders compared to controls. In the only study of patients specifically diagnosed with panic disorder, Uhde et al. (1984) found that the amount of time asleep (sleep time) and percentage of time in bed asleep (sleep efficiency) were not significantly different from those of controls. In this study, however, sleep may have been more restless in the panic disorder patients as evidenced by increased movement time during sleep. This variable is a measurement of arousals with movement artifact occurring during sleep. Moreover, in this study, there was a significant negative correlation between total sleep time and global anxiety measures.

In a second, separate study conducted by the Section on Anxiety and Affective Disorders at NIMH, we have found significantly decreased sleep time and sleep efficiency and increased sleep latency (the time from "lights out" to the onset of sleep) in 13 panic patients compared to normal controls. In this study, there were several significant correlations between these measures and ratings of anxiety (Table 22–1) (Mellman and Uhde, 1989).

In summary, the majority of studies of both subjective reports and laboratory monitoring with EEG document that difficulty initiating and maintaining sleep is common among patients with both panic and generalized anxiety disorders. How insomnia is related to the course of illness and treatment response in these disorders is also an important issue for future investigations.

Sleep Panic

Until recently, few clinicians or investigators have systematically evaluated the type

TABLE 22–1.
Correlation Coefficients of Behavioral Measures vs. Sleep Variables in Panic Disorder Patients

	Total sleep time	Sleep efficiency	Sleep latency	REM latency	REM density	REM percent	Stage 1 (%)	Stage 2 (%)	Delta (%)	Movement time
Age	−.11	−.60**	.06	.48*	.18	−.34	.65**	.26	−.41	−.36
Years ill	.13	−.65**	.19	.45*	.50*	.58**	.76***	.19	−.12	−.08
Panic attacks[a]	−.67***	.35	.74***	.18	.28	.11	.16	−.27	−.18	.08
Global anxiety	−.57**	−.49*	.83***	−.47*	.29	.25	.24	−.52*	.30	.09
Global depression	−.46	−.34	.79***	−.55**	.07	.43	−.36	−.57**	.34	.28
Spielberger anxiety	−.28	−.54*	.62**	−.23	.49*	.17	.34	−.44	.20	.11
Hamilton depression	−.13	−.47	.54*	−.57**	−.07	.64**	−.03	−.72***	.29	.28

[a]Number of panic attacks in the past month.
*P < 0.10.
**P < 0.05.
***P < 0.01.

and frequency of sleep panic in the assessment of patients with anxiety disorders. For example, no mention of sleep panic is made in the DSM III-R classification of anxiety disorders. However, increasing evidence suggests that sleep panic attacks may be a common feature of panic disorder (Lesser et al., 1985; Mellman and Uhde, 1987, 1988; Taylor et al., 1986; Uhde, 1986; Uhde and Mellman, 1987; Uhde et al., 1984). In fact, we suspect that the study of sleep panic attacks will provide new and useful information regarding the core neurobiology and physiology of panic disorder. In this section, we review our preliminary findings regarding the prevalence, phenomenology, and physiological correlates of sleep panic attacks.

PREVALENCE AND PHENOMENOLOGY OF SLEEP PANIC ATTACKS

We assessed the prevalence of sleep-related panic in 45 ambulatory panic disorder patients who were being treated in private, "anxiety" specialty clinics. Sixty-nine percent of the panic disorder patients reported a lifetime history of having had a sleep panic attack. Regarding frequency of these events, 38% reported sleep-related panic attacks as "rare" events, and 33% reported sleep panic as a "common"

event. In contrast, 92% of a population of healthy controls reported never having experienced a sleep panic attack.

We have also evaluated the symptoms associated with sleep panic attacks. Nine panic disorder patients with both daytime and sleep panic completed a panic attack symptom inventory following all panic episodes. The mean symptoms of sleep-related attacks were compared to symptoms of typical daytime episodes in these nine subjects. Overall, there was considerable overlap in daytime vs. sleep-related panic attacks. All attacks featured the sudden onset of intense fear or apprehension. The other most common symptoms of sleep panic were palpitations (100%), followed by dyspnea (56%) and flushing (56%). This compares to symptoms of palpitations (100%); fear of dying, going crazy, or losing control (89%); sweating (78%); and trembling and shaking (78%) in daytime panic episodes. The most discrepant difference in symptoms between sleep and awake panic attacks were fear of dying (33% in sleep panic vs. 89% in day panic), sweating (44% vs. 78%), and trembling and shaking (44% vs. 78%) (see Table 22–2). In general, the sleep panic episodes featured a smaller number of symptoms than correspond-

TABLE 22–2.
Symptoms of Typical Daytime Panic Attacks and Sleep Panic

	Typical panic (%)	Sleep panic (%)
Sudden onset of intense fear or apprehension	100	100
Dyspnea	33	56
Palpitations	100	100
Chest pain or discomfort	44	56
Choking or smothering feeling	33	44
Dizziness or unsteadiness	67	33
Feelings of unreality	56	56
Paresthesias	56	33
Hot or cold flushes	67	56
Sweating	78	44
Trembling or shaking	78	44
Fear of dying, going crazy, or losing control	89	33

ing day panic and often resolved more rapidly. They were further characterized by patients as originating suddenly during sleep ("like a jolt") and were not associated with dream recall. This type of symptom cluster in sleep vs. daytime panic attacks is similar to the pattern of symptoms noted by Adler et al. (1987) in their descriptions of sleep-related and relaxation-induced panic attacks.

PHYSIOLOGICAL CORRELATES OF SLEEP PANIC ATTACKS

As part of our ongoing sleep research, we have now investigated the sleep EEG correlates of six sleep-related panic attacks occurring in six different patients from a group of 13 patients diagnosed with panic disorder. The sleep EEG of these panic disorder patients was compared to the sleep physiology of seven normal controls. In the patients, sleep panic attacks occurred within 24–225 min of sleep onset and within 65 min before (n = 2) or 48 min following (n = 4) the first REM period. The epoch of sleep preceding awakenings with panic was scored as stage 3 for four of the episodes and stage 2 for two of the episodes. In all the stage 3 awakenings, delta sleep had only recently been established, and in the stage 2 awakenings some slowing of EEG activity preceded the awakenings. This pattern of awakening was distinct from sleep stages preceding nonpanic spontaneous awakenings. As is illustrated in Table 22–3, nonpanic awakenings appeared to occur somewhat randomly through the sleep cycle. Nonpanic awakenings from

delta sleep, however, were very infrequent. Electrocardiograms (EKG) were monitored in three subjects and revealed marked increases in heart rate prior to or simultaneous with sleep-panic-awakenings. Chest wall movement was monitored in one subject, and the pattern was stable before, during, and after awakening with panic. The clinical phenomenology of these events is also not suggestive of apneic episodes; they were nonrecurrent through the night; were associated with full arousal, and occurred in a nonobese, predominantly female population.

Although sleep was generally more disturbed in patients than in controls (i.e., patients had increased sleep latency, decreased sleep efficiency, and decreased total sleep time), these variables were not different on panicking vs. nonpanicking nights within the patient group. In fact, there was a trend toward increased movement time on nonpanic nights among sleep panicking subjects. There was also an association of increases in REM latency on the nights when sleep panic occurred that was not simply an artifact of awakening (see Tables 22–4 and 22–5). The increase in REM latency on nights of sleep panic was found both in comparing nights with and without sleep panic within patients and in comparing panic patients who did or did not experience sleep panic during the study. These findings appear to be consistent with the report of Lesser et al. (1985), who found stage 3 sleep preceding a panic awakening in one subject with an REM latency of 191 min. Hauri et al.

TABLE 22–3.
Stage of Sleep Preceding Awakenings and Sleep-Related Panic Attack

	Stage (%)				
	1	2	3	4	REM
Awakenings					
Controls[a]	6	73	6	—	15
Patients[b]	7	68	—	—	25
Panic attacks[c] from sleep	—	33	67	—	—

[a]Seven subjects, 21 nights recorded, 71 awakenings.

[b]Thirteen subjects, 34 nights recorded, 114 awakenings.

[c]Six episodes in six patients.

TABLE 22–4.
Sleep Panic vs. Nonpanicking Patients and Normal Subjects

Variable	Sleep panic (N = 6)	Nonpanic (N = 7)	Normal subjects (N = 13)	Overall significance (P)
Age of subjects (years)	44.8 ± 9.7[a]	32.2 ± 9.2	37.0 ± 9.4	NS
Hamilton depression	13.0 ± 8.7	15.3 ± 4.9		NS
Global depression	3.6 ± 2.4	5.3 ± 1.0		<0.10
Total sleep time (min)	368.8 ± 40.7	359.6 ± 39.4	439.6 ± 45.3	<0.005
Sleep efficiency (%)	81.3 ± 6.9	82.0 ± 9.7	91.2 ± 4.7	<0.05
Sleep latency (min)	27.8 ± 20.3	36.7 ± 22.3	14.1 ± 5.6	<0.10
REM latency (min)	101.2 ± 40.4	57.0 ± 19.5	71.1 ± 17.9	<0.05
REM percentage	20.7 ± 6.6	25.7 ± 8.4	27.5 ± 5.1	NS
Delta percentage	7.0 ± 7.4	9.6 ± 6.6	7.2 ± 6.6	NS
Movement time (min)	10.2 ± 7.6	16.0 ± 12.2	11.2 ± 8.3	NS

[a]Mean ± SD.

TABLE 22–5.
Sleep EEG Variables for Nights With Panic vs. Comparison Nights for the Same Patients

Variable	Night of panic	Nonpanic nights	Significance (P)
Total sleep time	368.8 ± 40.7[a]	369.3 ± 69.4	NS
Sleep efficiency	81.3 ± 6.9	82.2 ± 11.6	NS
Sleep latency (min)	27.8 ± 20.3	24.0 ± 22.7	NS
REM latency (min)	101.2 ± 40.4	69.9 ± 18.9	<0.05
REM percent	21.8 ± 7.5	23.6 ± 9.3	NS
Delta percent	7.0 ± 7.4	7.9 ± 9.4	NS
Movement time (min)	10.2 ± 7.6	14.1 ± 12.0	<0.10

[a]Mean ± SD.

(1986) also noted sleep panic episodes to arise primarily in non-REM sleep.

Thus sleep panic appears to be a not uncommon feature of panic disorder and has implications regarding the nature of panic attacks. Our physiological data lend support to the clinical observation that panic attacks occur unpredictably or spontaneously and may be physiologically triggered. It is difficult to invoke cognitive factors as primary to events that appear typically to arise from non-REM sleep in that it is REM sleep that is associated with the most vivid and affectively laden mentation (Dement and Kleitman, 1957; Foulkes, 1962). The specificity of sleep panic to a transition toward delta sleep and the association of sleep panic attacks with delayed REM onset needs further confirmation. An additional theoretically interesting and clinically relevant issue regarding sleep panic is the question of treatment response. Although anecdotal at this time, our preliminary experience suggests that recurrent sleep panic attacks respond to a similar pharmacological profile as panic attacks occurring during wake time in panic disorder patients.

An issue raised by these findings is the phenomenological overlap of sleep panic and night terrors (pavor nocturnus). Night terrors are also sudden arousals from non-REM sleep and more commonly occur in children (Fisher et al., 1973). Children typically are amnestic for these events. Kales et al. (1980) described a population of adults experiencing night terrors and noted several features that clinically overlap with panic disorder patients. Thus the relation of panic attacks and night terrors is a matter worthy of further investigation.

SLEEP DEPRIVATION: PANIC DISORDER AND MAJOR DEPRESSION

Because there is ample evidence that disrupted sleep, including sleep panic, frequently occurs in panic disorder, it would be worthwhile investigating what effects direct sleep deprivation has on symptoms of the illness. This research strategy would allow one to address, in part, the cause-effect relation between panic disorder and insomnia. That insomnia is simply a secondary complication of panic disorder is the most obvious possibility. However, it is theoretically possible that primary disturbances of sleep might "trigger" panic attacks or maintain pathological states of generalized or free-floating anxiety in the panic-prone individual. An additional reason for interest in sleep deprivation has to do with further elucidating the relation between panic disorder and major depression. A number of reports have documented that one night's total sleep deprivation produces an acute but usually transient antidepressant effect in one-third to one-half of depressed patients (Gerner et al., 1979; Pflug and Tolle, 1971; Roy-Byrne et al., 1986; Van den Berg and van den Hoofdakker, 1975). There is also evidence that response to sleep deprivation may predict response to antidepressant medications (Wirz-Justice et al., 1979), although this remains controversial and requires more systematic study with prospective methodologies. To determine whether panic disorder patients have a behavioral response to sleep deprivation similar to patients with major depression, our group investigated the effects of one night's total sleep deprivation in 12 panic disorder patients. These panic disorder patients were compared to ten depressed patients and ten normal controls previously studied at NIMH. Description of this technique has been given in greater detail elsewhere (Roy-Byrne et al., 1986). Briefly, as was expected, symptoms of anxiety and depression improved in the depressed sample. In contrast, the panic disorder patients as a group did not differ from the controls. In fact, a subgroup experienced a worsening of anxiety symptoms, with 40% experiencing a panic attack the next day. This observation is consistent with data recently collected from our survey of panic patients regarding sleep patterns. Fifty-six percent (25 of 45) of panic patients reported not getting enough sleep as a "common" precipitant of panic attacks. Therefore, the sleep disturbances associated with panic disorder may have a role in perpetuating or exacerbating symptoms of the illness and perhaps, in a vicious cycle, also further exacerbate the disruption of sleep. We have also seen cases in which the occurrence of sleep panic attacks appears to "condition" initial insomnia or, more specifically, a fear and avoidance of sleep. In addition to these clinically relevant implications of the effects of sleep deprivation in panic disorder, the phenomenon may provide clues to neurobiological mechanisms of the disorder. It would seem that sleep deprivation may have activating effects that lead to improvement in depression while exacerbating panic disorder symptoms. Further delineation of neuroendocrine parameters and physiological mechanisms underlying the behavioral responses to sleep deprivation would be of considerable interest for understanding both of these disorders.

SLEEP EEG STUDIES: MAJOR AFFECTIVE AND ANXIETY DISORDERS

Despite the disparate findings regarding sleep deprivation, many clinical and epidemiological studies in panic disorder suggest at least a partial overlap with depression. The clinical and biologic overlap of these disorders is discussed in greater detail elsewhere in this volume. Briefly, depressive episodes can occur in up to half of panic disorder patients (Uhde et al., 1985). Some but not all family studies show overlap of depression and panic disorder. With the exception of the dexamethasone suppression test (Curtis et al., 1982; Roy-Byrne et al., 1985), most neuroendocrine parameters that are abnormal in depression also have been shown to overlap with findings in panic disorder (Uhde et al., 1986). The biological relation between generalized anxiety disorder and depression has not been as intensively investigated; however, Breslau and Davis (1985) reported that, among a group of patients meeting the 6 month duration criteria for generalized anxiety disorder, 73% also met DSM III criteria for major depression.

Several investigations support a familial distinction between panic disorder and generalized anxiety disorder. For example, the concordance for panic disorder is five times greater in monozygotic than in dizygotic twins (Torgerson, 1983). Moreover, the rate of panic disorder in first-degree relatives of probands with panic disorder is 25%, which is significantly greater than the rate in control families (Crowe et al., 1983). The rate of generalized anxiety disorder, however, does not differ between panic and control families (Crowe et al., 1983). Despite these impressive data, the diagnostic validation of generalized anxiety disorder as a distinct entity from panic disorder or adjustment disorder has been questioned by several authors.

As a result, many questions regarding the nature and extent of the neurobiological overlap among these disorders remain unanswered. Although sleep EEG occupies only a small niche in the methodological armamentarium available to research psychiatrists, results from sleep EEG investigations may provide useful adjunct information relevant to theoretical issues regarding the nature of the overlap among these disorders. In particular, it would be valuable to distinguish whether patients with either panic disorder or generalized anxiety disorder have a sleep architecture similar to patients with major depressive disorder.

Sleep disturbance is one of the most common complaints of depressed patients, and a large number of studies have documented certain sleep EEG abnormalities that typically occur in major "endogenous" or "melancholic" depression (Gillin et al., 1979, 1984; Kupfer, 1976). Sleep in depression tends to be shallow as measured by reduced amounts of delta sleep. It is also often fragmented (more frequent stage changes) and inefficient (reduced percentage of time asleep while in bed). In fact, it has been suggested that some sleep EEG measures are more specifically linked to endogenomorphic and melancholic depressions. For example, the time period from the onset of sleep to the first REM period (REM latency) is often reduced, and the first REM period also tends to be of longer duration and more intense (more eye movements per minute) in depression. These REM-related findings have also been reported in other psychiatric disorders, although these syndromes, i.e., obsessive–compulsive disorders (Insel et al., 1982) and borderline personality disorder (Akiskal et al., 1985), are themselves frequently associated with depression of an endogenomorphic quality. Thus, although these sleep EEG parameters ultimately may have limited utility as diagnostic tests, they are of considerable theoretical interest in understanding the physiology of sleep disturbances in general and in generating new and specific hypotheses regarding psychiatric illnesses. Sleep research has contributed to the development and refinement of the "phase-advance" theories of depression (Papousek, 1975) and has highlighted the possibility that in the future sleep manipulations will play a role in the adjunct treatment of selective neuropsychiatric conditions. Included in these are the aforementioned observations that sleep deprivation can produce transient improvement in mood in some patients with major depression. For these reasons, comparative data regarding sleep architecture provide a method for delineating both distinct and overlapping features and mechanisms of anxiety and depression.

For example, reduced REM latency and increased REM percent have been found to discriminate depressed outpatients from those diagnosed with generalized anxiety disorder (Reynolds et al., 1983). Akiskal et al. (1984) found that reduced REM latency and increased REM percent distinguished a group of dysthymic patients from anxious depressives. Eight of 22 patients in the anxious group met criteria for panic disorder or agoraphobia with

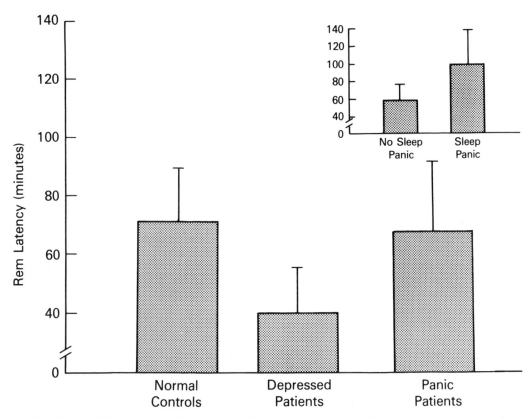

Fig. 22–1.   REM latency in depressed patients, panic disorder patients, and normal controls.

panic attacks. Sitaram et al. (1984) examined these same parameters, as well as sensitivity to cholinergic REM induction, in anxious patients and depressed patients and normal controls. REM abnormalities and increased sensitivity to REM cholinergic induction were present only in the depressed group. The anxious group was a mixture of patients with generalized anxiety disorder, agoraphobia, and panic disorder. Grunhaus et al. (1986) found that depressed patients who additionally experienced panic attacks had REM latencies approaching normal values in comparison to reduced values in depressed patients without panic attacks. Uhde et al. (1984) found a modest reduction in REM latency in panic disorder patients who were not acutely depressed. In this study, the panic disorder patients demonstrated *decreased* REM activity. In a separate study from the Section on Anxiety and Affective Disorders involving 13 panic patients, eight depressed patients, and

seven controls, REM latencies in the panic disorder population were more variable, with mean values comparable to those of controls and increased compared to the depressed group. Although none of the panic patients met concomitant criteria for major depression, there was a relation between depressive symptoms and some REM measures. Specifically, there was a significantly positive correlation between the percent of REM sleep and severity of depression ratings and a negative trend between depression ratings and REM latency (see Table 22–1). As was noted above, there also has been an association of increased REM latencies with the occurrence of sleep-related panic attacks that was not simply an artifact related to awakening. The REM latencies for our group of panic patients, including a subgroup who had sleep panic episodes during the sleep study compared to a group of normal controls and depressed patients, are presented in Figure 22–1, which illustrates that the mean REM latency for the panic disorder patients without sleep panic (57.0 ± 19.5 min) approached values seen in the depressed patients (40.2 ± 16.2), whereas the panic disorder patients with sleep panic had a mean value of 101.2 ± 40.4, which is greater than the REM latency of the normal controls (71.1 ± 17.9).

In summary, it appears the sleep EEG findings in depression (i.e., decreased REM latency, increased REM density) are not typically seen in panic disorder. Despite the overlap between panic disorder and major depressive disorder on many neuroendocrine measures, our sleep physiology observations underscore important differences across these mood and anxiety syndromes. The independent observations of a possible association of panic attacks with lack of reduction in REM latency in depression (Grunhaus et al., 1986) and findings of a positive correlation of daytime panic attack frequency and REM latency (Uhde et al., 1984) and our more recent finding of an association of sleep panic and relative increases in REM latency are intriguing. Mechanisms involving increased cholinergic sensitivity (Sitaram et al., 1984) and circadian phase advances (Papousek, 1975) have been proposed as relevant to the reduced REM latency finding in depression. To the extent that rhythm disturbances and cholinergic supersensitivity are relevant to the pathogenesis of affective disorders, it would be interesting to invetigate whether similar mechanisms apply to some panic disorder patients.

SUMMARY AND THEORETICAL IMPLICATIONS

Sleep disturbances have been documented in patients with panic and generalized anxiety disorders. In fact, complaints of insomnia appear to be quite prevalent in these anxiety disorders, and our data suggest that reports of frequent middle and late insomnia distinguish panic patients from controls. Despite the symptomatic overlap in the nature of subjective sleep complaints in panic disorder and depression, objective sleep EEG findings in both panic disorder and generalized anxiety disorder do not appear to overlap with the REM-related findings typically noted in endogenomorphic depression. Also, in contrast

to the case in many depressed patients with melancholic features, sleep deprivation appears to worsen anxiety symptoms in panic disorder.

Sleep-related panic attacks are a not uncommon feature of panic disorder. These appear to occur primarily in relation to non-REM sleep. Whether phenomena akin to sleep panic occur in the setting of generalized anxiety disorder is not known. One possible mechanism in the pathogenesis of sleep panic may be related to the observation that CO_2 inhalation can be panicogenic in panic disorder patients (Gorman et al., 1984). Relative degrees of hypoventilation occur during sleep, and this may play a role in the pathogenesis of sleep panic. Further investigation of the neurobiology of panic and sleep stages is needed to understand further the implications of these findings. An additional implication of these observations has to do with the relationship of panic to prepanic arousal. Challenge studies of panic, such as those utilizing sodium lactate (Liebowitz et al., 1985), have found an association of increased basal arousal with subsequent panic. Our findings, as well as those of Adler et al. (1987) documenting panic induced by relaxation techniques, suggest that increased basal arousal is not a prerequisite for panic. Thus some panic attacks appear to be associated with states of diminishing arousal and others appear to be triggered by situations that increase arousal above a critical threshold. Although speculative, our data together with previous observations suggest that the degree of arousal ("too little" or "too much") might be critical in terms of the panic disorder patient's risk of panic. That is, the maintenance of a critical range of arousal might be required to confer safety against panic; arousal levels above or below this hypothesized critical "window" would temporarily render the patient more vulnerable to an unprovoked panic attack. Such a homeostatic model is consistent with neurotransmitter models of panic in which dysregulatory abnormalities have been conceptualized within and across different neurotransmitter systems. Whether our proposed homeostatic model is itself an adaptive response or a pathologic component of panic disorder is an interesting theoretical question.

REFERENCES

Adler CA, Craske G, Barlow DH (1987): Relaxation-induced panic (RIP): When resting isn't peaceful. Integr Psychiatry 5:94–100.

Akiskal HS, Lemmi H, Dickson H, King D, Yerevanian B, Van Valkenburg C (1984): Chronic depression, Part 2. Sleep EEG differentiation of primary dysthymic disorders from anxious depression. J Affect Disorders 6: 287–295.

Akiskal HS, Yerevanian BT, Davis GC, King D, Lemmi H (1985): The neurological status of borderline personality: clinical and polysomnographic study. Am J Psychiatry 142:192–198.

Anderson DJ, Noyes R, Crowe RR (1984): A comparison of panic disorder and generalized anxiety disorder. Am J Psychiatry 141:572–575.

Breslau N, Davis GC (1985): DSM-III. Generalized anxiety disorder: An empirical investigation of more stringent criteria. Psychiatr Res 15:231–238.

Crowe RR, Noyes R, Pauls DL, Slymen D (1983): A family study of panic disorder. Arch Gen Psychiatry 40: 1065–1069.

Curtis CG, Cameron OG, Nesse RM (1982): The dexamethasone suppression test in patients with panic disorder and agoraphobia. Am J Psychiatry 139:1043–1045.

Dement W, Kleitman N (1957): The relation of eye movements during sleep to dream activity: An objective method for the study of dreaming. J Exp Psychol 53: 339–346.

Fisher C, Kahn E, Edwards A, Davis D (1973): A psychophysiological study of nightmares and night terrors. The suppression of stage 4 night terrors with diazepam. Arch Gen Psychiatry 28:253–259.

Foulkes WD (1962): Dream reports from different stages of sleep. J Abnormal Soc Psychol 65:14–25.

Gerner RH, Post RM, Gillin C, Bunney WE Jr (1979): Biological and behavioral effects of one night's sleep deprivation in depressed patients and normals. J Psychiatr Res 15:21–40.

Gillin JC, Duncan W, Pettigrew KD, Frankel BL, Snyder F (1979): Successful separation of depressed, normal and insomniac subjects by EEG sleep data. Arch Gen Psychiatry 36:85–90.

Gillin JC, Sitaram N, Wehr T, Duncan W, Post R, Murphy DL, Mendelson WB, Wyatt RJ, Bunney WE Jr (1984): Sleep and affective illness. In Post RM, Ballenger JC (eds): "Neurobiology of Mood Disorders." Baltimore: Williams & Wilkins, pp 157–189.

Gorman JM, Askanazi J, Lebowitz MR, Fyer AJ, Stein J, Kinmey JM, Klein DE (1984): Response to hyperventilation in a group of patients with panic disorder. Am J Psychiatry 141:857–861.

Grunhaus L, Rabin D, Harel Y, Greden JF, Feinberg M, Hermann R (1986): Simultaneous panic and depressive disorders: clinical and sleep EEG correlates. Psychiatry Res 17:251–259.

Hauri PJ, Ravaris CL, Friedman M (1986): Sleep in patients with panic attacks. Paper presented at 139th Annual Mtg, Am Psychiatric Assoc, Washington, DC.

Hoehn-Saric R (1981): Characteristics of chronic anxiety patients. In Klein DF, Rabkin JG (eds): "Anxiety: New Research and Changing Concepts." New York: Raven Press, pp 399–410.

Insel T, Gillin JC, Moore A, Mendelson WB, Lowenstein RJ, Murphy DL (1982): The sleep of patients with obsessive-compulsive disorder. Arch Gen Psychiatry 39: 1372–1377.

Kales JD, Kales A, Soldatos CR, Caldwell B, Charney DS, Martin ED (1980): Night terrors. Clinical characteristics and personality patterns. Arch Gen Psychiatry 37: 1413–1417.

Kupfer DJ (1976): REM latency—A psychobiological marker for primary depressive disease. Biol Psychiatry 11:159–174.

Lesser IM, Poland RE, Holcomb C, Rose DE (1985): Electroencephalographic study of nighttime panic attacks (single case study). J Nervous Mental Dis 173:774–746.

Liebowitz MR, Gorman JM, Fryer AJ, Levitt M, Dillon P, Levy S, Appleby IL, Anderson S, Palij M, Davies SO, Klein DF (1985): Lactate provocation of panic attacks. Arch Gen Psychiatry 42:709–722.

Mellman TA, Uhde TW (1987): Sleep panic. Paper presented at the Annual Scientific Mtg, Soc for Biol Psychiatry, Chicago, (Abstr 139), p 198.

Mellman TW, Uhde TW (1989): Electroencephalographic sleep in panic disorder: A focus on sleep related panic attacks. Arch Gen Psychiatry 46:178–184.

Papousek M (1975): Chronobiologische aspekte der zyklothymie. Fortschr Neurol Psychiatry 43:381–440.

Pflug B, Tolle R (1971): Therapie endogener depressionen durch schlafentugpraktische und theoretische konsequensen. Nervenarzt 42:117–124.

Reynolds CF, Shaw PH, Newton TF, Coble PA, Kupfer DJ (1983): EEG sleep in outpatients with generalized anxiety: A preliminary comparison with depressed outpatients. Psychiatry Res 8:81–89.

Roy-Byrne PP, Bierer LM, Uhde TW (1985): The dexamethasone suppression test in panic disorder: comparison with normal controls. Biol Psychiatry 20: 1237–1240.

Roy-Byrne PP, Uhde TW, Post RM (1986): Effects of one night's sleep deprivation on mood and behavior in panic disorder. Arch Gen Psychiatry 43:895–899.

Sheehan DV, Ballenger J, Jacobsen G (1980): Treatment of endogenous anxiety with phobic, hysterical and hypochondriacal symptoms. Arch Gen Psychiatry 37: 51–59.

Sitaram N, Dube S, Jones D, Pohl R, Gordon S (1984): Acetylcholine and alpha-adrenergic sensitivity in the separation of depression and anxiety. Psychopathology 17:24–39.

Taylor CB, Shreiber J, Agras WS, Roth WT, Margraf J, Ehlers A, Maddock RJ, Gossard D (1986): Ambulatory heart rate changes in patients with panic attacks. Am J Psychiatry 143:478–482.

Torgersen S (1983): Genetic factors in anxiety disorder. Arch Gen Psychiatry 40:1085–1092.

Uhde TW (1986): Treating panic and anxiety. Psychiatr Ann 16:536–541.

Uhde TW, Boulenger J-P, Roy-Byrne PP, Geraci MF, Vittone BJ, Post RM (1985): Longitudinal course of panic disorder: Clinical and biological considerations. Prog Neuro-Psychopharmacol Biol Psychiatry 9:39–51.

Uhde TW, Mellman TA (1987): Commentary on relaxation-induced panic (RIP): when resting isn't peaceful. Integr Psychiatry 5:101–104.

Uhde TW, Roy-Byrne PP, Gillin JC, Mendelsohn W, Boulenger J-P, Vittone BJ, Post RM (1984): The sleep of patients with panic disorder. Psychiatry Res 12: 251–259.

Uhde TW, Roy-Byrne PP, Post RM (1986): Panic disorder and major depressive disorder: biological relationship. In Shagass C, Josiassen RC, Bridger WH, Weiss KJ, Stoff D, Simpson GM (eds): "Biological Psychiatry, 1985 (Developments in Psychiatry, Vol 7)." Amsterdam: Elsevier, pp 463–465.

Van den Burg W, van den Hoofdakker RH (1975): Total sleep deprivation in endogenous depression. Arch Gen Psychiatry 32:1121–1125.

Wirz-Justice A, Puhringer W, Hale G (1979): Response to sleep deprivation as a predictor or therapeutic results with antidepressant drugs. Am J Psychiatry 136:1222–1223.

Index